Obstetrics & Gynecology Review 1994

NOTICE

Medicine is an ever-changing science. As new research and clinical experience broaden our knowledge, changes in treatment and drug therapy are required. The editors and the publisher of this work have checked with sources believed to be reliable in their efforts to provide information that is complete and generally in accord with the standards accepted at the time of publication. However, in view of the possibility of human error or changes in medical sciences, neither the editors, nor the publisher, nor any other party who has been involved in the preparation or publication of this work warrants that the information contained herein is in every respect accurate or complete, and they are not responsible for any errors or omissions or for the results obtained from use of such information. Readers are encouraged to confirm the information contained herein with other sources. For example and in particular, readers are advised to check the product information sheet included in the package of each drug they plan to administer to be certain that the information contained in this book is accurate and that changes have not been made in the recommended dose or in the contraindications for administration. This recommendation is of particular importance in connection with new or infrequently used drugs.

Obstetrics & Gynecology Review 1994

Harrison H. Sheld, M.D.

Associate Professor
Department of Obstetrics and Gynecology
University of Nevada
School of Medicine
Reno, Nevada

McGRAW-HILL, INC.
Health Professions Division
New York • St. Louis • San Francisco • Auckland • Bogotá • Caracas • Lisbon • London
Madrid • Mexico City • Milan • Montreal • New Delhi • San Juan • Singapore • Sydney • Tokyo • Toronto

Obstetrics & Gynecology Review 1994

Copyright © 1994 McGraw-Hill, Inc. All rights reserved. Printed in the United States of America. Except as permitted under the United States Copyright Act of 1976, no part of this publication may be reproduced or distributed in any form or by any means, or stored in a data base or retrieval system, without the prior written permission of the publisher.

1 2 3 4 5 6 7 8 9 0 MAL MAL 9 8 7 6 5 4

ISBN: 0-07-05644 2-6
ISSN: 1060-507X

This book was prepared camera-ready. The editors were Gail Gavert and Steven Melvin; the production supervisor was Gyl Favours. Malloy Lithographers was printer and binder.

CONTENTS

Preface . . . . *vii*

Gynecology 1

    Gynecology References 9

Reproductive Endocrinology 124

    Reproductive Endocrinology References 127

Gynecologic Oncology 177

    Gynecologic Oncology References 182

Obstetrics 267

    Obstetrics References 275

Perinatal Medicine 426

    Perinatal Medicine References 433

Index 559

PREFACE

Obstetrics and Gynecology Review 1994, the eighth volume in this series, is a compilation of abstracted articles from the *American Journal of Obstetrics and Gynecology* (Volumes 167-169) and *Obstetrics and Gynecology* (Volumes 81-83) presented in the framework of multiple choice questions used for medical education and evaluation. The questions have proven useful for board examination review as well as self-assessment. The 284 questions (from a data base of almost 500 questions) are representative of basic and timely information currently being published by scholars in obstetrics and gynecology. It is interesting to note how often divergent conclusions are drawn concerning a solution to a common problem. It is best to read the original article to reconcile and substantiate your knowledge and understanding of the information presented. At all times credit for the information belongs to the reporting investigators, and they are quoted liberally.

The same practical format has been used as in previous editions. Five topics have been chosen to expedite study: Gynecology, Reproductive Endocrinology, Gynecologic Oncology, Obstetrics, and Perinatal Medicine. Some editorial liberty has been taken in following this classification. For each topic there is a question and answer section.

Four basic types of questions that have proven popular have been retained. The authoring style conforms to that recomended by testing experts. In the answer section, there is an outline of the referenced article. In several instances a question has served as the basis for more than one abstract. For clarity, the outline is designed to have several parts: "Facts and Issues" bracketed as "F & I"; "Facts" noted by a solid bullet "•"; "Detail" noted by an open bullet "°", and "Issues" noted by a closing chevron "»". Facts are generally accepted statements; issues are suppositions or conclusions suggested by the investigators. Some information is at variance with standard or traditional concepts. The abstract may contain much more material than that pertaining to the question. In any case, for specific details of management refer to the original article or standard texts.

Intensive study and review of these questions should create an appreciation of the time, effort, and expense the scholars in our specialty have spent in pursuit of scientific accomplishment.

I wish to express my appreciation to Denise Gerner for her expert technical assistance in the preparation of this manuscript.

Harrison H. Sheld, M.D.
Las Vegas, Nevada
December 1993

Obstetrics & Gynecology Review 1994

GYNECOLOGY

Directions: Each of the questions or incomplete statements below is followed by several suggested answers or completions. Select the BEST answer in each case.

1. A post-menopausal patient not on estrogen replacement therapy had a benign D&C six months ago for uterine bleeding. Physical examination is within normal limits. She now reports 2½ weeks of bleeding per vaginam. The treatment of choice is

   A. GnRH agonist.
   B. hormonal replacement.
   C. hysterectomy.
   D. hysteroscopy.
   E. repeat D&C.

2. Which of the following is the most effective drug in eradicating bacterial vaginosis?

   A. Oral metronidazole.
   B. Intravaginal clindamycin.
   C. Intravaginal metronidazole.
   D. Oral clindamycin.
   E. Both oral metronidazole and oral clindamycin have about the same effect on eradicating bacterial vaginosis.

3. In the treatment of pelvic endometriosis, side effects from a 3.6 milligram subcutaneous implant of goserelin include

   A. acne.
   B. decreased libido.
   C. hirsutism.
   D. oily hair.
   E. weight gain.

4. A patient has a nonpalpable mammographically detected carcinoma of the breast. The chance of her having one or more positive axillary nodes is

   A. <1%.
   B. 5%.
   C. 10%.
   D. 20%.
   E. 25%.

5. The most sensitive method of detecting cervical infection by *Chlamydia trachomatis* is

   A. direct fluorescent antibody test.
   B. enzyme immunoassay.
   C. polymerase chain reaction.
   D. recovery on irradiated McConkey cells.
   E. serum detection of complement-fixing antibodies.

6. The most sensitive and specific method of diagnosing PID is

   A. C-reactive protein.
   B. culdocentesis.
   C. endometrial biopsy.
   D. history/physical examination.
   E. radionuclide scanning with labelled leukocytes.

7. Which of the following laboratory findings are most likely in the serum of a patient with an ectopic pregnancy? (↑=increased; ↓ = decreased)

   A. ↑ progesterone, ↑ HCG, ↑ estradiol, ↑ alpha-fetoprotein
   B. ↓ progesterone, ↓ estradiol and ↓ alpha-fetoprotein, ↑ HCG
   C. ↓ progesterone, ↓ HCG, ↓ estradiol and ↓ alpha-fetoprotein
   D. ↓ progesterone, ↓ HCG, ↓ estradiol and ↑ alpha-fetoprotein
   E. ↑ progesterone, ↑ estradiol, ↓ HCG and ↓ alpha-fetoprotein

8. Associated with an increased incidence of break-through bleeding:

   A. Demulen.
   B. O/N 7/7/7.
   C. Ovral.
   D. Triphasil.
   E. All have about the same incidence of break-through bleeding.

9. In planning for a post-coital test, within how many hours after the LH surge as detected by urinary assay should an evaluation of cervical mucus be made?

   A. 2
   B. 4
   C. 6
   D. 10
   E. 12

10. Patients who have a hysterectomy for benign disease have how much of a decrease in the risk of having ovarian cancer?

    A. 10%
    B. 25%
    C. 50%
    D. 75%
    E. less than 5%

11. Reasons for the removal of an otherwise asymptomatic myomatous uterus reaching the level of the symphysis pubis include

    A. if a uterus continued to enlarge it may compromise other structures; for example, ureters or lead to debilitating symptoms.
    B. if the uterus continued to enlarge surgical treatment becomes more difficult and carries greater risks.
    C. operating on a uterus before it enlarges further may improve a woman's chances for fertility and successful pregnancy.
    D. the ovaries cannot be adequately evaluated by bimanual evaluation.
    E. none of the above.

12. A patient has a conization for a pap test suggesting CIN III. The margins of the cone specimen show CIN. Six months later a repeat pap suggests CIN III. The treatment of choice is

    A. colposcopy.
    B. cryosurgery.
    C. hysterectomy.
    D. repeat conization.
    E. repeat pap.

13. At 12 weeks a pregnant patient has a Papanicolaou smear reported as satisfactory except that the evaluation is "limited by the lack of an endocervical component." The cervix appears grossly normal and the pregnancy is otherwise uncomplicated. The next best step in the patient's management is

    A. perform colposcopy and directed biopsies if needed at 28 weeks
    B. perform colposcopy and directed biopsies if needed now
    C. repeat the pap at 28 weeks
    D. repeat the pap in 12 months
    E. repeat the pap in two months

14. The maximum endometrial thickness observed during vaginal ultrasound for conservative management of a patient thought to have a complete abortion

    A. 3 millimeters
    B. 4 millimeters
    C. 5 millimeters
    D. 7.5 millimeters
    E. 1 centimeter

15. Leiomyosarcomas can be reliably diagnosed by

    A. intraoperative frozen section.
    B. preoperative computed tomography.
    C. preoperative endometrial sampling.
    D. preoperative magnetic resonance imaging.
    E. none of the above

16. The number of exfoliated cells of the uterine cervix is increased by

    A. age
    B. cigarette smoking
    C. phase of menstrual cycle
    D. presence of koilocytes
    E. use of oral contraceptives

17. Related to risks for the development of endometrial carcinoma

    A. gallbladder disease
    B. height
    C. later age at natural menopause
    D. more than two spontaneous abortions
    E. post menopausal hirsutism

18. A 26-year old patient is suspected of having PID. The most specific test in diagnosing her condition

   A. C-reactive protein
   B. endometrial biopsy
   C. erythrocyte sedimentation rate
   D. pelvic transvaginal ultrasound
   E. white blood cell

19. The rate of pregnancy loss after detection of a live embryo in the first trimester is approximately

   A. less 5%
   B. 10%
   C. 20%
   D. 25%
   E. 33%

20. A postmenopausal patient has developed bleeding per vaginam. An endometrial suction curettage used to obtain a tissue was reported as retrieving insufficient tissue for diagnosis. Physical evaluation finds a small uterus and nonpalpable ovaries. A pap test of the cervix shows only normal cells. A diagnostic ultrasound of the pelvis to estimate endometrial thickness is ordered. What is the minimal endometrial thickness which will allow the patient to be observed prospectively?

   A. Less than 5 millimeters.
   B. Less than 6 millimeters.
   C. Less than 7 millimeters.
   D. Less than 8 millimeters.
   E. The patient should have a formal curettage regardless of the endometrial thickness.

21. Cigarette smoking causes urinary incontinence by

   A. activating purinergic receptors
   B. depleting α adrenergic fibers
   C. interfering with collagen synthesis
   D. stretch injury to pudendal and intrapelvic nerves
   E. none of the above

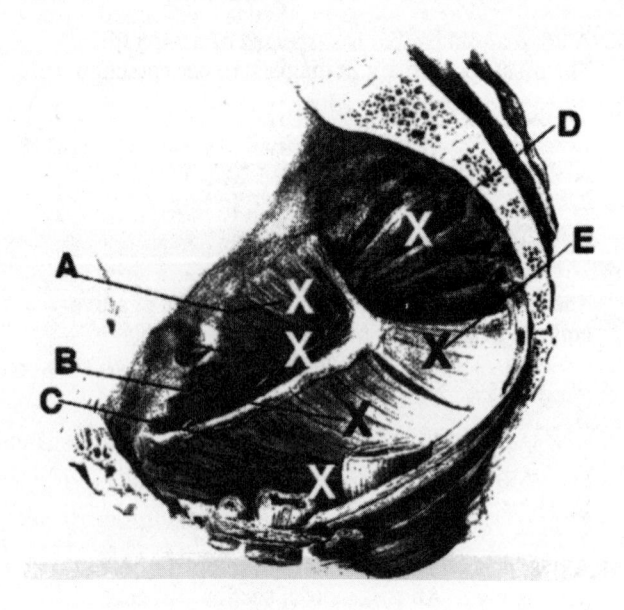

22. In the diagram above, which letter identifies the coccygeus muscle?

   A. A
   B. B
   C. C
   D. D
   E. E

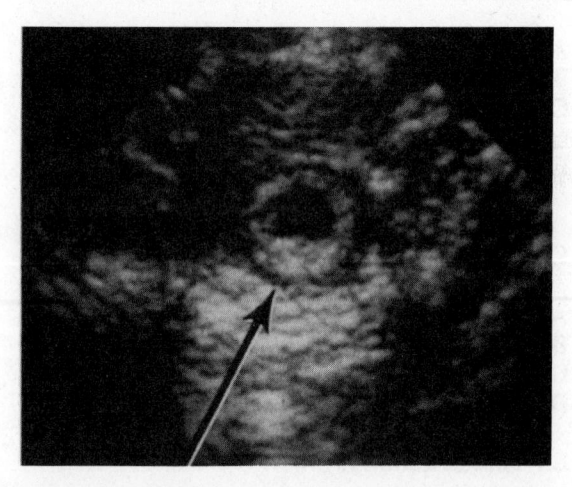

23. An asymptomatic patient six weeks pregnant by dates has a serum ß-hCG level of 2600 IU/ml and serum progesterone level of 50 ng/ml. The ultrasonogram of the involved adnexal region pictured above was obtained the same day the lab results were reported. The diagnosis is

   A. benign cystic teratoma.
   B. corpus luteum of pregnancy.
   C. ectopic pregnancy.
   D. endometrioma.
   E. hematosalpinx.

24. Associated with vulvar vestibulitis are all of the following EXCEPT

   A. erythema of minor vestibular glands.
   B. increased urethral pressure variability.
   C. interstitial cystitis.
   D. lactose intolerance.
   E. urethral syndrome.

25. Independent predictors of persistent ectopic pregnancy following salpingostomy include all of the following EXCEPT

   A. days of amenorrhea
   B. hematoperitoneum
   C. laparoscopic approach
   D. preoperative ß-hCG level greater 3000 international units per liter
   E. size of ectopic

26. True statements about the menopause include all of the following EXCEPT

   A. About half of menstruating women in the menopause experience vasomotor symptoms.
   B. Antidepressants are the therapy of choice to reduce vasomotor complaints.
   C. Regularly menstruating women with premenstrual tension are more likely to experience vasomotor symptoms in the premenopause.
   D. The severity of menopausal vasomotor complaints is related to the severity of bone loss.
   E. Women with a long premenopausal experience have vasomotor complaints more often than women with a short premenopause.

27. Drugs used for the prevention of pelvic adhesions from gonococcal salpingitis, all of the following EXCEPT

   A. colchicine
   B. Dextran 40
   C. Dextran 70
   D. nonsteroidal anti-inflammatory drugs
   E. progestins

Directions: Each set of lettered headings below is followed by a list of numbered words or phrases. For each numbered word or phrase select:

   A. if the item is associated with *(A) only*
   B. if the item is associated with *(B) only*
   C. if item is associated with *both (A) and (B)*
   D. if item is associated with *neither (A) nor (B)*

Items 28-30.

   A. severe dysplasia of uterine cervix
   B. invasive cervical carcinoma
   C. both
   D. neither

28. mean of age of occurrence younger than the mode age of occurrence.

29. mean of age of occurrence about 50.

30. mode age of occurrence about 40.

Items 31-33.

In the prophylaxis of deep venous thrombosis after gynecologic oncologic surgery:

   A. low-dose heparin (5,000 units every eight hours)
   B. intermittent pneumatic calf compression
   C. both
   D. neither

31. increased incidence of transfusion

32. increased incidence of wound separation

33. administration expense

Items 34-36.

   A. complete hydatidiform mole
   B. partial hydatidiform mole
   C. both
   D. neither

34. dispermy

35. malignancy potential 1:200

36. germline mutation

Items 37-39.

A. polycystic ovarian ovary
B. postmenopausal ovary in patients with endometrial cancer
C. both
D. neither

37. increased estrogen production

38. increased bioactive LH

39. decreased PSH

Items 40-42.

Effects of monophasic oral contraceptives containing:

A. ethinyl estradiol 20 micrograms plus desogestrel 150 micrograms
B. ethinyl estradiol 30 micrograms plus gestodene 75 micrograms
C. both
D. neither

40. increased levels of fibrinogen

41. increased fibrinolytic capacity

42. increased ceruloplasmin levels

Directions: For each of the questions or incomplete statements below, ONE or MORE of the answers or completions given is correct. In each case select:

A. if only 1, 2 and 3 are correct
B. if only 1 and 3 are correct
C. if only 2 and 4 are correct
D. if only 4 is correct
E. if all are correct

43. Complications of large loop excision of the transformation (LLETZ) for the treatment of cervical neoplasia includes

1. cervical stenosis.
2. immediate hemorrhage.
3. delayed hemorrhage.
4. inadequate tissue specimen for diagnosis.

44. Common side effects of sumatriptan when used for the treatment of menstrual migraine include

1. dizziness.
2. nausea and vomiting.
3. chest tightness.
4. photophobia.

45. In the evaluation of the endocervical canal, the endocervical curettage

1. has high false-positive rates.
2. has high false-negative rates.
3. interferes with the interpretation of subsequent cone biopsies.
4. has a large percentage of insufficient cellular material.

46. Treatments of chronic vulvar pruritus include

1. topical fluorinated hydrocortisones.
2. alcohol injection of affected tissue.
3. Mehring denervation.
4. subcutaneous injection of triamcinolone

47. Structures innervated by the pudendal nerve include

1. external anal sphincter.
2. urethral sphincter.
3. deep transverse perineal muscle.
4. bulbocavernosus.

48. Indications for conization of the uterine cervix include

1. endocervical curettage positive for intraepithelial neoplasia.
2. unsatisfactory colposcopy.
3. discrepant cytology.
4. squamous cell carcinoma reported on pap smear during pregnancy in the face of normal colposcopy.

49. Myomas cause infertility by

1. reducing the implantation space.
2. mechanical compression of the tube.
3. delaying sperm transport.
4. interference with endometrial blood supply.

50. Histological correlation of chromosomally normal conceptual tissue from spontaneous abortion includes

    1. a villous circulation indicating fetal life to 10 to 11 or more weeks.
    2. chronic intervillositis.
    3. villous infarcts.
    4. decidual vasculitis.

51. Medical management of an unruptured ectopic pregnancy can be considered if

    1. serum progesterone level is <5 nanograms.
    2. serum ß-hCG <2000 mIU/ml 48 hours apart.
    3. ultrasound shows an empty uterus.
    4. ultrasound shows a fetal heart rate and adnexal mass.

52. Factors associated with a favorable outcome when adnexal torsion is treated by untwisting include

    1. duration of symptoms.
    2. leukocytosis.
    3. fever.
    4. pregnancy.

53. Associated with toxic shock syndrome

    1. contraceptive sponge.
    2. diaphragm.
    3. tampon.
    4. LEEP excision of cervical neoplasia.

54. Mechanisms by which protein receptor mRNA is overexpressed in leiomyomata include

    1. alteration of estrogen receptors.
    2. anomalies in progesterone receptors.
    3. increase in insulin-like growth factor.
    4. overabundance of progesterone regulatory protein.

55. True statements about hormone replacement therapy and the risk of breast cancer include

    1. Synthetic estrogen is associated with an increased risk of breast cancer.
    2. Women who have ever used estrogen and stopped for two years are at increased risk.
    3. Use of estrogens for more than ten years is associated with an increased risk of breast cancer.
    4. The addition of progestins through estrogens reduces the risk of breast cancer.

56. Clinically effective in the treatment of Chlamydial cervicitis:

    1. amoxicillin
    2. erythromycin
    3. azithromycin
    4. clindamycin

57. Explanations for the absence of detectable levels of ß-hCG in the circulation of patients with ectopic pregnancies include

    1. trophoblastic degeneration.
    2. small volume of trophoblast.
    3. defect in ß-hCG biosynthesis.
    4. rapid clearance of the hormone from the circulation.

58. Predictive of successful anterior-posterior vaginal repair undertaken to relieve stress urinary incontinence

    1. increase in abdominal pressure transmission ratio
    2. increase in maximum urethral closure pressure
    3. increase in retrovesical angle during stress
    4. the presence of striated muscle in the levator ani

59. Clinically useful in maintaining bone mineral density during GnRH agonist treatment of endometriosis

    1. calcium carbonate
    2. medroxyprogesterone
    3. norethindrone
    4. sodium etidronate

60. Urodynamic measurements which respond to Kegel exercises in the successful treatment of stress urinary incontinence include

    1. maximal cystometric capacity
    2. urethral functional length
    3. Q-tip test
    4. urethral closure pressure

61. A woman's sexuality is reflected by

    1. multiplicity of orgasms
    2. cyclicity of arousability
    3. frequency of desire
    4. coital frequency

62. The clearance rate of 17ß-estradiol is related to

    1. fat mass
    2. fitness
    3. recent food intake
    4. thermal stress

63. Effective in decreasing complications in second trimester elective abortions

    1. antibiotic prophylaxis
    2. preoperative ultrasound
    3. laminaria tents
    4. intraoperative ultrasound

64. Inducers of cellular tissue factor activity include

    1. endotoxin
    2. interleukin-1
    3. tumor necrosis factor
    4. antiphospholipid antibodies

65. The effects of triphasic contraceptive use on hemostasis include

    1. tissue plasminogen activity is increased
    2. changes in coagulation factors are balanced by changes in anticoagulation factors
    3. they may be protective in relation to atherosclerosis and myocardial infarction
    4. the progestogen modifies the estrogenic effects on hemostasis

66. Treatments for an ovarian pregnancy include

    1. ipsilateral oophorectomy
    2. ovarian cystectomy
    3. ovarian wedge resection
    4. intramuscular methotrexate

67. Patients with Swyer syndrome have

    1. an XY karyotype
    2. female internal genitalia
    3. need to have gonadectomy
    4. the SRY gene preserved

68. Polycystic ovarian susceptibility allele is

    1. linked to HLA antigen location
    2. recessive
    3. involved with the cytochrome P450 steroid 21 hydrolyase
    4. immunologic in etiology

69. Markers of bone resorption include

    1. serum osteocalcin
    2. serum alkaline phosphatase
    3. urinary calcium excretion
    4. urinary hydroxyproline

70. Consistently present in the polycystic ovarian syndrome

    1. obesity
    2. hyperandrogenism
    3. hirsutism
    4. chronic anovulation

71. Increased in the hirsutism-hyperandrogenism syndrome

    1. LDL
    2. triglycerides
    3. DHEAS
    4. HDL

72. GnRH agonists are clinically useful in the treatment of

    1. endometriosis
    2. fibroids
    3. menorrhagia
    4. premenstrual syndrome

GYNECOLOGY REFERENCES

Directions: Each of the questions or incomplete statements below is followed by several suggested answers or completions. Select the BEST answer in each case.

1. A post-menopausal patient not on estrogen replacement therapy had a benign D&C six months ago for uterine bleeding. Physical examination is within normal limits. She now reports 2½ weeks of bleeding per vaginam. The treatment of choice is

   A. GnRH agonist.
   B. hormonal replacement.
   C. hysterectomy.
   *D. hysteroscopy.
   E. repeat D&C.

---

p. 419 (Townsend D E, Fields G, McCausland A, Kauffman K. Diagnostic and operative hysteroscopy in the management of persistent postmenopausal bleeding. Obstet Gynecol 1993; 82:419)

1. [F & I: •Background: Women who have postmenopausal bleeding usually undergo endometrial biopsy or D&C.

    •If the tissue is benign and the patient is taking hormones, the drug regimen is usually adjusted.

    •If she is not taking hormones, medication is often initiated.

    •Women who continue to bleed with or without hormone therapy become frustrated.

    •Many are subjected to additional D&Cs and even hysterectomy.

    •When hysteroscopy is performed for this indication, large numbers of women are found to have organic causes for their bleeding.

    • Over the past 4 years, 110 women with persistent postmenopausal bleeding (i.e., bleeding of more than 6 months in duration) have been evaluated and managed with diagnostic and operative hysteroscopy.

    •Objective: To describe experience in finding the causes for the bleeding and in managing the condition in these women.

    •Results: A benign organic cause (polyps in 42 and submucous myomas in 53) was noted in 95 women, 13 women had no disease, and two had early adenocarcinomas.

    •In those without an organic cause, adenomyosis was found on uterine biopsy in eight and atrophic changes were noted in five.

    •No neoplastic change was noted in the polyps or submucous fibroids.

    •Most patients with polyps had at least two or three lesions, which varied in size from at least 5 mm to those that filled the entire endometrial cavity.

    •All of the submucous myomas were solitary except in two cases.

      °The size varied at 1-to-6 cm.

      °In all cases, at least half of the myoma protruded into the endometrial cavity.

    • Both cases of cancer involved early lesions, grade 1 without invasion.

      °One was found behind a very large polyp, which had been observed along with other polyps when the patient had office video hysteroscopy.

°The malignancy, which was less than 1 cm in diameter, was missed in the office but discovered at the operative procedure.

°The lesion had the classic atypical vessels and irregular surface and fronds that are found with endometrial cancer.

•The other patient had a small raised tumor (less than 1 cm) in the right cornual area, which had been missed with an aspiration biopsy.

•Both patients are disease-free 2 years after hysterectomy.

• The mean operative time in these cases was 18 minutes (range 6-to-45).

•The average amount of irrigating fluid used was 9000 ml (range 1500-to-15,000).

•Fluid balance was noted to be within 300 ml in all cases.

•There were no complications during or after surgery.

•Half of the study population was back to their normal activities within 24 hours.

•The remaining patients required 3-to-5 days to recover completely from the effects of surgery.

• One hundred four of the 108 women who underwent resection of polyps or myomas with or without ablation had either amenorrhea or minimal bleeding on cyclic hormone replacement therapy (15) or were amenorrheic on continuous hormone replacement therapy (89) over a follow-up period of at least 24 months.

•Two of the 13 patients who had **endometrial ablation** alone had persistent bleeding.

• Among the patients who had polyps or fibroids—of whom half had resection alone and the others had resection and ablation—the success rates were virtually identical; i.e., one in each group had a recurrence of abnormal bleeding.

•This experience emphasizes the importance of direct visualization of the uterine cavity in any patient who has had abnormal uterine bleeding.

•Although there were two cases in which endometrial cancer was not noted preoperatively, one missed by endometrial aspiration and the other by diagnostic hysteroscopy, both women had early lesions and were managed appropriately.

•A surprisingly high number of women had organic causes for their postmenopausal bleeding, higher than that reported in the past.

°This may represent a skewed population because only patients who had persistent bleeding for at least 6 months were included.

•Pelvic vaginal ultrasound, used in four cases, **missed** the organic cause of bleeding.

•It may not be necessary to ablate the entire endometrial cavity after removing the polyp or myoma, as the success rates were the same in those who had resection alone or resection and ablation.

•The presence of **adenomyosis** did not appear to influence the results.

•Compared to premenopausal women with abnormal uterine bleeding, results in postmenopausal women with bleeding are equal or superior.

•The benefits of hormone therapy in the postmenopausal patient have been well documented.

•The cessation of hormone therapy because of bleeding is not uncommon, particularly when there is no good explanation for the cause of the bleeding.

•Bleeding is the primary reason women stop hormone replacement therapy.

•Diagnostic and operative hysteroscopy appears to provide a safe and easily performed technique to manage patients with such bleeding problems.]

---

2. Which of the following is the most effective drug in eradicating bacterial vaginosis?

    A. Oral metronidazole.
    B. Intravaginal clindamycin.
    C. Intravaginal metronidazole.
    D. Oral clindamycin.
  *E. Both oral metronidazole and oral clindamycin have about the same effect on eradicating bacterial vaginosis.

p. 966 (Hillier S L, Lipinski C, Briselden A M, Eschenbach D A. Efficacy of intravaginal 0.75% metronidazole gel for the treatment of bacterial vaginosis. Obstet Gynecol 1993; 81:963)

2. [F & I: •Background: Oral metronidazole is currently one of the two regimens recommended by the Centers for Disease Control for treatment of bacterial vaginosis.

•The dose having the greatest efficacy is 500 mg orally twice daily for 7 days, which has a 61-to-82% cure rate.

•Shorter therapy has been advocated to increase compliance and decrease the side effects associated with systemic metronidazole use.

•A single 2-g dose has a 69-to-72% cure rate assessed at 4 or more weeks after therapy.

•Bacterial vaginosis results from replacement of *Lactobacillus* by *Gardnerella vaginalis, Mycoplasma hominis,* and anaerobic bacteria.

•Because bacterial vaginosis is a localized syndrome with no apparent inflammation of the vaginal epithelium, topical treatment provides an appealing alternative to systemic antimicrobial use.

•Intravaginal metronidazole tablets were shown to be 79% effective, and vaginal sponges containing 1000 mg of metronidazole used for 3 days were 88% effective.

•Intravaginal 2% clindamycin cream used once a day for 7 days was also found to be 72-to-94% effective for the treatment of bacterial vaginosis.

•Objective: To evaluate 0.75% metronidazole gel, formulated at pH 4.0, for the treatment of bacterial vaginosis in a double-blind, placebo-controlled crossover trial.

•Results: Intravaginal metronidazole gel is clinically and microbiologically effective against bacterial vaginosis.

•Forty-seven of 53 women (89%) had a favorable response to metronidazole gel 4-to-16 days after completion of therapy.

•The response to therapy was similar among those who reported having had bacterial vaginosis previously (91%) and those without a history of this syndrome (81%).

•This frequency of clinical response immediately after therapy is similar to that reported for oral metronidazole (87-to-96%), oral clindamycin (94%), and intravaginal clindamycin (72-to-94%).

- Recurrence of bacterial vaginosis 1 month after treatment is 9-to-11% for oral metronidazole and 0-to-9% for intravaginal clindamycin.

- Bacterial vaginosis recurred in 15% of the women 1 month after treatment.

- The frequency of recurrence was similar for those with (two of 18, 11%) and without (two of 12, 17%) a history of bacterial vaginosis.

- **These data suggest that treatment with intravaginal metronidazole twice daily for 5 days results in cure rates similar to those observed with other oral and topical regimens.**

- Women who used the placebo gel had only a 17% cure rate based on clinical criteria and a 14% cure rate based on Gram stain criteria.

- Placebo-controlled trials are somewhat difficult to interpret when a topical placebo is used in a microbiologically complex ecosystem such as the vagina, as the use of nearly any product in the vagina will exert some effect on the vaginal flora.

- There was a statistically significant decrease in vaginal colonization by high concentrations of *G vaginalis* following use of the placebo gel.

- Preservatives in the placebo gel may have had some antibacterial effect against *G vaginalis*.

- Two of the four women who were initially cured by placebo developed recurrent bacterial vaginosis, suggesting that the cure achieved by placebo was incomplete.

- This is supported by microbiologic data showing persistence of more than 10^5 colony-forming units per milliliter of *G vaginalis* in both of the placebo-treated women who were considered clinical cures.

- Three of the four women who initially failed to respond clinically to intravaginal metronidazole were cured upon re-treatment using the identical formulation.

- The used tubes from the first treatment were weighed to ascertain whether the appropriate amount of medication had been used, and the residual drug was assayed to assure metronidazole potency.

- All four women stated that they had used the drug as instructed, and all four tubes were verified to contain active metronidazole.

- A second course of identical medication could be successful when the first course did not result in either clinical or microbiologic improvement if

    ° a longer duration of therapy is necessary for some women.

    ° sexual intercourse during intravaginal treatment effectively dilutes the drug.

- Poor compliance with instructions to use condoms during intercourse was noted.

    ° Nearly half of the women who stated that they had used condoms had sperm detected by vaginal smear.

- Vaginal intercourse during therapy could reduce the success of this or any other intravaginal therapy.

- Metallic taste, headache, and gastrointestinal distress are all frequent side effects of oral metronidazole.

- Intravaginal metronidazole was well tolerated.

•Yeast vulvovaginitis, a common sequel of treatment of bacterial vaginosis, was reported in 8-to-22% of women using oral metronidazole and 0-to-24% of women using intravaginal clindamycin for treatment of bacterial vaginosis.

•Symptomatic yeast vaginitis occurred in only two of the 53 women (4%) treated with metronidazole gel, despite a transient increase in vaginal colonization by yeast immediately after treatment.

•This acceptably low frequency of yeast vaginitis is comparable to the levels seen after use of other treatments for bacterial vaginosis.

•Optimally, any treatment regimen should eradicate the pathogens associated with bacterial vaginosis and restore a *Lactobacillus-predominant* flora.

•Lactobacilli that produce hydrogen peroxide appear to provide the primary microbiologic defense mechanism for the vaginal ecosystem.

•Whereas facultative lactobacilli were recovered from 83% of the women immediately after therapy, only 65% had lactobacilli in the vagina 1 month after treatment.

•Antibiotic therapy alone may not be sufficient to reestablish a Lactobacillus-predominant flora, and the dearth of them after therapy may contribute to the high frequency of bacterial vaginosis recurrence.]

---

3. In the treatment of pelvic endometriosis, side effects from a 3.6 milligram subcutaneous implant of goserelin include

   A. acne.
*B. decreased libido.
   C. hirsutism.
   D. oily hair.
   E. weight gain.

---

p. 202 (Rock J A, Truglia J A, Caplan R J. Zoladex (goserelin acetate implant) in the treatment of endometriosis: A randomized comparison with Danazol. Obstet Gynecol 1993; 82:198)

3. [F & I: •Background: Endometriosis, a condition affecting 2.5-to-15% of women of reproductive age, depends on cyclical ovarian steroids, especially estradiol (E2), and is associated with debilitating symptoms.

•The primary sequelae of endometriosis include pelvic pain, endometrial implants, dysmenorrhea, and dyspareunia.

•Endometriosis is associated with infertility.

•Goals of therapy include relief of symptoms, resolution of existing lesions, and prevention of new lesions.

•Among the available treatments for endometriosis, only extirpative therapy offers the possibility of a permanent cure.

•Although various therapies have provided clinical benefit, danazol, which has androgenic and anabolic properties, has been used most widely.

•Because of the troublesome side effects associated with danazol, the search for effective and safe alternatives has continued.

• The ability of GnRH agonists to produce amenorrhea and anovulation by inducing hypoestrogenism through down-regulation of pituitary GnRH receptors has led to their use in the treatment of endometriosis.

•Given by injection, infusion, or via the nasal mucosa, GnRH agonists have efficacy at least equivalent to that of danazol in the treatment of endometriosis in premenopausal women.

• Recent studies have focused on Zoladex (goserelin acetate implant; ICI Pharmaceuticals, Wilmington, DE), a newer, potent synthetic GnRH agonist.

•This agent, in a biodegradable, sustained-release, subcutaneous implant formulation, effectively suppresses serum concentrations of E2 to postmenopausal levels within 2 weeks, reduces the size of endometrial implants, decreases the revised American Fertility Society (AFS) score (an indicator of the degree of endometriosis), and improves the subjective symptoms associated with endometriosis.

•In addition, this implant formulation is convenient for the patient because it requires administration only once a month.

•Objective: To compare the efficacy and safety of Zoladex implant and oral danazol in premenopausal women with endometriosis.

•Danazol (Danocrine; Winthrop Laboratories, New York, NY) was chosen for comparison because it is approved for the treatment of endometriosis and is commonly used in clinical practice.

•Methods: Three hundred fifteen premenopausal women, 20-to-42 years of age, with stages I-to-IV endometriosis (revised AFS classification) confirmed by laparoscopy or laparotomy were randomized into a multicenter, open parallel study.

•The revised AFS score had to be 2 or more for active peritoneal and ovarian implants to be included.

•Other inclusion criteria required symptomatic (total pelvic symptom score 3 or more) or asymptomatic disease, with or without infertility.

• The women were randomized in a 2:1 ratio (208 Zoladex:107 danazol, to gain more experience with the new Zoladex treatment) to receive 24 weeks of therapy.

•A 3.6-mg dose of Zoladex was administered subcutaneously as an implant into the anterior abdominal wall every 28 days beginning on day 2 or 3 of the menstrual cycle; dose adjustment was not permitted.

•The initial danazol dose of 400 mg orally twice daily could be adjusted to 200 mg thrice daily, 200 mg twice daily, or followed by any one of these three regimens if clinically indicated.

•Therapy with danazol was initiated on day 2 or 3 after the commencement of menstruation.

•Patients are more tolerant of the symptoms of medical menopause due to GnRH agonists (e.g., hot flushes and vaginal dryness) than they are of those associated with danazol (e.g., acne, weight gain).

•In this comparative trial, Zoladex was better tolerated than danazol, as evidenced by fewer patient withdrawals due to adverse events (3 versus 12%, respectively).

•As a potent GnRH agonist, Zoladex provides rapid and complete suppression of E2.

•The subcutaneous route of administration provides a more consistent biologic efficacy profile than daily intranasal administration, and the implant formulation provides a convenient (once a month), effective dosing regimen.

•Of concern is that prolonged use of GnRH agonists may lead to clinically significant **bone loss**.

•Results: Treatment with Zoladex resulted in a mean bone mineral density loss of 5.4% over the 24-week treatment period, which is comparable to that reported for other GnRH agonists.

•Although statistically significant, this loss is similar to that observed in various physiologic conditions.

•Although bone mineral is lost after the full 24 weeks of treatment, the degree of loss at 24 weeks after discontinuing treatment (week 48) is considerably lower compared to baseline than is that seen at the end of treatment.

•This suggests the possibility of bone mineral density recovery and is consistent with expectations.

•In the small number (n = 11) of Zoladex-treated subjects who had bone mineral density determinations at week 72, 48 weeks after the completion of treatment, the mean loss level was higher than the mean of the larger group (n = 38) at the end of treatment.

•The reasons for this are not known.

°The pool of subjects was small and the variation large, and consequently a valid statistical comparison with the change from the pretreatment baseline cannot be made with any degree of confidence.

•Dietary and hormonal manipulations may retard bone mineral density loss in patients with endometriosis.]

---

4. A patient has a nonpalpable mammographically detected carcinoma of the breast. The chance of her having one or more positive axillary nodes is

   A. <1%.
   B. 5%.
   *C. 10%.
   D. 20%.
   E. 25%.

p. 1679 (Hall J A, Murphy D C, Hall B R, Hall K A. Mammographic abnormalities and the detection of carcinoma of the breast. Am J Obstet Gynec 1993; 168:1677)

4. [F & I: •Background: Approximately 5% of the results of screening mammograms are classified as abnormal, and 66% result in an excisional biopsy.

•Cancer is present in 13.8% to 37% of patients with nonpalpable mammographically detected abnormalities.

•Attempts have been made to investigate different types of mammographically detected abnormalities so as to reduce the number of negative-result or "unnecessary" biopsies.

•Objective: To report on the outcome of 169 patients with abnormalities as indicated by mammogram.

•The rates with which biopsy indicates cancer where there are mammographically detected abnormalities range from 10% to 20%.

•Attempts have been made to analyze mammogrpahically detected abnormalities to decrease the number of biopsies performed that show no signs of cancer.

•Mammographically detected abnormalities that result in a recommendation for biopsy are:

°a dominant mass,

°a mass with abnormal calcification,

°abnormal calcification alone, or

•Fact   °Detail   »issue   *answer

°asymmetric density.

•There was a **low yield** with asymmetric densities in this series.

•There is a lack of uniformity of descriptions of mammographically detected abnormalities that are not classic indicators of carcinoma.

»The gynecologist should review the films and be comfortable with the radiologist's method of reading.

•Omitting the biopsy with asymmetric density would have resulted in 55 fewer biopsy procedures and would have delayed the diagnosis in only one patient.

°This patient had one cancerous axillary node at the time of diagnosis, and the effect of further delay of diagnosis is unknown.

•Removing 55 biopsies on asymmetric densities raises the yield of biopsy to 15%.

»It would seem practical and permissible to defer immediate biopsy on many asymmetric densities in favor of follow-up films at a later date, given the very low yield of discovered carcinoma.

•The high rate of metastatic disease (50%) of nonpalpable mammographically discovered breast cancer may be because of the small size of this series.

•Mammographic screening is an effective diagnostic test to aid in the early discovery of breast carcinoma.

•A significant number of patients will have metastatic disease despite discovery of tumor by a mammogram.

•Some tumors are nonpalpable only because of clinical factors such as the size of the breasts, depth of the tumor, or density of surrounding breast tissue.

•It is not known how many nonpalpable breast cancers diagnosed by means of mammography are truly occult and how many are nonpalpable only because of clinical circumstances.

•Aside from the group of patients with asymmetric densities, it would seem wise to continue to recommend immediate biopsy for standard mammographic detection of an abnormal mass, an abnormal mass with calcification, and abnormal calcifications without a mass.]

---

5. The most sensitive method of detecting cervical infection by *Chlamydia trachomatis* is

    A. direct fluorescent antibody test.
    B. enzyme immunoassay.
 *C. polymerase chain reaction.
    D. recovery on irradiated McConkey cells.
    E. serum detection of complement-fixing antibodies.

---

p. 1441 (Witkin S S, Jeremias J, Toth M, Ledger W J. Detection of *Chlamydia trachomatis* by the polymerase chain reaction in the cervices of women with acute salpingitis. Am J Obstet Gynec 1993; 168:1438)

5. [F & I: •Background: 10% to 15% of reproductive age women in the United States have had at least one episode of salpingitis and approximately 1 million new cases occur annually.

•Salpingitis is a major cause of chronic pelvic pain, ectopic pregnancy, and infertility resulting from tubal occlusion.

- The most common causes of salpingitis are *Chlamydia trachomatis* and *Neisseria gonorrhoeae* infections, although other organisms have also been implicated.

- In general, women with gonococcal salpingitis have acute symptoms and are more easily identified and treated than are women with nongonococcal salpingitis.

- Although they often cause more extensive tubal abnormality than gonococcal infections, *C. trachomatis* infections are often only mildly symptomatic.

- A major reason for the lack of understanding of the epidemiologic nature and pathogenesis of salpingitis is difficulty in detecting chlamydial infections.

- The **obligate intracellular growth** of *C. trachomatis* makes its detection by culture a time-consuming and technically difficult procedure.

- Although currently the "gold standard," false-negative chlamydial cultures can occur as the result of inadequate inoculum size, poor sampling technique, problems in sample transport or storage, or the presence of factors in the sample that are inhibitory to the growth of *C trachomatis* or its host tissue culture cells.

- Newer, more rapid tests for detection of *C. trachomatis* involving the direct examination of specimens with an antichlamydial monoclonal antibody or a *Chlamydia*-specific deoxyribonucleic acid (DNA) probe have a sensitivity **no better than that of cultures** and can be falsely positive because of cross-reactivity with other bacteria.

- Use of the **polymerase chain reaction** to detect *C. trachomatis* may offer a significant advance over these other methods.

- With the use of oligonucleotide DNA primers specifically targeted to a region of the *C. trachomatis* genome and a heat-stable DNA polymerase, any *Chlamydia-specific* DNA present in a clinical sample can be amplified 1 million times in a few hours and can then be easily detected on an agarose or acrylamide gel.

- With the application of the polymerase chain reaction, the presence of as few as one or two chlamydial genomes per 10^5 host cells could be detected.

- When a woman infected with *C. trachomatis* had a negative culture for that organism after treatment, she also had a negative polymerase chain reaction response.

- In this study DNA primer pairs were used that amplify a 144 bp fragment of the *C trachomatis* major outer membrane protein gene present in all 15 *Chlamydia* serovars.

- Results: The polymerase chain reaction may be **more sensitive** than culture in detecting *C. trachomatis* in cervical samples from women with acute salpingitis.

- In many cases of salpingitis, as has been true for cervicitis, **no causative microorganism** can be identified.

- This lack of sensitivity of diagnosis, coupled with the limited ability to identify women at risk of chlamydial infections, greatly diminishes the capacity to understand both the epidemiologic nature and the pathogenesis of this infection and, in addition, limits the ability to initiate specific treatment to infected women and their sexual partners.

- The most likely explanation for these findings is that *C. trachomatis* was residing in the cervices of these women at a level below that required to yield a positive culture.

- Independent confirmation that these women may be harboring *C. trachomatis* was obtained by measurement of the cell-mediated immune response to *C. trachomatis*.

- A positive **lymphocyte response** to purified *C. trachomatis* elementary bodies was detected in 8 of 14 women whose test results were positive with the polymerase chain reaction; none of the women whose test results were negative with the polymerase chain reaction had a positive lymphocyte response to *C. trachomatis*.

•The cell-mediated immune response to *C. trachomatis* greatly declines after successful antibiotic treatment and detection of a positive lymphocyte proliferative response to this organism is a good indicator of a **current** chlamydial genital tract infection.

•The loss of a detectable lymphocyte proliferative response to *C. trachomatis* after antibiotic treatment of all the patients further supports the value of the **lymphocyte assay** as a measure of current infection.

•The presence of a cervical chlamydial infection at a level insufficient to sensitize a significant percentage of lymphocytes and allow the detection of an in vitro response to this organism is also the most likely explanation for the negative lymphocyte proliferative response in six of the women who had positive polymerase chain reaction results.

•Aside from its value as a sensitive, noninvasive method to detect *C. trachomatis* in the cervices of women with salpingitis, the biologic significance of a PCR positive cervical *C. trachomatis* infection that is culture negative remains to be definitively established.

•If left untreated, this organism is capable of evading immunologic defense mechanism and to persist in the cervix for long periods.

•Changes in the status of the host as the result of pregnancy, endocrine alterations, transient immunosuppression, or genital tract infection with some other microorganism could trigger the *Chlamydia* to proliferate and eventually to ascend farther up the genital tract.

•**A gonococcal genital tract infection can reactivate a latent chlamydial cervical infection.**

•Similarly, cortisone-induced immune suppression led to the reemergence of *C. trachomatis* from infected mice who had become culture negative.

•The detection of *C. trachomatis* with the polymerase chain reaction in the cervices of two culture-negative women with unexplained recurrent spontaneous abortions suggests that chlamydial reactivation may also be involved in the etiologic characteristics of this disorder.

•An association between recurrent abortion and antichlamydial antibodies in women who had cervical cultures that were negative for *C. trachomatis* has been made previously.

•*C. trachomatis* can persist in a nonculturable form that continues to induce inflammatory responses.]

---

6. The most sensitive and specific method of diagnosing PID is

    A. C-reactive protein.
    B. culdocentesis.
    C. endometrial biopsy.
    D. history/physical examination.
  *E. radionuclide scanning with labeled leukocytes.

p. 799 (Mozas J, Castilla J A, Alarcon J L, Ruiz J, Jimena P, Herruzo A J. Diagnosis of pelvic inflammatory disease with 99mTechnetium-hexamethylpropylenamine-oxime-labeled autologous leukocytes and pelvic radionuclide scintigraphy. Obstet Gynecol 1993; 81:797)

6. [F & I: •Background: The clinical picture of pelvic inflammatory disease (PID) is variable.

•Depending on the nature and severity of the disease, patients can complain of abdominal pain with or without signs of peritonitis or can present with silent disease, which is more difficult to diagnose and for which suitable treatment is often delayed.

- Because of the risk of complications and sequelae from PID, and because clinical symptoms are unreliable indicators of the disease, there is still a need for a precise, reliable method of diagnosis.

- A growing number of clinicians are using direct visualization of the internal reproductive organs with diagnostic laparoscopy.

- PID is clinically confirmed in only 65% of the cases in which laparoscopy is done.

- Laparoscopy and the anesthesia it requires both involve risks and are costly.

- Relatively noninvasive imaging techniques, including echography, computed tomography, and radionuclide scintigraphy, are available for the diagnosis and observation of suspected PID.

- Objective: To evaluate pelvic radionuclide scintigraphy after the injection of ^{99m}technetium-hexamethylpropylenamine-oxime labeled autologous leukocytes as a noninvasive method of differential diagnosis.

- Results: The pelvic diseases most frequently confused with acute salpingitis are ovarian cysts, endometriosis, ectopic pregnancy, and acute appendicitis.

- Many patients examined with laparoscopy because of a provisional diagnosis of ovarian tumor, appendicitis, or ectopic pregnancy are found to have PID.

- These observations show that the clinical diagnosis of PID is often mistaken and that some patients suspected of having other pelvic diseases actually have PID.

- The error rates in the diagnosis of PID have led clinicians to depend increasingly on laparoscopy, despite the risks inherent in the technique itself and in general anesthesia, and despite the cost of the procedure, which limits its use to carefully selected patients.

- Laparoscopy is justified when the diagnosis is unknown; when a differential diagnosis is required between PID and appendicitis, ectopic pregnancy, or rupture of a pelvic abscess; or when the response to antibiotics is unsatisfactory.

- Several methods have been proposed to improve the accuracy of the clinical diagnosis without resorting to laparoscopy, including the injection of ^{99m}technetium-hexamethylpropylenamine-oxime-labeled autologous leukocytes followed by pelvic radionuclide scintigraphy.

- This method has been used to detect intra-abdominal abscesses and several inflammatory processes.

- Radionuclide scintigraphy with labeled leukocytes, recognized by the Food and Drug Administration as a low-risk procedure, is highly accurate in diagnosing localized infections, abscesses, and inflammatory lesions involving leukocyte infiltration.

- In 40 women, the sensitivity was 95% and specificity was 85%; thus 90% of subjects were classified correctly with the technique.

- Compared with other methods of diagnosis used in PID, such as endometrial biopsy, C-reactive protein, or erythrocyte sedimentation rate, the injection of labeled autologous leukocytes followed by pelvic radionuclide scintigraphy was the most sensitive and specific method, correctly identifying the greatest proportion of patients.

  ° The three false-positives reflected acute appendicitis, tubal ectopic pregnancy, and pelvic endometriosis.

- Although the clinical entity identified was not PID, all three patients nonetheless benefited from laparoscopy.

Obstetrics and Gynecology: Review 1994-Gynecology References

•The false-positive findings may have been due to the inflammatory processes associated with these entities.

•The positive-PID subject whose pelvic radionuclide scintigraphy gave false-negative results was found to have mild PID on laparoscopy.

•Nevertheless, microbiologic cultures of the peritoneal exudate were positive for aerobic and anaerobic organisms.

•Clinicians should be aware that mild signs of PID may be beyond the resolution of the technique used.

•Because only in-patients were studied, the usefulness of this technique for the more subtle forms of PID which might be treated on an outpatient basis cannot be determined.]

---

7. Which of the following laboratory findings are most likely in the serum of a patient with an ectopic pregnancy? (↑=increased; ↓ = decreased)

   A. ↑ progesterone, ↑ HCG, ↑ estradiol, ↑ alpha-fetoprotein
   B. ↓ progesterone, ↓ estradiol and ↓ alpha-fetoprotein, ↑ HCG
   C. ↓ progesterone, ↓ HCG, ↓ estradiol and ↓ alpha-fetoprotein
 *D. ↓ progesterone, ↓ HCG, ↓ estradiol and ↑ alpha-fetoprotein
   E. ↑ progesterone, ↑ estradiol, ↓ HCG and ↓ alpha-fetoprotein

---

p. 709 (Grosskinsky C M, Hage M L, Tyrey L, Christakos A C, Hughes C L. hCG, progesterone, Alpha-fetoprotein, and estradiol in the identification of ectopic pregnancy. Obstet Gynecol 1993; 81:705)

7. [F & I: •Background: The determination of serial quantitative hCG levels for the diagnosis of ectopic pregnancy may delay treatment.

•A single serum progesterone determination has been used as an adjunct in the rapid diagnosis of ectopic pregnancy.

•In addition to hCG, a serum estradiol (E2) level, with or without progesterone determination, may be helpful in the early diagnosis of ectopic pregnancy.

•Objective: To correlate a group of biochemical markers of pregnancy with clinical outcome and thus to differentiate among healthy pregnancies, ectopic pregnancies, and otherwise compromised gestations.

°In addition to hCG, progesterone, and E2, alpha-fetoprotein (AFP), a product of the yolk sac and fetal liver was also measured.

•Clinically, those pregnancies resulting in a viable outcome or spontaneous abortion were associated with less adnexal tenderness than ectopic pregnancy.

•There was less vaginal bleeding with viable pregnancy than with any other outcome.

•Levels of E2, progesterone, and hCG were highest in viable pregnancy and lowest in ectopic pregnancy and in patients who were not pregnant.

•The scatter of **hCG and E2** values was so extensive that if used separately, they could **not** reliably predict outcome.

•In contrast, **progesterone** levels in viable pregnancy overlapped in less than 20% of cases with those in ectopic pregnancy.

°No viable pregnancy was associated with a progesterone level of less than 8 ng/mL, and no ectopic pregnancy with a level greater than 15 ng/mL.

°This "gray zone" from 8-to-15 ng/mL compares fairly well with that described elsewhere (10-to-25 ng/mL)

°**Alpha-fetoprotein** followed a different pattern from hCG, progesterone, and E2.

°Ectopic pregnancies tended to have **higher** AFP levels than any of the other outcome groups.

°°This could be due to abnormal placentation or other placental anomalies.

•**Elevated** progesterone, hCG, and E2 are very strongly associated with **viable pregnancy.**

•**Low** progesterone and **elevated** AFP are also strongly associated with **ectopic** pregnancy, although the scatter of AFP data limits the usefulness of this test.

•A single progesterone value could differentiate between ectopic pregnancy and viable pregnancy in more than 80% of patients in the current group and outperformed the accuracy of both clinical diagnosis and a panel of categorical clinical data employed in a multivariate logistic analysis.

•Finally, when specific biochemical marker level cutoffs were used in a multivariate logistic analysis of all four assays, an accuracy of 94.5% and specificity of 98.5% were achieved in the diagnosis of ectopic pregnancy.]

---

8. Associated with an increased incidence of break-through bleeding:

   A. Demulen.
   B. O/N 7/7/7.
   C. Ovral.
   D. Triphasil.
   *E. All have about the same incidence of break-through bleeding.

---

p. 730 (Krettek J E, Arkin S I, Chaisilwattana P, Monif G R G. *Chlamydia trachomatis* in patients who used oral contraceptives and had intermenstrual spotting. Obstet Gynecol 1993; 81:728)

8. [F & I: •Background: "Breakthrough bleeding" or spotting in oral contraceptive (OC) users has been attributed to failure of synthetic steroids to provide adequate support for endometrial integrity.

•Most packages for birth control pills carry specific information concerning breakthrough bleeding (bleeding that occurs during the usual nonbleeding part of the menstrual cycle) or spotting between periods.

•This information is usually reassurance that these benign phenomena, which tend to occur more often in the first few cycles than in later cycles, are usually temporary and have no clinical significance.

•What is poorly perceived in the literature is that intermenstrual spotting in patients taking OCs for two or more closely related cycles is a possible sign of chronic **endometritis**.

•Objective: To compare the prevalence of chlamydial antigen among OC users with and without intermenstrual spotting or bleeding.

•Oral contraceptives increase **cervical ectropion** and so theoretically facilitate detection of chlamydia because of more efficient specimen collection.

•Cervical ectropion may do more than simply enhance diagnostic accuracy.

•Whether OCs predispose to a chronic endometritis due to *C trachomatis* or other organisms is speculative.

•In this study, the population used six different OCs: Demulen; Ortho-Novum 7/7/7, 1/35, and 1/50; Ovral; and Triphasil.

•Both monophasic and triphasic, and low and high-dose-estrogen OCs were involved in late intermenstrual bleeding.

•The irregularity of sample sizes precluded meaningful statistical analysis.

•**Superficially, no one specific type of OC appeared to be uniquely associated with breakthrough bleeding.**

•Six of the eight endometrial biopsies exhibited a lymphocytic-plasma cell stromal infiltrate, which is found in endometrial biopsies obtained from women with chlamydial endocervicitis.

•In most instances, the etiology of the breakthrough spotting is probably the underlying chronic endometritis.

•An almost threefold increase in the number of positive Microtrak tests was detected in OC users with intermenstrual spotting versus women without breakthrough bleeding, and an almost fivefold increase over matched non-users without breakthrough bleeding.

•These results support previous studies that identified an increased prevalence of chlamydial infection in OC users.

•This study goes beyond this observation and suggests that for women previously well regulated on OCs, **breakthrough bleeding is an additive marker for potential chlamydial infection.**]

---

9. In planning for a post-coital test, within many hours after the LH surge as detected by urinary assay should an evaluation of cervical mucus be made?

   A. 2
   B. 4
   C. 6
   D. 10
   *E. 12

---

p. 738 (Corsan G H, Blotner M B, Nohrer M K, Shelden R, Kemmann E. The utility of a home urinary LH immunoassay in timing the postcoital test. Obstet Gynecol 1993; 81:736)

9. [F & I: •Background: An abnormality in the sperm-cervical mucus interaction is present in 10-to-15% of infertile couples.

•Poor postcoital test results associated with decreased rates of oocyte fertilization in in vitro fertilization programs, impaired zona-free hamster egg penetration, and lower conception rates in infertile couples; the validity of the postcoital test as a test of fertility has been questioned.

•Appropriate timing of the postcoital test is critical.

•This test should be performed in the immediate preovulatory period, when the effect of estradiol (E2) on the cervical mucus-producing cells or crypts is optimized.

•Home urinary LH immunoassay kits are used for timing both artificial insemination and coitus.

•Performing the postcoital test soon after the detection of the LH surge may identify a time in the cycle when cervical mucus quality is maximized.

•This may avoid doing a postcoital test too early in the cycle, when the estrogen effect on the cervical mucus is insufficient, or too late, when progesterone secretion alters cervical mucus quality.

•Objective: To determine whether use of a home LH kit improves the results of cervical mucus and postcoital test scores when compared to traditional timing methods in a group of normally ovulatory infertile women.

•Ovulation prediction kits are useful to time the postcoital test because they identify a time just before ovulation when the effect of estrogen on cervical mucus should be maximal.

•The day of the serum LH surge coincides with maximal cervical mucus scores.

°Maximal cervical mucus scores occur within 1 day of the serum LH surge in 97% of cycles.

•Cervical mucus scores decline rapidly after detection of the urinary LH surge; the postcoital test should be performed **within 12 hours of its detection.**

•The timing of the postcoital test by means of an ovulation prediction kit may be important to minimize false-negative results.

•In theory, LH-timed postcoital tests may reduce the number of patient office visits required to obtain optimally timed postcoital tests and avoid unnecessary medical treatment for cervical factor infertility.

•Results: An LH surge kit produced **similar** postcoital test and cervical mucus scores when compared with usual timing methods.

•Serum E2, LH, and progesterone values did not differ significantly between groups, suggesting that LH kits do **not** identify the preovulatory period better than traditional timing in ovulatory infertile women.

•There are several possible explanations for these findings.

•Although the BBT is an inaccurate prospective predictor of the precise day of the serum LH surge, it does provide a reasonably accurate estimate of the 2-to-3-day period on either side of the LH surge.

•This degree of accuracy may be adequate for satisfactory timing of the postcoital test in most ovulatory patients.

•Once-daily LH testing may not be as precise in identifying the preovulatory period as is commonly believed, and may only approximate the timing of the serum LH surge and ovulation.

•The failure of urinary LH kits to improve pregnancy rates in women undergoing donor insemination also questions whether LH kits can more reliably identify the ovulatory period than can BBT graphs.

•The onset of the urinary LH surge occurs after follicle rupture in 9% of the women, suggesting that once-daily LH testing to time periovulatory events may lack precision in some patients.]

---

10. Patients who have a hysterectomy for benign disease have how much of a decrease in the risk of having ovarian cancer?

    A. 10%
    B. 25%
    *C. 50%
    D. 75%
    E. less than 5%

---

p. 365 (Parazzini F, Negri E, La Vecchia C, Luchini L, Mezzopane R. Hysterectomy, oophorectomy, and subsequent ovarian cancer risk. Obstet Gynecol 1993; 81:363)

10. [F & I: •Background: Hysterectomy and unilateral oophorectomy may reduce the risk of subsequent ovarian cancer.

•These findings are interpreted in terms of selective mechanisms, as occult ovarian disease may be detected during surgery.

•Alternatively, hysterectomy may lower the risk of ovarian cancer by preventing exposure of the ovary to potential carcinogens from the perineum or vagina, or by altering ovarian blood flow and ovulation or other hormonal activities.

•Objective: To analyze this issue further, data from a case-control study on ovarian cancer was examined.

•Results: Previous hysterectomy about **halves** the risk of subsequent development of ovarian cancer.

•Hysterectomy and unilateral oophorectomy performed together had no apparent difference in ovarian cancer risk relative to either one alone.

•A reduced risk of ovarian cancer in women who have undergone hysterectomy has been reported.

•The Cancer and Steroid Hormone Study including women aged 20-to-54 years, found an RR of ovarian cancer of 0.6 in women who had hysterectomy with or without unilateral oophorectomy.

•The inverse association between hysterectomy and ovarian cancer risk was still present 10 years after surgery (RR = 0.6), but disappeared after 2 decades.

•The protective effect of hysterectomy is due to the "screening effect"; ie, hysterectomy provides an opportunity for examination of the ovaries.

•The risk of ovarian cancer did not appear to level off with time in women who had had a hysterectomy, supporting a biologic explanation of the effect of hysterectomy on ovarian cancer risk.

•Hysterectomy may alter ovarian blood flow, and this protective mechanism should take some time to come into effect and be more pronounced several years after surgery.]

---

11. Reasons for the removal of an otherwise asymptomatic myomatous uterus reaching the level of the symphysis pubis include

    A. if a uterus continued to enlarge it may compromise other structures; for example, ureters or lead to debilitating symptoms.
    B. if the uterus continued to enlarge surgical treatment becomes more difficult and carries greater risks.
    C. operating on a uterus before it enlarges further may improve a woman's chances for fertility and successful pregnancy.
    D. the ovaries cannot be adequately evaluated by bimanual evaluation.
    *E. none of the above.

p.751 (Friedman A J, Haas S T. Should uterine size be an indication for surgical intervention in women with myomas? Am J Obstet Gynec 1993; 168:751)

11. [F & I: •Background: Surgical intervention may be recommended when the size of the uterus exceeds that at 10 to 12 weeks of gestation in women presumed to have myomas.

•Hysterectomy is recommended for women with enlarged uteri except for those younger than 40 years who want to preserve their reproductive potential; the latter women are considered candidates for myomectomy.

•Reasons frequently cited for the necessity for surgical intervention in asymptomatic women with enlarged uteri include the following:

    °1. The ovaries cannot be adequately evaluated by bimanual examination.

Obstetrics and Gynecology: Review 1994-Gynecology References

°2. Malignancy cannot be ruled out in an enlarged pelvic mass.

°3. If a uterus continues to enlarge, it may compromise other structures (e.g., the ureters) or lead to debilitating symptoms.

°4. If a uterus continues to enlarge, surgical treatment becomes more difficult and carries greater risks.

°5. Operating on a uterus before it enlarges further may improve a woman's chances for future fertility and successful pregnancy.

°6. It may be difficult or impossible for a postmenopausal woman with myomas to take estrogen replacement therapy because of the potential for continued growth of these tumors with such therapy.

•**Inability to assess ovaries.** When the uterus is sufficiently enlarged to preclude an adequate physical examination of the adnexa, ultrasonography may be used as a surrogate for the adnexal examination.

•Ultrasonography is superior to bimanual examination in identifying ovarian enlargement, regardless of uterine size.

•When uterine enlargement makes it impossible to observe the ovaries by pelvic ultrasonography, magnetic resonance imaging may be used.

•**There are no data to support the contention that a reduction in uterine size by hysterectomy or myomectomy increases the probability of early detection of ovarian cancer.**

•This condition is rare before age 50, yet the number of hysterectomies performed for fibroids peaks in the 35 to 44-year age group and myomectomies are rarely performed after age 40.

•Because of the relatively young age of the patients involved, ovarian conservation is usually recommended even when hysterectomy is undertaken.

•Thus hysterectomy or myomectomy for the indication of "inadequate pelvic examination" subjects a women in the 30s or 40s to potentially serious risks with no proved benefit.

•**Inability to rule out malignancy in an enlarged pelvic mass.** By means of high-resolution ultrasonography the structure or origin of the pelvic mass can usually be determined.

•If the mass arises from the ovary, then the age of the patient, the ultrasonographic characteristics of the mass, and any changes in the mass over time will aid the gynecologist in deciding whether surgical intervention is warranted.

•If the enlarged pelvic mass is the uterus and the ovaries are examined ultrasonographically and appear normal, the overwhelming likelihood is that the uterine enlargement is caused by a benign condition such as a myoma or adenomyosis.

•In cases of uterine enlargement a hysterectomy may be performed to obtain a tissue diagnosis.

°Because uterine size is a poor predictor of malignancy evaluation; other diagnostic tests should precede surgical intervention.

•Endometrial carcinoma, the most common uterine malignancy, is predominantly a disorder of postmenopausal women; in most cases the uterus is **normal** in size.

°Vaginal bleeding is the presenting complaint in >90% of cases.

°An endometrial biopsy or a curettage will usually establish the diagnosis.

•Fact   °Detail   Page 25   »issue   *answer

- Uterine sarcomas are less common than uterine carcinomas.

  ° Leiomyosarcoma is the most common uterine sarcoma, with an incidence of 0.13% to 0.29%.

  ° Although in cases of leiomyosarcoma the uterus is often quite large, its size at diagnosis ranges from <6 to >20 weeks of gestation.

  ° The absolute size of the uterus is not reliably useful in the early or preoperative diagnosis of leiomyosarcoma.

  ° In addition to absolute uterine size, the **rate of uterine growth** is a finding commonly used to guide treatment decisions.

  ° A perception exists that a rapidly enlarging uterus is more likely to be malignant.

    ° **"Rapid uterine growth" has not been adequately defined or characterized; thus this hypothesis remains unstudied and untested.**

  ° The presence of a new or enlarging uterine mass in a postmenopausal woman should be viewed with concern, with an emphasis on definitive diagnosis and treatment.

  ° The entire uterus decreases in size, as do individual myomas, after estrogen withdrawal after natural or surgical menopause.

  ° When an enlarging uterus is associated with vaginal bleeding in a postmenopausal woman who is not receiving hormone replacement therapy, the urgency of diagnosis cannot be overemphasized.

  ° More than 50% of women with leiomyosarcomas are first seen with abnormal vaginal bleeding, yet endometrial sampling does not reliably confirm the diagnosis.

  ° Thus **menopausal status** has a profound impact on clinical decision making in this situation.

- **Compromise of other structures by an enlarging uterus.** An enlarged uterus may cause extrinsic bladder and bowel compression, leading to urinary frequency or urgency and to constipation.

  - A myomatous uterus extending out to the pelvic sidewalls may also compress one or both ureters; such compression may lead to hydroureter, hydronephrosis, and, potentially, compromised renal function, even in the absence of pain or other symptoms.

  - **The prevalence of these conditions in the presence of an enlarged myomatous uterus is not documented in the literature.**

    ° **The likelihood of irreversible organ damage in these cases is extremely low.**

  - Stable, asymptomatic **mild** hydroureter does not increase the likelihood of urinary tract infection or renal damage and should **not** be considered an absolute indication for surgical intervention.

  - **Moderate to severe** degrees of hydroureter or hydronephrosis **are** indications for surgical intervention.

  - The presence and degree of ureteral compression are easily evaluated with pelvic ultrasonography, which may be performed once or twice annually in patients who require close monitoring.

  - In selected instances (i.e., perimenopausal women) a short course (i.e., ≤6 months) of treatment with a gonadotropinreleasing hormone (GnRH) agonist may reduce uterine size, decreasing the degree of ureteral obstruction and allowing the patient to pass through menopause without surgical intervention.

  - **Increased surgical risk caused by an enlarging uterus.** One concern is that both surgical ease and surgical risk are correlated with uterine size.

- A corollary to this assumption is that if surgical intervention is inevitable, it is wise to intervene early, before a uterus with myomas has a chance to enlarge.

- **Uterine size has not been shown to correlate with morbidity in women undergoing hysterectomy.**

  ° Location and number of fibroids are probably more important variables influencing surgical difficulty than is absolute size, especially when myomas are positioned on the cervix or near the uterine blood supply.

  ° If a physician is concerned about the possibility that uterine enlargement will increase the severity of symptoms or the difficulty of a future operation, the patient can be examined every 3 to 6 months to closely monitor changes in uterine size and symptoms.

  ° If uterine enlargement leads to disabling symptoms, surgical intervention may then be planned.

- **Compromise of future fertility by myomectomy on a "large" uterus.** Myomectomy may decrease fertility, presumably because of postoperative adhesion formation.

- A common belief is that the likelihood of impaired fertility after myomectomy is positively correlated with preoperative uterine size.

  ° Although some investigators have reported lower conception rates after myomectomies in women with uteri >10 gestational weeks in size, others have found no correlation of fertility with the size or number of tumors removed.

- **Growth of the uterus and myomas caused by postmenopausal hormone replacement therapy.** No data suggest that significant uterine enlargement occurs in postmenopausal women taking the doses of estrogen and progestin generally used in hormone replacement therapy.

- Postmenopausal women with known myomas who are receiving hormone replacement therapy could be evaluated 3 months after the initiation of such treatment and then at intervals of 6 months to 1 year thereafter.

- If significant growth occurs during standard hormone replacement therapy, surgical intervention would be appropriate.

- **Risk of surgery for myomas. Mortality** varies with age, indication for surgery, and comorbidity.

- The overall death rate is 12 to 16 per 10,000 hysterectomies.

  °° It represents a sixfold relative risk compared with the death rate for women of the same age.

  °° When deaths from pregnant or cancer-related hysterectomies are excluded, the hysterectomy death rate drops to five to six per 10,000 operations.

- **It is estimated that more than 300 deaths occur annually in the United States from hysterectomy for benign conditions.**

- **Morbidity** from hysterectomy is significantly greater than is commonly appreciated.

  ° Morbidity can range from 25% to 50% of patients.

  ° The largest category, febrile morbidity, encompasses respiratory and urinary tract infections, wound and cuff infections and their sequelae, and fever without an identified source.

  ° Hemorrhage is difficult to study and is generally measured by its proxy, transfusion.

  ° Transfusion rates for hysterectomies performed at nine institutions between 1978 and 1981 ranged between 8% and 15%.

°Other major morbidities include damage to adjacent organs and such life-threatening sequelae as pulmonary embolus.

°°Rates for these complications are bladder injury, 0.3% to 0.8%; ureter injury, 0.1% to 0.5%; bowel injury, 0.1%; and pulmonary embolus, 0.2% to 0.3%.

°°The literature on adverse psychologic or sexual effects of hysterectomy is mixed, confusing, and changing.]

---

12. A patient has a conization for a pap test suggesting CIN III. The margins of the cone specimen show CIN II. Six months later a repeat pap suggests CIN III. The treatment of choice is

   *A. colposcopy.
   B. cryosurgery.
   C. hysterectomy.
   D. repeat conization.
   E. repeat pap.

p. 442 (Lapaquette T K, Dinh T V, Hannigan E V, Doherty M G, Yandell R B, Buchanan V S. Management of patients with positive margins after cervical conization. Obstet Gynecol 1993; 82:440)

12. [F & I: •Background: Although there are standard indications for cervical conization in the evaluation and treatment of cervical intraepithelial neoplasia (CIN), there is controversy regarding the management of CIN extending to the resection margins of a conization specimen.

•Following such a report there are three options:

°1) continued follow-up by Papanicolaou smears and endocervical curettage (ECC), with colposcopic evaluation if cytology indicates;

°2) repeat cervical conization; or

°3) hysterectomy, if other indications for hysterectomy exist.

•Conservative management is potentially complicated by later occult progression of CIN or patient loss to follow-up.

•Repeat surgery also has inherent risks and complications.

•The second cervical resection margin may again reveal residual disease, future fertility may be impaired, or no detectable residual disease in the second surgical specimen may suggest overtreatment.

•The methods of performing cervical conization include various laser instruments, the loop electro-excision procedure, and cold knife excision.

•They do not differ in their ability to eradicate CIN, but the types and frequency of perioperative and postoperative complications vary considerably.

•Objectives: To clarify the natural history of CIN at a cervical resection margin and to propose a management plan, by retrospectively reviewing the outcomes of patients treated for CIN in whom conization specimens were noted to have disease extending to the cervical margins.

•This study includes a large number of patients followed for a long period.

•The incidence of resolution of CIN after conization with positive margins was 58% (i.e., 42% of the patients had persistent CIN).

- There was no significant difference in persistence of CIN between patients managed conservatively and those managed surgically (P = .59).

- Histology revealed resolution of dysplasia in women having hysterectomy.

- In the group of patients having conization only, the negativity of successive Papanicolaou smears for at least 2 years (every 4 months the first year and every 6 months the second year) was also considered as reliable.

- Weaknesses in the current analysis concern the high proportion of patients lost to follow-up (14%) and bias in selecting higher grades of CIN for hysterectomy.

- Patient attrition is a significant management consideration in patients who travel long distances after referral, but prefer local follow-up once evaluation and initial treatment are complete.

- Because of the retrospective nature of this study, selection bias in treatment planning was not adjustable, but was minimal.

- In the group managed conservatively (47 patients, or approximately one-half the study population), 80% had CIN III at conization, compared to 91% CIN III in the remaining patients managed surgically (46 patients).

- In this study, the **best predictors of persistence of dysplasia with conservative management were location of the positive resection margin and degree of CIN in the conization specimen.**

- There was 47% CIN persistence with positive endocervical margins versus 13% persistence with positive ectocervical margins, and 45% CIN persistence in the CIN III population compared with 23% for CIN II.

- Among all patients with persistent CIN (39), 87% (34) had CIN III and 5% (two) had CIN II noted at the endocervical margin.

- There are several potential explanations for spontaneous resolution of CIN extending to the resection margins after conization alone (64%) or after delayed hysterectomy (33%) and for the absence of CIN after immediate hysterectomy (57%):

    ° destruction of CIN at surgery via tissue necrosis from resecting the tissue or establishing hemostasis,

    ° destruction of tissue at the margins from postsurgical inflammatory reaction, or

    ° severing of the conization at the exact boundary between CIN and normal tissue.

- Cervical conization is integral to the evaluation and treatment of CIN under well-defined circumstances.

- In the event that pathologic analysis reveals extension of disease to the resection margins, conservative follow-up with frequent Papanicolaou smears could be used to delay, or entirely avoid, repeat conizations or hysterectomy in 58% of patients.

- Those with the highest risk of CIN persistence had CIN III at the endocervical resection margins; these patients deserve the closest and most aggressive follow-up after conization.

- No invasive cancer occurred in the present series.

- The number of subjects was statistically insufficient to provide assurance that the risk of invasion is negligible.

- This emphasizes the need for close cytologic follow-up.

»The management plan for a cone specimen with positive margins consists of repeat Papanicolaou smears every 4 months for 1 year, every 6 months the following year, and then annually.

•In case of an abnormal smear 4 months after conization, the smear in 4 months for a low-grade squamous intraepithelial lesion was repeated.

•The complete work-up was repeated, consisting of colposcopy, biopsies, and ECC, if the Papanicolaou smear shows a high-grade or a low-grade squamous intraepithelial lesion on two occasions.

•Further conservative management or surgery depends on the results of colposcopy and histology.]

---

13. At 12 weeks a pregnant patient has a Papanicolaou smear reported as satisfactory except that the evaluation is "limited by the lack of an endocervical component." The cervix appears grossly normal and the pregnancy is otherwise uncomplicated. The next best step in the patient's management is

   A. perform colposcopy and directed biopsies if needed at 28 weeks
   B. perform colposcopy and directed biopsies if needed now
   C. repeat the pap at 28 weeks
   *D. repeat the pap in 12 months
   E. repeat the pap in two months

---

p. 130 (Kost E R, Snyder R R, Schwartz L E, Hankins G D V. The "less than optimal" cytology: Importance in obstetric patients and in a routine gynecologic population. Obstet Gynecol 1993; 81:127)

13. [F & I: •Background: The occurrence of unacceptably high false-negative rates and deficient quality assurance measures for cervical-vaginal cytology have resulted in efforts to improve both the quality and the efficiency of the cytologic screening process.

•In 1988, a multidisciplinary group met in Bethesda, Maryland to revamp the nomenclature for reporting cervical and vaginal cytologies.

•The group specifically noted the need for "communication of the cytopathologic findings to the referring physician in unambiguous diagnostic terms that have clinical relevance."

•The "less than optimal" category, which was created to provide a statement about the adequacy of any given cytologic specimen, is the focus of the present study.

•Multiple reasons were possible for a cytologic smear to qualify as less than optimal, including the lack of an endocervical component.

•This is analogous to the term "absence of endocervical cells" in the old nomenclature; the Bethesda System appropriately specifies that this terminology be used only in premenopausal women with a cervix.

•The system broadened the definition of an adequate endocervical component to include endocervical cells, and endocervical mucus or squamous metaplastic cells.

•Despite the new additions provided by the Bethesda System, several deficiencies exist.

•Most important, no quantifiable, specific microscopic criteria were provided to distinguish satisfactory from unsatisfactory or less than optimal smears.

•In 1991, a second National Cancer Institute workshop (Bethesda II) convened to address these issues.

•One result of this was elimination of the less than optimal terminology, which was replaced by the phrase "satisfactory for evaluation but limited by...."

   °This category would include those smears that are satisfactory but limited by the absence of an endocervical component.

•Fact   °Detail   »issue   *answer

- The 1991 report specifically acknowledged the need for guidelines and for clinical trials to resolve the questions regarding management, but none have since been issued.

- The observation of an inordinately high rate of less than optimal tests in the obstetric population prompted this clinical investigation.

- Objective: To determine whether an otherwise normal cytology specimen that lacks an endocervical component safely constitutes an adequate screening test.

- Many providers believe it medicolegally imprudent to allow "less than optimal" terminology in a patient's medical record as the sole cervical cancer screen pending their next routine examination.

- Although Bethesda II eliminated the terminology "less than optimal," it substituted the disclaimer "but limited by . . ."; the issue of how to manage these tests remains to be resolved.

- Results: A significant difference in the percentages of less than optimal tests in obstetric versus gynecologic patients was found.

- Several factors may explain this 1.8-fold increase in less than optimal tests among the obstetric patients.

- First, the sampling techniques differed between obstetric and gynecologic patients.

  ° The prenatal smears were performed with a wooden spatula and cotton-tip applicator, whereas all other gynecologic and postpartum cytologic tests were collected with a wooden spatula and nylon brush.

  ° Endocervical cell retrieval is increased with the use of a nylon brush; reported retrieval with a cotton-tip applicator ranges from 81-to-88%, compared with 98-to-98.6% using a nylon brush.

  ° Theoretically, the physiologic cervical eversion commonly occurring in pregnancy should make retrieval of endocervical components easier, thus decreasing the incidence of less than optimal tests.

  ° Health care providers may hesitate to perform the same rigorous sampling in obstetric patients for fear of inducing bleeding.

- The management of less than optimal tests centers on the question: Do these tests constitute adequate cervical cancer screening or are they inadequate cytologies requiring immediate repeat evaluation?

- The absence of an endocervical component has been proposed as evidence of inadequate sampling of the squamocolumnar junction.

- This theory is based on data in nonpregnant women showing that patients whose Papanicolaou tests contained an endocervical component had an increased rate of dysplasia.

- When the frequency of dysplasia was stratified in these studies by the presence of endocervical cells, a two- to fourfold increase was found in those smears that contained endocervical cells.

- The assumption underlying the recommendation for an early test is that cervical cancer precursors may be missed on tests that lack an endocervical component.

- Several longitudinal studies performed in women whose entry smears lacked an endocervical component failed to find a higher frequency of abnormalities in later smears.

- **It may well be that the presence of endocervical cells is a marker of a slightly higher probability of cervical intraepithelial neoplasia.**

°The abnormal squamocolumnar junction may more easily shed endocervical cells.

•There was essentially no difference between cytologies repeated 12 months after a less than optimal test (performed at the postpartum visit) versus those performed in routine gynecologic patients with adequate cytologies.

•Clearly, postpartum women with a prenatal less than optimal smear do not constitute a high-risk group due to prior inadequate sampling.

»Consequently, early rescreening of obstetric patients based on lack of an endocervical component is **not** recommended.

•Early rescreening of gynecologic patients with a less than optimal test is a low-yield procedure.

°The pickup of dysplasia in this group was only one case (0.3%, one of 305).]

---

14. The maximum endometrial thickness observed during vaginal ultrasound for conservative management of a patient thought to have a complete abortion

    A. 3 millimeters
    B. 4 millimeters
    C. 5 millimeters
    D. 7.5 millimeters
    *E. 1 centimeter

---

p.15 (Rulin M C, Bornstein S G, Campbell J D. The reliability of ultrasonography in the management of spontaneous abortion, clinically thought to be complete: A prospective study. Am J Obstet Gynec 1993; 168:12)

14. [F & I: •Background: When patients are seen in the first trimester of pregnancy with vaginal bleeding, a history of cramps, and passage of tissue or clots, the diagnosis of spontaneous abortion is usually apparent.

•If the cervix is open or tissue is present in the cervical os, the abortion is incomplete, and curettage is carried out.

•When the cervix is closed and bleeding is not heavy, distinguishing between complete and incomplete abortion can be difficult.

•Management has been either empiric or based on clinical findings.

•Ultrasonography is used in the diagnosis of ectopic pregnancy and the evaluation of threatened abortion, but documentation of its ability to identify retained products of conception after spontaneous abortion is needed.

•Objective: To test a management protocol based on the hypothesis that patients with an ultrasonographic examination showing no retained products of conception could be safely managed without curettage.

•Results: The basic hypothesis and management protocol were supported by an uneventful spontaneous resolution in 48 of 49 (98%) women with negative ultrasonographic examinations.

•Two criteria were used to decide that the ultrasound examination was positive, **collection of echogenic material or a thickened endometrium**.

•The standard for the minimum positive value was based on the finding that single-layer endometrial thickness in the late secretory phase of the menstrual cycle measured between 3 and 5.5 mm.

•Because the two opposing layers are included in the description of endometrial thickness, actually a double layer, **1.0 cm as the maximum thickness for conservative management** was chosen.

°One patient whose endometrium measured 1.1 cm had a negative curettage.

°Five of seven endometria between 2.0 and 2.4 cm contained villi.

°Nine of 13 patients with a positive result on ultrasonography had retained products of conception proved by curettage, for a positive predictive value of 69%.

•Conclusion: The spontaneous resolution rate was 98% when the endometrial stripe was <1.0 cm in thickness.

°It is quite likely that a number of patients with a few undetectable chorionic villi will have a good outcome without curettage.]

---

15. Leiomyosarcomas can be reliably diagnosed by

   A. intraoperative frozen section.
   B. preoperative computed tomography.
   C. preoperative endometrial sampling.
   D. preoperative magnetic resonance imaging.
   *E. none of the above.

---

p.180 (Schwartz L B, Diamond M P, Schwartz P E. Leiomyosarcomas: Clinical presentation. Am J Obstet Gynec 1993; 168:180)

15. [F & I: •Background: Uterine leiomyosarcoma is an uncommon malignancy with an estimated yearly incidence of 0.67 per 100,000 women aged ≥20 years.

•It represents 1.3% of all uterine malignancies and about 25% of uterine sarcomas.

•The incidence ratio between benign and malignant leiomyomas is estimated to be 800 to 1.

•Distinguishing between these two possibilities continues to be difficult because presenting symptoms of leiomyosarcomas resemble those of benign leiomyomas and most commonly include uterine bleeding, pelvic pain, and/or a pelvic mass.

•Preoperative diagnosis of leiomyosarcoma is unreliable in spite of diagnostic imaging and endometrial sampling.

•Intraoperative frozen sections are not always decisive.

•The inclination is to treat two subsets of patients conservatively: young women wishing to preserve fertility and perimenopausal women wishing to postpone definitive therapy with the hope of eventual uterine shrinkage after menopause.

•Some patients do not wish to have a hysterectomy, and others are treated with gonadotropin-releasing hormone (GnRH) agonists to shrink myomas (and increase hematocrit) before definitive therapy.

•GnRH agonists are used to decrease uterine size in an effort to convert a potential abdominal hysterectomy into a vaginal hysterectomy.

•By decreasing uterine size, GnRH agonists may allow for a Pfannenstiel incision rather than a midline vertical skin incision often required for removal of large myomas.

•Use of newer, more conservative approaches such as GnRH agonists, hysteroscopic resection of presumed submucosal leiomyomas, and Nd:YAG laser endometrial ablation could delay more optimal evaluation and treatment of a patient with a leiomyosarcoma.

•Objective: To explore radiologic, surgical, and clinicopathologic characteristics of leiomyosarcomas in an effort to better understand their features and maximize preoperative interpretation of findings.

•Results: Leiomyosarcomas can be located at virtually any uterine site.

•GnRH analogs are frequently administered to women with myomas to achieve shrinkage of the myoma and to allow correction of anemia before initiation of surgery.

•Close monitoring of myomas during conservative evaluation and treatment is warranted.

•The finding that 95% of leiomyosarcomas present as the **largest or only** uterine mass is a unique and clinically pertinent factor.

»The largest myoma (especially when one myoma is significantly larger than the rest) should be monitored most closely during conservative management or GnRH analogue therapy.

•The actual location of the myoma within the uterus seems to be of less clinical significance, although collectively at least 26 of 49 (53%) leiomyosarcomas reported were **submucosal**.

°Although these submucosal tumors would seem to be more readily diagnosed by biopsy, in only 33% of cases did endometrial sampling correctly diagnose the leiomyosarcoma.

•For the incidentally suspicious myoma seen at the time of laparotomy, frozen section does **not** provide a reliable diagnosis (only 3 of 16 patients in combined studies were correctly diagnosed this way).

•This is of special interest to the gynecologist who encounters patients presenting with uterine bleeding, pain, or infertility and an enlarging uterus, especially when conservative therapy is initiated.

•Definitive surgery and staging in the presence of a rapidly growing uterine mass and, of course, with a positive endometrial biopsy should be undertaken.

•Diagnostic imaging can be used to differentiate myomas from leiomyosarcomas.

•Characteristic of tumor vascularity has been described with Doppler ultrasonography.

•Vaginal ultrasonography, with its increased resolution, and magnetic resonance imaging are both promising in terms of providing more detailed structural patterns of leiomyosarcomas.

•These improving imaging techniques should focus on the dominant leiomyoma during conservative management.

•A possible association between **uterine leiomyosarcoma and primary breast cancer** is suggested from the presence of both tumors in the Hutterite population, which is a highly inbred genetic isolate in North America, past reports of similar stromal giant cells identified in both tumors, and induction of both mammary carcinomas and uterine leiomyosarcomas in rats after oral administration of ethyl methanesulfonate, which is a potent mutagenic alkylating agent.

•The possible relationship between uterine leiomyosarcoma and breast cancer noted needs further investigation.

»Women with uterine leiomyosarcomas should participate in breast cancer screening programs.]

16. The number of exfoliated cells of the uterine cervix is increased by

    A. age
*B. cigarette smoking
    C. phase of menstrual cycle
    D. presence of koilocytes
    E. use of oral contraceptives

p. 1908 (Basu J, Mikhail M S, Palan P R, Payraudeau P H, Romney S L. Factors influencing the exfoliation of cervicovaginal epithelial cells. Am J Obstet Gynec 1992; 167:1904)

16. [F & I: •Background: Cigarette smoking is a risk for the development of cervical cancer.

•The mechanism(s) whereby smoking exerts its carcinogenic effect(s) is unknown.

•Smoking, in normal women, increases the number of exfoliated cervicovaginal epithelial cells.

•Objective: To investigate the association of smoking and exfoliation of cervicovaginal epithelial cells while controlling for other factors that may potentially influence cell exfoliation (e.g., the presence of cervical intraepithelial neoplasia, the presence of koilocytes, the use of oral contraceptives, age, and the phase of the menstrual cycle).

•Results: In normal healthy women smoking significantly **increases** the number of exfoliated cervicovaginal epithelial cells.

•The presence of cervical intraepithelial neoplasia is an additional independent factor associated with an acceleration of the exfoliation of cervicovaginal epithelial cells.

•The stimulatory effects of smoking and the presence of cervical intraepithelial neoplasia on the exfoliation of cervicovaginal epithelial cells are comparable.

•These two factors in combination were found **not** to have any additive effect.

•The number of exfoliated epithelial cells was not influenced by age, phase of the menstrual cycle, use of oral contraceptives, or the presence of koilocytes.

•Although the presence of koilocytes in cervical biopsy tissues often correlates with an infection with human papillomavirus, the relationship is not specific and **koilocytosis can be present in other conditions.**

•A number of epidemiologic studies have shown an increased risk for both preinvasive and invasive cervical cancer among smokers.

•The carcinogenic effect(s) of cigarette smoke on the cervix has been implicated by studies that have detected cotinine, nicotine, and mutagenic activity in the cervical mucus of smokers.

•The mechanism(s) whereby tobacco constituents exert their carcinogenic effect(s) still remain poorly understood.

•Nicotine and cotinine are selectively accumulated in the cervical mucous against a serum concentration gradient.

•Although nicotine does not have carcinogenic properties, the presence of high local concentrations of nicotine in cervical mucous membrane may lower the immunologic defense(s) of the cervix and render it more susceptible to human papillomavirus infection.

•Cigarette smoking significantly **decreases** plasma levels of antioxidant nutrients, particularly that of ascorbic acid and ß-carotene.

•Antioxidants possibly protecting the cells from free radical mediated lipid peroxidation are **deficient** in women with cervical dysplasia and invasive cervical cancer.

•Finding of increased exfoliation of cervicovaginal epithelial cells in smokers and in women with cervical intraepithelial neoplasia suggests that smoking or the presence of cervical intraepithelial neoplasia may induce an acceleration in the exfoliation of cervicovaginal epithelial cells.

•The increased rate of epithelial exfoliation may reflect a disorder in cell maturation.

•Such cumulative adverse effects of smoking persisting over a prolonged period of time may be a component of the oncogenic process.]

---

17. Related to risks for the development of endometrial carcinoma

    A. gallbladder disease
    B. height
    C. later age at natural menopause
    D. more than two spontaneous abortions
    *E. post menopausal hirsutism

p. 1321 (Brinton L A, Berman M L, Mortel R, Twiggs L B, Barrett R J, Wilbanks G D, Lannom L, Hoover R N. Reproductive, menstrual, and medical risk factors for endometrial cancer: Results from a case-control study. Am J Obstet Gynec 1992; 167:1317)

17. [F & I: •Background: Many risks for endometrial cancer appear to be correlated.

•For example, the woman at risk for developing the disease is "fat, forty, and infertile," but the relative importance of these factors has not been defined.

•Women with **diabetes, hypertension, gallbladder disease, and thyroid disease** may experience elevated risks, but whether these effects are independent of the association of endometrial cancer with obesity is unresolved.

•Different **menstrual and reproductive characteristics** affect the risk of endometrial cancer, but the exact nature of these relationships is unknown.

•**Multiparity** is associated with reduced risk, but the role of miscarriages and spontaneous abortions has not been determined.

•Objective: To clarify the significance of these factors in the etiology of endometrial cancer.

•Results: Nulligravidity is a major risk for endometrial cancer, with the absence of a previous pregnancy being associated with a nearly threefold elevation in risk.

°The protective effect of pregnancy appeared to be dependent on the pregnancy being carried to term, because prior miscarriages and induced abortions had no independent effects.

°The occurrence of one or more births was associated with about a 60% decrease in risk compared with no prior births, with risk decreasing somewhat further with additional births.

•Unlike the relationship with breast cancer, the **age at which a woman first gave birth** did **not** appear related to risk.

•**Breast-feeding** did **not** appear to alter the risk of endometrial cancer.

•**Infertility** emerged as a risk only when examined in relation to parity.

°Among nulliparous women, difficulty conceiving or ever having sought advice for infertility were associated with relative risks of 1.8 and 7.6, respectively.

- Age at **menarche** had a significant effect on risk.

    ° Age at menarche persisted after adjustment for a variety of risks, including weight and parity.

    ° Because early menarche reflects early onset of regular periods and longer exposure to circulating hormones, it was of interest to examine endometrial cancer risk in relation to histories of menstrual irregularities.

- **Amenorrhea** leading to physician consultation has been associated with a substantial excess risk of endometrial cancer in young women.

- There was no relationship of risk to either regularity of menstrual cycles or histories of amenorrhea, but subjects reporting **longer days of flow** were at a significant excess risk.

- Endometrial cancer was **not** associated with late age at natural menopause, an effect that has been hypothesized to reflect prolonged exposure of the uterus to estrogen stimulation in the presence of an ovulatory (progesterone-deficient) cycles.

    ° This failure to find a relationship of risk with age at menopause may reflect the difficulties in distinguishing natural cessation of menopause from abnormal bleeding preceding the diagnosis of endometrial cancer, especially among older women.

- **Weight** was strongly related to endometrial cancer risk.

- Relationships were stronger with weight than for measures of obesity, such as **Quetelet's index**.

- Heavy women (notably those weighing >200 pounds) had a disproportionately high risk.

    ° Adipose tissue is the primary site in postmenopausal women for conversion of adrenal androstenedione to estrone.

- Obesity has also been related to **lower levels of sex hormone-binding globulin,** leading to greater bioavailability of estrogens.

- In premenopausal women obesity may increase risk through more frequent anovulatory cycles, leading to lower levels of progesterone.

    ° Endometrial cancer risk might vary not only by the amount of body fat but also by its distribution.

- There was **no** relationship of risk to **hypertension**.

- A history of **diabetes** was associated with a significant twofold excess in risk, which persisted over time and was independent of effects of weight.

- There was an increased risk among women reporting histories of **hirsutism**.

    ° An association would appear plausible, given recognized endogenous hormonal influences on the development of hirsutism.

- The results support a function for hormones in the etiology of endometrial cancer.

- Use of unopposed estrogens greatly enhanced risk, whereas oral contraceptive use resulted in substantially reduced risks, presumably reflecting the antiestrogenic effects of progestins.

- Further implicating a role for hormones were substantially elevated risks among obese women, who have been found to have greater conversion rates and bioavailability of estrogens.

•Although the biologic mechanisms underlying the effects of nulliparity (early age at menarche, extended days of menstrual flow, history of diabetes, and hirsutism developing at older ages) remain inapparent, it is possible that they may also operate through hormonal mechanisms, leading to a unifying scheme as the etiology of this disease.]

18. A 26-year old patient is suspected of having PID. The most specific test is diagnosing her condition

    A. C-reactive protein
    B. endometrial biopsy
    C. erythrocyte sedimentation rate
*D. pelvic transvaginal ultrasound
    E. white blood cell count

p. 915 (Cacciatore B, Leminen A, Ingman-Friberg S, Ylostalo P, Paavonen J. Transvaginal sonographic findings in ambulatory patients with suspected pelvic inflammatory disease. Obstet Gynecol 1992; 80:912)

18. [F & I: •Background: Post-inflammatory tubal scarring and peritubal adhesions cause infertility.

•The diagnosis of PID based on pelvic examination and laboratory tests is often incorrect.

•Laparoscopy can confirm suspected PID.

•Endometrial biopsy is an alternative to laparoscopy, particularly in the outpatient diagnosis of PID, is a simple office procedure that can be performed without anesthesia.

•Transabdominal ultrasound is also useful in identifying complicated PID (e.g., tubo-ovarian abscess), but has not been evaluated extensively for the outpatient diagnosis of uncomplicated PID.

•Endovaginal probes have improved the accuracy of ultrasound imaging of the pelvic organs.

•Transvaginal sonography is a noninvasive office procedure that can easily be combined with bimanual examination and may be useful in the diagnosis of acute gynecologic problems, including PID.

•Objective: To evaluate transvaginal sonographic findings in ambulatory patients with suspected PID.
•PID is diagnosed visually by laparoscopic examination.

•Most PID cases are mild or subclinical and do not necessitate hospitalization.

•It is important to develop strategy that would augment the outpatient diagnosis of PID.

•Endometrial biopsy is an office test for the outpatient diagnosis of PID.

•A biopsy showing **plasma cell endometritis** has a sensitivity of 89% and specificity of 67% for the diagnosis of laparoscopically proven PID.

•Transvaginal sonography is another office procedure that is noninvasive and relatively simple, and can be performed with an empty bladder.

•Proximity to the pelvic organs allows the use of high-frequency transducers, which significantly increase the image resolution of sonography.

•Methods: 51 outpatients with low abdominal pain and suspected PID, were evaluated with transvaginal sonography in relation to endometrial biopsy findings.

•Overall, only 25% of the women with low abdominal pain and clinically suspected PID had plasma cell endometritis on endometrial biopsy.

- There was **no** correlation between laboratory tests (white blood cell count, erythrocyte sedimentation rate, C-reactive protein) and the presence of plasma cell endometritis.

- Transvaginal sonography performed well in the outpatient diagnosis of PID.

- None of the patients with normal sonograms had plasma cell endometritis.

- Other causes of acute pelvic pain not necessarily associated with pelvic infection, such as ovarian cysts, were easily detected by vaginal ultrasound.

- A sonogram consistent with PID, i.e., a thickened and fluid-filled tube with or without free pelvic fluid, was detected in 85% of patients with plasma cell endometritis.

- The fallopian tube is usually not visible on sonography unless it is filled with fluid or there is abundant fluid in the cul-de-sac.

- **Abdominal scanning** has **not** been very effective in detecting small changes and discriminating PID from other conditions such as ovarian cysts or endometriosis.

- Transvaginal sonography detected findings consistent with salpingitis with a specificity of 100%.

- **Free pelvic fluid** was also detected in 21% of patients without histopathologic evidence of plasma cell endometritis.

  ° The specificity of this sign alone in the diagnosis of PID was lower (79%) than that of the other selected ultrasound findings.

- In the cases with plasma cell endometritis, the tubes were generally dilated and fluid-filled with a thickened wall, suggesting an active inflammatory process.

- Similar sonographic findings might be associated with late sequelae of an earlier PID episode, such as chronic sactosalpinx.

  ° Repeat sonography was performed after 4 weeks, and showed normal findings in 60% of the cases with proven plasma cell endometritis.

- An interesting finding was the high prevalence (47%) of **polycystic-like ovaries**.

- Not all women with polycystic ovaries have endocrinologic abnormalities characteristic of polycystic ovary disease.

- Polycystic-like ovaries have been found in up to 22% of unselected populations and in more than half of women with chronic pelvic pain.

- A reactive polycystic change of ovarian texture is associated with PID.

- Oophoritis probably increases the volume of the ovaries by producing inflammatory exudate and edema in the vascular pole, leading to an increased stromal component as well.

- A thickened ovarian capsule might prevent normal follicular growth, thus causing multifollicular degeneration.

- Because a vast majority of patients with tubal infertility have no history of frank PID, the accuracy of the diagnosis of PID needs to be improved.]

19. The rate of pregnancy loss after detection of a live embryo in the first trimester is approximately

   *A. less 5%
   B. 10%
   C. 20%
   D. 25%
   E. 33%

p. 113 (van Leeuwen I, Branch D W, Scott J R. First-trimester ultrasonography findings in women with a history of recurrent pregnancy loss. Am J Obstet Gynec 1993; 168:111)

19. [F & I: •Background: Among normal women the presence of a live embryo detected by first-trimester ultrasonography predicts a >96% rate of successful pregnancy.

   •These data might be used in counseling patients with **recurrent** pregnancy loss.

   •Among women with recurrent pregnancy loss the rate of live birth after the confirmation of a viable embryo in the first trimester is unknown.

   •Objectives: To document first-trimester ultrasonographic findings in women with recurrent pregnancy loss and to determine the rate of subsequent pregnancy loss and live births after the identification of a live embryo in the first trimester.

   •Forty-three (64%) of the patients had primary recurrent pregnancy loss (three or more pregnancy losses and no live birth).

   •The median number of pregnancy losses in this group was four (range 3 to 33).

   •A complete evaluation for recurrent pregnancy loss, which consisted of an endometrial biopsy, parental chromosome analysis, hysterosalpingogram, testing for antiphospholipid antibodies, and endocervical cultures for chlamydia and mycoplasma or empirical antibiotics given to patient and spouse, was performed in 25 of the 43 patients (58%).

   •The causes of recurrent pregnancy loss in these patients were the following:

   °(1) abnormal parental karyotype, two patients (5%),

   °(2) uterine abnormality, six patients (14%),

   °(3) luteal phase defect, four patients (9%),

   °(4) antiphospholipid syndrome, one patient (2%), and

   °(5) idiopathic, 25 patients (58%).

   •In five patients (12%) the evaluation was incomplete and no diagnosis was ascertained.

   •Many of these patients underwent specific treatments before or during a subsequent pregnancy including:

   °leukocyte immunization (22 patients),

   °uterine surgery (four patients),

   °treatment with progesterone (two patients) or low-dose aspirin (one patient), and

   °treatment with a combination of prednisone and low-dose aspirin (one patient).

•Results: Approximately three fourths of pregnancies in patients with recurrent pregnancy loss will have a live embryo at first-trimester ultrasonography.

•In these pregnancies neither maternal age nor the number of previous pregnancy losses was associated with any particular first-trimester ultrasonography finding.

•Also, there was no obvious relationship between the cause of recurrent pregnancy loss and the ultrasonography findings, although the numbers in each diagnostic category were small.

•The rate of loss was <4%, regardless of what gestational age the ultrasonographic examination was performed.

•These data can be quite reassuring when used to counsel such patients about the chance of miscarriage or fetal death.

•The prospective study of patients with recurrent pregnancy loss indicates that the rate of pregnancy loss after the identification of a live embryo is **four to five times higher**.

•Conclusion: A relatively high proportion of pregnancies in patients with recurrent pregnancy loss will exhibit a live embryo at the time of first-trimester ultrasonography.

•The rate of spontaneous abortion or fetal death in these patients is higher than in an unselected group of obstetric patients.]

---

20. A postmenopausal patient has developed bleeding per vaginam. An endometrial suction curettage used to obtain a tissue was reported as retrieving insufficient tissue for diagnosis. Physical evaluation finds a small uterus and nonpalpable ovaries. A pap test of the cervix shows only normal cells. A diagnostic ultrasound of the pelvis to estimate endometrial thickness is ordered. What is the minimal endometrial thickness which will allow the patient to be observed prospectively?

   *A. Less than 5 millimeters.
   B. Less than 6 millimeters.
   C. Less than 7 millimeters.
   D. Less than 8 millimeters.
   E. The patient should have a formal curettage regardless of the endometrial thickness.

---

p. 730 (Goldchmit R, Katz Z, Blickstein I, Caspi B, Dgano R. The accuracy of endometrial pipelle sampling with and without sonographic measurement of endometrial thickness. Obstet Gynecol 1993; 82:727)

20. [F & I: •Background: Although D&C is generally accepted as the standard method for endometrial sampling, safer, less expensive, and well-tolerated techniques may replace curettage while maintaining diagnostic accuracy.

•The Vabra aspirator (Berkeley Medevices, Berkeley, CA) is safe and inexpensive, but has the disadvantages of causing considerable discomfort to the patient and requiring an electric vacuum pump.

•The Pipelle endometrial suction curette (Unimar, Inc., Wilton, CT) may be more convenient for both physician and patient because cervical dilation is usually unnecessary.

•Compared to the Vabra aspirator, the Pipelle curette showed the same efficacy but better patient tolerance.

•Similar results were observed in randomized clinical trials when the Pipelle curette was compared with the Novak curette and with the Tis-U-Trap (Milex Products, Chicago, IL).

•Comparison of the Pipelle sampler to formal curettage suggested that Pipelle aspiration should be the first measure in cases of menstrual disturbance.

- •To enhance the diagnostic yield, sonography is frequently used to investigate the endometrium.

- •An endometrial thickness less than 6 mm is associated with insufficient tissue for histologic examination in postmenopausal women.

- •Sonography may not distinguish proliferative from hyperplastic endometrium, and in one case from low-grade carcinoma, when the endometrial thickness was 5-to-8 mm.

- •Objective: To evaluate the efficacy of Pipelle endometrial sampling with and without the addition of sonographic measurement of endometrial thickness and to compare it to subsequent curettage.

- •The utility of endometrial sampling and sonographic measurement of endometrial thickness has not been established in the evaluation of endometrial cancer.

- •Curettage is the technique most often used for endometrial sampling, but sensitivity and specificity are difficult to assess.

- •This study assumed that curettage is the criterion standard used to compare the accuracy of other sampling methods.

- •Other techniques include disposable suction devices, which are convenient to both patient and physician.

- •Curettage, the Vabra aspirator, and the Novak curette had equal diagnostic accuracy rates in 619 patients undergoing hysterectomy.

- •The Pipelle, a newer device, was equally accurate while causing less discomfort.

- •Results: Cases of carcinoma were identified by Pipelle aspirator and curettage.

- •In unmatched results, ten cases of insufficient tissue in the Pipelle aspirates were found, including two cases of endometrial polyp found by curettage, all attributable to technical errors (negative pressure gradient not created, device not moved or rotated enough).

- •The subsequent management in cases with insufficient tissue is unknown.

- •Although the data may imply that a result with insufficient tissue should be followed by curettage, other studies have found no significant undiscovered abnormality when curettage was performed after an endometrial biopsy technique.

- •Patient follow-up has an important function, but was not performed.

- **•In cases in which Pipelle aspiration and sonography of the endometrium do not reveal existing disease, the patients should be reexamined and curettage avoided unless bleeding recurs.**

- •Sonographic endometrial thickness in postmenopausal women was evaluated to exclude endometrial abnormality.

- •In patients with postmenopausal bleeding and endometrial thickness of 5 mm or less, follow-up without endometrial sampling was suggested.

- •The case of grade 1 adenocarcinoma in a woman with postmenopausal bleeding and an endometrial thickness of 4 mm shows early identification of endometrial cancer without significant sonographic endometrial changes.

- »Endometrial sampling should be performed on all postmenopausal patients regardless of the sonographic endometrial thickness.

- • This is the first study in which sonography was added to endometrial biopsy by Pipelle and compared to D&C for evaluation of abnormal uterine bleeding.

- Using a cutoff value of **5 mm**, over 90% sensitivity and over 95% specificity was achieved as compared to formal curettage in the whole population, and sensitivity and specificity of 100% in the subset of 19 postmenopausal patients admitted for bleeding.

- The data suggest that normal Pipelle aspirates in premenopausal patients with abnormal uterine bleeding are highly accurate.

» Although the subgroup of postmenopausal patients was relatively small, sonographic endometrial thickness of 5 mm or less and normal Pipelle aspirates may safely replace curettage in this group.]

---

21. Cigarette smoking causes urinary incontinence by

    A. activating purinergic receptors
    B. depleting α adrenergic fibers
    C. interfering with collagen synthesis
    D. stretch injury to pudendal and intrapelvic nerves
 *E. none of the above

p. 1217 (Bump R C, MCClish D K. Cigarette smoking and urinary incontinence in women. Am J Obstet Gynec 1992; 167:1213)

21. [F & I: Objective: To examine the relationship between cigarette smoking and urinary incontinence in adult women.

- The data from this case-control study of 322 incontinent and 284 continent adult women establish a strong statistical relationship between cigarette smoking and urinary incontinence.

- Women who previously smoked had a 2.2-fold increase and women who currently smoked had a 2.5-fold increase in the risk of genuine stress incontinence.

- The risk of genuine stress incontinence was positively correlated with both the current intensity of cigarette consumption and the magnitude of the lifetime exposure to cigarette smoking.

    °Former and current smokers also had a twofold to threefold increase in the risk of motor incontinence, although the magnitude of this risk showed no correlation with current intensity or lifetime exposure.

- The increased prevalence of incontinence is independent of other risks for incontinence, such as older age, increased parity, greater weight, or higher prevalence of estrogen deprivation.

- A limitation of any case-control study is the potential for bias in the selection of the control group.

- The prevalence of smoking in the normal continent group was 26.9%.

- The normal continent group was not subjected to urodynamic testing.

- None of the normal continent subjects fulfilled the International Continence Society definition for incontinence: "the involuntary loss of urine which is socially or hygienically objectionable to the patient and which is objectively demonstrable."

    °The International Continence Society also states than an abnormal urodynamic test result in an asymptomatic patient does not warrant a diagnosis of incontinence.

- In contrast, all of the incontinent subjects did have objectionable incontinence; urodynamic testing simply objectively documented it and identified its cause.

- There are several plausible explanations for a smoking woman's increased risk of incontinence.

•The most obvious is the smoker's stronger, more frequent, and more violent cough, which may damage components of the urethral sphincteric mechanism, promoting the development of incontinence, and may worsen the frequency and severity of existing incontinence.

•In addition, products of the tobacco smoke itself (e.g., hypoxia, carbon monoxide, nicotine), the antiestrogenic hormonal effects of smoking, and processes known to be associated with smoking (e.g., vascular disease, smoker's cough, asthma, obstructive pulmonary disease) may also have direct and indirect effects on the function of the bladder and urethra.

°For example, smoking has been shown to directly interfere with **collagen synthesis**.

°**Antiestrogenic** hormonal effects could adversely affect the quality of collagen and also decrease smooth muscle tone through depletion of α-adrenergic receptor activity.

°Downward bulging of the pelvic floor because of violent or prolonged coughing attacks may cause repeated stretch-induced injury to the pudendal and intrapelvic nerves supplying skeletal muscles, adding to the progressive denervation that seems to be an important part of the pathogenesis of genuine-stress incontinence.

°**Nicotine**, an important and addictive component of cigarette smoke, has extremely complex neuropharmacologic actions that are still being defined.

•Adenosine 5'-triphosphate-stimulated **purinergic receptors** are found in the human bladder; further, nonadrenergic, noncholinergic nerves have been estimated to be responsible for 50% of the contractile response of the human female bladder.

•The current study does not suggest which, if any, of these mechanisms may be responsible for the increased risk of incontinence in smokers.

•The data do not demonstrate a decreased risk of incontinence from smoking cessation.

•There are several plausible explanations for this finding.

•First, there is no information regarding the relative timing of the onset of incontinence and the cessation of smoking.

°It is possible that some women stopped smoking, either on their own or on the advice of their physician, in an effort to diminish urine loss.

•Second, it is likely that many of the anatomic and neuromuscular changes that could result from smoking and contribute to incontinence may not be reversible.

•Smoking cessation is an important approach to the management of incontinence.

•Some effects of smoking (e.g., antiestrogenic effects, the strength and frequency of coughing) are reversible and their consequences are progressive.

•Diminishing these effects may help lessen the severity of incontinence or prevent its recurrence after successful treatment.

•With the attributable risk of urinary incontinence in women caused by cigarette smoking estimated at 28%, strategies designed to discourage women from starting to smoke or to encourage smoking women to stop smoking could have a significant impact on the overall prevalence of incontinence in women.

•Because urinary incontinence has a profound psychosocial impact and is viewed by many younger women as a more immediate threat, more stigmatizing and more humiliating than cancer or heart disease, the realization that incontinence is yet another consequence of smoking may prove an effective deterrent and help combat the converging smoking prevalence rates among men and women.]

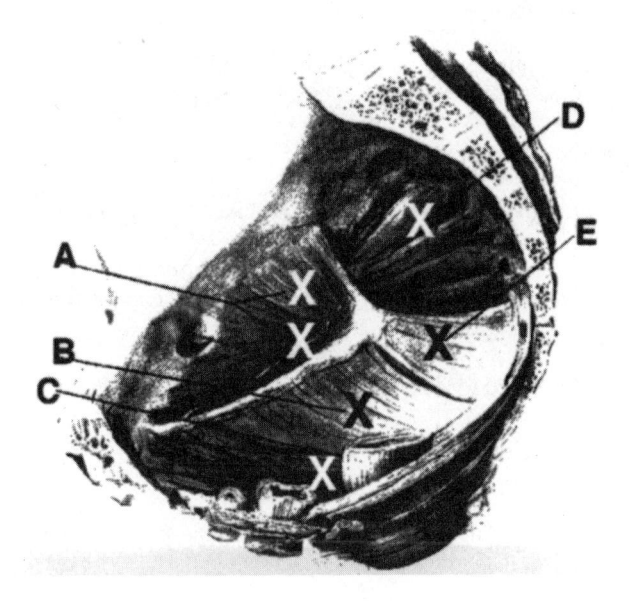

22. In the diagram above, which letter identifies the coccygeus muscle?

   A. A (Obturator internus)
   B. B (Iliococcygeus)
   C. C (Pubococcygeus)
   D. D (Pyriformis)
   *E. E (Coccygeus)

p. 1670 (Shull B L, Capen C V, Riggs M W, Kuehl T J. Bilateral attachment of the vaginal cuff to iliococcygeus fascia: An effective method of cuff suspension. Am J Obstet Gynec 1993; 168:1669)

22. [F & I: •Background: Standard surgical texts emphasize the use of the cardinal uterosacral ligament complexes at the time of hysterectomy to reduce the likelihood of posthysterectomy vaginal cuff prolapse.

•Posthysterectomy vaginal cuff prolapse is a complex dilemma, one whose management requires versatility by the reconstructive surgeon.

•The surgical approaches described by Symmonds and Pratt, Symmonds et al., Nichols, Addison et al., and by Zacharin and Hamilton are effective in providing successful suspension of the prolapsed cuff.

•Objective: To determine the anatomic success, defined as no peristent or recurrent support defects, of suspension of the vaginal cuff to the iliococcygeus muscle.

•Methods: The posterior colporrhaphy and cuff suspension are approached by excising a diamond-shaped section of tissue from the perineum and introitus, freeing the vaginal epithelium from the rectum and rectovaginal fascia.

•The dissection is carried cephalad to the cuff and laterally to the levator fascia.

•The fascia overlying iliococcygeus muscle is identified lateral to the rectum and anterior to the ischial spine.

•The bowel is retracted medially and a suture placed in the iliococcygeus fascia just anterior to the ischial spine.

- Nonabsorbable sutures may be used and a pulley stitch placed in the undersurface of the vaginal epithelium at the ipsilateral angle of the cuff.

- If absorbable sutures are used, the suture should be placed full thickness through the apex of the vaginal epithelium into the vault and then returned from the vault into the pararectal space.

- A similar suture is placed on the opposite side.

- These sutures are left untied until the perirectal fascia has been approximated in the midline.

- Once the defect in perirectal fascia has been corrected, the cuff sutures are securely tied, bringing the vaginal axis into a posterior position and the vaginal epithelium into direct apposition over iliococcygeus fascia.

- The iliococcygeus fascia has been used to suspend the vaginal cuff since 1963.

- **Patients with pelvic support defects require meticulous preoperative and intraoperative identification of all areas requiring repair.**

- Ideally, all defects should be identified at the preoperative examination; experienced surgeons should recognize that the intraoperative findings dictate the ultimate procedures to be performed.

- Reports on pelvic reconstructive procedures fail to compare specific preoperative clinical and intraoperative surgical findings, and also do not report specific postoperative anatomic findings.

- There is controversy over what is therapeutic versus what is prophylactic, as is the case of sacrospinous ligament suspension of the vaginal cuff.

- Results: 17% of the study group were thought to have normal support for the cervix or cuff preoperatively; it became clear intraoperatively that the use of the uterosacral cardinal ligaments pedicles would **not** offer optimal support for the vaginal cuff.

- In these women attachment of the vaginal cuff to the iliococcygeus fascia provided an effective addition to the planned procedure.

- Long-term anatomic success depends on more than cuff suspension.

- Each fascial defect must be precisely identified and specifically repaired.

- Iliococcygeus fascia attachment is a valuable procedure because the tissue used for suspension is easily accessible and not directly adjacent to any major nerves or vessels.

- The fascia provides a strong anchor bilaterally, allowing the apex to rest posteriorly over the sacrum.

- In patients with inadequate uterosacral ligaments or with vaginal length too short to reach the ischial spines, the use of iliococcygeus fascia permits the surgeon to use the vaginal approach but does not commit the patient to sacrospinous ligament suspension or colpocleisis.

- Suspension of the vaginal cuff is the most successful part of the reconstructive procedure, but the anterior segment (bladder and urethra) is more likely to show long-term evidence of support defects.

- The exaggerated retroversion of the vagina accompanying sacrospinous ligament suspension may predispose the anterior segment to excess pressure and subsequently to support defects in much the same way retropubic urethropexy predisposes to posterior cul-de-sac hernias.

- Iliococcygeus fascial attachment produces less of the exaggerated vaginal retroversion.

- Additionally, bilateral attachment provides symmetry and dual points for support.

• These mechanisms and properly performed repair of all support defects should help minimize persistent or acquired anterior segment defects.

• Reconstructive surgeons should possess the flexibility, versatility, and dexterity to individualize each operative procedure depending on surgical findings.

• In follow-up from 6 weeks to 5 years there were two patients with persistent or recurrent cuff prolapse.

• Two of the 42 patients have required further surgery: one an enterocele and rectocele repair and the other an enterocele repair and sacrospinous ligament suspension of the vaginal cuff.]

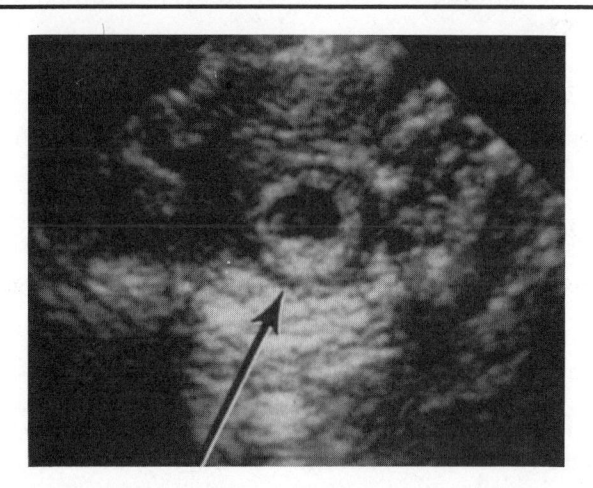

Reproduced with written permission from the publisher, C.V. Mosby Company, St. Louis, Mo.
Burry K A, Thurmond A S, Suby-Long T D, Patton P E, Rose P M, Jones M K, Choffel J K, Nelson D W. Transvaginal ultrasonographic findings in surgically verified ectopic pregnancy. Am J Obstet Gynec 1993; 168:1796

23. An asymptomatic patient six weeks pregnant by dates has a serum ß-hCG level of 2600 IU/ml and serum progesterone level of 50 ng/ml. The ultrasonogram of the involved adnexal region pictured above was obtained the same day the lab results were reported. The diagnosis is

   A. benign cystic teratoma.
   B. corpus luteum of pregnancy.
 *C. ectopic pregnancy.
   D. endometrioma.
   E. hematosalpinx.

p. 1797 (Burry K A, Thurmond A S, Suby-Long T D, Patton P E, Rose P M, Jones M K, Choffel J K, Nelson D W. Transvaginal ultrasonographic findings in surgically verified ectopic pregnancy. Am J Obstet Gynec 1993; 168:1796)

23. [F & I: •Background: The combination of serum ß-hCG and vaginal ultrasonography has a high sensitivity and specificity for the diagnosis of ectopic pregnancy.

• Many women at risk for an ectopic pregnancy have adnexal masses seen by transvaginal ultrasonography.

• In 40% to 65% of cases there is a 1 to 2 cm cystic area surrounded by an echogenic ring.

• **This finding has been described as a tubal or adnexal "ring," "doughnut," or "bagel."**

• A protuberant corpus luteum may have similar characteristics and has been mistaken for an ectopic pregnancy, resulting in unnecessary laparoscopy.

• Women with tubal gestations were observed to have a tubal ring surrounded by a thin hypoechoic area, or "**halo.**"

Obstetrics and Gynecology:Review 1994-Gynecology References

•Objective: To determine the prevalence, sensitivity, and specificity of this halo sign in women with an adnexal mass.

•Most ectopic pregnancies can be diagnosed within 2 weeks of a missed period and treated before tubal rupture.

•Many are treated while asymptomatic.

•Early diagnosis may even allow medical management only.

•Serial serum ß-hCG assays and transvaginal ultrasonography are routinely performed in women who are at risk for an ectopic pregnancy.

•52% of the women with ectopic pregnancy had an adnexal ring.

•A living fetus or yolk sac in an extrauterine location in seven women (10%) is less than the reported incidence of 13% to 21%.

°This difference may be because of an earlier diagnosis of tubal pregnancy in the current study.

•A thin, circumferential, sonolucent rim or halo was identified in 24 of 36 (67%) women with an adnexal ring.

•The cause of the halo sign is uncertain.

°In one case, tubal anatomy after excision was distorted, limiting the examination; the findings suggested that the halo results from **subserosal edema**.

•A second patient was scanned endovaginally while undergoing laparoscopic linear salpingostomy.

•The adnexal ring with a surrounding halo persisted after evacuation of the products of conception, suggesting that the halo is subserosal edema and the echogenic ring is the edematous wall of the tube.

•The sensitivity of the halo sign for diagnosing a tubal gestation was low (44.4%).

•The specificity of this sign was high (95.1%), with a positive predictive value of 92.3%.

•The sensitivity and specificity of the adnexal ring with a halo sign for ectopic pregnancy needs to be prospectively determined in women at risk for ectopic pregnancy.

•If the halo sign occurs in corpora lutea in a normal 4 to 5-week intrauterine gestation or if it occurs with endometriosis, hydrosalpinx, or other pelvic pathologic condition that can coexist with pregnancy, this would decrease the specificity of this sign as determined in this selected retrospective population.

•The presence of a halo around the adnexal ring may be an early positive ultrasonographic finding of an ectopic pregnancy that indicates intervention when other clinical or ultrasonographic findings are equivocal.

•When the clinical findings are compelling for an ectopic pregnancy, laparoscopy is still indicated regardless of the ultrasonographic findings.]

24. Associated with vulvar vestibulitis all of the following EXCEPT

    A. erythema of minor vestibular glands.
    B. increased urethral pressure variability.
    C. interstitial cystitis.
*D. lactose intolerance.
    E. urethral syndrome.

p. 112 (Foster D C, Robinson J C, David K M. Urethral pressure variation in women with vulvar vestibulitis syndrome. Am J Obstet Gynec 1993; 169:107)

24. [F & I: •Background: Vulvar vestibulitis syndrome is a chronic condition characterized by severe focal pain to touch of the vaginal vestibule and associated with insertional dyspareunia.

•Vulvar vestibulitis syndrome does not include symptoms associated with acute inflammatory conditions nor with the immediate postoperative state.

•Typically, the patient describes painless coitus for >1 year before the abrupt development of insertional dyspareunia.

•The patient commonly undergoes a multitude of therapies, often without improvement.

•A visible abnormality limited to erythema of the minor vestibular glands has been identified.

•The cause of this abnormality has been considered multifactorial.

•Urinary tract complaints of urgency, frequency, and dysuria without bacteriuria, commonly found in urethral syndrome, and interstitial cystitis are associated with vulvar vestibulitis syndrome.

    °The association of vestibulitis and interstitial cystitis is called "urogenital sinus syndrome," because of the common embryologic origin of bladder trigone, urethra, and vulvar vestibule.

•In normal women continuous recording of intraurethral pressure shows a rhythmic variation ranging from 0.001 to 0.03 Hz.

•Urethral smooth muscle may be the source of this pressure variability.

•Several factors associated with variation in urethral pressure include maximum urethral pressure, level of arousal (sleeping, awake at rest, or performing mental calculations), and presence of urologic problems such as urethral syndrome.

•"Urethral instability" means abnormally large short-term variations in the urethral pressure not associated with increases in intraabdominal pressure or urethral vascular pulsations.

•"Normal" and "abnormal" urethral pressure variability is undefined by the International Continence Society.

•Objective: To report on urodynamic characteristics of patients with vulvar vestibulitis syndrome, particularly the measurements of urethral pressure variability.

•Methods: Attempts were made to place patients in a standard level of arousal by requiring each to perform a mini-mental status examination during urethral pressure recording.

•Under a similar level of arousal patients with vulvar vestibulitis syndrome should have a **greater** urethral pressure variability than asymptomatic patient or patients with chronic pelvic pain.

•Results: A significantly greater urethral pressure variability was found in patients with vulvar vestibulitis syndrome compared with patients with chronic pelvic pain and asymptomatic patients.

- The cause-effect relationship of the current observation is unknown.

- A possible confounding effect of coexisting urinary tract dysfunction in patients with vulvar vestibulitis syndrome was not evident, given the lack of a significant difference in proportion of urinary tract complaints between groups.

- The covariate "age" was considered to have a greater chance of confounding results.

- **Increasing** age is associated with a decrease in urethral closure pressure, a decrease in urethral pressure variability, and a lower chance of suffering from vulvar vestibulitis.

- Patients with vulvar vestibulitis syndrome, commonly between 20 and 40 years old, will have a younger mean age than the general urodynamic patient.

- For this reason, age group matching was performed for patients with vulvar vestibulitis syndrome and chronic pain.

- Although race did not affect urodynamic findings, patients with vulvar vestibulitis syndrome are exclusively white and vulvar vestibulitis syndrome patients and patients with chronic pain were group-matched for race.

- Multiple regression analysis showed a significant difference of urethral pressure variability by diagnostic group, controlling for age, race, and parity, proving that vulvar vestibulitis syndrome as a diagnostic group was acting independently on urethral pressure variability.

- Factors contributing to intraurethral pressure, including thickness of urothelium, periurethral vascularity, relative anatomic position of urethra, quality of periurethral connective tissue, and variations in smooth and striated muscle tone.

- The minute-by-minute variability in urethral pressure results from vascular pulsation and variation in muscular tone.

- Urethral striated muscle may contribute 20% to 84% to urethral pressure variability compared with urethral smooth muscle.

- Urethral electromyographic variability does not correlate with urethral pressure variability and that urethral pressure variability is only partially inhibited by pudendal blockade.

  ° Changes in states of arousal (sleep vs wake state) **increase** urethral pressure variability.

  ° An increase in urethral pressure variability was found during a mental status examination.

- Whether this is because of an increase of stress on the individual or is a function of a greater time of observation cannot be determined.

- Previous evaluations of 1 hour in length, in contrast to a 16-minute length in this study, have shown higher pressure variability.

- This suggests that overall time of observation may be an important variable to control.

- The study suggests a **functional**, in contrast to a structural, component to vulvar vestibulitis syndrome.

- Whether reduction of muscular tonus at the vestibule and the urethral sphincter by biofeedback or by antispasmodic drugs might be effective in pain relief remains to be determined.

- The association of increased urethral pressure variability may link vulvar vestibulitis syndrome to "sympathetically maintained" pain.

- Such chronic pain disorders are characterized by burning, vasomotor instability, and muscle spasm.

•Pharmacologic blockade of ß-receptors for "sympathetically maintained pain" may ameliorate vulvar vestibulitis syndrome.

•The development of a topical therapy directed toward alteration of smooth muscle tonus might be an alternative to the **perineoplasty**, the most effective therapy to date.]

---

25. Independent predictors of persistent ectopic pregnancy following salpingostomy include all of the following EXCEPT

    A. days of amenorrhea
    B. hematoperitoneum
    C. laparoscopic approach
    *D. preoperative ß-hCG level greater 3000 international units per liter
    E. size of ectopic

p. 378 (Seifer D B, Gutmann J N, Grant W D, Kamps C A, DeCherney A H. Comparison of persistent ectopic pregnancy after laparoscopic salpingostomy versus salpingostomy at laparotomy for ectopic pregnancy. Obstet Gynecol 1993; 81:378)

25. [F & I: •Background: Clinical experience has suggested an occurrence of persistent ectopic pregnancy after laparoscopic treatment ranging at 3-to-20%.

•Objective: To examine the past 5 years' experience for the occurrence of persistent ectopic pregnancy after laparoscopic salpingostomy versus salpingostomy at laparotomy for the treatment of intact ampullary ectopic pregnancy.

•This retrospective cohort study compared two surgical treatments of intact ampullary ectopic pregnancy, demonstrating a **higher** occurrence of persistent ectopic pregnancy following laparoscopic salpingostomy than after salpingostomy performed through a laparotomy incision.

•Significant clinical factors identified as independent predictors of persistent ectopic pregnancy following salpingostomy included a **laparoscopic approach, fewer days of amenorrhea, and smaller size of the ectopic**.

•Other factors associated with persistent ectopic pregnancy in the laparoscopic group, but not independent predictors of persistent ectopic pregnancy, included more frequent absence of products of conception at salpingostomy and less frequent hemoperitoneum noted at the initial salpingostomy.

•Clinical factors seemingly incidental to the occurrence of persistent ectopic pregnancy following salpingostomy performed by either laparoscopy or laparotomy included a history of risks for ectopic pregnancy, history of previous ectopic, preoperative ß-hCG titers of at least 3000 IU/L, and presence of pelvic adhesions.

•The greater use of vasopressin or laser in the laparoscopy group is most likely related to the nature of the surgical approach itself.

•Vasopressin is more likely to be used by a laparoscopist to create a cleavage plane to help expel the products of conception as well as to obtain hemostasis.

°These methods are often unnecessary at salpingostomy by laparotomy because the surgeon is able to palpate and, if necessary, excise the products of conception from the implantation site.

•**Days of amenorrhea and size of the ectopic** had been identified previously as independent predictors of persistent ectopic pregnancy after laparoscopic salpingostomy for ectopic pregnancy.

•The present study corroborates this and identifies the laparoscopic approach as an additional independent predictor of persistent ectopic pregnancy.

•Incomplete surgical removal of trophoblastic tissue may be due to poorly defined cleavage planes between trophoblast and the implantation site of an early gestation secondary to reduced hemorrhage around the eccyesis.

•Earlier ectopics are probably smaller in size, which may result in less hemorrhage with less bleeding from the fimbriated end of the tube and thus less hemoperitoneum.

•This combination of events may be responsible for the greater challenge to the laparoscopist who wants to obtain and remove products of conception from these relatively early ectopics.

•Other risks for persistent ectopic pregnancy include preoperative and postoperative ß-hCG titers.

•Persistent ectopic pregnancy can occur following linear salpingostomy regardless of whether laparotomy or laparoscopy is performed.

°The risk of persistent ectopic pregnancy is greater after laparoscopic salpingostomy than after salpingostomy at laparotomy.

•The advantages of laparoscopy (e.g., avoidance of an abdominal incision, less postoperative discomfort, and shorter convalescence with reduced time away from work and family) are accompanied by an increased risk of persistent ectopic pregnancy.

•Methotrexate offers significant promise for this complication, with minimal morbidity.

•The availability of methotrexate as second-line therapy for persistent ectopic pregnancy following laparoscopic salpingostomy allows laparoscopy to remain the preferred surgical approach for the treatment of intact ampullary ectopic pregnancy.]

---

26. True statements about the menopause include all of the following EXCEPT

    A. About half of menstruating women in the menopause experience vasomotor symptoms.
    *B. Antidepressants are the therapy of choice to reduce vasomotor complaints.
    C. Regularly menstruating women with premenstrual tension are more likely to experience vasomotor symptoms in the premenopause.
    D. The severity of menopausal vasomotor complaints is related to the severity of bone loss.
    E. Women with a long premenopausal experience have vasomotor complaints more often than women with a short premenopause.

---

p. 779 (Oldenhave A, Jaszmann J B, Haspels A A, Everaerd W T. Impact of climacteric on well-being. Am J Obstet Gynec 1993; 168:772)

26. [F & I: •Background: The climacteric is associated with atypical complaints such as flushes, sweating, and vaginal dryness, which leads to dyspareunia.

•These complaints are termed **atypical** because they are considered to be related to climacteric hormonal changes.

•Flushes and sweating are atypical but **not** specific for the climacteric, occurring also during fright and in the presence of diseases not known to be related to the climacteric, such as carcinoid, pheochromocytoma, basophilic chronic granulocytic leukemia, systemic mastocytosis, pancreatic tumor, medullary carcinoma of the thyroid, and diffuse toxic goiter.

•Other more general complaints are not considered to be atypical for the climacteric because they also occur in nonclimacteric persons and because there is so far no evidence that they are related to climacteric hormonal changes.

•These complaints are labeled atypical; no reference is intended as to their actual prevalence in climacteric women.

•Atypical complaints have a higher prevalence in irregularly menstruating women (at least one menstruation in the preceding year) than in either regularly menstruating or postmenopausal women.

•Objective: To study the relation between the severity of vasomotor complaints (flushes and sweating) and atypical complaints.

•Results: (1) vasomotor complaints in different degrees of severity are already present in a substantial percentage of menstruating women aged ≥39 years (41.1%), reaching the highest prevalence around the menopause (85%) to decline only slowly in the postmenopause (57% LMP >10 years),

•(2) a substantial percentage of menstruating women with vasomotor complaints experience sweating in absence of flushes,

•(3) with increasing severity of vasomotor complaints there is an increase in the severity of all atypical complaints in menstruating and nonmenstruating women, indicative of an overall reduced well-being,

•(4) menstruating women report several atypical complaints more often than nonmenstruating women with a similar severity of vasomotor complaints, and

•(5) there is virtually no effect of age on atypical complaints in nonmenstruating women after adjustment for vasomotor complaints.

•The severity of vasomotor complaints is related to the severity of atypical complaints, which may mimic nonpsychotic psychiatric disturbances.

•The highest prevalence of vasomotor complaints and the highest rate of bone loss occur in the late premenopause and early postmenopause.

°The severity of vasomotor complaints may be a marker of the rate of climacteric bone loss.

•Vasomotor complaints in menstruating women may be related to elevated gonadotropin levels, because follicle-stimulating hormone levels increase with age in ovulating women, whereas estradiol levels remain unchanged and menstruating women experiencing flushes have higher follicle-stimulating hormone levels than those who do not.

•In menstruating women sweating in the absence of flushes may point at a milder or earlier disturbance of the thermoregulation than when full-blown flushes are experienced.

•Because during the premenopause the length of the menstrual cycles are highly variable, it is conceivable that vasomotor complaints may occur in waves when longer menstrual cycles occur.

°Proof of this is only possible in prospective studies.

•The estimated mean length of the phase with irregular menstrual cycles was 5.5 years.

•Premenopausal women with a multiple atypical complaints often also have a high level of atypical complaints when menstruation ceases.

•Regularly menstruating women with premenstrual tension complaints or with vasomotor complaints are more likely to experience vasomotor complaints in the premenopause and postmenopause.

•Women with a long premenopausal phase experience vasomotor complaints more often than those with a shorter premenopause.

°This may indicate that women with complaints related to the menstrual cycle are also more at risk for more severe vasomotor complaints later in the climacteric.

•Flushes, although the most typical climacteric complaint, are not considered by many women to be their most distressing complaint.

•For most women flushes are in fact relatively easy to cope with, because they are characteristic, short-lived (duration approximately 3 minutes) and occur relatively infrequently in most women.

•Many women are bothered more by the atypical complaints for which they often do not have an explanation and for which they seek medical care.]

27. Drugs used for the prevention of pelvic adhesions from gonococcal salpingitis, all of the following EXCEPT

   *A. colchicine
   B. Dextran 40
   C. Dextran 70
   D. nonsteroidal anti-inflammatory drugs
   E. progestins

p. 120 (Marcovici I, Brill A I, Scommegna A. Effects of colchicine on pelvic adhesions associated with the intrauterine inoculation of *Neisseria gonorrhoeae* in rabbits. Obstet Gynecol 1993; 81:118)

27. [F & I: •Background: Pelvic inflammatory disease, with resultant pelvic adhesive disease, is responsible for as many as 50% of cases of female infertility.

•More than 25% of patients with acute salpingitis are less than 25 years old, and 75% are nulliparous.

•Treatment for pelvic inflammatory disease involves a combination of bed rest and antibiotics.

•Despite different antibiotic regimens, infertility following acute salpingitis may be as high as 12.8% after the first episode, 35.5% after two episodes, and up to 75% after three or more episodes.

°Antibiotic therapy alone does not ensure preservation of fertility.

•Many agents besides antibiotics have been proposed for prevention of adhesions including corticosteroids, nonsteroidal anti-inflammatory agents, low-molecular-weight dextran (dextran 40), high-molecular-weight dextran (dextran 70), and progestins.

•Colchicine has been advocated for the treatment of many diseases in which inflammation or fibrosis is prominent and reduces postsurgical peritoneal adhesions in a rat model.

•Objective: To study the effect of colchicine on adhesion formation following intrauterine gonococcus inoculation in a rabbit model.

•Colchicine is used for the treatment of many diseases in which inflammation or fibrosis is prominent, including familial Mediterranean fever, amyloidosis, scleroderma, Behçet disease, and psoriasis.

•Colchicine is an antiinflammatory agent for acute gouty arthritis and prolongs survival in patients with mild to moderate biliary cirrhosis of the liver.

•By binding to tubulin, colchicine blocks mitosis, interferes with transcellular movement of collagen, stimulates the production of collagenase in vitro, and inhibits the secretion of histamine from mast cells and the chemotactic reaction of the leukocyte.

•Side effects from therapeutic dosages are usually mild and include abdominal pain, diarrhea, and vomiting.

•The mechanism by which infection causes adhesions has not been established clearly.

•Bacterial enzymes may damage tissue and produce a substantial inflammatory response.

•Such substances may alter tissue blood flow and attract inflammatory cells, leading to formation of fibrinous attachments.

•If these attachments persist for 3 or more days, fibroblastic proliferation occurs.

•Because the gonococcus is present only transiently, the antibiotic was given 2-to-4 hours after inoculation to help ensure the presence of the medication during the livelihood and presumptive period of damage by the organism.

•Results: The antibiotic alone did **not** prevent adhesion formation.

•Colchicine alone or in combination with antibiotics was useful in preventing adhesions associated with inoculation of the gonococcus.

•Colchicine may offer a novel approach to the prevention of inflammation-induced pelvic adhesions in women.]

Directions: Each set of lettered headings below is followed by a list of numbered words or phrases. For each numbered word or phrase select:

    A. if the item is associated with *(A) only*
    B. if the item is associated with *(B) only*
    C. if item is associated with *both (A) and (B)*
    D. if item is associated with *neither (A) nor (B)*

Items 28-30.

    A.   severe dysplasia of uterine cervix
    B.   invasive cervical carcinoma
    C.   both
    D.   neither

28. mean of age of occurrence younger than the mode age of occurrence.   Ans: D

29. mean of age of occurrence about 50.   Ans: B

30. mode age of occurrence about 40.   Ans: B

---

p. 431 (Carson H J, Demay R M. The mode ages of women with cervical dysplasia. Obstet Gynecol 1993; 82:)

28-30. [F & I: •Background: Many women seem to have Papanicolaou smears with dysplasia at younger ages than the reported mean ages.

•This discrepancy suggested that the mean may not be the best statistic to describe the ages of these women.

•The mean is most useful when a population is normally or symmetrically distributed; the bell-shaped (gaussian) curve is formed around the mean, with the majority of the population under the middle of the curve.

•The mean is influenced by extreme values; thus, a small number of elderly women could offset the mean age of a large number of young women.

•Objective: To determine whether other measures of central tendency for age, i.e., the median or mode, might more appropriately describe the ages of women with dysplasia or carcinoma.

•The mean, median, and mode ages of women with smears showing dysplasia or squamous cell carcinoma were determined.

- The age distribution was plotted for each population, and the various measures of central tendency were assessed.

- Results: The ages of women with no disease, dysplasia, and CIS are **not** normally distributed; they are asymmetrically skewed to younger ages.

- One of the other measures of central tendency, i.e., the median or mode, might better describe the ages of these women.

- Like the mean, the median is unique for a population and, by definition, is in the middle of the population; the advantage of using the median is that it is **less sensitive** to the effect of extreme values than is the mean.

- In these populations, the median approximated the mean so closely that this measure of central tendency for age did not resolve the discrepancy that observed clinically.

- The mode, by contrast, is a **qualitative measure of central tendency** that states which age occurs most frequently.

- The advantage of using the mode is that it is **not affected by extreme values** and reflects peaks when they occur.

- The disadvantage, as evidenced in the population of CIS, is that the mode may not be unique.

- The nondiseased comparison population was also not normally distributed.

- Like the populations with dysplasia, the nondiseased population was skewed to younger women.

- The asymmetry of the nondiseased population suggests that the reason the populations with dysplasia were skewed to the younger ages was simply that **the entire clinic population was young**.

- The Kruskall-Wallis one-way analysis of variance with multiple comparisons found that the nondiseased population was older than the groups with mild and moderate dysplasia at a statistically significant level ($P < .05$).

- This result is not surprising because the nondiseased population represented women of all ages, including older women, with unremarkable Papanicolaou smears.

- In fact, the age of this population was indistinguishable from that of the older populations with severe dysplasia and CIS.

- For dysplasia, using the mode resolves the discrepancy based on the clinical impression that dysplasia occurs in women younger than the reported mean ages would lead one to expect.

- The mode ages are generally less than the reported mean ages and also lower than mean ages for dysplasia.

- Because the ages of women with carcinoma are normally distributed, the mean appropriately describes them.

- This study does not definitively document the true or universal ages of all women with dysplasia or cancer.

- There are regional, institutional, and methodologic differences that will cause similar statistics from other centers to be different for these populations.

- The value of this study is that it shows why the distribution of the ages of women with dysplasia is generally younger than the mean lead one to expect.

•Appropriate descriptive statistics help the clinician evaluate individual patients in the true context of the disease.

•For example, if a 19-year-old woman presents with mild dysplasia, she would seem unusually young compared to the mean (29 years), but not compared to the mode (22 years); the gravity of this finding can be assessed appropriately in the correct clinical context.

•Likewise, it is useful to know that the mean age of women with carcinoma (52.8 years) appropriately reflects that population.

•This information aids the cytologist, who can be alerted to search more carefully for carcinoma when any evidence of dysplasia is present in the specimen of an older woman.

•It is also helpful to the clinician to know the usual age of women with carcinoma, so they can plan appropriate follow-up and care of older patients.]

Items 31-33.

In the prophylaxis of deep venous thrombosis after gynecologic oncologic surgery:

    A. low-dose heparin (5,000 units every eight hours)
    B. intermittent pneumatic calf compression
    C. both
    D. neither

31. increased incidence of transfusion   Ans: A

32. increased incidence of wound separation   Ans: D

33. administration expense   Ans: B

---

p. 1154 (Clarke-Pearson D L. Synan I S, Dodge R, Soper J T, Berchuck A, Coleman R E. A randomized trial of low-dose heparin and intermittent pneumatic calf compression after the prevention of deep venous thrombosis after gynecologic oncology surgery. Am J Obstet Gynec 1993; 168:1146)

31-33. [F & I: •Background: In women with gynecologic malignancies low-dose heparin given over 12 hours postoperatively is **ineffective** in preventing deep venous thrombosis.

•Intermittent pneumatic calf compression used intraoperatively and for 24 hours postoperatively did **not** prevent deep venous thrombosis.

•Gynecologic oncology patients benefit from either low-dose heparin when given as three doses every 8 hours preoperatively and every 8 hours postoperatively or intermittent pneumatic calf compression applied intraoperatively and maintained for the first 5 postoperative days.

•Methods: Regimen 1 (low-dose heparin) was given in the following manner: 5000 units of heparin was given subcutaneously at 2 PM, 10 PM, and 6 AM before starting surgery at 8 AM.

•Postoperatively the patient received 5000 units of heparin subcutaneously every 8 hours for 7 postoperative days.

°If the patient was not fully ambulatory by the seventh postoperative day, heparin was continued until full ambulation was established.

°If the patient was discharged from the hospital before the seventh postoperative day, the heparin was discontinued at the time of hospital discharge.

- Patients assigned to regimen 2 had intermittent pneumatic calf compression initiated at the induction of anesthesia and continued while the patient was in the operating room, recovery room, and recumbent in her hospital bed.

- The pneumatic compression sleeves were removed while the patient ambulated postoperatively.

- Intermittent pneumatic calf compression was continued for 5 postoperative days.

  ◦ If the patient was not fully ambulatory by the fifth postoperative day, intermittent pneumatic calf compression continued until the patient ambulated completely.

  ◦ If the patient was discharged from the hospital before the fifth postoperative day, pneumatic calf compression was terminated at the time of hospital discharge.

- History and physical examination were performed at the time of the hospital admission, with specific attention to coexisting risks for thromboembolic complications.

- Patients also underwent laboratory testing, including evaluation of hematocrit, platelet count, activated partial thromboplastin time, and prothrombin time.

- Deep vein thrombosis was assessed by means of the fibrinogen uptake test, on the basis of identification by scintillation counting of iodine-125-labeled fibrinogen incorporated into acute thrombi forming in the leg veins.

- The accuracy of this test, when correlated with venography, has been established, and criteria for diagnosis have been described; I^{125} fibrinogen counting was performed at 2 inch intervals over the deep veins of the calf and thigh.

- Oral supersaturated potassium iodine was given preoperatively to block thyroid uptake of I^{125} iodide.

- I^{125} fibrinogen (100 µCi) was administered intravenously to all patients immediately after surgery.

- Beginning on the first postoperative day, the fibrinogen uptake test was performed daily until the patient was discharged.

- **Deep vein thrombosis** was diagnosed when I^{125} counts were increased >20% over counts in the adjacent scan site or in the same site on the contralateral leg or over the previous days' counts at the same location, with persistence for 2 consecutive days.

- If the fibrinogen study suggested thrombus formation in the popliteal region or thigh, **ascending venography** was used to confirm deep vein thrombosis.

- Patients were followed by the fibrinogen uptake test throughout their hospitalization and were followed clinically for the first 30 days postoperatively.

- Signs and symptoms of deep vein thrombosis and pulmonary embolism were also evaluated daily.

- Symptoms of deep vein thrombosis were evaluated by impedance plethysmography, duplex Doppler ultrasonography, and ascending contrast venography, if clinically indicated.

- Symptoms and signs of **pulmonary embolism** were assessed further by **ventilation-perfusion lung scan and pulmonary arteriography**.

- Deep vein thrombosis and pulmonary embolism continue to be significant complications after major surgery and are particularly prevalent in high risk patients, such as women with gynecologic cancers.

- 17% to 45% of patients develop deep vein thrombosis after surgery for gynecologic cancer and 1% to 2.5% will die from a postoperative pulmonary embolism.

•Results: The presence of varicose veins, age, and history of deep vein thrombosis were significant factors associated with postoperative deep vein thrombosis.

•Some previously identified risks such as race, cancer diagnosis, prior radiation therapy, and weight were **not** significantly associated with deep vein thrombosis.

•These factors may have been negated by the beneficial effect of thrombosis prophylaxis.

•Low-dose heparin and intermittent pneumatic calf compression can significantly reduce the incidence of postoperative deep vein thrombosis.

•In separate trials the reduction in the incidence of deep vein thrombosis was approximately threefold when an effective prophylactic regimen was used.

•The incidence of deep vein thrombosis in the two groups of patients is consistent with prior studies and would suggest a reduction in postoperative deep vein thrombosis compared with historic controls, in which the incidence of postoperative deep vein thrombosis was approximately 18%.

°Statistical analysis of the results does not demonstrate a significant difference between the two prophylactic methods (P = .54).

°Such a low incidence of deep vein thrombosis would have required 1780 patients to have sufficient statistical power to demonstrate a reduction in the incidence of deep vein thrombosis from 7% to 4%.

•Because low-dose heparin and pneumatic compression are equally effective in reducing the incidence of deep vein thrombosis, the current study was designed to determine whether there is a significant difference in morbidity associated with these two methods.

•In prior studies there have been no serious complications caused by intermittent pneumatic compression.

•Complications associated with low-dose heparin include an increased frequency of wound hematoma, injection site necrosis, intraoperative bleeding complications, increased transfusion requirements, and formation of retroperitoneal lymphocysts.

°These complications may be seen more frequently in particular subgroups of patients who are more sensitive to low-dose heparin.

•Previous trials that have included patients with gynecologic malignancies have shown that 10% to 15% of patients receiving 5000 units of heparin subcutaneously will have an activated partial thromboplastin time prolonged >1.5 times the control value.

•**Thrombocytopenia** has also been associated with the use of low-dose heparin.

•25 patients (23%) had prolonged activated partial thromboplastin times.

•Low-dose heparin patients had significantly higher maximum and final activated partial thromboplastin time values.

•Patients treated with low-dose heparin who underwent pelvic and paraaortic lymphadenectomy had significantly larger volumes of retroperitoneal suction drainage.

•Three of four lymphocysts occurred in the low-dose heparin group.

•32% of patients who received low-dose heparin patients required **blood transfusions** postoperatively, compared with 17% in the intermittent pneumatic calf compression group (P = .03).

•Patients on the low-dose heparin also received significantly more units of blood postoperatively (P = .02).

•Patients receiving low-dose heparin had no significant difference in their final hematocrit compared with the intermittent pneumatic calf compression group.

°This would suggest that the low-dose heparin group was appropriately transfused to maintain their hematocrits in a similar range as the intermittent pneumatic calf compression group.

»Because of the complications associated with low-dose heparin, intermittent pneumatic calf compression has a better therapeutic index and should be considered the prophylactic regimen of choice in gynecologic oncology patients.

»If intermittent pneumatic calf compression is not available, the alternative therapy, low-dose heparin, should be used.

•Four of 11 deep vein thromboses diagnosed in the first 30 days postoperatively occurred after prophylaxis was discontinued.

»It may be reasonable to consider continuing prophylaxis for longer periods of time in selected high risk patients.]

Items 34-36.

   A. complete hydatidiform mole
   B. partial hydatidiform mole
   C. both
   D. neither

34. dispermy   Ans: C

35. malignancy potential 1:200   Ans: B

36. germline mutation   Ans: C

---

p. 568 (Fisher R A, Newlands E S. Rapid diagnosis and classification of hydatidiform moles with polymerase chain reaction. Am J Obstet Gynec 1993; 168:563)

34-36. [F & I: •Background: Approximately 8% of patients with hydatidiform mole require subsequent chemotherapy for gestational trophoblastic tumor.

•It is important to distinguish hydatidiform moles from other types of fetal wastage.

•Pathologically, hydatidiform moles may be of two types, complete hydatidiform moles or partial hydatidiform moles.

•Generally, complete hydatidiform moles have higher malignancy potential, with the incidence of chemotherapy after complete hydatidiform moles being 8.6% in the United Kingdom and after partial hydatidiform moles in the order of 1 in 200.

•This risk is still significant; in the United Kingdom all patients with hydatidiform moles are routinely monitored by measurement of human chorionic gonadotropin levels after evacuation of the molar pregnancy.

•Complete hydatidiform moles can be further divided genetically on the basis of their mechanism of origin.

•The relative risk of a gestational trophoblastic tumor developing after the less common **dispermic** complete hydatidiform mole compared with the more usual **monospermic** complete hydatidiform mole has not yet been resolved.

- Although a complete hydatidiform mole can generally be identified pathologically, a partial hydatidiform mole may be difficult to identify because it has features in common with both normal placentae and complete hydatidiform moles.

- Dispermic and monospermic complete hydatidiform moles are two genetically distinct entities; they cannot be distinguished on the basis of pathologic characteristics alone.

- The unusual genetic constitution of hydatidiform moles makes it possible to identify hydatidiform moles and distinguish between a partial hydatidiform mole, a monospermic complete hydatidiform mole, and a dispermic complete hydatidiform mole by using genetic analysis.

- Cytogenetic polymorphisms, enzyme polymorphisms, and restriction fragment length polymorphisms of deoxyribonucleic acid (DNA), in particular the variable number tandem repeat sequences, have been examined to identify parental contributions to the genome and diagnose and classify hydatidiform moles.

- The time required and the complexity of these techniques makes them inappropriate for routine use.

- Variable number tandem repeat sequences can be identified in DNA by using the polymerase chain reaction.

- By using appropriate primers polymerase chain reaction can be used to detect Y chromosome-specific sequences in DNA and identify the sex of an individual.

- Objective: To determine whether the polymerase chain reaction can be used to diagnose the gestational trophoblastic disease and distinguish between the various forms of molar disease.

- Hydatidiform moles are distinguished pathologically from other types of abnormal pregnancies by **cyst formation and, more particularly, the presence of trophoblastic hyperplasia.**

    ° Genetically these pathologic characteristics are associated with the presence of **two paternal contributions** to the nuclear genome.

- In complete hydatidiform moles no maternal contribution is present, the diploid conceptus being androgenetic in origin.

- Complete hydatidiform moles may be monospermic if they arise by doubling of a haploid sperm, in which case they will be genetically homozygous.

- More rarely they may arise by dispermy, in which case they may be homozygous or heterozygous for any informative paternal marker.

- Partial hydatidiform moles are **triploid**, having one maternal and two paternal contributions to the nuclear genome.

    ° They generally arise by dispermy.

- Triploids with two maternal contributions to the nuclear genome do not generally have the pathologic characteristics of a hydatidiform mole.

- Occasional tetraploid partial hydatidiform moles have been described; an excess of paternal contributions (for example, three sets of paternal chromosomes) are present in these cases.

- Two paternal contributions to the genome are associated with specific pathologic characteristics and with the high malignancy potential of molar pregnancies.

- **A pregnancy with a hydatidiform mole is about 1000 times more likely to progress to choriocarcinoma than a normal pregnancy.**

- Among hydatidiform moles, those that progress to gestational trophoblastic tumors are generally complete hydatidiform moles.

- It is important to identify hydatidiform moles and to distinguish between complete hydatidiform moles and partial hydatidiform moles.

- The relative risk of a dispermic or a monospermic complete hydatidiform mole progressing to a gestational trophoblastic tumor has yet to be established, although dispermic complete hydatidiform mole may have a higher malignancy potential.

- This makes it desirable to distinguish between monospermic and dispermic complete hydatidiform moles so that the relative risk can be assessed.

- To determine the genetic origin of a hydatidiform mole, genetic polymorphisms need to be examined in parental and molar tissue.

- Early studies used cytogenetic polymorphisms; these techniques are time-consuming and are dependent on successful culture of molar cells and production of suitable metaphase spreads for analysis.

- Studies with **enzyme polymorphisms** provide a more rapid method of analysis but are often insufficiently informative for a complete diagnosis.

- With the development of polymerase chain reaction, a technique that amplifies small amounts of DNA, the potential for rapid diagnosis of hydatidiform mole has become feasible.

- Comparison of parental and molar polymorphisms can be made after amplification of DNA containing a polymorphic restriction site or a variable number tandem repeat, the latter polymorphisms being preferred because analysis of these can be carried out in a single-step reaction and requires only a few hours to perform compared with the >4 days generally required for Southern blot analysis of DNA.

- Complete hydatidiform moles and partial hydatidiform moles can be distinguished by using polymerase chain reaction.

- All results with polymerase chain reaction were compatible with those already obtained with other types of polymorphic analysis in these cases.

- In partial hydatidiform moles both maternal and paternal contributions could be identified in 5 of 7 cases, distinguishing them from the androgenetic complete hydatidiform moles.

- The remaining two cases were uninformative for this polymorphism.

- Partial hydatidiform moles are generally triploid with two paternal alleles.

  ° They arise by dispermy and the two paternal alleles may be identical and only a single paternal band observed.

  ° The more efficient amplification of smaller alleles makes quantitative analysis of variable sized polymerase chain reaction products difficult.

- Confirmation of two paternal contributions can be made by amplification with primers for other variable number tandem repeat sequences.

  ° Four of the partial hydatidiform moles were positive for Y chromosome-specific sequences.

  ° All four had been shown to have Y chromosome-specific sequences by other techniques.

  ° Polymerase chain reaction can be used to accurately determine the sex of hydatidiform moles.

- The polymerase chain reaction was used to distinguish between monospermic and dispermic complete hydatidiform moles.

•Because two thirds of dispermic complete hydatidiform moles are theoretically 46,XY, these should be identified by the presence of a Y chromosome-specific sequence alone.

°Two such cases were identified in series.

°Both had been shown to be Y-positive by other techniques.

•By using a panel of primers for variable number tandem repeats it should be possible first to examine sufficient samples to assess the risk of gestational trophoblastic tumor after dispermic complete hydatidiform mole, and second to make possible a distinction between monospermic and dispermic complete hydatidiform moles should this prove to have prognostic significance.

•Polymerase chain reaction has the added advantage of requiring only small amounts of DNA.

°It is used for diagnosis of very small samples of tumor tissue or trophoblast cells extracted from the blood of patients with suspected gestational trophoblastic tumor.

•Alleles were not identified in any of the hydatidiform moles that were not found in the parental DNA.

°Alleles inconsistent with parental origin may sometimes occur in molar tissue as the result of a spontaneous new mutation or because of nonpaternity of the parental DNA sample.

°New germline mutations arise at relatively high frequencies in variable number tandem repeat sequences and have been described in cases of hydatidiform mole.

°An occasional allele inconsistent with parental origin might be expected in a large series.

°A distinction between a new mutation and nonpaternity can be made by examining several different polymorphic sequences.

•On the basis of a single test with one set of primers, diagnosis between partial hydatidiform mole or complete hydatidiform mole could be made in 14 of 19 cases of hydatidiform mole.

•By using sex chromosomespecific sequences, 2 of 3 dispermic complete hydatidiform moles could be identified.]

Items 37-39.

        A.   polycystic ovarian ovary
        B.   postmenopausal ovary in patients with endometrial cancer
        C.   both
        D.   neither

37. increased estrogen production   Ans: C

38. increased bioactive LH   Ans: C

39. decreased PSH   Ans: A

---

p. 1830 (Nagamani M, Doherty M G, Smith E R, Chandrasekhar Y. Increased bioactive luteinizing hormone levels in postmenopausal women with endometrial cancer. Am J Obstet Gynec 1992; 167:1825)

37-39. [F & I: •Background: The postmenopausal ovary secretes significant amounts of androstenedione and testosterone and minimal amounts of estrogen.

•Ovaries of postmenopausal women with endometrial cancer are steroidogenically more active than those of women without endometrial cancer.

•Ovarian vein steroid levels in postmenopausal women with endometrial cancer are significantly higher than those in women without endometrial cancer.

•Ovarian stromal tissue of postmenopausal women is responsive to luteinizing hormone (LH) with an increase in the release of androstenedione.

•The increase in ovarian steroid secretion that is seen in postmenopausal women with endometrial cancer is due to an increase in LH secretion.

•Objective: To investigate the secretion of immunoactive and bioactive LH in postmenopausal women with endometrial cancer.

•Results: A more biologically active form of LH is secreted in postmenopausal women with endometrial cancer.

•A significant positive correlation between **free estradiol and the mean bioactive LH levels** was found.

•Most of the postmenopausal women with endometrial cancer studied were **obese**.

•Obesity is associated with **lower** sex hormone-binding globulin levels; free estradiol levels in these women were significantly higher.

•In a hyperestrogenic environment the pituitary gland secretes a more biologically active form of LH.

•The bioactive/immunoactive LH ratios are increased in the late follicular phase of the menstrual cycle, when the serum estradiol concentrations rises significantly.

•Increased unbound estradiol levels that are present in obese postmenopausal women with endometrial cancer could result in selective amplification of bioactive LH secretion.

•The results indicate a link between obesity, free estradiol, bioactive LH, increased ovarian steroid production, and endometrial cancer.

•Bioactive LH levels are in fact increased in postmenopausal women with endometrial cancer.

•The cancer patients studied were heavier than the controls, so it is possible that the increase in bioactive LH is related to obesity.

•The menopausal ovary is the site of gonadotropin action.

•Ovarian androgen synthesis in postmenopausal women is gonadotropin dependent.

•The ovarian stroma of postmenopausal women with endometrial cancer is responsive to LH with release of androstenedione and testosterone.

•Increased bioactive LH secretion could lead to increased ovarian androgen production, thus resulting in increased prehormone availability for estrogen formation from peripheral conversion.

•A "vicious cycle" may exist in postmenopausal women with endometrial cancer, probably initiated by obesity: increased free estradiol levels resulting from a decrease in sex hormone-binding globulin → increase in bioactive LH secretion → increased production of aromatizable androgens by the ovary → increased estrogen production from peripheral conversion and free estradiol levels.

•The hormonal milieu in obese postmenopausal women with endometrial cancer appears to be somewhat similar to that observed in premenopausal women with polycystic ovarian disease.

°Unlike polycystic ovarian disease, the FSH levels in postmenopausal women with endometrial cancer are **not** decreased, probably because of the absence of follicles in the postmenopausal ovary and the lack of inhibin.]

Items 40-42.

Effects of monophasic oral contraceptives containing:

    A.   ethinyl estradiol 20 micrograms plus desogestrel 150 micrograms
    B.   ethinyl estradiol 30 micrograms plus gestodene 75 micrograms
    C.   both
    D.   neither

40.   increased levels of fibrinogen   Ans: C

41.   increased fibrinolytic capacity   Ans: C

42.   increased ceruloplasmin levels   Ans: C

p. 37 (Petersen K R, Sidelmann J, Skouby S O, Jespersen J. Effects of monophasic low-dose oral contraceptives on fibrin formation and resolution in young women Am J Obstet Gynec 1993; 168:32)

40-42. [F & I: •Background: Cardiovascular disorders in women using combined oral contraceptives have been linked to alterations in hemostatic function and in lipoprotein and carbohydrate metabolism.

•In the coagulation system the concentrations of the vitamin-K-dependent coagulation factors tend to increase with decreased, increased, or unchanged concentrations of the inhibitors of coagulation.

•Also within the fibrinolytic system a number of changes have been seen, in particular increased capacity.

•Because the influence of oral contraceptives on the two systems primarily depends on estrogen dose, changes in hemostatic variables and the occurrence of thromboembolism may be associated because vascular morbidity decreases with reduced estrogen dose.

•Progestogens only exert **minor** effects within the **hemostatic** system, although they may influence the magnitude of the changes related to the dose-dependent effects of estrogens.

•This minor influence is in contrast to the **profound** influence of progestogens of **lipoprotein and carbohydrate metabolism**.

•Along with a reduction of estrogen dose, development of new progestogens with reduced androgenic properties has been part of the strategy to reduce the side effects of oral contraceptives.

•Objective: To evaluate the influence on coagulation and fibrinolysis of two combined oral contraceptives containing ethinyl estradiol in monophasic combination with the newly developed progestogens desogestrel and gestodene.

•Results: In this assessment of the hemostatic function during intake of low-dose oral contraceptives, the balance between generation and resolution of fibrin seemed to be maintained after 12 months of treatment with both compounds.

°Disturbances were indicated when molecular markers of in vivo activation of coagulation and fibrinolysis were applied.

•**Coagulation variables.**

•The finding that both hormonal compounds induced **elevation** in **Factor VIIc and fibrinogen** is consistent with other studies on the ethinyl estradiol plus gestodene combination and other oral contraceptives but differs from values of fibrinogen previously obtained with the ethinyl estradiol plus desogestrel preparation.

•The assumption of a causal relationship between elevated levels of plasma fibrinogen and Factor VIIc and **arterial** thromboembolic disease has **never** been established; increase in these factors observed in oral contraceptive users seem to parallel estrogen dose, which has primarily been associated with **venous** thromboembolism.

•The concept of increased coagulative capacity in oral contraceptive users caused by increased levels of fibrinogen and vitamin K-dependent procoagulants has been questioned, and clot promoting and inhibiting factors should also be evaluated when discussing hypercoagulability.

•Recurrent thromboembolic disease occurs in hereditary states of deficiencies of inhibitors of coagulation, antithrombin III and protein C and S, and decreased antithrombin III activity in users of oral contraceptives with high estrogen content has been noted.

•Newer oral contraceptives do not seem to affect antithrombin III levels, but relevant interindividual differences do exist because low levels of antithrombin III in oral contraceptive users with a family history of thromboembolism have been described.

•Decreased levels of protein C have not been found with oral contraception.

•About 40% of total protein S in plasma exists in its free form, and the remainder forms a complex with complement component C4B-binding globulin.

•The levels of total protein S, which in the heterozygous state of deficiency are reduced to about 50% of normal, seem to correlate better with the occurrence of thrombotic attacks than do levels of free protein S.

•The unchanged antithrombin III levels observed during treatment with both compounds have been found previously, but increased levels of protein C during treatment with the ethinyl estradiol plus gestodene compound contrasts earlier findings.

•Longitudinal evaluation of thrombin formation by means of thrombin-antithrombin III complexes has not previously been performed in oral contraceptive users.

•The finding of unchanged levels of thrombin-antithrombin III contrast earlier studies measuring fibrinopeptide A, a cleavage product of the polymerization of fibrinogen.

•The increased activity in the ethinyl estradiol plus gestodene group was ascribed to the higher estrogen to progestogen ratio as compared with the desogestrel group where unchanged activity was found.

•The marked estrogenic effect of both preparations (indicated by increased **ceruloplasmin** levels) did not result in increased thrombin formation; this finding raises the question as to whether estrogenicity is solely responsible for the influence of oral contraceptives on clotting activity.

•**Fibrinolytic variables.**

•Oral contraceptives primarily affect the extrinsic (tissue plasminogen activator-plasminogen activator inhibitor) pathway of fibrinolysis.

•The increase in systemic tissue plasminogen activator activity, along with elevated levels of plasminogen, may indicate an increased fibrinolytic capacity as assessed in vitro during intake of both compounds.

°Decreased levels of plasminogen activator inhibitor type I might be responsible for the increased tissue plasminogen activator activity because the antigen level of tissue plasminogen activator decreased during hormonal intake.

°Increased fibrinolytic activity has been described during treatment with the gestodene-containing formulation.

•Tissue plasminogen activator activity reflects the systemic balance between tissue plasminogen activator and plasminogen activator inhibitor type 1.

•Another steroid-sensitive regulatory mechanism of fibrinolysis is provided by **histidine-rich glycoprotein,** which inhibits the binding of plasminogen to fibrin by blocking the lysine-binding sites of the plasminogen molecule.

•When the efficacy of the fibrinolytic system was estimated by fibrin degradation products, an increase after 3 and 6 months of treatment with the gestodene-containing preparation was observed.

°This finding may reflect the more pronounced decrease in plasminogen activator inhibitor activity.

•Changes in the coagulation and fibrinolytic system were noted in both treatment groups, but only minor fluctuations in the molecular markers of the overall dynamic balance between formation and resolution of fibrin were observed.

•Adverse effects of oral contraceptives on hemostatic function cannot necessarily be ruled out because the markers applied do not assess the local interaction between blood and the vessel wall.

•The influence of oral contraceptives on lipid and carbohydrate metabolism and the interactions between these systems and hemostatic function must be included when the biochemical mechanisms underlying any cardiovascular event in oral contraceptive users are elucidated.]

Directions: For each of the questions or incomplete statements below, ONE or MORE of the answers or completions given is correct. In each case select:

A. if only 1, 2 and 3 are correct
B. if only 1 and 3 are correct
C. if only 2 and 4 are correct
D. if only 4 is correct
E. if all are correct

---

43. Complications of large loop excision of the transformation (LLETZ) for the treatment of cervical neoplasia includes

    1. cervical stenosis.
    2. immediate hemorrhage.
    3. delayed hemorrhage.
    4. inadequate tissue specimen for diagnosis.

p. 734   Ans: A   (Spitzer M, Chernys A E, Seltzer V L. The use of large-loop excision of the transformation zone in an inner-city population. Obstet Gynecol 1993; 82:731)

43. [F & I: •The characteristics of the ideal therapeutic modality for cervical lesions include:

　°1) an outpatient modality under local anesthesia,

　°2) a rapid and easy technique,

　°3) few complications and side effect,

　°4) highly effective treatment,

　°5) a modality that could be used as both an "ablation equivalent" and a "cone biopsy equivalent,"

　°6) a "conservative" modality (removing the smallest amount of tissue necessary to effect a diagnosis and cure), and

　°7) a modality that can be done during a routine colposcopy clinic visit without the need for special scheduling and without reducing the number of women who can be cared for in a clinic session.

　•Objectives: To see whether LLETZ could be used successfully to treat patients in a routine colposcopy clinic without the need for special scheduling or reduction in the number of women seen during a clinic session, and to compare these results to laser surgery.

　•Using most currently available therapeutic modalities for CIN, a cure rate of 90-to-95% can be expected after one treatment in selected patients.

　•Before this LLETZ series, the cure rate in an inner-city population was reduced because 26.9% of those patients scheduled to have laser surgery never returned for treatment despite repeated attempts to locate them.

　°Consequently, only 65.8% of the women with known disease actually achieved a cure.

　•These numbers point to the benefits of treating these patients at the time they are counseled regarding their biopsy findings rather than scheduling therapy for some future date.

　•Many therapies can be done in an outpatient facility, but each has certain drawbacks.

　•**Laser surgery** requires considerable training and expertise, expensive equipment, greater time to perform, and adequate ventilation to disperse the smoke created by the procedure.

°Although laser surgery can be done in an outpatient facility, it is often scheduled separately and may be limited to laser ablations.

•Although **cryotherapy** is easily performed with inexpensive equipment, its use is limited in many instances.

°Several groups of patients are **not** candidates for cryotherapy: those with large lesions, high-grade lesions, or lesions with glandular extension; those in whom the transformation zone was not fully visualized; and those with a discrepancy between cytology and pathology.

°In this population, that would exclude at least 136 of 236 patients (57.6%) from this technique.

•**Large-loop excision of the transformation zone** can be done under local anesthesia.

°It is easily learned and can be applied to most situations, including patients with high-grade lesions and those whose transformation zone is not fully visualized.

•LLETZ was used to treat women needing "ablation equivalents" as well as "cone biopsy equivalents."

•All procedures were well tolerated using only local anesthesia, including the cone biopsy equivalents.

»Patients were no more likely to have an unsatisfactory colposcopic examination after LLETZ than before the procedure.

•Complications such as bleeding and cervical narrowing were uncommon.

•The cure rate of 91.3% (95% CI 87.1-95.5) was comparable to that of other methods and significantly higher than the 65.8% actual cure rate achieved using laser surgery.

•The equipment is inexpensive and the technique is rapid; the modality is well suited to use in a routine colposcopy clinic.

•The patients do not need to return on another day or to a different location.

•LLETZ meets more of the criteria for the ideal therapeutic modality in an inner city population than do any other options.

•The decrease in the actual cure rate due to poor compliance among patients who are scheduled for treatment at a later date suggests that it may often be preferable to treat patients when they are told of the diagnosis.

»A "see and treat" approach without the benefit of pre-treatment colposcopy and biopsy for patients in an inner city population is **not** advocated.

•In the two largest series on the use of LLETZ for the treatment of CIN, the majority of patients were treated on the first visit, without prior histologic confirmation of disease.

•Ninety-five percent of these women were found subsequently to have evidence of disease.

•An important benefit of LLETZ is that it provides a histologic specimen in each case.

•The unexpected discovery of cervical cancer on a cone specimen is unusual in the private sector, but it has been reported in up to 1% of LLETZ specimens.

•In this inner city population, 1.7% of the patients were found to have cancer (0.84% microinvasive and 0.84% frankly invasive).

•The reason for this difference may be found in the nature of an inner city population.

•The ease of LLETZ should not lead to overtreating women who ultimately are unlikely to have evidence of disease on the LLETZ specimen.]

---

44. Common side effects of sumatriptan when used for the treatment of menstrual migraine include

   1. dizziness.
   2. nausea and vomiting.
   3. chest tightness.
   4. photophobia.

p. 769   Ans: E   (Solbach M P, Waymer R S. Treatment of menstruation-associated migraine headache with subcutaneous Sumatriptan. Obstet Gynecol 1993; 82:769)

44. [F & I:•Background: Of approximately 18 million women in the United States who suffer from migraine, many experience attacks that are worse at the time of menses, improve during pregnancy, and cease after menopause.

•These migraines are typically more severe and disabling than other migraines and are less responsive to drug and nonpharmacologic treatments.

•The pathogenesis of migraine is unknown, although distention and inflammation of cranial blood vessels may be the source of pain.

•Sumatriptan, a 5-HT receptor agonist, is effective for the acute treatment of migraine.

•Its proposed mechanism of action is vasoconstriction of cranial blood vessels.

•Another mechanism may be its ability to block extravasation of plasma proteins and neuropeptides into the walls of dural blood vessels.

•Sumatriptan reduced severe or moderate pain to mild or no pain in 70-to-72% of migraine patients within 1 hour of subcutaneous injection.

•Objectives: To determine whether sumatriptan is more effective in treating menstruation-associated migraine than is placebo and whether it is as effective in treating menstruation-associated migraine headache as it is for migraine not associated with menses.

•Current treatment for patients with menstruation-associated migraine do not differ from other migraine modalities.

•It is difficult to compare the effectiveness of sumatriptan for menstruation-associated migraine with other acute treatments; there have been few rigorous, well-controlled trials in this subset of the migraine population.

•Conventional acute therapy has included analgesics alone or in combination with narcotics, ergots, and nonsteroidal anti-inflammatory drugs.

•These treatments are not specific to the menstrual migraine, and their effectiveness is variable.

•Prophylactic treatment of menstruation-associated migraine is popular because of the presumed predictability of the timing of attacks.

•There is evidence that these techniques are less likely to succeed in treating the menstrual migraine.

•For example, propranolol and nadolol have been reported as effective prophylaxis for all migraine attacks except those associated with menses.

•Prolonged use of sumatriptan in patients given relatively unrestricted access over 1 year showed no evidence of dose escalation, abuse, or increase in migraine frequency.

•In addition, sumatriptan worked well whether taken early in an attack (less than 4 hours) or after the attack had been ongoing (more than 4 hours).]

---

45. In the evaluation of the endocervical canal, the endocervical curettage

　　1. has high-false positive rates.
　　2. has high-false negative rates.
　　3. interferes with the interpretation of subsequent cone biopsies.
　　4. has a large percentage of insufficient cellular material.

p. 575　　Ans: E　　(Hoffman M S, Sterghos Jr S, Gordy L W, Gunasekaran S, Cavanagh D. Evaluation of the cervical canal with the endocervical brush. Obstet Gynecol 1993; 82:573)

45. [F & I: •Background: Colposcopy of the cervix with directed biopsy is the standard method of investigating an abnormal Papanicolaou test.

•The role of endocervical curettage (ECC) in this process is controversial.

•Other methods of sampling the endocervical canal, including cytologic techniques, also are used.

•An ECC is often performed as part of the initial investigation and triage of the nonpregnant patient with an abnormal Papanicolaou test.

•The chief disadvantages of routine ECC are patient discomfort, cost, and a large percentage of false-positive and false-negative results.

•The endocervical brush is an instrument devised to sample the endocervical canal cytologically.

•This device has proven efficacy superior to that of the cotton-tipped applicator when used for the Papanicolaou test.

•Objectives: To evaluate and compare the cytologic information obtained from the endocervical brush and the histologic information obtained from the standard ECC used to evaluate the endocervical canal in patients with an abnormal Papanicolaou test.

•Problems with the ECC include high false-positive and false-negative rates, a large percentage of insufficient samples, interference with histologic interpretation of a subsequent cone biopsy, and the discomfort and expense associated with the procedure.

•To reduce the false-positive rate of the ECC, colposcopic evaluation has been recommended following curettage to assess contamination by an ectocervical lesion.

•To reduce the false-negative rate of the ECC, evaluation of the amount of endocervical material obtained in each case has been recommended.

•When the colposcopic examination is satisfactory, evaluation of the endocervical canal is aimed at uncovering a "skip" area of squamous abnormality or an endocervical epithelial abnormality.

•Endocervical sampling is controversial because these abnormalities appear to be uncommon, and false-positive results lead to unnecessary conization.

•The concern is that omission of the ECC may lead to inadequate treatment of dysplasia or a missed diagnosis of invasive cancer.

- Results: 19 of 65 patients (29%) with a satisfactory colposcopy had disease in the endocervical canal according to interpretation of the cone biopsy or hysterectomy specimen; 15 of the 19 had CIN.

- Of the 65 patients with satisfactory colposcopy, none had occult "skip" dysplasia or invasive carcinoma in the endocervical canal.

- The explanation for this high percentage of squamous intraepithelial abnormalities in the endocervical canal is most likely that colposcopy was considered satisfactory if the entire transformation zone could be visualized, regardless of whether the lesion or transformation zone extended up the endocervical canal.

- A better indicator of the potential value of endocervical evaluation in the patient with "satisfactory colposcopy" would be to examine a large series of cone biopsies in patients with no visible abnormality above the external cervical os.

- Most of the studies that have evaluated ECC against a cone biopsy or hysterectomy specimen have analyzed the ECC results only in relation to whether the colposcopy was satisfactory or unsatisfactory.

- The false-positive rate is one of the chief difficulties with the ECC for the patient with a satisfactory colposcopy.

- In this study there was a greater problem with the endocervical brush.

- An exclusionary guard or sheath added to the brush could markedly decrease the false-positive rate.

- The false-positive rate for these two techniques cannot be calculated accurately for the present study population of "satisfactory colposcopy" patients.

- The false-positive rate was calculated by looking at the ECC and brush results compared to the entire group of specimens interpreted as containing no endocervical abnormality on the cone biopsy or hysterectomy specimen.

- This methodology does not account for the number of results that were positive as a result of ectocervical contamination, regardless of the presence of disease in the endocervical canal.

- The false-positive rate was 18% for the ECC and 75% for the brush.

- The false-positive rate remains a significant weakness, especially for the brush, in evaluation of the endocervical canal.

- From the results of the ECC and brush presented, differences between correct positive or negative results for these two methods are less apparent in the patients with an unsatisfactory colposcopy.

- The brush in this group is superior to the ECC in some aspects.

- The results also suggest that the ECC may be better than the brush in diagnosing invasive carcinoma in the endocervical canal.

- These numbers are clearly too small to draw conclusions, and the importance of this finding in this small subgroup certainly does not speak strongly against the brush as compared to the ECC.

- When considering the total study group in this series, the brush was a more sensitive indicator than ECC for disease in the endocervical canal, with a greater negative predictive value.

- The ECC, on the other hand, was a more specific test although the positive predictive value was not statistically significantly different.

- **The low specificity of the brush makes it too unreliable for diagnosing endocervical disease.**

•If studies using a protective sheath demonstrate improved results, then a role for the brush in the diagnosis of endocervical disease may be reconsidered.

•Given its greater sensitivity, the brush might be used as initial screening for endocervical disease.

•If the brush is positive, then an ECC, with its greater specificity, could be performed.

•The brush might also be of value when following the patient (without treatment) with low-grade squamous intraepithelial neoplasia.

•Use of the ECC for backup evaluation of the endocervical canal is also suboptimal in both its sensitivity and specificity.

•A technique that deserves further study is loop excision of the transformation zone, which has the advantage of diagnosis and treatment in one step and in an office setting.

•The operator may remove variable amounts of the endocervical canal, and the procedure may be particularly cost-effective for the patient with a high-grade squamous intraepithelial lesion that extends a visible distance up the canal.

•Despite these developments, the optimal way to evaluate the endocervical canal is unknown.]

---

46. Treatments of chronic vulvar pruritus include

    1. topical fluorinated hydrocortisones.
    2. alcohol injection of affected tissue.
    3. Mehring denervation.
    4. subcutaneous injection of triamcinolone

---

p. 568   Ans: E   (Kelly R, Foster D C, Woodruff D. Subcutaneous injection of triamcinolone acetonide in the treatment of chronic vulvar pruritus. Am J Obstet Gynec 1993; 169:568)

46. [F & I:•Background: Chronic vulvar pruritus is a most distressing physical and sociologic symptom for many patients, as well as for their physicians.

•The superior surfaces of the labia majora extending from the mons to the anal orifice are most involved.

•During the acute phase of scratching, these tissues are erythematous.

•Later, after continued injury by the fingernail, the vulvar skin often takes on the leathery, lichenified appearance of chronic dermatitis.

•The most common treatment of chronic vulvar pruritus is the use of topical steroids, often without the benefit of a biopsy-confirmed diagnosis.

•With failure of topical therapy, alternative surgical approaches such as alcohol injection or the Mehring procedure have been advocated.

•Unfortunately, both procedures require conduction or general anesthesia and both run the risk of subsequent infection and tissue sloughing.

•Objectives: To report on the subcutaneous vulvar injection of triamcinolone acetonide as an alternative to standard therapies.

•To demonstrate that subcutaneous corticosteroid injection, an office procedure, provides prolonged relief of vulvar pruritus with little or no tissue trauma.

- Methods: If topical steroids alleviated the symptom for a period of 30 to 60 minutes during the 2 week trial, then a subcutaneous injection of triamcinolone acetonide 10 mg/ml was recommended.

- The focus for injection was massaged with a local anesthetic agent to decrease the discomfort.

- A small wheal of local anesthetic was produced at the upper margin of the labium majus on either side corresponding to the areas of concern.

- A 25-gauge needle with local anesthetic was then inserted at these sites.

- Subsequently 15 to 20 mg of triamcinolone acetonide 10 mg/ml (1 ml is equal to 10 mg) was then slowly injected as the needle was directed posteriorly, toward the anal orifice.

- A total of 15 to 20 mg of triamcinolone acetonide or 1.5 to 2 ml of the preparation was injected on either side.

- The area was massaged thoroughly so that the agent was diffused throughout the labia.

- The patient was instructed to use a cool sitz bath the following evening for about 10 to 15 minutes.

- The patient was also instructed that it would take approximately 24 to 48 hours for the agent to be effective.

- Therapy for pruritus has included topical application of steroids or one of several surgical procedures.

- Local irritants, such as the use of detergents in washing the underclothes and hygiene sprays to the vulva, must be eliminated.

- Systemic disease such as diabetes mellitus must be identified and treated.

- Although the use of fluorinated hydrocortisones for a long period can result in dermal fibrosis, such formulations are more effective in alleviating the local symptom than are the nonfluorinated variety.

- Topical steroids are helpful in alleviating the local problem in many cases, often the application of such medication controls the symptoms for only short periods of time.

- Since the patient cannot and should not persistently apply such local agents, she will continue to scratch and thus lacerate the tissue with the introduction of a variety of irritants through the fingernail.

- Furthermore, most medications are prepared in a petrolatum base, which may produce local reactions.

- Alcohol injection of the affected tissue can control the symptoms.

    ° The procedure does necessitate regional or general anesthesia, and on occasion, there is sloughing of the vulvar skin.

    ° It is usually used after failure of local medications.

- The **Mehring denervation** is an even more extensive procedure that requires incisions through the skin and underlying tissues from the level of the clitoris to the level of the fourchette.

    ° It is not commonly used.

- An alternative approach to treatment is reported in this article.

- A large majority of patients experienced prolonged relief of the pruritus with a mean duration of relief of approximately 6 months.

•In 10 cases the procedure was repeated with success.

•The patient must be informed that even with subcutaneous injection of corticosteroids, on occasion there may be focal slough of tissue because of interruption of the blood supply.

•Because the injection is subcutaneous and not into the skin, breakdown is not a common complication.

•As a matter of fact, in this series of 45 patients that complication did not occur in any case.

•Persistent irritation with associated breakdown of the local tissue, proliferation, and repair may be the most common sequence of events in patients who eventually have a malignancy.

•In contrast to that of cervical carcinoma, the pathogenesis of vulvar carcinoma is poorly understood.

•Older women with vulvar squamous cell carcinoma often have a history of pruritic disorders ranging from squamous hyperplasias to lichen sclerosis.

•A recent histopathologic study found squamous hyperplasia adjacent to vulvar squamous cell cancer in 74% of cases (14/19).

•All of the squamous hyperplasia-associated squamous cell cancers of the vulva were negative for human papillomavirus by in situ hybridization and polymerase chain reaction for human papillomavirus.

•Although a cause effect relationship between vulvar pruritus *per se* and invasive carcinoma cannot be made at this time, inflammation, pruritus, and the accompanying excoriation may ultimately be shown to be a precursor to malignancy.

•The described office procedure may alleviate the distressing symptom of chronic itching for long periods of time and may prevent the development of more aggressive neoplastic problems.]

---

47.   Structures innervated by the pudendal nerve include

   1. external anal sphincter.
   2. urethral sphincter.
   3. deep transverse perineal muscle.
   4. bulbocavernosus.

---

p. 389   Ans: E   (Benson J T, McClellan E. The effect of vaginal dissection on the pudendal nerve. Obstet Gynecol 1993; 82:387)

47. [F & I: •Background: Pudendal neuropathy is a clinically significant component of female pelvic floor disorders, i.e., urinary incontinence, fecal incontinence, and prolapse.

• Pudendal neuropathy is mainly caused by obstetric vaginal delivery, but other causes may be contributory.

•Vaginal dissection, as employed in anterior and posterior colporrhaphy and needle urethropexy, may produce pudendal neuropathy by disrupting pudendal nerve branches.

•Pelvic floor surgery performed by the abdominal route, without vaginal dissection, should not produce pudendal neuropathy because dissection does not involve the area of distribution of the pudendal nerve branches.

•Objectives: To test the hypothesis that the vaginal route of female pelvic floor surgery produces neuropathy of the pudendal nerve, as measured by pudendal nerve and perineal nerve terminal motor latencies.

•To compare terminal motor latencies in women having surgery with and without vaginal dissection.

- •Methods: All patients had clinically significant pelvic floor prolapse with or without urinary and fecal incontinence.

- •Pelvic floor prolapse was defined as vaginal vault or uterine descent of at least 50% (descending more than 4 cm below the ischial spines) accompanied by grade III or greater cystocele or rectocele (protruding beyond the introitus in the upright position with Valsalva maneuver).

- •The mean age was 62 years in the vaginal group and 65 years in the abdominal group.

- •All were estrogenized.

- •Fifty-nine percent of the vaginal subjects and 70% of the abdominal subjects had undergone previous pelvic floor surgery.

- •The surgical approach used in the vaginal group consisted of vaginal-paravaginal cystocele repair and sacrospinous vault suspension with or without needle urethropexy.

- •The surgical procedures in the abdominal group included abdominal paravaginal cystocele repair and colposacral suspension with or without retropubic urethropexy.

- • Right and left pudendal nerve and right and left perineal nerve terminal motor latency studies were performed before and at least 6 weeks after surgical intervention.

- • The method for measuring the pudendal nerve terminal motor latency was developed at St. Mark's Hospital in London from the technique of electroejaculation described by Brindley.

- • Terminal motor latency studies involve depolarizing a nerve by electrical stimulation while recording the response from the muscles it innervates.

- •This response is termed a compound muscle action potential.

- •The latency of the response is defined as the time elapsed between the onset of the stimulus and the onset of the response.

- •Pathologic processes in nerves can increase the latency of the compound muscle action potential.

- • For the pudendal nerve terminal motor latency, stimulation was delivered transrectally to the pudendal nerve at the ischial spine.

- •Surface electrodes at the external anal sphincter measured the resulting compound muscle action potential.

- •The stimulation was supramaximal (level of stimulus intensity producing no further amplitude enhancement of the response).

- •Surface ring electrodes around a Foley catheter recorded the response of the compound muscle action potential at the proximal urethra.

- • These two tests study the pudendal nerve in its two terminal branches: the inferior hemorrhoidal branch supplying the external anal sphincter and the perineal branch innervating the musculature surrounding the vagina and urethra.

- •Two major conclusions may be drawn from this study.

- •One is that preoperative pudendal and perineal nerve terminal motor latencies are similarly prolonged in patients with prolapse and pelvic relaxation, supporting a previous report linking pudendal neuropathy with pelvic floor prolapse.

•The second is that the vaginal route of pelvic floor surgery appears to produce neuropathy of the pudendal nerve.

•Clinically significant neuropathy is assumed when terminal motor latency studies increase more than 2 SDs.

•Is the neuropathy created by vaginal dissection of clinical importance? Denervation is recognized as a cause of female pelvic floor dysfunction, including urinary and fecal incontinence and pelvic relaxation.

•Perhaps the accentuation of pudendal neuropathy produced by vaginal dissection affects the surgical outcome.]

---

48. Indications for conization of the uterine cervix include

    1. endocervical curettage positive for intraepithelial neoplasia.
    2. unsatisfactory colposcopy.
    3. discrepant cytology.
    4. squamous cell carcinoma reported on pap smear during pregnancy in the face of normal colposcopy.

p. 397   Ans: E   (Hoffman M S, Collins E, Roberts W S, Fiorica J V, Gunasekaran S, Cavanagh D. Cervical conization with frozen section before planned hysterectomy. Obstet Gynecol 1993; 82:394)

48. [F & I: •Background: Women with cervical intraepithelial neoplasia (CIN) III may elect to have definitive treatment with hysterectomy.

•In some, outpatient evaluation does not satisfactorily rule out invasive cancer or, less frequently, fails to make a definitive diagnosis of CIN III, and cervical conization is necessary before hysterectomy.

•Objective: To report experience with the accuracy and usefulness of cervical conization with frozen section before hysterectomy.

•Methods: Patients in whom hysterectomy was planned for or with a concomitant or suspected diagnosis of CIN underwent preliminary conization with frozen section for any of the following indications:

°1) unsatisfactory colposcopy,

°2) endocervical curettage (ECC) positive for any degree of CIN,

°3) cytology suggestive of malignancy or CIN III without histologic explanation,

°4) an extensive CIN III lesion, and

°5) microinvasion detected on colposcopically directed cervical biopsy.

•Cone biopsy was performed with a scalpel, taking care to avoid trauma to the specimen, and sent it immediately to the pathologist for frozen section.

•The pathologist inked the peripheral margins of the cone and then cut the cone radially into slices approximately 1-to-2 mm thick.

•The pieces were prepared in water-soluble embedding material, and 4-to-5 μ sections were prepared with the cryostat.

•Sections were stained with polychrome and/or hematoxylin and eosin and were examined.

•The remaining tissue was processed for permanent sections in the usual manner.

- The frozen sections were correlated with the permanent sections at a later date.

- The sensitivity, specificity, and positive and negative predictive values for the frozen section compared with the final histopathologic diagnosis were calculated.

- **Microinvasion** in the cone biopsy was defined as stromal invasion to a depth of 3 mm or less from the basement membrane, with no capillary or lymphatic space involvement by tumor.

- When hysterectomy is planned for CIN, it is important to be reasonably certain that invasive carcinoma does not exist.

- Despite outpatient evaluation with cytology, colposcopy with directed biopsy, and ECC, diagnosis is not always possible without a cone biopsy.

- Cervical conization alone is highly effective treatment for CIN III, but its efficacy in the treatment of early microinvasive cervical cancer is unknown.

- Prior studies have reported a reasonably high degree of accuracy for frozen-section interpretation of cervical conization specimens.

- Providing appropriate treatment is given, cone biopsy with frozen section followed by hysterectomy has a number of advantages, including reduced costs and inconvenience to the patient, the need for only one anesthetic, and the potential for reduced infection and technical difficulty associated with delayed hysterectomy.

- Results: Frozen-section evaluation of a cone biopsy specimen carries a degree of accuracy that enables the surgeon to make an immediate decision about definitive therapy.

- In the case of an adequate colposcopic examination with a directed biopsy showing CIN III, there is no uniform agreement on the necessity for cone biopsy before proceeding with hysterectomy.

- If the **Papanicolaou smear suggests malignancy** in such patients, a cone biopsy certainly should be performed.

- A **positive ECC** may also influence this decision.

  ° An ECC positive for CIN has been another indication for conization of the cervix before definitive hysterectomy.

  ° Much of the controversy surrounding the role of ECC involves its use in the triage of patients for outpatient therapies.

  ° Its place for the patient who is planned for definitive hysterectomy is somewhat different in that the main concern is to rule out invasive cancer.

  ° In the present study, when this was the indication for conization, only one invasive cancer was found.

  ° In some earlier studies, the degree of CIN found on ECC predicted somewhat the risk of finding invasive cancer on final pathology.

  ° The presence of severely dysplastic or questionably invasive tissue on ECC indicates the need for preliminary cone biopsy before proceeding with hysterectomy.

- **Unsatisfactory colposcopy** is another classic indication for cone biopsy in patients with CIN, but the role of cone biopsy in these women who are planned for definitive hysterectomy for CIN is uncertain.

  ° Twenty-one patients in the present study underwent cone biopsy with frozen section for this indication, and seven of them had invasive cancer.

°This number is too small to allow conclusions to be drawn, and this issue is not well addressed in the literature.

•**Discrepant cytology** is another indication for cone biopsy and was listed as the sole indication in 25 of subjects.

°Biopsy did not reveal invasive cancer in any of these women.

°Nine patients had CIN III diagnosed accurately on frozen section of the cone biopsy done as a result of discrepant cytology; they were then able to have hysterectomy under the same anesthesia.

•Few data exist on the use of cone biopsy with frozen section before cesarean hysterectomy.

•Cervical conization is indicated before planned cesarean hysterectomy when an entire CIN III lesion cannot be seen colposcopically or when there is any suspicion that occult invasive cancer may be present (such as a class V Papanicolaou smear or a biopsy suggesting possible microinvasion).

»Preliminary cone biopsy with frozen section before cesarean hysterectomy should be performed only when clearly indicated; vaginal delivery followed by evaluation 6-to-8 weeks later may be preferable in some patients.

•When **microinvasion** is found on colposcopically directed biopsy or is reported on the frozen section of a cone biopsy, proceeding with definitive surgery based on the frozen-section report is considered **controversial**.

•Ideally, the diagnosis of microinvasive carcinoma of the cervix is based on careful review of the permanent sections taken from a cone biopsy.

•Twelve women had a diagnosis of microinvasion based on frozen section, and all proceeded directly to definitive therapy.

•For most of these women, the surgeon reviewed the slides with the pathologist at the frozen section once a diagnosis of microinvasion was made.

•Based on this combined review, two patients were treated with radical hysterectomy after it was noted that there were multiple foci of microinvasion.

•Even though both of these patients met the Society of Gynecologic Oncologists' definition of microinvasion, the presence of **multiple foci** of microinvasion was believed to signify a volume of invasive cancer substantial enough to require radical hysterectomy.

•The one patient who had a cone biopsy immediately after cesarean delivery had the depth of invasion underestimated on the frozen section this section was not reviewed by the surgeon despite some uncertainty expressed by the pathologist.

•Few data exist in the literature on the accuracy of frozen section in the diagnosis of microinvasive carcinoma of the cervix.

•Frozen section was accurate for the nonpregnant subjects, but the small number precludes a definitive conclusion.

»When microinvasion is reported on frozen section of the cone biopsy, the surgeon should review the slides immediately with the pathologist.

•This allows clear communication between the two and gives the surgeon a much better idea of the exact nature of the invasive process.

•The role of frozen section in the diagnosis of microinvasive carcinoma of the cervix requires further study.

•None of the subjects who underwent hysterectomy for CIN or microinvasive carcinoma had residual invasive carcinoma in the final hysterectomy specimen.

•The cone biopsy margins were not analyzed on either the frozen sections or permanent sections.

•Conclusion: The use of cone biopsy with frozen section appears to be accurate and useful in the management of selected patients with dysplastic and early neoplastic lesions of the cervix who have elected definitive surgical treatment.

•For certain groups of patients, such as those with mildly dysplastic cells on the ECC and certain patients with an unsatisfactory colposcopy, preliminary cone biopsy with frozen section may be unnecessary.

•More experience is needed to assess the role of cone biopsy with frozen section in other groups of women such as those with microinvasive cancer and those who are pregnant.]

---

49. Myomas cause infertility by

 1. reducing the implantation space.
 2. mechanical compression of the tube.
 3. delaying sperm transport.
 4. interference with endometrial blood supply.

p. 215   Ans: E   (Tulandi T, Murray C, Guralnick M. Adhesion formation and reproduction outcome after myomectomy and second-look laparoscopy. Obstet Gynecol 1993; 82:213)

49. [F & I: •Background: Myomectomy is sometimes indicated for infertile women with leiomyoma uteri.

• This procedure often causes adhesion formation, which may further decrease fertility.

•A second-look laparoscopy has been advocated to liberate these post-myomectomy adhesions.

•Objective: To evaluate adhesion formation after myomectomy and the reproductive outcome of infertile women with a large leiomyomatous uterus after myomectomy and second-look laparoscopy.

•Results: Myomectomy is often associated with adhesion formation.

•Most of the adhesions are found between the uterine incision and omentum or intestines.

•Intra-abdominal adhesions may cause bowel obstruction and abdominal pain, whereas adnexal adhesions may inpair fertility.

•Myomectomy with a **posterior uterine incision** is associated with more and a higher degree of **adnexal adhesions** than that with a fundal or anterior uterine incision.

»When performing a myomectomy, one should attempt to avoid a posterior uterine incision.

•The site of uterine incision that allowed removal of as many myomas as possible was chosen.

•Usually, myomas on the posterior uterine wall can be removed using a fundal incision.

•When they cannot, a second-look laparoscopy to liberate the adhesions should be considered.

•Whether the pregnancy rate in these women is superior to that in women who do not undergo a second-look laparoscopy and lysis of adhesions remains to be seen.

•**The most favorable incision is one that is located anteriorly.**

•Postoperative adhesions are usually found only between the bladder and the anterior wall of the uterus, and the adnexa are free from adhesions.

•Myomectomy with fundal incision causes intra-abdominal adhesions, but it is associated with a mild degree of adnexal adhesions.

•Clearly, the worst adnexal adhesions occur following posterior incision.

•The pregnancy rate (66.7%) at 12 months of follow-up compares favorably to those previously reported.

•The association between myoma and infertility is not fully understood, but may involve **reduction of the implantation space, mechanical compression of the fallopian tube, delay in sperm transport because of increased uterine surface, and interference with uterine vascularization causing endometrial impairment of implantation.**]

---

50. Histological correlation of chromosomally normal conceptual tissue from spontaneous abortion includes

    1. a villous circulation indicating fetal life to 10 to 11 or more weeks.
    2. chronic intervillositis.
    3. villous infarcts.
    4. decidual vasculitis.

---

p. 295   Ans: E   (Salafia C, Maier D, Vogel C, Pezzullo, Burns J, Silberman L. Placental and decidual histology in spontaneous abortion: Detailed description and correlations with chromosome number. Obstet Gynecol 1993; 82:295)

50. [F & I: •Background: Spontaneous pregnancy loss is the most common complication of pregnancy.

•50% of spontaneous abortions occur because of chromosomal abnormalities in the conceptus.

•Though this statistic is helpful in counseling a patient who has had a pregnancy loss, it would be even more helpful to know specifically if that patient's abortion was caused by a chromosomal abnormality.

•If the karyotype was abnormal, the cause for that pregnancy loss is then known.

•Alternatively, if the karyotype was normal, investigation of possible maternal factors could be initiated if the woman has had other pregnancy losses.

•For cases in which the woman has undergone therapy for a diagnosed cause of habitual abortion but pregnancy loss has occurred again, knowledge of the fetal karyotype helps decide whether the treatment failed or whether that particular pregnancy would have been lost despite treatment.

•Unfortunately, information on the karyotype of an abortus is usually not available.

•Routine karyotyping is expensive, inconvenient, and requires specialized laboratory facilities and personnel.

•Even when attempts are made to karyotype abortus material, the tissue may fail to grow or there may be significant contamination with maternal cells.

•Finally, karyotyping can only be done on fresh tissue, but the need for that information may not become apparent until months or years after the pregnancy loss.

•When a patient has had subsequent pregnancy losses and presents for evaluation of recurrent abortion, she could be evaluated and counseled in a more rational manner if there were a way to determine retrospectively her abortuses' karyotypes.

- One possible way to determine retrospectively the chromosomal status might be careful histologic examination.

- Previous histologic studies of spontaneous abortions have correlated specific **villous morphologies** with particular karyotypic abnormalities, such as trisomy 13 and monosomy.

- The specific morphologic distinctions are difficult to make in a routine laboratory during evaluation of the products of miscarriage.

- It would be far more useful clinically to be able to use histologic data to distinguish between normal and abnormal karyotypes.

- In addition to data regarding the abortus' karyotype, careful examination of the products of conception might provide insight into the etiology of chromosomally normal losses.

- Objectives: To assess easily evaluated villous and decidual histologic markers in spontaneous abortions in a large group of women with no history of recurrent pregnancy loss, to examine their relationships to normal versus abnormal chromosome number, and to determine the ability of histologic and clinical data to predict chromosome number.

- The present population consisted of highly motivated couples who chose cytogenetic evaluation of their first or second failed pregnancy.

- These patients may differ from their peers by socioeconomic, age, and other demographic features.

- The distribution of chromosomally normal and abnormal conceptions is generally consistent with unselected series of abortions showing at least half of all spontaneous abortions to be chromosomally abnormal.

- Results: The data indicate significant associations between specific histologic markers and normal or abnormal chromosome number, although definitive karyotypic diagnosis is not possible using any one histologic feature.

- Features that can be routinely recognized by histologic examination of the products of conception in pregnancy loss and knowledge of maternal age and duration of pregnancy from the LMP can be used to solve a regression equation.

- From this solution, one can calculate a probability of as great as 97% for a normal chromosome. number or 88% for an abnormal chromosome number, depending on the specifics of an individual case.

- The two factors most significant in predicting chromosome number were **the duration of pregnancy from the LMP and the duration of embryo/fetus viability, as assessed by circulatory characteristics**.

- Though LMP dating of pregnancy may be inaccurate, the present data show that the embryo/fetus appears to be viable to within approximately 2 weeks of pregnancy loss in 42% of chromosomally normal gestations but in only 19% of chromosomally abnormal gestations.

- There are different periods of intrauterine retention after death in conceptions with normal versus abnormal chromosome number.

- Two possible explanations for this difference are as follows.

- In a chromosomally abnormal gestation, abnormal embryonic development and death may precede death of placental tissue, as placental tissue can function normally despite chromosomal abnormalities (hydatidiform moles are an example).

- The decline in placental hormone production and consequent uterine bleeding and contractions would occur as later events, so that there would be a delay between embryo death and clinical signs of abortion.

- In a chromosomally normal gestation in which pregnancy loss is caused by maternal factors, **placental damage may be the initial event**, and the sequelae of embryo death and uterine bleeding would occur closer in time to each other.

- Alternatively, in chromosomally abnormal conceptions, there may be a delay in the appearance of anucleated red blood cells, and the methodology used to judge the duration of fetal viability in elective terminations may not be applicable to chromosomally abnormal spontaneous abortions.

- There is generally normal villous morphogenesis in chromosomally normal abortions.

- These data suggest that, when maternal age and duration of pregnancy from the LMP are considered as confounders, no decidual or placental lesion is characteristic of chromosomally abnormal pregnancy loss, i.e., when pregnancy failure is the direct result of embryo/fetal pathology.

    º For example, **hydropic changes** involving more than 50% of the villi were significantly more frequent in cases with abnormal chromosome number.

- The multiple logistic regression shows that the more important features of losses with abnormal chromosome number are **advanced maternal age** and shorter duration of pregnancy from the LMP.

- Gestations lost at younger gestational age, and lost from older mothers, are more likely to have hydropic changes.

- In chromosomally normal losses, when the cause of pregnancy loss is not so readily apparent, the observations of specific significant lesions may clarify the mechanisms involved.

- An increased prevalence of chronic inflammatory lesions (chronic intervillositis and decidual vasculitis) was identified in chromosomally normal pregnancies.

- These lesions may indicate a role of the maternal immune response in certain cases of early pregnancy loss.

- Another lesion found more often in chromosomally normal losses is **villous infarct**.

- Although villous infarcts are not infrequent in placentas delivered at term, they are distinctly unusual in early pregnancy.

- The finding that **infarcted villi were significantly related to chromosomally normal losses** suggests possible decidual vaso-occlusion in certain cases of early pregnancy loss.

- Although the frequency of decidual thrombosis alone did not differ between chromosomally normal and abnormal losses, this may be due to decidual vascular occlusion occurring as a final degenerative change of failed pregnancy, regardless of cause.

- Overall, these data support a role for underlying defective maternal-fetoplacental interaction in early pregnancy failure.

- Defective decidua-trophoblast interaction may be a primary process in many forms of pregnancy compromise.

    º This was **not** found in this series.

- The tissue sampling and histologic criteria were developed with an eye to the daily practical utility in the routine laboratory setting.

- Tissue sampling effects may have contributed to this discordance.

•Focus was on distinctions between genetically abnormal but non-molar abortions and those in which chromosome number was normal.

•The findings of this study are important in three ways.

•First, they allow construction of a formula that can predict karyotypic normality or abnormality from clinical data and pathologic examination of tissue.

°This formula should have significant clinical usefulness as it enables the clinician to inform the patient of the likelihood of abortal chromosomal normality or abnormality with more precision than the "50-50 chance" provided by epidemiologic studies.

•Second, the presence of these findings may provide clues as to the underlying pathophysiology of chromosomally normal pregnancy losses.

•Finally, this study provides baseline data for the investigation of villous and decidual histology in recurrent abortion.]

---

51. Medical management of an unruptured ectopic pregnancy can be considered if

    1. serum progesterone level is <5 nanograms.
    2. serum ß-hCG <2000 mIU/ml 48 hours apart.
    3. ultrasound shows an empty uterus.
    4. ultrasound shows a fetal heart rate and adnexal mass.

---

p. 1761   Ans: E   (Stowall T G, Ling F W. Single-dose methotrexate: An expanded clinical trial. Am J Obstet Gynec   1993; 168:1759)

51. [F & I: •Background: If the necessity for laparoscopy to diagnose ectopic pregnancy is eliminated, treatment with intramuscular methotrexate can offer the advantages of decreased cost, avoidance of anesthetic and laparoscopic-related morbidity, and less time lost from the patient's daily activities.

•In 1989 and 1991 an individualized dosing regimen of methotrexate (1 mg/kg) and citrovorum (0.1 mg/kg) factors was reported, in which patients received one to four doses until the quantitative human chorionic gonadotropin (hCG) titers declined by 15% on two consecutive days.

•Subsequently experience with a single-dose (50 mg/m^2) intramuscular methotrexate regimen in a group of 30 patients was reported.

•Objective: To expand experience with minimally invasive diagnostic techniques combined with a single-dose methotrexate treatment protocol for selected unruptured ectopic pregnancies.

•Methods: All patients were diagnosed as having an ectopic pregnancy by means of a nonlaparoscopic diagnostic algorithm that combines the use of serial hCG titers, serum progesterone, transvaginal ultrasonography, and curettage.

•Patients with a serum progesterone level <5.0 ng/ml or an hCG level ≥2000 mIU/ml that was persistently rising abnormally (<50% increase over 48 hours) underwent curettage and were followed according to the previously published nonlaparoscopic algorithm.

•Patients with a rising hCG titer ≥2000 mIU/ml without an associated intrauterine sac visualized by transvaginal ultrasonography did not require pretreatment curettage, nor did those patients with an ectopic pregnancy with cardiac activity demonstrated by transvaginal ultrasonography.

•This method of ectopic pregnancy diagnosis precludes intervention in cases of viable pregnancy and was 100% accurate in a randomized trial.

•Patients were eligible for study inclusion if

°(1) they were hemodynamically stable,

°(2) the hCG titers increased after curettage, if performed,

°(3) transvaginal ultrasonography demonstrated an unruptured ectopic pregnancy ≤ 3.5 cm in greatest dimension,

°(4) the patients desired future fertility, and

°(5) they signed an informed written consent.

- Patients were excluded from the study if

    °(1) they had declining hCG titers after curettage,

    °(2) transvaginal ultrasonography demonstrated an ectopic pregnancy > 3.5 cm in greatest dimension,

    °(3) they were hemodynamically unstable at presentation,

    °(4) they did not desire future fertility, and

    °(5) there was evidence of hepatic dysfunction (aspartate aminotransferase greater than two times normal), blood dyscrasia (white blood count <2000 cells/cm), thrombocytopenia (platelet count <100,000), or renal disease (serum creatinine >1.5 mg/dl).

- A blood type, Rh, and antibody screen were obtained on all patients.

    °Those who were Rh negative were given Rh immunoglobulin (300 μg) at treatment initiation.

- All women were treated as outpatients with an intramuscular injection of methotrexate (50 mg/m^2) without citrovorum factor rescue.

- Patients were instructed to refrain from alcohol and intercourse and to avoid vitamin preparations containing folic acid until complete resolution of the ectopic pregnancy.

- Patients with hematocrits <35% were given 325 mg of ferrous sulfate twice daily.

- Patients were instructed to use either oral contraceptive pills or barrier contraception for at least 2 months after treatment completion.

- Patients were further instructed that they might experience an increase in abdominal pain during the first several days after treatment initiation.

- An hCG titer was obtained on day 1 (treatment initiation) and on days 2 (patients 1 through 30), 4 and 7.

- The first 30 patients had an hCG titer study on day 2, but this was eliminated in subsequent patients.

- A complete blood cell count and aspartate aminotransferase level were repeated on day 7 (patients 1 through 30).

- These were not repeated in any of the remaining patients because there were no changes noted in these tests as previously reported.

- Patients with a ≥15% decline in the hCG titers between days 4 and 7 were followed up weekly until the hCG titer was ≤12 mIU/ml.

- If there were a <15% decline or a rise in the hCG titer between days 4 and 7, patients were given a second intramuscular dose of methotrexate (50 mg/m^2) on day 7.

- A second treatment course was also given if the hCG titer plateaued between the weekly levels.

- Repeat transvaginal scanning was performed to rule out ectopic pregnancy rupture if the patient had increasing abdominal pain.

- If the ectopic pregnancy had cardiac activity at treatment initiation, transvaginal scanning was performed on alternate days until cardiac activity disappeared.

- Repeat pelvic examinations were not performed in any patients after treatment initiation, to avoid the potential of iatrogenic tubal rupture.

- A hysterosalpingogram was requested of all patients on day 6 to 9 after the second menstrual cycle after treatment completion (hCG <12 mIU/ml).

- Patients were contacted by telephone or letter every 6 months to seek information regarding any conception that had occurred after treatment.

- Single-dose methotrexate appears to be as effective as the previously published multidose regimen but has the advantages of requiring less methotrexate, not requiring citrovorum recovery, reducing patient follow-up, and being associated with less cost.

- Like the previously published multidose protocols, single-dose methotrexate can be safely accomplished on an outpatient basis.

- Single-dose methotrexate virtually eliminates side effects, thereby increasing the safety and patient acceptance of this form of treatment.

- Reported methotrexate side effects such as gastritis, stomatitis, elevated hepatic transaminase levels, leukopenia, or thrombocytopenia were not encountered in this series, thus reinforcing the safety of methotrexate when used for ectopic pregnancy.

- Only one patient had nausea with vomiting lasting 24 hours, which may or may not have been a drug-induced side effect.

- All patients in this study had the diagnosis of ectopic pregnancy confirmed by means of a diagnostic algorithm that does not require laparoscopy.

- For other physicians to achieve the clinical advantages reported here, implementation of this diagnostic method with strict adherence to the diagnostic algorithm is imperative.

- By doing so, inadvertent administration of methotrexate to an intrauterine pregnancy and performance of curettage on a viable intrauterine pregnancy are avoided.

- Early in this trial all patients underwent curettage before treatment initiation to ensure that a viable intrauterine pregnancy was not interrupted.

- Because viable intrauterine pregnancies can be visualized at an hCG <2000 mIU/ml on transvaginal ultrasonography, these patients no longer need to undergo curettage.

- Also, it is **not** necessary to perform a pretreatment diagnostic curettage on patients with an empty uterus and cardiac activity in the adnexa seen on vaginal ultrasonography.

- Such use of contemporary ultrasonography technology assumes a well established system of reliable radiologic personnel and equipment support.

- The presence of cardiac activity was not considered a contraindication to methotrexate initiation.

•Of seven treatment failures two had cardiac activity.

•Treatment failure in the presence of cardiac activity (2/14, 14.3%) is higher than the failure rate in the absence of cardiac activity (5/106, 4.7%).

•Although not an absolute contraindication to methotrexate, the presence of cardiac activity in the ectopic pregnancy continues to represent a relative contraindication.

•Resistance to implementation of intramuscular methotrexate as primary treatment for ectopic pregnancy has been tied to its potential associated side effects, failure rates, required follow-up, and uncertain reproductive outcome.

•Physicians who continue to rely on laparoscopy to diagnose ectopic pregnancy rightfully treat the ectopic pregnancy surgically at the time of diagnosis; the patient thereby does not require medical treatment.

•Although this was not a randomized comparison of methotrexate with laparoscopic surgery, the methotrexate failure rates were similar to previously reported laparoscopic surgical series.

•The follow-up required after methotrexate therapy and the reproductive outcomes were similar to those after a conservative laparoscopic procedure.]

---

52. Factors associated with a favorable outcome when adnexal torsion is treated by untwisting include

   1. duration of symptoms.
   2. leukocytosis.
   3. fever.
   4. pregnancy.

p. 1749   Ans: D   (Zweizig S, Perron J, Grubb D, Mishell Jr. D R. Conservation management of adnexal torsion. Am J Obstet Gynec 1993; 168:1791)

52. [F & I: •Background: Adnexal torsion has been treated by salpingo-oophorectomy without untwisting the adnexa to avoid the potential complication of thrombotic emboli from the ovarian vein.

•Objectives: To evaluate postoperative morbidity in patients who underwent conservative therapy (ovarian cystectomy) for adnexal torsion compared with those who had salpingo-oophorectomy.

•to determine predictors that might be associated with the ability to perform conservative surgery.

•Concern about untwisting of the adnexa precipitating thrombotic events such as pulmonary embolus has meant that most women with adnexal torsion are treated by salpingo-oophorectomy.

•Four series from outside the United States report 97 cases of adnexal torsion treated by untwisting followed by salpingo-oophorectomy, cystectomy, or cyst aspiration.

•No thrombotic complications were reported in these series, although the issue was not always specifically addressed.

•The incidence of fatal pulmonary emboli in women <40 years old undergoing all types of pelvic surgery is between 0.1% and 0.5%.

•Eighty-two patients in this series underwent untwisting of the adnexa, and in 61 of these the ovary was saved.

•No thrombotic complications were seen, so the risk of pulmonary embolus in reproductive-age patients who had conservative surgery was 0% with a 95% confidence interval that reached 6%.

- The sample size series is too small to show a lack of increased morbidity from pulmonary embolus when adnexa are untwisted in appropriate patients.

- Patients who had conservative treatment were compared with those who had extirpative treatment to evaluate whether patients with retained adnexa who had had transient ischemia would have more postoperative complications than those who had complete adnexectomy.

- No difference in length of **hospital stay** was found between the two groups; **postoperative febrile morbidity** was observed in 12% of the women treated by salpingo-oophorectomy compared with 3% of the women who had conservative surgery.

  ° This increase in morbidity may reflect **pyrogen release** by necrotic tissue from the ovary that had to be removed.

- No significant differences were seen between the two groups in comparing other complications such as **wound seromas**, and the incidence of complications was no greater than that in the general population of women undergoing gynecologic surgical procedures.

- No **complications of pregnancy** were seen postoperatively in the pregnant patients who were treated by conservative surgery.

- The occurrence of postoperative morbidity was also examined in patients who underwent untwisting of the adnexa with or without cystectomy; it was not found to differ from those patients whose adnexa were not untwisted.

- Several factors evaluated in this study may be useful for counseling patients preoperatively.

- Pregnant patients were found to have a 60% **decrease** in the risk of requiring extirpative surgery, whereas patients with leukocytosis or fever had more than twice the risk of requiring salpingo-oophorectomy.

- Of interest was that **duration of symptoms** was **not** found to be predictive of eventual management.

- In spite of the presence or absence of these preoperative factors the results indicate that untwisting of the adnexa and ovarian cystectomy can be performed in reproductive-age women with adnexal torsion in the absence of a grossly necrotic adnexa.

- None of the patients in this series were found to have **ovarian vein thrombi** in the absence of total ovarian necrosis.

- If ovarian vein thrombi are identified in otherwise viable appearing adnexa, it may be possible to ligate the vessel above the thrombus and proceed with untwisting of the adnexa.

- Although patients who required salpingo-oophorectomy were found to have larger masses and a greater degree of torsion, conservative management was used to treat masses up to 22 cm in diameter and with as many as 900 degrees of torsion.

- **Fluorescein** was found to be useful when adequacy of tissue perfusion could not be determined by gross inspection after untwisting of the adnexa; in the majority of cases gross visual evidence of vascular perfusion was sufficient.

- Untwisting of potentially viable adnexa followed by cystectomy in patients with adnexal torsion appears to be a safe procedure that is well tolerated.

- This conservative approach should be encouraged in women of childbearing age to reduce the possibility of premenopausal loss of ovarian function when the contralateral ovary has to be subsequently removed because of another pathologic entity.]

53. Associated with toxic shock syndrome

   1. contraceptive sponge.
   2. diaphragm.
   3. tampon.
   4. LEEP excision of cervical neoplasia.

p. 203   Ans: A   (Rosen D J D, Margolin M L. Menashe Y, Greenspoon J S. Toxic shock syndrome after loop electrosurgical excision procedure. Am J Obstet Gynec 1993; 169:202)

53. [F & I: •Background: Toxic shock syndrome occurs in menstruating women and in postsurgical patients.

•The incidence of menstrual toxic shock syndrome is approximately 1 in 100,000.

•In 1986 nonmenstrual toxic shock syndrome accounted for about 55% of the total cases reported.

•The loop electrosurgical excision procedure is used increasingly to treat cervical intraepithelial neoplasia.

•Objective: To report a case of toxic shock syndrome that developed after loop electrosurgical excision procedure for cervical intraepithelial neoplasia.

•Menstrual toxic shock syndrome was described in 1980.

•Since withdrawal of the Rely tampon from the marketplace, cases of menstrual toxic shock syndrome have decreased, although the incidence of nonmenstrual toxic shock syndrome cases has remained constant.

•The **criteria** for diagnosis include a temperature of ≥38.9° C, a diffuse erythematous macular rash, hypotension, and multiple system involvement.

•The rash desquamates 1 to 2 weeks after the onset of illness.

•Although the patient did not have hypotension, there was a significant orthostatic decrease in blood pressure.

•The patient probably had toxic shock syndrome, although the *S. aureus* organism was not available for toxic shock syndrome toxin-1 testing.

•A penicillinase-resistant penicillin is the drug of choice to eradicate *S. aureus*.

•Patients with toxic shock syndrome are less likely to have a recurrent episode if they are treated with a penicillinase-resistant penicillin.

•In this case a quinolone—ciprofloxacin—was selected to empirically treat a "traveler's diarrhea" but coincidentally had activity against *S. aureus*.

•The patient did not receive additional therapy because the organism was eradicated.

•Toxic shock syndrome should be included in the differential diagnosis of every case of high fever, rash, and hypotension in a seriously ill patient.

•If toxic shock syndrome is suspected, supportive treatment and administration of a semisynthetic penicillin or cephalosporin with activity against *S. aureus* should be initiated.

•The loop electrosurgical excision procedure is becoming a popular and effective surgical therapy for cervical intraepithelial neoplasia.

•Physicians should be aware that toxic shock syndrome may occur after any surgical procedure, including the loop electrosurgical excision procedure.

•Approximately 5% of healthy women harbor *S. aureus* as part of the normal vaginal flora.

•*S. aureus is* an infrequent cause of infection in obstetrics and gynecology patients.

»This single case does not justify pretreatment vaginal cultures for *S. aureus* because of the rarity of this complication.

»Prophylactic antibiotic therapy to prevent toxic shock syndrome is not advised because the incidence of serious allergic reactions to the antibiotic may approximate the incidence of toxic shock syndrome after loop electrosurgical excision procedure.

»Patients undergoing loop electrosurgical excision procedure should be counseled to seek medical care if they have a fever, rash, or diarrhea with or without the other symptoms of toxic shock syndrome.]

---

54. Mechanisms by which protein receptor mRNA is overexpressed in leiomyomata include

   1. alteration of estrogen receptors.
   2. anomalies in progesterone receptors.
   3. increase in insulin-like growth factor.
   4. overabundance of progesterone regulatory protein.

---

p. 84 Ans: E   (Brandon D D, Bethea C L, Strawn E Y, Novy M J, Burry K A, Harrington M S, Erickson T E, Warner C, Keenan E J, Clinton G M. Progesterone receptor messenger ribonucleic acid and protein are overexpressed in human uterine leiomyomas. Am J Obstet Gynec 1993; 169:78)

54. [F & I: •Background: Leiomyomas, the most common uterine tumor in women, are associated with infertility, cause significant morbidity, and are one of the most frequent indications for hysterectomy.

•The mechanism of conversion of normal myometrial tissue to leiomyoma and the factors that orchestrate abnormal growth of leiomyoma cells are poorly understood.

•These tumors occur only after puberty, are most common in women >30 years old, and regress with the menopause.

•This suggests that leiomyoma growth is dependent on ovarian steroids.

• Leiomyoma growth is affected by progesterone, because these tumors can rapidly increase in size during pregnancy, a time when progesterone levels are markedly elevated.

•Increased mitotic activity in leiomyomas during the secretory phase of the menstrual cycle further suggests that these tumors are affected by progesterone.

•Because RU 486, a potent antiprogestin, can cause marked regression of uterine leiomyomas suggests that progesterone receptors may control leiomyoma growth.

•Objective: To identify molecular abnormalities that underlie the aberrant growth response of leiomyomas to steroid hormones, the expression of the progesterone receptor gene and the proliferation-associated antigen Ki-67 was analyzed.

•To control for variations in hormonal status between individuals, leiomyoma tissue was compared with adjacent normal myometrium from the same patient.

•Results: Increased progesterone receptor messenger ribonucleic acid (mRNA) and progesterone receptor protein was found in uterine leiomyomas.

• Progesterone receptor mRNA and progesterone receptor protein are overexpressed in human uterine leiomyomas compared with normal adjacent myometrium.

• This is not likely to be caused by a difference in cell type, because histologic studies have shown that both tumor and myometrial tissues consist almost exclusively of smooth muscle cells.

• Women served as their own controls.

• Another possibility is that measurement of progesterone receptor levels by ligand binding assays can be influenced by endogenous steroid.

• To control for variation in the hormonal milieu, progesterone receptor mRNA and protein concentrations in uterine leiomyomas and adjacent normal myometrium from the same patient was examined.

• Several established methods to quantify progesterone receptor gene expression were used, including Northern blot analysis, enzyme immunoassay, immunohistochemistry, and Western blot analysis.

• Western blot analysis indicated that the progesterone receptor A protein is **overexpressed** in leiomyoma compared with adjacent normal myometrium.

• Analyses of additional patient samples will be required to determine if the progesterone receptor A, B, or both are most often overexpressed in tumors.

• The human A and B isoforms are believed to be translated from distinct mRNA transcripts that originate from alternate transcription initiation from a single progesterone receptor gene.

• These receptor isoforms can differentially stimuate transcription from chimeric reporter genes constructed with different progestin response elements.

• Further studies will be necessary to determine if progesterone receptor A or B-specific mRNA transcripts are aberrantly expressed in uterine leiomyomas.

• A correlation between progesterone receptor overexpression and cell proliferation (indicated by increased levels of the proliferative antigen Ki-67) suggests that enhanced progesterone receptor concentrations may be related to abnormal growth of leiomyoma cells.

• For this reason, it will be important to determine if cultured leiomyoma cells have an increased growth response to progesterone compared with cultured myometrial cells.

• There are several possible mechanisms by which progesterone receptor mRNA could be overexpressed in leiomyomas.

• Because expression of progesterone receptor is regulated by estrogen, it is possible that the increased amount of progesterone receptor is caused by alteration of estrogen or estrogen receptors in leiomyomas.

• Alternatively, progesterone receptor may have escaped normal regulation by estrogen receptors.

• Anomalies in progesterone receptor regulation are found in breast carcinomas where progesterone receptor is expressed in the absence of estrogen receptors and, in some cases, not expressed in the presence of estrogen receptors.

• Progesterone receptor levels in leiomyomas could also be enhanced because of alterations in the level of growth factors or other serum factors.

° For example, insulin-like growth factor-1 can stimulate progesterone receptor production in uterine cells.

•Gene amplification or mutation of the regulatory region of the progesterone receptor gene, resulting in increased transcription is also a possibility.

•An overabundance of progesterone receptor protein, a transcription regulator, may cause an imbalance in the amount of other growth regulatory genes such as protooncogenes or growth factors, which, in turn, could contribute to aberrant leiomyoma growth.

•Further studies will be necessary to determine which, if any, of these mechanisms underlie enhanced progesterone receptor expression in leiomyomas.]

---

55. True statements about hormone replacement therapy and the risk of breast cancer include

   1. Synthetic estrogen is associated with an increased risk of breast cancer.
   2. Women who have ever used estrogen and stopped for two years are at increased risk.
   3. Use of estrogens for more than ten years is associated with an increased risk of breast cancer.
   4. The addition of progestins through estrogens reduces the risk of breast cancer.

p. 1479   Ans: B   (Coldtiz G A, Egan K M, Stampfer M J. Hormone replacement therapy and risk of breast cancer: Results from epidemiologic studies. Am J Obstet Gynec 1993; 168:1473)

55. [F & I: •Background: The increased risk of breast cancer associated with early menarche, pregnancy, and late menopause points to a potential role of ovarian hormones in its cause.

•In some studies urine or plasma estrogen levels have been positively related to breast cancer risk.

•Among postmenopausal women obesity, which increases estrogen levels, has been associated with higher risk of breast cancer incidence and mortality.

•These data suggest that estrogen levels influence the risk of disease among postmenopausal women.

•Although exogenous estrogens have been suspected of increasing the risk for breast cancer, no relation has been observed in most studies.

•With few exceptions, previous case-control and follow-up studies, as well as studies using population rates for comparison, have focused primarily on **ever use**, without making a distinction between current and past use of postmenopausal estrogens.

•Because of the promoting effect of estrogen in animals, one may expect a different relation between breast cancer among current or recent-past users of estrogens as opposed to more remote use.

•In a meta-analysis the combined estimate of relative risk from 23 studies was 1.01 (95% confidence interval 0.95 to 1.08), indicating **virtually no relation** between ever using (predominantly past use) estrogens and risk of breast cancer.

•More recently, techniques of meta-analysis have been used to combine data addressing the question of duration of use and risk of breast cancer.

•Objectives: To look at the combined data with the addition of recently published new studies, to address the role of **current** compared with **past** use of replacement therapy, and to examine the relation of estrogen plus progestin compared with estrogen therapy alone.

• to examine the relation between duration and risk of breast cancer by means of all available data.

•In this meta-analysis, **no** association was observed between ever-use of postmenopausal hormone therapy and risk of breast cancer and little evidence to support any latency effect.

•Women who had used estrogens in the past and stopped replacement therapy for more than 2 years were **not** at increased risk.

- There was a suggestion of a modest **increase** in risk associated with **synthetic estrogens** (as reflected in the European studies) compared with conjugated estrogens, in which no increase in risk for ever-use was observed.

- This may reflect higher circulating estrogen levels among women taking synthetic estrogens.

- No strong evidence was found to support a linear increase in risk with **longer duration** of estrogen use; few studies have evaluated very long-term use (≥20 years).

- Use for **more than 10 years** was associated with a slight but significant **increase** in risk.

- Some of the effect of long duration of use may be caused by an increased proportion of current users in the long-duration categories.

- No evidence was observed to support a differential effect of estrogen therapy among women with a family history of breast cancer compared with those without a family history, nor among women with a prior history of benign breast disease.

- Although ever-use does not appear related to risk of breast cancer, **current use may be associated with increased risk.**

- Current users must see a physician to renew prescriptions and hence are more likely to be screened for breast cancer.

- Because some detection bias cannot be ruled out contributing to this elevated risk, additional data on survival among women who use replacement hormone therapy are needed.

- Data from three studies suggest that survival among cases detected while women are using replacement hormone therapy may be improved compared with those detected among never-users.

- The summary relative risk for **combination therapy** was 1.13, similar to that for estrogen alone (1.05).

- These combined data provide evidence that addition of progestins will **not** reduce risk of breast cancer.

- Breast cancer appears to respond differently than uterine cancer, where estrogens raise the risk several fold, and progestins are protective.

- These data do **not** support the use of progestins among hysterectomized women.

- Given the adverse effect of progestins in high doses on the lipid profile, this combination may attenuate the reduction in total mortality observed for estrogen therapy alone.

- The higher risk of breast cancer among women using combination therapy than those using unopposed estrogens may reflect the greater proportion of current users among women taking estrogens and progestins.

- Conclusions: Women who have used estrogen in the past are **not** at increased risk of breast cancer.

- **Current use** may be associated with an **increased** breast cancer incidence, but the relation with mortality is less clear.

- **Long-term use** may lead to **slight increases** in risk, but this needs to be substantiated in further studies.

- **Family history** of breast cancer and personal history of **benign breast disease** do **not** appear to modify the relation between replacement therapy and risk of breast cancer]

56. Clinically effective in the treatment Chlamydial cervicitis:

    1. amoxicillin
    2. erythromycin
    3. azithromycin
    4. clindamycin

p. 748   Ans: E   (Magat A H, Alger L S, Nagey D A, Hatch V, Lovchik J C. Double-blind randomized study comparing amoxicillin and erythromycin for the treatment of *Chlamydia trachomatis* in pregnancy. Obstet Gynecol 1993; 81:745)

56. [F & I: •Background: *Chlamydia trachomatis* is the most common sexually transmitted bacterial pathogen in the United States and the most likely to be encountered in obstetric populations.

    •Left untreated, an affected woman may

    °1) transmit the organism to her offspring at delivery,

    °2) develop endometritis-salpingitis postpartum,

    °3) experience an adverse obstetric outcome such as premature rupture of membranes or premature labor, and

    °4) serve as a horizontal vector for continued spread of the disease in the community.

    •Pregnant women have the greatest risk of developing serious complications from the infection and are epidemiologically crucial in both vertical and horizontal transmission.

    •Until recently, the only drug recommended for treatment of chlamydial infections during pregnancy was erythromycin.

    •Some patients are unable to complete a therapeutic course of erythromycin because of undesirable side effects, specifically nausea and gastrointestinal distress.

    •Recognizing the need for alternative therapy, the most recent Centers for Disease Control (CDC) guidelines for the treatment of sexually transmitted diseases recommend the use of **amoxicillin** for women intolerant of erythromycin.

    •Objectives: To determine the relative efficacies of amoxicillin and erythromycin in eradicating *C. trachomalis* from the lower genital tract of pregnant women.

    •A secondary goal was to evaluate whether amoxicillin is better tolerated and, hence, promotes patient compliance and cure rates superior to those for erythromycin.

    •Each year, 155,000 infants are born to mothers with genital chlamydia, with vertical transmission frequently resulting.

    •Chlamydial conjunctivitis develops in approximately 30-to-40% of exposed infants, whereas pneumonia has been estimated to occur in 10-to-20%.

    •There may also be an association between maternal cervical infection with *C. trachomatis* and preterm delivery.

    •Erythromycin can eradicate antenatal *C. trachomatis* from the maternal genital tract.

    °At the recommended dosage of 500 mg orally four times daily, a significant number of patients experience undesirable gastrointestinal side effects and are unable to complete a therapeutic course.

°An alternative to erythromycin is needed.

•Several antibiotics have been effective in the treatment of chlamydial cervicitis in the nonpregnant patient but are generally considered contraindicated during pregnancy.

•**Clindamycin** has been suggested as an alternative.

°The cost of a 7-day course of clindamycin remains ten times that of erythromycin, which discourages routine use.

•Beta-lactam antibiotics, such as amoxicillin, were initially thought to be ineffective against chlamydial infections.

•Results: Equivalent success rates in treating maternal cervical infection (98.4 versus 94.8%) for amoxicillin and erythromycin.

•The amoxicillin regimen showed a comparable incidence of side effects but a significantly lower incidence of intolerance compared to erythromycin.

•Amoxicillin 500 mg three times daily for 7 days is an effective and well-tolerated antimicrobial agent for the treatment of antenatal cervical chlamydial infection.

•Approximately 86% of the patients who completed 21 doses of therapy were cured.

•When compared with erythromycin, there was no significant difference in efficacy.

°Although more than twice as many patients remained infected after treatment with amoxicillin as did after completing a course of erythromycin, this was not statistically significant ($P = .14$).

•Using the 500-mg preparation of erythromycin, a large number of women experienced side effects, and 23.1% of the total developed symptoms that caused them to discontinue treatment.

•Amoxicillin was better tolerated, with a sixfold reduction in the number of complaints; discontinuation was required in only one patient (1.5%).

•Of interest is that of the 15 patients intolerant to erythromycin, 12 were successfully treated subsequently with amoxicillin.

•Because almost one-quarter of the patients assigned to receive erythromycin were unable to complete their course of therapy, the actual success rates of the regimens were 84.6 versus 72.3% for amoxicillin and erythromycin, respectively.

•The success rate more accurately reflects the effectiveness of a drug regimen in the clinical setting.

°Although these differences were not statistically significant, additional studies are warranted to determine whether amoxicillin is in fact superior to erythromycin in clinical practice.

•Results: Amoxicillin is a reasonable alternative for those intolerant to erythromycin.

•In view of the sizeable failure rates for both regimens, a test-of-cure culture appears indicated when treating chlamydial infections in pregnancy.]

57. Explanations for the absence of detectable levels of ß-hCG in the circulation of patients with ectopic pregnancies include

   1. trophoblastic degeneration.
   2. small volume of trophoblast.
   3. defect in ß-hCG biosynthesis.
   4. rapid clearance of the hormone from the circulation.

p. 878   Ans: E   (Maccato M L, Estrada R, Faro S. Ectopic pregnancy with undetectable serum and urine ß-hCG in the ectopic trophoblast by immunocytochemical evaluation. Obstet Gynecol 1993; 81:878)

57. [F & I: •Background: The steady rise in the incidence of ectopic pregnancy and the need for rapid and definitive diagnosis of this condition has led to the development of diagnostic algorithms based on the use of immunoassays sensitive for ß-hCG in both urine and blood.

•The most common explanation for ectopic pregnancies associated with undetectable levels of serum ß-hCG is the absence of viable trophoblastic tissue.

•Ectopic trophoblast cells can be deficient in ß-hCG production.

•Objective: To report a case of a ruptured ampullary ectopic pregnancy associated with intra-abdominal hemorrhage and undetectable levels of ß-hCG in serum and urine, in the presence of trophoblastic tissue producing ß-hCG as demonstrated by immunohistochemistry.

•Four theoretical mechanisms can explain the absence of detectable levels of ß-hCG in the circulation of patients with ectopic pregnancy:

   °1) trophoblast degeneration with absent hormone production,

   °2) small volume of trophoblastic tissue,

   °3) defective ß-hCG biosynthesis, and

   °4) rapid clearance of the hormone from the circulation.

•The ability of trophoblastic tissue to produce ß-hCG was shown by the immunohistochemical stain.

•Although the volume of ectopic trophoblast cannot be estimated accurately, chorionic villi and trophoblast cells were found in several histologic sections from the affected fallopian tube, suggesting that the amount of tissue present should have produced a detectable level of hormone.

•A normal serum creatinine value suggests that the patient had a normal glomerular filtration rate.

•The possibility of an abnormally high ß-hCG clearance rate is unlikely, unless an error in the patient's ß-hCG biosynthesis produced a modified molecule with very high clearance.

•This biosynthetic defect could involve the glycosylation steps.

•Increases in the ß-hCG clearance rate were noted when the carbohydrate portion of the molecule was absent.

•Another possible explanation is that different epitopes of the ß-hCG subunit may be identified by the two different antibodies used for the serum immunoassay and tissue staining.

•The mechanism responsible for the negative urine and serum pregnancy tests in this patient remains unknown.

• The clinical significance of this case is that an ectopic pregnancy, including a ruptured tubal ectopic pregnancy, may occur even though the serum and urine pregnancy tests are negative.

• ß-hCG levels must be high enough to be detected in serum or urine, or these tests may not be useful.

» One should not delay in using additional diagnostic aids such as culdocentesis or vaginal and abdominal ultrasound scans when evaluating the patient suspected of having an ectopic pregnancy.]

---

58. Predictive of successful anterior-posterior vaginal repair undertaken to relieve stress urinary incontinence

    1. increase in abdominal pressure transmission ratio
    2. increase in maximum urethral closure pressure
    3. increase in retrovesical angle during stress
    4. the presence of striated muscle in the levator ani

---

p. 428   Ans: E   (Hanzal E, Berger E, Koelbl H. Levator ani muscle morphology and recurrent genuine stress incontinence. Obstet Gynecol 1993; 81:426)

58. [F & I: •Background: The urethral closure mechanism has been studied in anatomical, urodynamic, and radiologic investigations.

• The importance of extraurethral factors such as the pelvic floor muscles is a matter of increasing interest, especially in patients with genuine stress incontinence.

• There are morphologic differences in biopsy specimens of the pubococcygeal muscle obtained during posterior vaginal repair in women with both prolapse and genuine stress incontinence.

• In one group of patients, striated muscle tissue could be identified in the specimens; these patients had significantly **higher** abdominal pressure transmission ratios during preoperative urodynamics as compared with a second group of patients who lacked striated muscle tissue in the pubococcygeus muscle.

• Objective: To evaluate the impact of levator ani muscle morphology on the outcome of anteroposterior vaginal repair.

• Methods: According to the results of this evaluation, two groups of patients were identified: 11 (36.7%) showed striated muscle fibers in their biopsy specimens (group A) whereas specimens of the remaining 19 patients (63.3%) contained only connective tissue, smooth muscle, or fat tissue (group B).

• Anteroposterior repair attempts to correct pelvic floor anatomy and improve support to the urethrovesical unit.

• The basic concept of the procedure does not take into consideration the preoperative condition of the pelvic floor muscles; on the contrary, this procedure is thought to be particularly beneficial in patients with marked pelvic floor relaxation.

• According to the results, levator ani muscle morphology is an important preoperative factor in the outcome of anteroposterior vaginal repair.

• All patients with striated muscle-positive biopsy specimens were continent after a follow-up period of up to 44 months, whereas patients without evidence of striated muscle tissue had a 53% recurrence rate of genuine stress incontinence.

• This finding indicates that women with deteriorated levator morphology have an increased risk of recurrent genuine stress incontinence and may not benefit from vaginal surgery performed as a single procedure to treat genuine stress incontinence.

• Detachment of the periurethral vagina from the levator ani may contribute to genuine stress incontinence.

•This concept of reconstructive surgery of the pelvic floor has emphasized posterior vaginal repair.

•Orientation of the vagina in the erect position is oblique or even horizontal and the levator plate lies directly beneath, adjacent to the bladder and urethra, thus lending support to these structures under normal circumstances.

•Anterior colporrhaphy, as performed on the study subjects, included repair of a cystocele and raising of the bladder neck by approximating the paravaginal fascia.

•Posterior vaginal repair aimed at reformation of the levator plate in a way that the pubococcygeus muscles on both sides were sutured together in the midline, thus forming a new support structure for the pelvic viscera.

•Biopsies were taken from the posterior part of the pubococcygeal muscle, so no reliable statement can be made from the data about muscle morphology in the anterior segment of the levator.

•It is likely that degeneration occurs in all muscles of the pelvic floor.

•This degeneration may result in a reduced density of striated muscle fibers, leading to failure of identification of striated muscle tissue in biopsy specimens of the pubococcygeus muscle.

•Anteroposterior vaginal repair resulted in an increase in abdominal pressure transmission ratios in both groups of patients.

•Accordingly, all patients in group A were continent.

•As regards group B, this observation suggests that even in patients with impaired muscle condition, anteroposterior repair is capable of elevating the urethrovesical unit above the levator plate.

•Group B patients had a significantly lower abdominal pressure transmission ratio than group A, indicating a possible correlation of this urodynamic index with pelvic floor muscle morphology.

•The greater the difference between pre- and postoperative pressure transmission ratios, the more likely is a cure.

•In addition, compared with group B, postoperative perineal sonography in group A disclosed a significantly smaller retrovesical angle during straining, which indicates that an intact levator muscle maintains better support of the pelvic viscera during stress than a damaged one.

•Comparing preoperative and postoperative values of the retrovesical angle during straining within each group, a significant decrease of this measurement in group A patients, versus an increase in group B was noted.

•This finding suggests a more active role of the pelvic floor muscles during an intra-abdominal pressure rise when muscle morphology is unimpaired.

•These observations indicate that a comparison of both pre and postoperative abdominal pressure transmission ratios and retrovesical angles during stress is helpful in determining the adequacy of surgical correction of the anatomical defect associated with genuine stress incontinence.

•**A decrease of the maximum urethral closure pressure at rest** in group B patients, which was associated with a higher recurrence rate of genuine stress incontinence was found.

•This urodynamic index remained unchanged in group A.

•At the beginning of the study, all patients were incontinent and a vast majority had mild degrees of prolapse.

•It seems unlikely that some of the urethral function before surgery was a result of the prolapse, due to torsion and partial obstruction, and once the prolapse was reduced this compensatory mechanism was lost.

•Deterioration in postoperative urethral resting pressure must be due to other factors associated with vaginal surgery, which remain to be elucidated.

°One possible reason might be **surgical damage to the paraurethral tissue**, resulting in partial denervation of the urethral sphincter.

°This provides an additional explanation for the high percentage of recurrences in group B patients.

•At follow-up, there were no differences in the distance between the transducer head and the urethrovesical junction (distance A) between group A and group B patients.

°Both groups showed a significant increase of distance A after surgery.

°This confirms that anteroposterior repair elevates the urethrovesical unit regardless of levator ani muscle morphology.]

---

59. Clinically useful in maintaining bone mineral density during GnRH agonist treatment of endometriosis

    1. calcium carbonate
    2. medroxyprogesterone
    3. norethindrone
    4. sodium etidronate

p. 581   Ans: E   (Surrey E S, Fournet N, Voigt B, Judd H L. Effects of sodium etidronate in combination with low-dose norethindrone in patients administered a long-acting GnRH agonist: A preliminary report. Obstet Gynecol 1993; 81:581)

59. [F & I: •Background: GnRH agonists are effective in the therapy of symptomatic endometriosis.

•Safety and compliance for long-term continuous administration may be limited by bone mineral density loss and vasomotor symptoms due to the hypoestrogenic state induced by these agents.

•Treatment of postmenopausal women with progestins alone in the absence of exogenous estrogens inhibits vasomotor symptoms, and both metabolic and radiologic evidence of bone mineral density loss.

•The administration of various progestins in conjunction with GnRH agonists as a form of "add-back" therapy is an attempt to maintain effectiveness while eliminating side effects.

•The addition of **medroxyprogesterone** acetate eliminated secondary vasomotor symptoms and preserved bone mineral density but **failed to relieve painful symptoms or to reduce endometriotic implants**.

•The addition of **norethindrone**, a 19-nor-testosterone-derived progestin, **decreased the extent of disease-associated symptoms while essentially eliminating hot flushes** in maximal mean doses of 2.04 mg/day.

°**Bone mineral density was still noted to decrease reversibly.**

•Increasing the daily norethindrone dose to 10 mg both prevented bone loss and preserved the effectiveness of a long-acting GnRH agonist on symptomatic disease.

°**Potentially detrimental changes in circulating lipoproteins were noted.**

- Sodium etidronate is an organic bisphosphonate compound that inhibits osteoclast-mediated bone resorption in the appropriate doses.

- This agent has minimal side effects.

- It has proven effectiveness in the treatment of Paget disease and in short-term retardation of postmenopausal osteoporosis in the absence of estrogen replacement.

- Objective: To assess the efficacy of combining sodium etidornate with low dose norethindrone on bone mineral density, vasomotor symptoms, and lipid profiles given to patients treated with a long-acting GnRH agonist preparation.

- Methods: Eleven patients with symptomatic endometriosis, documented laparoscopically, were randomized into two treatment groups.

- All subjects received the depot preparation of the GnRH agonist leuprolide acetate, 3.75 mg intramuscularly (IM) every 28 days for 6 months.

- Therapy was initiated in the midluteal phase.

- Six patients (group I) also received sodium etidronate (Didronel) in an oral dose of 400 mg/day for 2 weeks followed by a 6-week course of oral calcium carbonate, 500 mg/day.

- This cycle was repeated three times during the 6-month trial.

- In addition, norethindrone (Norlutin) was self-administered in a 2.5-mg/day oral dose.

- Five patients (group II) received norethindrone only in a 10-mg/day oral dose in addition to the agonist.

- Persistent hypoestrogenemia was induced after administration of GnRH agonist alone or in combination with either high-dose norethindrone or a lower dose of norethindrone supplemented by cyclic sodium etidronate.

- Estrogen levels achieved were well within the range observed in postmenopausal women in all three treatment groups.

- Results: The addition of norethindrone in doses as low as 2.5 mg/day significantly reduced these symptoms despite maintenance of a persistent hypoestrogenic state.

- These findings were confirmed by objective monitoring of vasomotor instability.

- This beneficial effect was also maintained with the use of higher daily doses of norethindrone.

- **The addition of either norethindrone 10 mg/day or norethindrone 2.5 mg/day in combination with cyclic sodium etidronate appeared to prevent the bone loss from the lumbar spine demonstrated in patients receiving GnRH agonist alone over a similar 24-week interval.**

- Changes in bone density with the two "add-back" regimens were indistinguishable from the changes seen over 6 months in untreated, regularly cycling control subjects.

- Changes in bone density over time in normal cycling women as measured by serial dual-energy x-ray absorptiometry scans have not been previously reported.

- The effectiveness of lower doses of norethindrone has not been consistently found in preventing bone loss.

- Norethindrone doses of 5-to-10 mg/day retard osteoporotic change in postmenopausal women receiving no exogenous estrogens.

•The addition of sodium etidronate cycled with calcium carbonate to low-dose norethindrone appeared to prevent the bone loss seen with administration of agonist alone.

•Sodium etidronate is an organic bisphosphonate compound that acts at low doses to inhibit osteoclast-mediated bone resorption and has been successfully used in the management of Paget disease of bone.

•Although chronic continuous use may be associated with the development of osteomalacia, recent studies of short-term use (14 days) cycled with calcium carbonate (70 days) in doses similar to those in the current investigation have demonstrated prevention of bone loss and reduction of vertebral fractures in postmenopausal women treated for 2 years.

•The present investigation did not assess the effects of cyclic sodium etidronate and calcium alone on bone mass.

•The additional treatment group was not included in this study design given the extremely unlikely possibility that sodium etidronate would exert a beneficial effect on vasomotor symptoms induced by agonist therapy.

•Norethindrone exerts a potentially deleterious effect on circulating lipid profiles when chronically administered.

•Patients assigned to group II and receiving a 10-mg/day dose of this progestin experienced significant rises in LDL/HDL cholesterol over the course of therapy.

°This result was not found among patients receiving lower doses (group I).

•Although the clinical significance of these short-term lipoprotein changes has not been established, elimination of this effect with reduction in progestin dose is reassuring.]

---

60. Urodynamic measurements which respond to Kegel exercises in the successful treatment of stress urinary incontinence include

    1. maximal cystometric capacity
    2. urethral functional length
    3. Q-tip test
    4. urethral closure pressure

---

p. 285   Ans: D   (Elia G, Bergman A. Pelvic muscle exercises: When do they work? Obstet Gynecol 1993; 81:283)

60. [F & I: •Background: Urinary incontinence affects more than half of the elderly female population.

•Increasing attention has been directed toward the quality of life in the older population, and urinary incontinence has been defined as a condition that causes psychosocial impairment.

•Surgical therapy results in the highest cure rate in women with genuine stress urinary incontinence; in an elderly population, it may not be the treatment of choice.

•Surgical correction may also be a problem for young working women affected by genuine stress urinary incontinence because of the relatively long period of inactivity needed for postoperative recovery.

•Originally described by Kegel, pelvic muscle exercise has proved to be a method of conservative treatment of genuine stress urinary incontinence for women who cannot or wish not to undergo surgery for medical or social reasons.

•Objectives: To compare urodynamic and clinical findings before and after a program of pelvic muscle exercise to identify predictors of successful outcome.

- The International Continence Society defined urinary incontinence as "loss of urine that becomes a social or hygienic problem to the patient."

- By this definition, more than 55% of incontinent women did not consider themselves incontinent 3 months after finishing a bladder training program of Kegel exercise.

- Proper instruction in the Kegel exercise is a long and time-consuming process requiring a well-trained and devoted team.

- Brief verbal instruction leads to inadequate results.

- Women with severe stress incontinence respond less favorably to conservative treatment including Kegel exercise than do women with mild incontinence.

- Results: Kegel exercise results can be predicted with reasonable accuracy in women with either a mild or severe clinical manifestation of stress incontinence.

- Six of seven patients with mild incontinence responded favorably to Kegel exercise, whereas 13 of 15 women with severe stress incontinence did not.

- Static urodynamic measurements were unchanged by Kegel exercise.

- Bladder function tests, such as cystometry, and urethral function measurements, such as urethral functional length, were **unchanged** even when Kegel exercises resulted in good clinical outcome.

- Support to the bladder base (by the cotton swab test) was also **unchanged** by Kegel exercise.

- The only urodynamic indices **changed** by Kegel exercise were **abdominal pressure transmission to the proximal and middle urethra during stress and the urethral closure pressure**.

- Successful operations for stress urinary incontinence result in urodynamic change of the pressure transmission ratio between the bladder and urethra on cough, while all other static measurements remain unchanged.

- Kegel exercises, when successful, resulted in urodynamic changes similar to those following surgery; when the exercises were unsuccessful, no urodynamic index was significantly changed.

- In women with **mild** stress incontinence, Kegel exercise has a **reasonable chance** of being helpful.

- In those with **severe** stress urinary incontinence, it has **limited** benefit, although some patients may respond favorably.

- Although clinical assessment of severity of symptoms seems to be related to the urodynamic findings, it is a very subjective and limited index.

- Most women fall into the category of moderate stress urinary incontinence, which is subject to personal bias.

  ° In this group, clinical evaluation may have limited value in predicting who will respond favorably to Kegel exercise, and urodynamic evaluation may be beneficial.

  ° If abdominal pressure transmission to the urethra on cough is **80% or more**, these patients are likely to respond favorably to Kegel exercise, and it may be cost-effective to place them in a long training program.

- It is premature to conclude that patients with severe stress incontinence and/or a pressure transmission ratio of less than 80% should undergo surgery as the first line of treatment.

  » Recommendation: Every woman with stress incontinence should be offered a trial of Kegel exercise followed by reassessment of symptoms.]

61. A woman's sexuality is reflected by

1. multiplicity of orgasms
2. cyclicity of arousability
3. frequency of desire
4. coital frequency

p. 361   Ans: A   (Helstrom L, Lundberg P O, Sorbom D, Backstrom T. Sexuality after hysterectomy: A factor analysis of women's sexual lives before and after subtotal hysterectomy. Obstet Gynecol 1993; 81:357)

61. [F & I: •Background: Sexual functioning after hysterectomy has been evaluated together with psychiatric health.

•In studies in which patients were asked specifically whether their sexual relations had changed after hysterectomy, the incidence of diminished sexual functioning, usually measured as diminished sexual desire and frequency of sexual intercourse, varied from 38% to 10%.

•Uterine smooth-muscle contractions may be part of the female orgasm.

•Disturbance of the innervation of the uterus and upper vagina after total hysterectomy could result in disturbed sexual function, such as problems with lubrication and orgasm.

•A study comparing subtotal and total hysterectomy reported better libido and more frequent sexual activity in women who had undergone the less radical operation.

°More postoperative sequelae after total than after subtotal hysterectomy were reported, suggesting that the effect on the women's sexuality might result from the surgical technique.

•Objectives: To examine a group of women before and after subtotal hysterectomy to determine the effect of removal of the body of the uterus on subsequent sexuality.

•Underlying preoperative factors for sexuality to use as predictors or indices for postoperative sexuality were also assessed.

•Results: Half of the women answered "better" when asked about their postoperative sexuality and another 29% reported no change.

•This may reflect the success of the operation in giving these women a feeling of health and freedom from symptoms.

•The surgical method used also produced few postoperative sequelae.

•The finding that 21% experienced poorer sexuality after the operation corresponds to other findings in the literature.

•Only small changes in most indices of sexuality were found.

•With the use of latent factors, these changes could be evaluated more easily.

•Coital frequency, frequency of desire, cyclicity of arousability, and multiplicity of orgasm before the operation had the strongest relation to sexuality after surgery.

•**Coital frequency is partner-related and does not measure only the sexual interest of the woman herself.**

•Multiplicity of orgasm, cyclicity of arousability, and frequency of desire better reflect a woman's sexuality.

- Cyclicity of arousability shows that the woman is able to feel aroused and that she is also practicing sexual activity as "arousability" is defined as physical signs of being sexually aroused.

- The variables of preoperative cyclicity were interpreted as reflecting cyclicity in sexual activity induced by the bleeding pattern, and not only by hormonal changes.

- After the hysterectomy, a large number of women still described cyclicity in desire and arousability.

- Women who do feel desire for sex and are able to be sexually aroused despite the symptoms that lead to hysterectomy are more likely to remain sexually active after hysterectomy.

- This explains why these factors have a high correlation to postoperative sexuality.

- Many women reported variables that reflect the negative influence of the disease on sexuality before surgery.

- Women with less sexual interest or diminished coital frequency might be expected to improve after experiencing relief of symptoms, but neither deterioration nor improvement of sexuality were found in this group.

- It is surprising that occurrence of and relief from deep dyspareunia have a low relation to postoperative sexuality.

- The explanation might be that among women with sexual dysfunction and pain, there is a hidden group with a psychological vulnerability to psychosomatic disorders.

- Such a vulnerability might also result in a higher "risk" of being offered or demanding hysterectomy.

- Women were studied before and after subtotal hysterectomy.

- This procedure produces less frequent postoperative sequelae than total hysterectomy.

- Studying only women who underwent subtotal hysterectomy reduced the negative effects that these postoperative sequelae might have on sexuality.

- The results describe the importance of factors that can be generalized for all women.

- Relief from dyspareunia causes a positive change in the self-esteem and sexual feelings of many women.

- The importance of preoperative sexuality for predicting postoperative sexuality after hysterectomywas examined.

- Over the year of observation, single variables of sexuality did not change much, and neither did the profile of sexuality expressed as the latent factors.

- When counseling a woman before hysterectomy, it is appropriate to use the factors that indicate the latent factors as predictors of sexuality after surgery.

- These factors were frequency of intercourse, existence of cyclicity of desire, frequency of desire, and frequency and multiplicity of orgasm.]

62. The clearance rate of 17ß-estradiol is related to

   1. fat mass
   2. fitness
   3. recent food intake
   4. thermal stress

p. 584   Ans: E   (Clapp III J F, Capeless E L, Little K D. The effect of sustained exercise on follicular phase levels of 17ß-estradiol in recreational athletes. Am J Obstet Gynec 1993; 168:581)

62. [F & I: •Background: This study was designed to examine the possibility that acute changes in the circulating levels of 17ß-estradiol could be used as an indirect measure of the magnitude of the exercise-induced decrease in splanchnic blood flow.

•ß-estradiol and progesterone are rapidly cleared from the circulation by the liver, implying that their metabolic clearance rate may be flow dependent.

•Hepatic clearance of both ß-estradiol and progesterone is decreased by factors that reduce splanchnic blood flow (anesthesia, quiet standing, exercise) indicated that this was indeed the case.

•During sustained exercise circulating levels of both progesterone and ß-estradiol increase, with a greater increase at higher exercise intensities.

•During sustained exercise there is a redistribution of blood flow away from the splanchnic circulation to the exercising muscle and skin, with a resultant fall in splanchnic blood flow.

•The magnitude of the fall in splanchnic blood flow during exercise is directly proportional to the intensity of the exercise above the threshold level of 25% of maximal aerobic capacity ($\dot{V}O_2$max).

•A fall in splanchnic blood flow during exercise should produce a proportional fall in the hepatic clearance of ß-estradiol with a commensurate rise in its circulating level.

°During recreational exercise the magnitude of the increase in the circulating levels of ß-estradiol should be a valid index of both exercise intensity and the magnitude of the decrease in splanchnic blood flow.

•Results: Regularly cycling recreational athletes experience an intensity-dependent increase in the circulating levels of 17ß-estradiol during moderate duration, continuous, antigravitational exercise.

•The primary route of clearance for 17ß--estradiol in the human is hepatic, and, because it is virtually cleared in one pass by the liver in animal models, it is likely that its clearance is flow limited.

•Because exercise also produces an intensity-dependent decrease in splanchnic blood flow, it is probable that the magnitude of the exercise-induced increase in the circulating levels of 17ß-estradiol reflects the magnitude of the exercise-induced fall in splanchnic blood flow.

•The fact that similar changes in the level of cortisol were not observed also supports this interpretation.

•Because a much greater fraction of cortisol (89% vs 20%) is tightly bound to globulin, its hepatic uptake and clearance should not vary with fairly wide variations in splanchnic blood flow.

•The relationship between exercise intensity and endogenous levels of 17ß-estradiol was present over a wide range of intensities and levels.

•This relationship may provide a noninvasive estimate of changes in splanchnic blood flow in women during experimental perturbations other than exercise.

•The variability in the relationship indicates that it is undoubtedly influenced by a host of other variables, which include fat mass, volume of distribution, and training status, recent food intake, fitness, level of hydration, thermal stress, exercise type, and duration of exercise.

•Although pulses in 17ß-estradiol release did not appear to play a major role over this time interval, it is possible that endogenous hormonal production rates may also be influenced by these and other exercise variables.

•Indeed, this possibility has been recently used to explain the different responses seen in 17ß-estradiol and progesterone levels during exercise in fasting women and in women taking oral contraceptives.

•The exogenous infusion data clearly demonstrate that exercise decreases the metabolic clearance rate of 17ß-estradiol.

•Conclusions: Sustained exercise acutely increases the circulating levels of ovarian steroids and provide evidence that the magnitude of the increase is linearly related to exercise intensity.

•This is interpreted as primarily reflecting a flow-limited decrease in hepatic clearance caused by the exercise-induced decrease in splanchnic blood flow.

•Although the scatter in the data suggest that confounding variables are present, it appears that it may prove to be a useful tool for the noninvasive assessment of changes in splanchnic blood flow in women.]

---

63. Effective in decreasing complications in second trimester elective abortions

   1. antibiotic prophylaxis
   2. preoperative ultrasound
   3. laminaria tents
   4. intraoperative ultrasound

p. 636   Ans: E   (Jacot F R M, Poulin C, Bilodeau A P, Morin M, Moreau S, Gendron F, Mercier D. A five-year experience with second-trimester induced abortions: No increase in complication rate as compared to the first trimester. Am J Obstet Gynec 1993; 168:633)

63. [F & I: •Background: Large surveys done in the late 1970s found a several fold increase in the complication rate of second-trimester induced abortions when compared with that of first-trimester abortions.

•The risk of second-trimester abortions can be 11 times greater than the risk of first-trimester procedures.

•This risk was still increased to the fourfold range when concurrent sterilizations and saline solution or prostaglandin inductions of labor were excluded.

•The United States Centers for Disease Control also found a complication rate for second-trimester dilation-and-evacuation procedures three to four times greater than that for first-trimester suction curettages.

•Since then several large studies have shown very low complication rates for dilation and evacuation, but their diagnostic criteria have varied.

•None compare first and second-trimester complication rates in the same clinical setting, and few have a high rate of follow-up.

•Objectives: To report results comparing the complication rate of late second-trimester with first-trimester abortions, and describe the techniques used.

•Methods: Local anesthesia was used in all cases.

- Supplementary nitrous oxide inhalation (40% to 60% mixed with oxygen) was available and was used by most patients.

- The gases are delivered through a safety device that ensures a minimum 20% oxygen content and shuts off the flow if the oxygen supply fails.

- Nitrous oxide used this way induces mild conscious sedation and analgesia.

- Full general anesthesia is not desired or achieved.

- For supplementary analgesia, intravenous fentanyl, 50 to 100 ug, was also available for dilation and evacuation and was used in approximately half of those cases.

- Paracervical blocks consisted of 20 ml of 1% **lidocaine** to which 3 or 4 U of vasopressin was added.

- Constant support is offered by a sympathetic nurse.

- Preoperative cervical cultures for gonorrhea and Chlamydia were taken from all patients, usually on the same day as the surgery.

- Treatment for positive cases was begun as test results became available, 3 to 7 days later.

- Routine hemograms, blood typing, and pregnancy tests were performed, as were tests for rubella in nulliparous patients.

- Prophylactic doxycycline, 100 mg twice a day for 3 days, was given in all cases where cervical laminaria tents were used for >24 hours (gestational age ≥17 weeks) and in other cases when a history of pelvic inflammatory disease was elicited.

- Prophylactic amoxicillin was prescribed preoperatively when proved or strong suspicion of cardiac valvulopathy existed.

- Laminaria tents were used starting at 13 weeks' gestation; for 13 and 14 weeks a single large laminaria japonica was applied overnight; for 15 and 16-week gestations one or two synthetic dilator tents (Dilapan, Gynotec, Lebanon, NJ) were applied for 18 to 24 hours; for 17 to 20 weeks a single Dilapan was applied on day 1 and replaced by three to six Dilapan and japonica combinations on day 2, with surgery being performed on day 3.

- Preoperative ultrasonographic examinations were performed in all cases of ≥15 weeks' gestation and in earlier cases when the gestational age was doubtful.

- Results: The lower complication rate in later gestations was a surprising observation.

- Possible explanations include the routine use in this group of antibiotic prophylaxis, preoperative ultrasonography, and laminaria application and the smaller number of surgeons involved in dilation-and-evacuation cases.

- The dilation-and-evacuation technique has been refined since the 1970s.

- Authors have already shown the importance of local anesthesia, serial laminaria application, appropriate use of oxytocin and vasopressin, prophylactic antibiotics, and ultrasonography.

- The combined and systematic use of all these measures and the progressive incremental training of the surgeons result in even safer procedures.

- **Intraoperative ultrasonographic guidance**, used only occasionally, is recommended on a routine basis by some surgeons.

» Late induced abortions can be performed as safely as early ones.]

Obstetrics and Gynecology: Review 1994-Gynecology References

64. Inducers of cellular tissue factor activity include

   1. endotoxin
   2. interleukin-1
   3. tumor necrosis factor
   4. antiphospholipid antibodies

p. 207   Ans: E   (Branch D W, Rodgers G M. Induction of endothelial cell tissue factor activity by sera from patients with antiphospholipid syndrome: A possible mechanism of thrombosis. Am J Obstet Gynec 1993; 168:206)

64. [F & I: •Background: Patients with circulating antiphospholipid antibodies have a thrombotic predisposition that may result in intravascular thrombosis or fetal death resulting from placental insufficiency.

•The mechanism of the thrombotic predisposition is unknown.

•**Tissue factor,** a latent membrane lipoprotein of inducible cells, is the major initiator of coagulation in vivo.

°It is expressed in a variety of cells (e.g., endothelial cells, monocytes) after the cells are exposed to appropriate stimuli.

•Inducers of cellular tissue factor activity include endotoxin, interleukin-1, and tumor necrosis factor.

•Expression of tissue factor activity results in formation of a tissue factor-Factor VII complex on the cell surface, which activates Factor X.

•Activated Factor X converts prothrombin to thrombin, the major serine protease leading to fibrin formation and platelet activation.

•Objective: To investigate the possibility that antiphospholipid antibodies might induce the expression of tissue factor in human endothelial cells.

•The mechanism(s) of thrombosis and fetal death in patients with antiphospholipid antibodies is a matter of continuing controversy.

•Antiphospholipid antibodies may lead to thrombosis and fetal death by impairing vascular tissue prostacyclin production.

•Antiphospholipid antibodies do not impair prostacyclin production by perturbed or thrombin-stimulated human umbilical vein endothelial cells.

•Inhibition of vascular tissue prostacyclin production is a possible pathophysiologic mechanism because of the high frequency of fetal growth impairment and preeclampsia in the antiphospholipid syndrome.

•Both fetal growth impairment and preeclampsia are associated with impaired prostacyclin production.

•Antiphospholipid antibodies predispose to thrombosis and fetal loss by interfering with the activation of protein.

•Under normal circumstances, activated protein C exerts its antithrombotic effect primarily by inactivating Factors Va and VIIIa.

•Activation of protein C occurs on the endothelial cell surface and depends on the presence of thrombin and its endothelial cell receptor, thrombomodulin.

•Fact   °Detail   Page 108   »issue   *answer

- Phospholipids are important in the activation of protein C and antiphospholipid antibodies may interfere with the thrombin-thrombomodulin-protein C interaction by binding to endothelial cell membrane phospholipids.

- Lupus anticoagulant decreases or abolishes the protein C-mediated inactivation of activated Factor V.

- Unlike antiphospholipid syndrome, inherited protein C deficiency is **not** prominently associated with fetal growth retardation, preeclampsia, fetal death, or arterial thrombosis, suggesting that impaired activation or dysfunction of protein C is not an important pathophysiologic mechanism of antiphospholipid antibodies.

- Results: Antiphospholipid sera induce tissue factor activity in human endothelial cells and tissue factor induction activity resides, at least in part, in the IgG fraction of the antiphospholipid serum.

- Sera and IgG from patients with systemic lupus erythematosus stimulate the expression of endothelial cell procoagulant activity characteristic of tissue factor.

- Although half of antiphospholipid-negative systemic lupus erythematosus sera induced endothelial cell tissue factor expression, >90% of antiphospholipid-positive sera did so.

- The factor(s) responsible for the induction of tissue factor was, in part, heat sensitive.

- Induction or enhancement of endothelial cell tissue factor expression may be a mechanism by which antiphospholipid antibodies promote thrombosis in vivo in the systemic circulation.

  ° Tissue factor expression predisposes to thrombotic lesions of the venous and arterial circulation.

  ° Unlike the common inherited predispositions to thrombosis (e.g., antithrombin III deficiency, protein C deficiency, protein S deficiency), antiphospholipid antibodies are associated with both venous and arterial thrombotic episodes.

  ° The finding that antiphospholipid antibodies induce tissue factor expression correlates with the clinical observation that antiphospholipid antibodies are associated with thrombosis in both the venous and arterial systems.

- Tissue factor is richly expressed by placenta, suggesting that tissue factor affect placentation.

- The data indirectly support the hypothesis that induction of tissue factor by antiphospholipid antibodies initiate the thromboses and subsequent vascular damage in the spiral arterioles at the trophoblast-decidual interface.

- Actual tissue factor activity cannot be easily measured in vivo; investigation of this procoagulant property may provide information about the pathogenesis of antiphospholipid-induced thrombosis.

- The mechanism of antiphospholipid antibody induction of tissue factor activity is unknown.

- Tissue factor requires phospholipid interactions for function in the cell membrane, and tissue factor activity is enhanced by phosphatidylserine.

- One possibility is that antiphospholipid antibodies interact with tissue factor through adjacent phospholipids, enhancing (rather than inhibiting) the influence of the phospholipids on tissue factor activity.

- The time requirement of several hours for induction of tissue factor activity would support an antiphospholipid-induced increased tissue factor protein synthesis.

•Conclusion: Antiphospholipid sera enhance tissue factor expression by human umbilical vein endothelial cells, another possible mechanism by which antiphospholipid antibodies may cause thrombosis and fetal loss.]

---

65. The effects of triphasic contraceptive use on hemostasis include

   1. tissue plasminogen activity is increased
   2. changes in coagulation factors are balanced by changes in anticoagulation factors
   3. they may be protective in relation to atherosclerosis and myocardial infarction
   4. the progestogen modifies the estrogenic effects on hemostasis

p. 1255   Ans: A   (Notelovitz M, Kitchens C S, Khan F Y. Changes in coagulation and anticoagulation in women taking low-dose triphasic oral contraceptives: A controlled comparative 12-month clinical trial. Am J Obstet Gynec 1992; 167:1255)

65. [F & I: •Background: Minimization of risks for cardiovascular disease, including thromboembolic events, is a continuing concern in the use of oral contraceptives.

•Changes in the concentration of coagulation factors and the incidence of venous thromboembolism are primarily related to the estrogen component and are dose related.

•The low-dose oral contraceptives currently used carry less cardiovascular risk than previous higher-dose formulations.

   °There may be a cardioprotective effect associated with oral contraceptive use, particularly in relation to atherosclerosis and myocardial infarction.

   °Although there is no conclusive evidence that progestogens alone affect hemostatic parameters, the progestogen component of oral contraceptives does have a dose-related effect on arterial vascular disorders.

   °The progestogen component may modify the estrogenic effects of an oral contraceptive on hemostatic parameters.

•Objective: To evaluate the effects of two commonly used triphasic preparations, Triphasil (levonorgestrel plus ethinyl estradiol) and Ortho Novum 7/7/7 (norethindrone plus ethinyl estradiol) on both coagulation and anticoagulation factors.

•Studies evaluating the effect of sex steroids on hemostasis all have the same deficiencies.

•The factors measured are remote from the site of thrombosis; there are no known tests that reliably predict coagulation; some of the factors (e.g., factor XII) may initiate both coagulation and fibrinolysis; and the changes that occur may be statistically significant but, with few exceptions, the mean values do not exceed the reference laboratories' normal ranges.

   °Any hemostatic effect by these agents is theoretically doubtful.

•Given these limitations, the results of tests for coagulation and anticogulation factors in the current study indicated **no significant difference** between the levonorgestrel plus ethinyl estradiol and norethindrone plus ethinyl estradiol combination triphasic oral contraceptives.

•The progestogens in these oral contraceptives do not differ significantly in their effect on these factors, either by direct impact on hemostasis or by influencing estrogen's effects on hemostasis.

•Results: Do **not** support the suggestion that the progestogen modifies the effect of estrogen on hemostasis.

- Although both oral contraceptives induced changes in coagulation and anticoagulation factors (that were often statistically significant), mean values usually remained within normal reference ranges, with the exception of their effect on **plasminogen** activity.

- The prothrombin time is a clinical marker of activation of the **extrinsic** compartment of the coagulation cascade, because it reflects factor VII activity.

  ° Higher levels of factor VII and fibrinogen may be associated with an increased tendency to arterial disease and thrombosis.

  ° Mean prothrombin time levels **decreased** significantly for both oral contraceptive groups after 6 and 12 months.

  ° The clinical significance of changes in prothrombin time is questionable because the mean prothrombin time for the control group also was significantly decreased after 12 months and there were no statistically significant differences between the control and treatment groups.

  ° All values were within the laboratory range.

- The **partial thromboplastin time** is reflective of a more complex interaction of segments of the **intrinsic** system leading eventually to the activation of factor X.

- The partial thromboplastin time values for the control group remained constant, which suggests the validity of oral contraceptive-induced shortening of the partial thromboplastin time.

- These decreases also are consistent with the results of an earlier evaluation of contraceptives containing norethindrone; these findings need to be interpreted within the context of the wide biologic range of partial thromboplastin time function and the simultaneous changes in anticoagulation and fibrinolysis.

- For example, factor XII (which stimulates the intrinsic system) and fibrinogen antigen values increased significantly with both oral contraceptives; in contrast, factor XII activity decreased significantly in the control group.

- Factor XII stimulates fibrinolysis as well.

- **Fibrinogen** is the substrate that is converted by thrombin to fibrin and is increased in most (if not all) studies evaluating exogenous estrogen.

  ° Although an increased fibrinogen level is an epidemiologic risk for arterial disease and thrombosis it is important to differentiate endogenous evaluations in untreated subjects with exogenously stimulated values in response to oral contraceptives.

  ° The latter response is pharmacologically balanced by enhanced fibrinolysis.

- Decreases in **antithrombin III** are associated with estrogen use; the values for antithrombin III antigen and activity in this study generally remained unchanged.

- The unchanged antithrombin III activity levels in both oral contraceptive-treated groups are (theoretically at least) capable of inhibiting any increase in coagulability, as suggested by the partial thromboplastin time change.

- Prime actions among the actions of antithrombin III is inhibition factor Xa activity.

- Increases in concentration of other anticoagulation factors may also compensate for the increases in coagulation factors; for example, values for plasminogen activity increased significantly with both oral contraceptives.

- The increase in plasminogen activity is especially encouraging.

66. Treatments for an ovarian pregnancy include

1. ipsilateral oophorectomy
2. ovarian cystectomy
3. ovarian wedge resection
4. intramuscular methotrexate

p. 1307   Ans: E   (Shamma F N, Schwartz L B. Primary ovarian pregnancy successfully treated with methotrexate. Am J Obstet Gynec 1992; 167:1307)

66. [F & I: •Background: The incidence of primary ovarian pregnancy is one in 7,000 pregnancies, which is an increase from one in 25,000 to one in 40,000 pregnancies in the 1950s.

•Risks include a history of pelvic inflammatory disease, prior pelvic surgery, or use of an intrauterine contraceptive device or progestin-only minipill.

•Presenting symptoms are similar to those of tubal pregnancies.

•The Spiegelberg pathologic criteria for the diagnosis of ovarian pregnancy include: an intact ipsilateral tube separate from the ovary, a gestational sac occupying the position of the ovary, ovary and sac connected to the uterus by the uteroovarian ligament, and ovarian tissue histologically demonstrated in the sac wall.

•Conservative treatment is of paramount importance because these patients are usually young, healthy, and fertile and desire future childbearing.

•The treatment for an ovarian pregnancy was ipsilateral oophorectomy.

•Conservative ovarian surgery, such as cystectomy or wedge resection, at both laparotomy and laparoscopy has been successful.

•**Methotrexate** is a therapy for small, unruptured tubal pregnancies.

•Treatment with methotrexate should also be advantageous in preserving the ovary in patients with unruptured ovarian pregnancies.

°The limiting factor is that it is difficult to diagnose an ovarian pregnancy preoperatively, and the diagnosis is often retrospective.

•In this case not only was methotrexate an effective therapeutic intervention for a laparoscopically documented unruptured ovarian pregnancy, but its use also allowed avoidance of more interventional surgery, thereby preventing possible complications such as hemorrhage, ovariectomy, or subsequent pelvic adhesive disease.

•Conclusion: Single-dose intramuscular methotrexate is an effective therapeutic option in the management of the patient with an early unruptured ovarian pregnancy.]

67. Patients with Swyer syndrome have

   1. an XY karyotype
   2. female internal genitalia
   3. need to have gonadectomy
   4. the SRY gene preserved

p. 1802   Ans: E   (Tho S P T, Layman L C, Lanclos K D, Plouffe L, Byrd J R, McDonough P G. Absence of the testicular determining factor gene SRY in XX true hermaphrodites and presence of this locus in most subjects with gonadal dysgenesis caused by Y aneuploidy. Am J Obstet Gynec 1992; 167:1794)

67. [F & I: •Background: The best candidate for the testicular determining factor gene is located within a region that is 35 kilobases (kb) proximal to the Y pseudoautosomal boundary and is named SRY for sex-determining region on Y.

•The SRY gene is defined by the probe pY53.3, is located approximately 8 kb proximal to the Y pseudoautosomal boundary, and is conserved in mammals.

•The SRY gene encodes a testis-specific transcript.

•De novo mutation of SRY reported in two XY females with gonadal dysgenesis further supported that SRY is a testicular determining factor.

•A mouse 14 kb DNA fragment containing SRY introduced into mouse embryos was able to induce sex reversal in three of the 11 XX transgenic animals.

•When the same experiments were applied to the 25 kb human genomic DNA carrying SRY, no sex reversal occurred despite expression of the transgene into the mouse urogenital ridge at 11.5 to 12 days of development.

•Although the mouse *Sry* gene seems to fulfill the requirements for testicular determination, further analysis of the human SRY gene and studies of phenotype-genotype correlations in subjects with disorders of primary sexual differentiation are necessary to clarify the role of this regulatory gene in the cascade of gonadal differentiation.

•Objective: To determine if the testicular determining factor gene SRY is present in XX true hermaphrodites and in gonadal dysgenesis caused by Y aneuploidy.

•The SRY gene was examined in two groups of subjects: (1) XX true hermaphrodites known to be negative for Y DNA, including the previous testicular determining factor candidate gene ZFY, and (2) individuals with 45,X/46,XY gonadal dysgenesis who mostly have the Y DNA preserved, a large number of whom completely lack testicular development.

•Results: The absence of the SRY gene in all five 46,XX true hermaphrodites who were previously shown to be negative for the other Y-specific sequences.

•The same Y sequences were present in most 45,X/46,XY gonadal dysgenesis subjects, including the 10 individuals who completely lacked testicular development.

•The hypothesis of an abnormal X:Y interchange during paternal meiosis as the origin of XX maleness, has been confirmed in approximately 80% of XX males with the advent of molecular techniques.

•The high frequency of recombination in the pseudoautosomal region seems to predispose to unequal crossover and transfer.

•It appears that most 46,XX true hermaphrodites would harbor some Y DNA sequences or at least the ZFY or SRY sequences.

- All five XX true hermaphrodites failed to carry Y DNA, including the best testicular determining factor candidate, SRY.

- To date only three XX true hermaphrodites harbored Y DNA material.

- Absence of the SRY gene in most 46,XX true hermaphrodites further supports the speculation that multiple genes contribute to testicular morphogenesis.

- As for the Y DNA-negative XX males, testicular formation in XX true hermaphrodites may be caused by activation of a mechanism downstream in the pathway from the testicular determining factor gene leading to the first switch of Sertoli cell differentiation.

- Testis differentiation may also be caused by mutations of genes on the X chromosome or an autosome that may normally function together with Y-located sequences for testicular determination.

- The possible role of X genes in testicular determination is suggested by the observation of kindreds with X-linked forms of 46,XY gonadal dysgenesis.

- Cases of absence of Y sequences in 45,X mixed gonadal dysgenesis and integrity of Y DNA in a nonmosaic 46,XY subject with unilateral streak and contralateral testis would suggest that mosaicism alone cannot account for a complete or partial failure of testicular differentiation.

- Approximately 50% of individuals with 45,X/46,XY constitution develop dysgenetic testes instead of ovotestes and that approximately the remaining 50% harbored only bilateral streak gonads in spite of intact SRY.

- This study reports the preliminary data of a molecular screen for presence or absence of the SRY gene in the first largest series of subjects with gonadal dysgenesis caused by Y aneuploidy.

- Sequence analysis of the SRY gene in these subjects with different gonadal phenotypes should be the subsequent step to clarify the role of SRY in initiating human testicular differentiation.

- Most individuals with 46,XY gonadal dysgenesis or Swyer syndrome were found to have the SRY sequence preserved.

- These patients may have an inactive SRY gene or a mutation elsewhere in the pathway of gonadal differentiation.

- Two XY gonadal dysgenesis females were first reported as showing de novo mutations in the SRY gene.]

---

68. Polycystic ovarian susceptibility allele is

    1. linked to HLA antigen location
    2. recessive
    3. involved with the cytochrome P450 steroid 21 hydrolyase
    4. immunologic in etiology

p. 1805   Ans: A   (Ober C, Weil S, Steck T, Billstrand C, Levrant S, Barnes R. Increased risk for polycystic ovary syndrome associated with human leukocyte antigen DQA1*10501. Am J Obstet Gynec 1992; 167:1803)

68. [F & I: •Background: Although familial clustering of polycystic ovary syndrome is not uncommon, the underlying genetic cause is unknown.

- An increased frequency of human leukocyte antigen (HLA) DRw6 in 75 English patients with polycystic ovary syndrome as compared with 110 reference panel controls has been found.

°A link between polycystic ovary syndrome and human leukocyte antigens in 16 polycystic ovary syndrome families was not found.

•The development of polycystic ovary syndrome may be associated with human leukocyte antigen region loci that lie proximal to the HLA-DR loci on chromosome 6.

•Objective: To identify genes that confer susceptibility to polycystic ovary syndrome by examining HLA-DQAl alleles in a well-defined cohort of patients with polycystic ovary syndrome.

•This locus was chosen because it is proximal to the HLA-DR loci and because alleles at this locus have linkage disequilibrium with alleles at the cytochrome P450 steroid 21-hydroxylase and other class III loci.

°If there are other loci in this region that are involved in steroidogenesis and are associated with polycystic ovary syndrome, an association with HLA-DQAl alleles would be expected.

•Results: An association between HLA-DQA1*0501 and polycystic ovary syndrome was found.

•An earlier study reported an association between HLADRw6 and polycystic ovary syndrome (defined by menstrual disturbances and hyperandrogenism, including hirsutism, and ultrasonographically detected polycystic ovaries.)

•Because of linkage disequilibrium, HLA-DRw6 is commonly found on a chromosome (or haplotyype) with HLA-DQA1*0101, *0102 or *0103, whereas HLA-DQA1~0501 is commonly associated with HLADR3 or -DR5.

•The frequency of the HLA-DQA1*0101, *0102, and *0103 alleles was 0.26 in polycystic ovary syndrome as compared with 0.43 in control subiects.

•Associations with different HLA alleles in different polycystic ovary syndrome populations could reflect genetic heterogeneity.

°That is, polycystic ovary syndrome in the English study may be genetically distinct from the polycystic ovary syndrome described in this sample.

°That both studies found an association with alleles at closely linked loci suggests that this is unlikely.

•Two alternative explanations for these observations are possible.

°The first is that HLA-DQAI*0501 is on the same haplotype as DRw6 in subjects with polycystic ovary syndrome.

°It is not uncommon for linkage relationships between HLA loci to differ in disease as compared with normal families.

°A second possibility is that there is one polycystic ovary syndrome susceptibility allele on chromosome 6, but it is in linkage disequilibrium with different HLA haplotypes in the two samples.

°In the English sample the susceptibility allele is on a DRw6 haplotype, and in the this sample it is on a DQA1*0501 haplotype; this implies that recombination occurs between HLA-DR/DQ loci and the polycystic ovary syndrome susceptibility locus more commonly than it occurs between the HLA-DR and HLA-DQ loci.

°For example, alleles at the HLA-DP loci, which map centromeric to the HLA-DQ loci, show less striking linkage disequilibrium with alleles at the HLA-DR and HLA-DQ loci in population studies.

»Because polycystic ovary syndrome does not appear to have an immunologic cause, the susceptibility locus is not an HLA locus per se.

°Rather, it is likely that HLA alleles are merely markers for the susceptibility allele.

°Observation of increased homozygosity in subjects with polycystic ovary syndrome further suggests that the susceptibility allele is recessive.

°Genes involved in the regulation of steroidogenesis in addition to the cytochrome P450 steroid 21-hydrolyase genes may be located in this region.]

---

69. Markers of bone resorption include

    1. serum osteocalcin
    2. serum alkaline phosphatase
    3. urinary calcium excretion
    4. urinary hydroxyproline

---

p. 119   Ans: E   (Field C S, Ory J, Wahner H W, Herrmann R R, Judd H L, Riggs B L. Preventive effects of transdermal 17ß-estradiol on osteoporotic changes after surgical menopause: A two-year placebo-controlled trial. Am J Obstet Gynec 1993; 168:114)

69. [F & I: •Background: Estrogen deficiency related to menopause is associated with significant loss of bone mineral in the spine, femur, radius, and metacarpal.

•In postmenopausal women estrogen replacement therapy effectively protects and augments existing bone mass and reduces the incidence of fractures of the distal radius and hip.

•**Orally** administered estrogen, the most frequently used replacement therapy, can stimulate the synthesis of hepatic proteins and increase the circulating levels of hormone-binding globulins and renin substrate.

•This effect has been credited to first-pass hepatic metabolism of the large bolus of estrogen that is absorbed by the intestine and delivered to the liver after an oral dose.

•**Transdermal** administration of estrogen avoids this first-pass hepatic effect and delivers estradiol to the general venous circulation at a continuous rate.

•In addition, transdermal administration raises concentrations of estradiol to levels corresponding to those of women in the early to midfollicular phase of their menstrual cycles.

•Objective: To evaluate the effects of three dosages of transdermally administered 17ß-estradiol on markers of bone loss in women who had recently undergone surgical menopause.

•Methods: After screening, which included physical examination, mammography, chemistry studies with complete blood count, differential, and cholesterol levels, 127 women were stratified by age (40 to 49 years or >50 years old) and randomly assigned to one of three 17ß-estradiol groups (0.025, 0.05, or 0.1 mg/day) or to a placebo control group matched to each dosage strength of 17ß-estradiol.

•Results: Transdermally administered 17ß-estradiol is comparable to oral conjugated estrogen in preventing the accelerated phase of postmenopausal bone loss that occurs after menopause.

•At all treatment doses, transdermal 17ß-estradiol retarded bone loss compared with the placebo.

•The lowest dosage of 0.025 mg/day reduced, but did not prevent, bone loss in the lumbar spine, whereas a dosage of 0.05 mg/day maintained bone mass and a dosage of 0.01 mg/day significantly increased it.

•These effects occurred in a dose-dependent manner.

- **Thus a dosage of 0.05 mg/day appears to be the minimal effective dose in preventing bone loss from the lumbar spine, the common site of fractures resulting from postmenopausal osteoporosis.**

- This dosage maintains serum estradiol in the range found in premenopausal women in the follicular phase of the menstrual cycle and appears to be roughly equivalent to the dosage of oral equine estrogen of 0.625 mg/day, which is the minimal effective dosage of oral estrogen required to prevent postmenopausal bone loss.

- The gain in bone density of the lumbar spine at the two higher dosages of 0.05 and 0.1 mg/day was transient and occurred almost entirely in the first year of treatment.

  ° Thereafter bone density was maintained.

- When bone turnover is high, as in the immediate postmenopausal period, an antiresorptive agent such as estrogen will increase bone mass only until a new steady state is reached.

  ° At steady state the decrease in bone resorption is matched by a decrease in bone formation; thereafter, bone mass is maintained but not increased.

  ° Increases in bone density have previously been found in postmenopausal women after treatment with oral estrogen, but increases in bone density after estrogen treatment of oophorectomized women were found to occur only in those women who started therapy within 3 years of menopause, when bone turnover is the highest.

- The effects of transdermal estrogen on the lumbar spine, which is predominantly cancellous bone, were substantially better than those at the midradius, which is composed almost entirely of cortical bone.

- Cancellous bone has a much higher rate of bone turnover and is more responsive to hormonal changes.

- There was bone loss from the mid-radius at all three dosage levels of estradiol, although less than occurred in the placebo group.

- During the second year of treatment bone loss from the mid-radius was prevented, but it continued in the placebo group.

- Both higher dosages of 17ß-estradiol were more effective than the 0.025 mg/day dosage at the mid-radius, but in contrast to the lumbar spine, it was not dose-dependent.

- In the placebo group there was substantial bone loss from predominantly cancellous bone of the lumbar spine 6.4% over 2 years) and from the predominantly cortical bone of the appendicular skeleton (4.9% over 2 years).

- These findings differ sharply from those obtained in epidemiologic studies made in women monitored through natural menopause when such large accelerations were not seen.

- During natural menopause ovarian production of sex steroids may begin to decline several years earlier and may continue after cessation of menstrual periods.

- This decline would lead to a blunting of the induction of rapid bone loss observed here after acute induction of estrogen deficiency.

- Women who entered the study had undergone abdominal hysterectomy with bilateral oophorectomy and had not been deprived of estrogen for >6 months since the loss of ovarian function.

- **The major effect of estrogen administration in postmenopausal women is to reduce bone turnover; bone resorption decreases more than bone formation.**

- The results obtained with the biochemical markers used are consistent with this mechanism.

•Serum concentrations of bone Gla protein {osteocalcin} and bone alkaline phosphatase are biochemical markers of bone formation.

•Compared with results in the placebo group, values for these markers decreased in all three treatment groups.

•The decrease was more apparent at the end of the second year than at the end of the first year, consistent with a delayed fall in bone formation in response to the decrease in bone resorption.

•Decreases in urinary hydroxyproline excretion, an index of bone **resorption**, were larger at 1 year for the 0.05 mg/day 17ß-estradiol group and at 2 years for the 0.1 mg/day 17ß-estradiol group.

•Although the primary effect of estrogen in postmenopausal women is to decrease bone resorption, the smaller decreases in urinary hydroxyproline as compared with decreases in serum bone Gla protein alkaline phosphatase probably is the result of the relatively poor specificity of this marker.

•Similarly, there are no significant changes in urinary calcium excretion after either 1 or 2 years; this index reflects both calcium absorption and bone resorption and is a relatively insensitive marker for bone turnover.

•No major side effects were found during 2 years of treatment with transdermal 17ß-estradiol.

•Local patch application irritation occurred in about 10% of the two higher dosage regimens but was not a significant problem in the 0.025 mg/day or in the placebo groups.

•The follow-up periods and the number of subjects in this clinical trial were too low to make a general comparison of the long-term risks and benefits of transdermal 17ß-estradiol as compared with oral estrogen.]

---

70. Consistently present in the polycystic ovarian syndrome

   1. obesity
   2. hyperandrogenism
   3. hirsutism
   4. chronic anovulation

---

p. 1807   Ans: C   (Carmina E, Koyama T, Chang L, Stanczyk, Lobo R A. Does ethnicity influence the prevalence of adrenal hyperandrogenism and insulin resistance in polycystic ovary syndrome? Am J Obstet Gynec 1992; 167:1807)

70. [F & I: •Background: Polycystic ovary syndrome is extremely heterogeneous.

•Because of this diversity in clinical and biochemical findings, the syndrome might be aptly called the syndrome of hyperandrogenic chronic anovulation on the basis of findings of the two cardinal features: hyperandrogenism and chronic anovulation.

•In studies of pathogenesis, no unifying hypothesis has been accepted.

•Also, the presence of previously held characteristic features are no longer necessary for the diagnosis.

°nonhirsute patients with polycystic ovary syndrome-hyperandrogenic chronic anovulation have been studied, and obesity need not be present.

•Adrenal hyperandrogenism and insulin resistance may be involved in the pathogenesis.

•Objectives: To determine the prevalence of adrenal hyperandrogenism and insulin resistance in patients with hyperandrogenic chronic anovulation in patients living in three countries.

- Three different ethnic groups in three different geographic areas were chosen for study to determine if genetic or environmental factors influence the prevalence of adrenal androgen excess or insulin resistance.

- If the occurrence of adrenal androgen excess or insulin resistance was found to be different in the three groups considered to have hyperandrogenic chronic anovulation-polycystic ovary syndrome, then some question would arise as to the relevance of these features in the diagnosis of hyperandrogenic chronic anovulation-polycystic ovary syndrome or alternatively that what has been considered to be polycystic ovary syndrome may, in fact, constitute several different disorders.

- Known similarities in these groups of patients with hyperandrogenic chronic anovulation were LH, testosterone, and estradiol levels.

- That obesity and the prevalence of hirsutism is variable in polycystic ovary syndrome has been known for some time.

- Japanese women had significantly lower ideal body weight and were not characteristically obese.

° In spite of similar levels of LH and serum androgen, Japanese women were not hirsute.

- What determines the manifestation of hirsutism in polycystic ovary syndrome are peripheral factors, specifically 5α-reductase activity.

- In keeping with this, serum 3α-androstanediol glucuronide, a marker of skin 5α-reductase activity, was significantly lower in Japanese women and was elevated in North American and Italian women, where the prevalence of hirsutism in this study was 60% to 75%, respectively.

- The prevalence of elevated levels of DHEA sulfate in polycystic ovary syndrome is at least 50% in this population.

- Of significance was the finding that the levels of DHEA sulfate and the prevalence of this elevation among Japanese and Italian women with hyperandrogenic chronic anovulation was very similar to that of the group in the United States.

- Serum 11 ß-hydroxyandrostenedione is an excellent marker of adrenal androgen excess and may have more specificity for the adrenal gland than the measurement of DHEA sulfate.

- These measurements were also similar in the three groups and suggest that in spite of differences in weight, diet, and genetic and environmental factors, **the prevalence of adrenal androgen excess in hyperandrogenic chronic anovulation is fairly constant** and occurs in up to two thirds of patients.

- Although fasting insulin levels were lower in Japanese compared with North American and Italian women, **insulin resistance**, as defined by the insulin tolerance test, **was similar** in the three groups.

- The lower fasting insulin levels in Japanese women may be explained by their lower body mass; a highly significant correlation existed between fasting insulin and ideal body weight in all groups.

- Fasting insulin levels alone may not be able to diagnose insulin resistance in hyperandrogenic chronic anovulation.

- **Insulin resistance**, as defined by the insulin tolerance test, **occurred in approximately 70%** of all patients and was similar in these three ethnic groups.

- Insulin resistance may be central to the pathogenesis of polycystic ovary syndrome and appears to be a characteristic of all patients with this diagnosis.

- Although androgen, estrogen, and gonadotropin levels are similar in different ethnic groups, body mass and the presence of hirsutism need not be.

°Further, in spite of these differences, adrenal androgen excess is fairly uniform, occurring in at least 50% of patients and insulin resistance is a characteristic of the majority of women with hyperandrogenic chronic anovulation.]

71. Increased in the hirsutism-hyperandrogenism syndrome

1. LDL
2. triglycerides
3. DHEAS
4. HDL

p. 1816   Ans: A   (Wild R A, Alaupovic, Givens J R, Parker I J. Lipoprotein abnormalities in hirsute women: II. Compensatory responses of insulin resistance and dehydroepiandrosterone sulfate with obesity. Am J Obstet Gynec 1992; 167:1813)

71. [F & I: •Background: Women with hirsutism-hyperandrogenism are biologic experiments in nature that illustrate hormonal determinants of cardiovascular risk.

•They have **unfavorable** lipoprotein and apolipoprotein lipid profiles compared with normal women; these unfavorable profiles are apparent even when matched for body weight.

•Interventional studies with gonadal suppression have followed-up cross-sectional observational studies to determine that insulin resistance common in women with hirsutism/hyperandrogenism whether or not they are obese has more of an effect on apolipoprotein metabolism than does endogenous testosterone.

•Insulin resistance may be the body's compensatory response to weight gain.

•Dehydroepiandrosterone sulfate (DHEAS) secretion-action may be a compensatory ameloriative response to insulin resistance that is reflected in apolipoprotein profiles.

•Objective: To define the interrelationships between insulin, androgens, obesity and apolipoprotein metabolism.

•Results: Women with hirsutism-hyperandrogenism have lipoprotein lipid profiles characterized by low levels of high-density lipoprotein-cholesterol and higher triglycerides than are found in normal women, and they have higher cholesterol and low-density lipoprotein-cholesterol concentrations.

•Although high cholesterol, particularly low-density lipoprotein-cholesterol, is the most widely recognized lipoprotein lipid risk, there is increasing evidence that the combination of low levels of high-density lipoprotein-cholesterol and higher-than-normal triglycerides is an atherogenic profile that accounts for much premature coronary vascular disease not accounted for by elevated cholesterol.

•The combination of low levels of high-density lipoprotein-cholesterol and high triglycerides (whose metabolisms are intimately related) may well reflect the effect of insulin resistance on lipoprotein lipid metabolism.

•Women with hirsutism-hyperandrogenism have insulin resistance whether or not they are obese; because they have endogenous androgen, estrogen excess, and insulin resistance, they are biologic experiments in nature that illustrate hormonal determinants that may impinge on risk factors that influence vascular atherogenicity and hence coronary vascular disease.

•Lessons learned from their evaluation may give insight into why men and women differ with respect to incidence and severity of cardiovascular disease.

•Insulin resistance has a more profound influence on lipoprotein lipid metabolism in patients with hirsutism-hyperandrogenism than does endogenous androgen.

•Although women with hirsutism-hyperandrogenism have insulin resistance even when they are not obese, they are often troubled with problems of excess body weight.

- Obesity aggravates insulin resistance; for that reason the confounding effects of obesity as they impinge on lipoprotein lipid metabolism in women with hirsutism-hyperandrogenism have been difficult to study.

- Lipoprotein lipid metabolism is influenced by a host of factors, not the least of which are hormonal influence, dietary fat and fiber content, exercise, and genetics.

- When contrasted with normal women, those with hirsutism-hyperandrogenism according to body mass index, some fascinating insights developed.

- The working hypothesis is that the unbound testosterone/DHEAS ratio is an indicator of adrenal androgen production and is a reflection of the ameliorative effect of DHEAS on insulin resistance and ovarian androgen production and metabolism in women with hirsutism-hyperandrogenism.

- There was a graded response of lipoprotein lipid profiles according to degree of obesity in parallel with a graded degree of insulin resistance.

- Interestingly, DHEAS (a reflection of adrenal androgen secretion) correlated negatively with fasting insulin (an indicator of insulin resistance) in the women with hirsutism-hyperandrogenism, reaching statistical significance in those who were most obese.

- When the unbound testosterone/DHEAS ratios are compared in those with body mass indexes 28 to 37 versus body mass indexes 37 to 61, as expected, greater ratios were seen in those most obese.

  ° The incremental increase was not as great as expected.

  » This is because of the effect of **adrenal DHEAS that may well improve insulin sensitivity**.

- The effect of insulin resistance is reflected at the site of the ovary by increased testosterone secretion from the stromal compartment and at the site of the liver, as reflected in lower sex hormone-binding globulin concentrations, which in turn affect androgen metabolic clearance.

  ° There is in vitro and in vivo evidence that DHEA improves insulin sensitivity in women with hyperandrogenism.

- There is some evidence that insulin inhibits adrenal 17,20-lyase activity and possibly augments tissue 5α–reductase activity.

  » Insulin resistance may be from one or more genetic defects (possibly the myriad of altered molecular mechanisms leading to insulin resistance may be evolutionary for the same reason), but it might also be a compensatory response of the body to weight gain.

  ° When the body is exposed to excess energy sources, the effects of insulin can be quite deleterious.

  ° Adrenal DHEAS production may be a response to the ravages of the effects of insulin resistance.

- Hyperinsulinemia reflects insulin resistance, and insulin resistance and its modulators are focal to the demonstrated lipoprotein lipid abnormalities.]

72. GnRH agonists are clinically useful in the treatment of

   1. endometriosis
   2. fibroids
   3. menorrhagia
   4. premenstrual syndrome

p. 104   Ans: E   (Leather A T, Studd J W W, Watson N R, Holland E F N. The prevention of bone loss in young women treated with GnRH analogues with "add-back" estrogen therapy. Obstet Gynecol 1993; 81:104)

72. [F & I: •Background: The continuous administration of GnRH agonist analogues by multiple daily insufflations, daily subcutaneous injections, or monthly subcutaneous implants induces amenorrhea by creating a hypogonadotropic hypogonadism, which results in suppression of ovulation.

•This property is effective in the treatment of endometriosis, fibroids, menorrhagia, and premenstrual syndrome (PMS).

•The long-term use of GnRH analogues for these benign problems is limited by the development of a pseudomenopausal state with hot flushes, vaginal dryness, and bone demineralization.

•The data on bone demineralization due to use of GnRH analogues are variable, with some studies showing no loss and others reporting a rapid loss of up to 6% in vertebral bone with 6 months' use.

•The hypoestrogenic side effects disappear shortly after the drug is stopped, and the bone loss appears to be at least partially reversible within 6 months of treatment cessation.

°The subsequent resumption of a normal menstrual cycle is usually associated with a return of the original gynecologic symptoms.

•Estrogen replacement therapy (ERT) in the postmenopausal woman treats menopausal symptoms effectively and prevents the associated bone loss.

•The effect of ERT on the bone density of postmenopausal women may be dose-dependent, with low-dose oral treatments preventing any further loss and transdermal patches or subcutaneous implants replacing lost bone density.

•Objective: To determine whether the addition of a low dose of oral estrogens in young women using a depot implant GnRH analogue could prevent the loss of bone density.

•Methods: This was a 6-month double-blind, placebo-controlled study of 60 women randomly allocated to one of three treatment groups:

°1) placebo plus placebo—placebo depot implant every 4 weeks and placebo ERT tablets daily,

°2) Zoladex plus placebo—goserelin 3.6 mg depot implant every 4 weeks and placebo ERT tablets daily, and

°3) Zoladex plus ERT—goserelin 3.6 mg depot implant every 4 weeks and estradiol valerate 2 mg/day, with the addition of norethisterone 5 mg on days 22-to-28 of each 28-day cycle.

•Results: The use of a depot implant of goserelin monthly for 6 months is associated with loss of bone density from both the proximal femur and lumbar spine.

•This hypoestrogenic bone loss is preventable by "add-back" estrogen therapy given concurrently over the same period.

•The low dose of estrogen used, thought to be the minimum required to prevent postmenopausal bone loss, was sufficient to prevent the GnRH analogue-induced loss.

- The concept of "add-back" therapy is promising because it may permit GnRH analogues to be used for a longer period than the presently accepted limit of 6 months.

- Progestogens have been used to prevent postmenopausal bone loss, but their effect on bone density and on the relief of menopausal symptoms is generally considered to be inferior to that of estrogen.

- Whether estrogen "add-back" will limit the effectiveness of GnRH analogues in the treatment of benign gynecologic conditions remains to be fully evaluated.

- The women in this study all had PMS, and those in the active ERT group who completed the study were satisfied with the treatment.

- There was a considerable dropout rate, which is partly explained by the difficulties in performing research in patients with PMS.

  ° The cyclic progestogen given with ERT to prevent endometrial hyperplasia in postmenopausal women causes problems with compliance because of mood swings, irritability, bloatedness, and breast tenderness, symptoms similar to those of PMS.

  ° These side effects may also partly explain the dropouts in the group taking active ERT.

- Although the use of estrogen "add-back" resulted in no net loss of bone over the 6 months of the study, three women still lost a significant amount of bone density (greater than twice the measured precision).

» It would be wise to perform bone density scans serially in women receiving long-term GnRH analogues and "add-back" estrogen therapy to identify the group that still loses bone density on this treatment.

- The problems of compliance with "add-back" estrogen therapy and progestogenic side effects may be reduced by using continuous combined low-dose estrogens and progestogens daily or the new gonadomimetic tibolone (Livial; Organon Laboratories, Cambridge, UK).

  ° These preparations should prevent withdrawal bleeding, and the symptomatic problems associated with the use of cyclic progestogens.]

REPRODUCTIVE ENDOCRINOLOGY

Directions: Each of the questions or incomplete statements below is followed by several suggested answers or completions. Select the BEST answer in each case.

1. What is the lowest motile sperm count from which success can be expected using hMG/IUI therapy?

   A. 1 million.
   B. 5 million.
   C. 10 million.
   D. 15 million.
   E. 20 million.

2. True statements about relaxin include

   A. elevated levels in the first trimester are a risk for preterm labor.
   B. hCG depressed relaxin secretion.
   C. it is necessary for spontaneous labor.
   D. it maintains uterine quiescence during pregnancy.
   E. there is diurnal variation in its secretion during pregnancy.

3. The "clomiphene challenge test" involves serial determinations of

   A. basal body temperature.
   B. serum 17-hydroxyprogesterone.
   C. serum estradiol.
   D. serum FSH.
   E. serum progesterone.

4. A patient who has experienced three consecutive spontaneous abortions with the same partner is to be treated with intradermal injection of 100 million irradiated paternal mononuclear cells. What result can be expected?

   A. Increased incidence of congenital anomalies.
   B. Increased incidence of twins.
   C. Pregnancy with small for gestational age infant.
   D. Spontaneous abortion.
   E. None of the above.

5. A patient who regularly smokes two packs of cigarettes per day is to be placed on estrogen replacement therapy. Considering serum levels of both estrogen and progestogen in such a patient compared to a nonsmoker, the replacement amount of

   A. estrogen and progestogen should be about the same as in a nonsmoking patient.
   B. estrogen and progestogen should be greater.
   C. estrogen should be greater; progestogen should be less.
   D. estrogen should be less; progestogen should be greater.
   E. estrogen and progestogen should be less.

6. The spontaneous abortion rate in donor insemination is likely to be highest in those cases where there is

   A. ejaculatory failure.
   B. genetic indication to use a donor.
   C. male infertility.
   D. male subfertility.
   E. reversed vasectomy.

7. Results to be expected from a 10-day course of naltrexone in obese women with polycystic ovarian syndrome include a **reduction** of serum

   A. androstenedione.
   B. DHEAS.
   C. FSH/LH.
   D. response to GnRH.
   E. testosterone.

8. In a population **not** predisposed to abnormal auto-immune function, IgA antibodies against phospholipids and histones are related to

   A. age.
   B. gravidity.
   C. history of fetal loss.
   D. life-style.
   E. marital status.

9. The major chorionic gonadotrophin component of early pregnancy found in urine is

   A. beta core.
   B. free α.
   C. free ß.
   D. nicked hCG.
   E. non-nicked hCG.

10. The condition most likely to require laparoscopic (vs transvaginal) oocyte retrieval for in vitro fertilization is

    A. male factor infertility.
    B. mild endometriosis.
    C. pelvic inflammatory disease.
    D. previous tubal ligation.
    E. unexplained fertility.

11. The immediate management of a patient undergoing ovulation induction with hMG and hCG who experiences the hyperstimulation syndrome manifested by enlarged ovaries, ascites and evidence of hemoconcentration is

    A. anticoagulation
    B. diuretics
    C. fluid restriction
    D. paracentesis
    E. salt restriction

12. A patient who is 10 weeks pregnant presents with a history of pulmonary embolism in her last pregnancy. Heparin prophylaxis is to be considered. The maximum effect of subcutaneous heparin is obtained how many hours after administration?

    A. ½-1
    B. 2-3
    C. 4
    D. 6
    E. 8

13. The majority of recurrent pregnancy losses are caused by

    A. anatomical factors
    B. endocrine disorder
    C. immunologic disorders
    D. infection
    E. none of the above

14. Which of the following is the best predictor of the ability of spermatozoa to bind to zona pellucida?

    A. sperm concentration
    B. sperm linearity
    C. sperm mobility
    D. sperm morphologic pattern
    E. sperm velocity

15. The addition of the IgG fraction derived from plasma containing antiphospholipid antibodies to normal placental tissue will produce

    A. a decrease in prostacyclin
    B. a decrease in thromboxane
    C. an increase in prostacyclin
    D. an increase in thromboxane
    E. no change in either prostacyclin or thromboxane because the placental doesn't respond to antiphospholipid antibodies

Directions: Each set of lettered headings below is followed by a list of numbered words or phrases. For each numbered word or phrase select:

A. if the item is associated with *(A) only*
B. if the item is associated with *(B) only*
C. if item is associated with *both (A) and (B)*
D. if item is associated with *neither (A) nor (B)*

Items 16-18.

In the treatment of endometriosis:

   A. danazol (800 mg BID) x 6 months.
   B. leuprolide (3.75 mg IM monthly) x 6 months.
   C. both
   D. neither

16. androgenic side effects.

17. increase in serum total cholesterol.

18. skin rash.

Items 19-21.

A. endometrium
B. breast epithelial cells
C. both
D. neither

19. unopposed estrogen enhances development of cancer

20. estrogen receptor declines during the luteal phase

21. progesterone receptor levels content are the same throughout cycle

---

Directions: For each of the questions or incomplete statements below, ONE or MORE of the answers or completions given is correct. In each case select:

A. if only 1, 2, and 3 are correct
B. if only 1 and 3 are correct
C. if only 2 and 4 are correct
D. if only 4 is correct
E. if all are correct

22. True statements about male fertility include

   1. Fertilization can occur in sperm without motility.
   2. Fertilization can occur in a seminal fluid specimen with less than 10% normal forms.
   3. Sperm with abnormal shapes have a normal genetic constitution.
   4. Under zona insemination results in unacceptable rates of polyspermy.

23. Operative in the pathophysiology of infertility caused by *Chlamydia trachomatis*

   1. induction of male antisperm antibodies.
   2. induction of female antisperm antibodies.
   3. inflammation of endometrium.
   4. direct embryotoxic effects.

24. True statements about the use of GnRH agonists during pregnancy include

   1. There are no known teratogenic effects on humans.
   2. Theoretically it could interfere with placental estrogen synthesis.
   3. GnRH is not found in the embryonic hypothalamus until 10 weeks of gestation.
   4. In the third trimester GnRH is present in high concentration in the placenta.

25. A patient with hyperandrogenic oligoamenorrhea is thought to have late onset adrenal hyperplasia. She is given a short-term ACTH stimulation test and subsequent 17-hydroxypregnenolone and DHEA levels were found to be twice normal levels. This is most likely due to

   1. increased activity of 17-hydroxylase.
   2. increased activity of 17,20-desmolase.
   3. 21-hydroxylase deficiency.
   4. 3ß-hydroxysteroid dehydrogenase deficiency.

26. Causes of reproductive failure in patients with mild to moderate endometriosis include

   1. oligo-ovulation
   2. luteal phase defect
   3. luteinized unruptured follicle
   4. aseptic peritonitis

27. Advantages of leuprolide over danazol for the treatment of endometriosis include

   1. more rapid onset
   2. less irregular bleeding
   3. more complete ovarian suppression
   4. decreases the disease process to a greater extent

REPRODUCTIVE ENDOCRINOLOGY REFERENCES

Directions: Each of the questions or incomplete statements below is followed by several suggested answers or completions. Select the BEST answer in each case.

1. What is the lowest motile sperm count from which success can be expected using hMG/IUI therapy?

   *A. 1 million.
   B. 5 million.
   C. 10 million.
   D. 15 million.
   E. 20 million.

p.784 (Nulsen J C, Walsh S, Dumez S, Metzger D A. A randomized and longitudinal study of human menopausal gonadotropin with intrauterine insemination in the treatment of infertility. Obstet Gynecol 1993; 82:780)

1. [F & I: •Background: Controlled ovarian hyperstimulation with human menopausal gonadotropin (hMG) and intrauterine insemination (IUI) has been advocated as an effective method of treating subfertile couples with patent fallopian tubes and presumably normal ovulatory function when more traditional therapy has failed.

•This treatment is used for male factor infertility, cervical factor infertility, unexplained infertility, and endometriosis.

•Cycle fecundity rates of approximately 13, 25, and 13% for male factor infertility, idiopathic infertility, and endometriosis, respectively, when controlled ovarian hyperstimulation was used.

•This compares with a cycle fecundity of approximately 5% with IUI alone.

•Evaluation of the efficacy of this technique is circumspect because studies addressing this treatment have been retrospective in nature.

•Retrospective studies have many inherent weaknesses, including heterogeneity of the treatment and control groups with respect to factors such as diagnosis, age, duration of infertility, and prior treatment.

•This heterogeneity brings into question the validity of the conclusions drawn from these studies.

•Objective: To evaluate in a randomized and longitudinal fashion the efficacy of controlled ovarian hyperstimulation combined with IUI versus well-timed IUI alone in the treatment of various causes of infertility in the presence of normal ovulation.

•Controlled ovarian hyperstimulation with IUI is advocated as an effective but untested method of treating subfertile couples with patent fallopian tubes and presumably normal ovulatory function when more traditional therapy has failed.

•Theoretical reasons for enhanced fertility include an increased density of motile sperm in the upper reproductive tract, an increased number of fertilizable oocytes, and correction of occult ovulatory dysfunction.

•The majority of studies supporting this method have been retrospective in nature.

•Ideally, the study design would have randomized patients to one of the two treatment modalities for the entire duration of the study.

•Previous attempts at such a study design were unsuccessful because of the subjects' unwillingness to receive a single treatment modality for the duration of the study that they perceived to be relatively ineffective (i.e., IUI alone).

- For this reason, the alternating treatment design was used and the results were analyzed in two steps: first by considering results for the initial randomized cycle alone and second by using modeling techniques to isolate the effect of hMG over time.

- IUI was combined with controlled ovarian hyperstimulation because retrospective work has found enhanced cycle fecundity with hMG/IUI versus hMG alone.

- During the initial cycle following randomization to the two treatment groups, hMG/IUI therapy was found to be significantly more effective than IUI alone when all diagnostic groups were combined.

- For the first treatment cycle alone, no comment can be made regarding the efficacy of hMG/IUI therapy within each individual diagnostic group because of relatively small numbers.

- When the couples were followed longitudinally as they alternated between treatment groups, and as the cycle numbers within individual diagnostic groups accumulated, the efficacy of hMG/IUI became apparent.

- For individuals with the diagnosis of endometriosis, hMG/IUI therapy was more effective than IUI alone.

- The results remained the same for minimal, mild, and moderate stages of disease.

- The observed cycle fecundity of 11.8% may be somewhat lower than that observed in individuals with the sole diagnosis of endometriosis, as 19% (11 of 57) of the couples included in this diagnostic group also had male factor contributing to their infertility.

- The average duration between surgical intervention and enrollment was 14 months.

- Thus, the majority of these patients were surgical treatment failures.

- There was an inadequate number of subjects enrolled to evaluate the efficacy of hMG/IUI therapy in the treatment of individuals with **severe** endometriosis.

- The efficacy of this treatment would be limited if significant pelvic adhesive disease were present.

- In the case of male factor infertility, hMG/IUI therapy appeared to be more effective than IUI alone, but these results only approached statistical significance.

- This result may constitute a type II error.

- The current result of a 13.0% cycle fecundity is similar to the retrospective studies, which found a cycle fecundity of 8-to-15%.

- There is a direct association between the number of motile sperm in the insemination and subsequent cycle fecundity.

- **hMG/IUI therapy is ineffective if the total motile sperm count per insemination is less than one million.**

- The effectiveness of this treatment for total motile sperm counts ranging between one and five million is less clear.

- With total motile counts greater than five million, cycle fecundity rates appeared to approach or exceed those observed with endometriosis and unexplained infertility.

- For unexplained infertility, hMG/IUI therapy was significantly more effective than IUI alone.

- These prospective data confirm previous retrospective data showing cycle fecundities with hMG ranging from 15-to-33%.

Obstetrics and Gynecology:Review 1994-Reproductive Endocrinology References

- With regard to "other" diagnoses, there was no significant enhancement in cycle fecundity.

  ° This group was not homogeneous, with pelvic factor being disproportionately represented relative to cervical factor.

  ° Further studies are needed to evaluate the role of hMG/IUI in the treatment of these two diagnoses, although retrospective studies have clearly suggested a role for hMG/IUI in the treatment of cervical factor infertility.

- A frequent criticism of hMG/IUI therapy is the increased risk of **multiple births**.

- The multiple-gestation rate observed in the present investigation was 16.7%, which is somewhat less than that observed for individuals undergoing in vitro fertilization (IVF) and similar to previous studies using hMG/IUI.

- This rate is higher than that observed in the general population.

- All multiple gestations were twins.

- Although multiple gestation remains a significant risk of hMG/IUI therapy, the availability of selective reduction provides an effective treatment modality for those couples who elect this option.

- A second frequent criticism of hMG/IUI therapy has been the risks associated with this procedure.

- In the current investigation, no patient experienced severe **ovarian hyperstimulation syndrome**, and there were no clinically detected cases of pelvic infection secondary to IUI.

- There were no hospitalizations due to adverse sequelae of hMG/IUI therapy.

- It remains to be determined in a large, randomized study how hMG/IUI therapy compares with assisted reproduction technologies such as IVF and gamete intrafallopian transfer (GIFT).

- The cycle fecundity rates achieved are similar to those achieved with IVF, though perhaps somewhat less than those achieved with GIFT.

- In principle, hMG/IUI therapy is similar to GIFT in that multiple gametes are introduced into the fallopian tubes.

- In the case of hMG/IUI, this occurs by IUI and natural retrieval of the oocytes by the fallopian tubes.

- In contrast, GIFT requires mechanical retrieval of eggs and surgical placement of the gametes into the fallopian tube.

- Considering the expense and risks associated with IVF and GIFT relative to hMG/IUI, a trial of hMG/IUI may be warranted before proceeding with the assisted reproduction technologies.

- What number of cycles of hMG/IUI determines an adequate trial cannot be answered conclusively.

- It appears that cycle fecundity remains relatively constant for the first five cycles and then declines.

- The number of individuals completing more than six cycles was relatively small, and the data must be interpreted with caution.

- In a similar retrospective analysis, 94% of the pregnancies occurred in the first four attempts; cycle fecundity rates dropped by 50% after completion of the first four cycles.

- It appears reasonable to restrict a trial of hMG/IUI therapy to four or five cycles, with the understanding that pregnancies may well be achieved with attempts in excess of four, but at a significantly lower success rate.]

•Fact   °Detail   »issue   *answer

2. True statements about relaxin include

   *A. elevated levels in the first trimester are a risk for preterm labor.
   B. hCG depressed relaxin secretion.
   C. it is necessary for spontaneous labor.
   D. it maintains uterine quiescence during pregnancy.
   E. there is diurnal variation in its secretion during pregnancy.

p. 827 (Weiss G, Goldsmith L T, Sachdec R, Von Hagen S, Lederer K. Elevated first-trimester serum relaxin concentrations in pregnant women following ovarian stimulation predict prematurity risk and preterm delivery. Obstet Gynecol 1993; 82:821)

2. [F & I: •Background: Relaxin, a peptide hormone, is detected in the peripheral circulation during pregnancy in an extensive number of mammalian species.

•Its major biologic action in mammals is **remodeling of the connective tissue** of the reproductive tract, allowing accommodation of the pregnancy and successful parturition.

•In women, relaxin is the best-characterized peptide hormone produced by the corpus luteum.

•The recent elucidation of the primary structure of human relaxin and the advent of sensitive assays for quantitation of the human hormone have allowed detailed characterization of the secretion pattern of this peptide hormone in women.

•Although the specific role of relaxin during human pregnancy is not precisely known, purified porcine relaxin administered to women either intravaginally or intracervically can advance cervical softening, effacement, and dilation and can decrease the time to delivery.

•Two conditions are associated with **increased** peripheral relaxin concentrations in women: **multiple gestation and ovarian stimulation**.

•Stimulation of ovarian follicular development with exogenous gonadotropin therapy is being performed in an increasing number of women to enhance fertility.

°For example, this therapy is now widely used to induce ovulation in anovulatory women and to synchronize follicular development as part of in vitro fertilization (IVF) protocols.

•Levels of circulating relaxin are higher in singleton pregnancies resulting from ovulation induction with exogenous gonadotropins than in spontaneous singleton pregnancies.

•Ovulation induction leads to the formation of multiple corpora lutea, which may lead to increased peripheral relaxin concentrations.

•Circulating relaxin levels are higher in multiple pregnancies and following IVF.

•Women who undergo IVF and those pregnant after ovarian hyperstimulation have an increased incidence of preterm delivery.

•Because relaxin can soften and ripen the human cervix and because conditions that are associated with hyperrelaxinemia (such as ovarian stimulation for ovulation induction) result in a greater incidence of prematurity, it was hypothesized that the hyperrelaxinemia caused by ovarian stimulation would result in an increased rate of premature labor or preterm delivery.

•It was further hypothesized that the increased relaxin levels resulting from ovarian stimulation would be detectable in the first trimester and would correlate with prematurity.

•Objective: To test these hypotheses by studying patients who achieved pregnancy after undergoing ovarian stimulation.

Obstetrics and Gynecology: Review 1994-Reproductive Endocrinology References

- Pregnancy outcome in women who had undergone ovarian stimulation and had elevated first-trimester peripheral relaxin concentrations was compared to pregnancy outcome in stimulated women who had normal first trimester peripheral relaxin concentrations.

- Results: Women who have highly elevated circulating relaxin concentrations in the first trimester are at **increased** risk for prematurity.

- This increased risk is in addition to any greater risk due to increased fetal number.

- This is the first direct association between prematurity and relaxin as an independent variable.

- Relaxin levels during early pregnancy can predict pregnancy outcome.

- Relaxin is a structural analogue of insulin, containing an A and B chain connected by inter-chain disulfide bridges.

- The gene for human relaxin resides on the **ninth** chromosome.

- Relaxin is present in the circulation throughout pregnancy, starting in the late luteal phase.

- Serum concentrations are highest during the first trimester.

- Levels at 6 and 12 weeks are similar.

- During this time, levels rise and fall by roughly 20%.

- After 12 weeks of pregnancy, the levels remain constant throughout the remainder of pregnancy.

- Although there is marked variability in concentrations between women, levels in a single individual tend to be fairly stable.

- There are no diurnal secretion patterns, pulsatility, or minute-to-minute variations in levels.

- Thus, first-trimester relaxin concentrations reflect the concentrations throughout pregnancy.

- The role of relaxin in human pregnancy has not been well established.

- Though relaxin is obligatory for cervical dilation and normal parturition in pigs and rats, it is **not essential in women**.

- Women who become pregnant using egg donation are aluteal and have no detectable circulating relaxin.

- Aluteal women without circulating relaxin do go into spontaneous labor, and their cervices dilate.

- Relaxin causes significant connective tissue changes in various mammalian species in vivo.

- Relaxin decreases incorporation of radiolabeled proline, an index of collagen synthesis, into cervical tissue.

- In human dermal fibroblasts, relaxin causes significant collagen turnover both by stimulating collagenase expression and by modulating collagen synthesis.

- Purified porcine relaxin administered either intravaginally or intracervically to women can advance cervical softening, effacement, and dilation and can speed delivery.

- These observations suggest that relaxin can contribute to cervical alterations that prepare for cervical dilation and delivery.

- Though relaxin is effective in reducing the amplitude of spontaneous and induced contractions in pig and rat myometrium, the effects of relaxin on human myometrium are not as clear.

- There is a lack of substantive effect of relaxin on strips of human myometrium obtained from pregnant uteri.

  ° This may be due to either an inherent unresponsiveness of pregnant human myometrium to relaxin or an already maximal effect of relaxin from intrauterine sources.

- Ovarian stimulation results in multiple simultaneous ovulations.

- The multiple corpora lutea thus formed can provide a greater mass of relaxin-secreting tissue, which may result in higher circulating relaxin concentrations.

- Multiple gestations can also result from ovarian stimulation.

- Multiple gestations produce higher circulating concentrations of hCG, a substance that **stimulates** relaxin secretion.

- In multiple gestations resulting from ovarian stimulation, hyperrelaxinemia probably results from both the increased mass of relaxin-secreting luteal tissue and the higher concentrations of the relaxin-secretion stimulant, hCG.

- Because relaxin can alter cervical connective tissue, it is likely that there is an association between hyperrelaxinemia and prematurity.

- The clinical usefulness of relaxin measurement during early pregnancy in women who conceive after spontaneous ovulation remains to be established.

- In women who become pregnant after ovarian stimulation, first-trimester hyperrelaxinemia identifies a group of high-risk women who can be monitored more closely to detect and potentially treat early cervical dilation of premature labor, perhaps with cervical cerclage.

- The mechanism of maintenance of uterine quiescence during human pregnancy and the causes of human labor are poorly understood.

- The present data suggest that relaxin may be one of the endogenous agents involved in this mechanism.

- The reasons that multiple human pregnancies deliver earlier than singleton pregnancies are likewise poorly understood.

- The increased relaxin concentrations resulting from the greater number of corpora lutea present in nonidentical multiple pregnancies may contribute to the earlier delivery of these pregnancies.

- Elevated relaxin levels can increase the risk of a poor outcome regardless of the number of fetuses.

- This increased risk appears to be additive to the elevated risk associated with greater fetal number.

- These results suggest that further understanding of the control of luteal secretion and function during pregnancy and of the relaxin receptor may lead to the development of new specific agents that may aid in the prevention of premature birth.]

3. The "clomiphene challenge test" involves serial determinations of

    A. basal body temperature.
    B. serum 17-hydroxyprogesterone.
    C. serum estradiol.
*D. serum FSH.
    E. serum progesterone.

---

p. 540 (Scott R T, Leonardi M R, Hofmann G E, Illions E H, Neal G S, Navot D. A prospective evaluation of clomiphene citrate challenge test screening of the general infertility population. Obstet Gynecol 1993; 82:539)

3. [F & I: •Background: The clomiphene citrate challenge test was described originally in 1987 as a means of assessing ovarian reserve.

•In the test's original description, women with elevated serum FSH concentrations either before or after administration of clomiphene citrate on cycle days 5-to-9 had diminished ovarian reserve.

•The diminished reserve was reflected by both a poorer response to ovulation induction with exogenous gonadotropins and lower long-term pregnancy rates.

•Some women with apparently normal ovulatory cycles have diminished ovarian reserve of a qualitative nature, which prevents them from conceiving.

•**The clomiphene citrate challenge test combines measurement of serum FSH levels** during the interval of recruitment in the early follicular phase (cycle day 3) and then 1 week later (cycle day 10) following 5 days of clomiphene citrate therapy (100 mg/day) given on cycle days 5-to-9.

•Patients with adequate ovarian function overcome the effects of the estrogen receptor blockade and suppress their FSH levels back into the normal range by cycle day 10.

•Because clomiphene citrate and its active metabolites persist far beyond cycle day 10, the postulated mechanism of the suppression is an increase in gonadal peptide production, such as inhibin, and/or an increase in circulating estradiol (E2) levels.

•Ultimately, the circulating FSH level on cycle day 10 reflects the endocrine feedback activity of the developing cohort of follicles, which appears to correlate well with both ovarian responsiveness and clinical outcome.

•The validity of the clomiphene citrate challenge test as a means of predicting ovarian function has been best studied in women attempting to conceive through assisted reproductive technologies.

•In these studies, women with abnormal tests responded poorly to ovulation induction with both production of fewer follicles and lower peak E2 levels.

•Subsequently, fewer oocytes and embryos were obtained, resulting in lower pregnancy rates.

•That the disorder related principally to oocyte quality was confirmed by finding that these patients achieved outstanding pregnancy rates through oocyte donation.

•Although the validity of clomiphene citrate challenge test screening in women planning to participate in assisted reproduction programs has been documented, those studies dealt with selected patient populations.

•The appropriate indications, if any, for screening the general infertility population have not been reported.

•Objective: To evaluate the use of clomiphene citrate challenge test screening in a totally unselected general infertility population.

- This long-term prospective study found that the clomiphene citrate challenge test predicts decreased pregnancy rates in women from a general infertility population.

- The pregnancy rates of women with abnormal results were reduced by approximately 80% compared to normal controls.

- These findings have a number of physiologic and clinical implications for women presenting for the evaluation of infertility.

- Direct extrapolation of the results of prior studies to the general infertility population is not straightforward.

- It was possible that an abnormal result reflected only that the overall cohort in any given cycle would respond poorly to ovulation induction with exogenous gonadotropins, or that the gametes would perform poorly within the nonphysiologic environment present during assisted reproduction cycles.

- Because circulating FSH levels on days 3 and 10 of a test cycle probably depend on the metabolic activity of more than one member of the developing cohort of follicles, it was possible that women with an abnormal clomiphene citrate challenge test could still produce a high-quality oocyte as a result of natural folliculogenesis.

- In fact, the results of this study indicate that these theoretical reservations were unfounded, and that an abnormal clomiphene citrate challenge test result predicts decreased pregnancy rates even outside assisted reproduction programs.

- This study was not designed to evaluate the mechanisms that lead to the decreased pregnancy rates in patients with abnormal tests.

- Nevertheless, given that circulating FSH levels reflect the metabolic activity of the developing cohort of follicles and that these patients respond poorly to controlled ovarian hyperstimulation, the most likely explanation is **diminished ovarian reserve with production of oocytes with poor reproductive potential**.

- That women could have significant qualitative differences in gamete production is not surprising.

- Analogous studies in the male have clearly shown that spermatozoa that appear equivalent at routine semen analysis may have dramatically different abilities to bind zonae (hemizona assay), produce fertilization (sperm penetration assay), or achieve pregnancies.

- Unfortunately, oocytes are not readily available for equivalent functional or qualitative evaluations without the use of costly and invasive techniques such as in vitro fertilization.

- The clomiphene citrate challenge test appears to provide an indirect and more practical means of assessing qualitative ovarian reserve.

- Perhaps the most significant finding of this study was the high prevalence of **unexplained infertility** in patients with abnormal clomiphene citrate challenge tests.

- In fact, half of the women with abnormal test results had no other explanation for their infertility.

- The association between unexplained infertility and abnormal tests was present in all age groups, and ranged from 29% in women 30-to-34 years of age to 50% in women over 40.

- Remarkably, both patients with abnormal clomiphene citrate challenge test results who were less than 30 years old had unexplained infertility.

- This suggests that diminished ovarian reserve may be a definable etiology for some patients previously considered to have unexplained infertility and that clomiphene citrate challenge test screening may be of particular value in this group.

- Clinical application of the results of this study will require the practicing clinician to decide who to screen, how to screen, and how to interpret the results from the laboratory.

- Because the test is relatively inexpensive and extremely safe, the decision regarding who to screen is based on where the greatest yield of positive results will be obtained.

- The incidence of abnormal tests in women less than 30 years of age was low (3%).

- The incidences of abnormal results in women who were 30-to-34, 35-to-39, and 40 years or greater were 7, 10, and 26%, respectively.

- These incidences are certainly in the range of a variety of disorders routinely screened for during general infertility evaluations.

» Women who are 30 years of age or older are routinely screened.

- Women with unexplained infertility are also screened, based on the high incidence of abnormal results within this subpopulation.

- Another issue relates to how best to perform the clomiphene citrate challenge test.

- It is interesting that only a single patient had an elevated FSH level on day 3, with a normal level found in the day-10 sample.

- The fact that the majority of women with abnormal results had elevated day-10 values and that only rarely was the day-3 value elevated in the absence of an elevation on day 10 are consistent with the central premise of the test.

- One could speculate that the endocrinologic activity of the developing cohort of follicles was able to maintain normal FSH concentrations in the early follicular phase, but was inadequate to overcome the antiestrogenic effects of the clomiphene citrate.

- Because screening with day-10 FSH concentrations alone would have detected 22 of the 23 abnormal patients, it is possible that day-10 screening alone might be adequate.

- This would have obvious advantages in reducing both cost and patient discomfort.

- Nevertheless, the literature reports a substantial number of patients who had abnormal basal day-3 FSH values with normal concentrations on day 10.

- Larger numbers of subjects must be screened before one can recommend that the day-3 sample be omitted.

- Having decided who and how to screen, the practicing clinician must make sure that he or she knows how to interpret the actual test results.

- Because of the large difference between the assay used in this study and those previously reported in the literature, extrapolation of results without reference to the specific assay and reference preparation is unwise.

- It is impractical to think that every laboratory could accumulate and evaluate a large enough clinical experience to define its own abnormal ranges.

- Before patient counseling or clinical application of the results, normal ranges should be compared by running the laboratory's assay in parallel with those reported in the literature.]

4. A patient who has experienced three consecutive spontaneous abortions with the same partner is to be treated with intradermal injection of 100 million irradiated paternal mononuclear cells. What result can be expected?

    A. Increased incidence of congenital anomalies.
*B. Increased incidence of twins.
    C. Pregnancy with small for gestational age infant.
    D. Spontaneous abortion.
    E. None of the above.

p. 651 (Aoki K, Kaijura S, Matsumoto Y, Yahami Y. Clinical evaluation of immunotherapy in early pregnancy with x-irradiated paternal mononuclear cells for primary recurrent aborters. Am J Obstet Gynec 1993; 169:649)

4. [F & I: •Immunotherapy's effect in preventing recurrent abortion is unknown

•Its effect might be due to a psychologic (placebo) effect more than a true immunologic effect, such as a maternal immunologic recognition of the conceptus.

•Objective: To evaluate the efficacy of immunotherapy for the treatment of recurrent abortion.

•Primary recurrent aborters were immunized in early pregnancy by intradermal injection of 100 to 200 million x-irradiated (50 Gy) paternal mononuclear cells and its effect was compared with that observed in patients immunized in the same manner but with only 1 million such paternal cells.

•A successful pregnancy requires a certain optimal level of maternal immunologic recognition of the conceptus, which produces a maternal immunologic response that blocks maternal killer cells and maintains pregnancy.

•Immunotherapy has been used for recurrent aborters in whom the abortions were caused by insufficient maternal immunologic recognition.

•The efficacy and safety of this treatment remains obscure, as does the immunologic mechanism by which pregnancy is maintained.

• The results of randomized, double-blind controlled studies are inconsistent.

•The current study is not a randomized placebo controlled trial but presents two advantages.

•First, because the intradermal immunization was performed at around 5 and again at around 7 weeks of gestation, the time elapsed from conception to immunization was very short.

•Second, the two treatment groups differed only in the number of paternal cells used in immunization, and there was no significant difference in mean age or mean number of prior abortions between the two groups.

•The finding that the pregnancy success rate was significantly higher (83.0%) in patients immunized with 100 to 200 million cells than in those immunized with 1 million cells (55.3%) reveals a dose-dependent response to the number of cells used for immunization.

•The improved pregnancy outcome observed after immunization with paternal mononuclear cells reflects a regulated immunologic response in patients.

•The pregnancy success rate in women immunized with 100 to 200 million cells was significantly increased when they were first immunized within weeks of gestation.

•The finding that this group also showed an extremely high (7.5%, 4/53) rate of birth of **twins** may support the postulate that the first immunization was effective in maintaining the pregnancy and that it even prevented the so-called vanishing twin phenomenon.

•Interestingly, there was not a single small-for-date baby among the 114 infants born, including the five pairs of twins, nor were any of the babies born with some kind of abnormality.

•This finding suggests a favorable immunotherapeutic effect of the x-irradiated paternal cells on the course of early pregnancy.

•Some of the subjects in this study would have maintained pregnancy and given birth without the immunotherapy.]

---

5. A patient who regularly smokes two packs of cigarettes per day is to be placed on estrogen replacement therapy. Considering serum levels of both estrogen and progestogen in such a patient compared to a nonsmoker, the replacement amount of

    A. estrogen and progestogen should be about the same as in a nonsmoking patient.
    B. estrogen and progestogen should be greater.
 *C. estrogen should be greater; progestogen should be less.
    D. estrogen should be less; progestogen should be greater.
    E. estrogen and progestogen should be less.

---

p. 1020 (Byrjalsen I, Haarbo J, Christiansen C. Role of cigarette smoking on the postmenopausal endometrium during sequential estrogen and progestogen therapy. Obstet Gynecol 1993; 81:1016)

5. [F & I: •Background: Hormone replacement therapy is widely prescribed to alleviate climacteric symptoms and to prevent postmenopausal bone loss.

•As estrogen monotherapy is associated with an increased risk of endometrial cancer, addition of an adequate dose of progestogen is generally recommended for women with an intact uterus to protect the endometrium from hyperplasia and cancer.

•Because this is currently the only indication for adding progestogen and because these compounds may have significant adverse effects, it is essential to prescribe the minimum effective dose.

•In a study assessing hormonal effects on the endometrium, the serum concentration of the secretory endometrial protein placental protein 14 mirrored the endometrial status.

•The status can also be assessed by histologic and biochemical examination of endometrial biopsy specimens.

•Theoretically, cigarette smoking may affect the concentration of placental protein 14 in serum and the biochemical markers in endometrial tissue.

•All the markers are sensitive to hormones, and smoking has been found to reduce the serum levels of both estradiol (E2) and estrone (E1) during oral hormone replacement therapy.

•In postmenopausal non-users of hormone therapy, **smokers** seem to have a **decreased** risk of **endometrial cancer** than non-smokers, despite comparable serum levels of estrogen.

•These findings indicate significant differences in the endometrial response to hormone replacement therapy of smokers and non-smokers.

•This may be important in prescribing the optimum treatment for the individual woman.

•Objective: To report the effect of cigarette smoking on the endometrial response to sequentially combined estrogen and progestogen therapy in postmenopausal women.

•During sequentially combined hormone replacement therapy, the postmenopausal endometrium undergoes cyclical changes comparable to those of premenopausal women.

- The secretory endometrial protein placental protein 14, which is synthesized in the glandular cells of the secretory-phase endometrium, reflects this variation.

- Serum placental protein 14 is an easy and noninvasive method of assessing the hormonal effects of treatment.

- In postmenopausal women receiving sequentially combined hormone replacement therapy, the increase of serum placental protein 14 was halved in smokers as compared to non-smokers.

- Part of the explanation lies in the **reduced level of serum E2**, which agrees with previous data demonstrating a comparable reduction in the serum concentrations of both E2 and E1 during oral hormone replacement therapy.

- The underlying mechanism is not completely understood, **but increased hepatic metabolism of estrogens in smokers may be important.**

- This was confirmed by the significantly larger proportion of smokers with an atrophic endometrium.

- The lower levels of endometrial E2 and isocitrate dehydrogenase among smokers could be explained by the lower serum levels of E2.

- The reduction was not statistically significant, perhaps because of a larger imprecision in the measurement of these markers, or because a representative biopsy is difficult to obtain.

- A non-E2 mediated reduction in serum placental protein 14 was also found in smokers.

- This has not been reported before, and the underlying mechanism is largely unknown.

- Theoretically, this could coincide with the decreased risk of endometrial cancer seen in smokers despite comparable serum E2 levels.

- Estrogen therapy is the drug of choice for prevention of bone loss in women after menopause.

- The recommended minimum fully effective oral dose of 17ß-E2 is 2 mg/day.

- Smokers receiving 2 mg of E2 valerate (equipotent to 1.5 mg 17ß-E2) lost bone mineral in comparison with corresponding nonsmokers.

- If women who smoke are to derive the same effects of treatment as those who do not, they may benefit from receiving a relatively higher dose of E2.

- Adequate doses of a progestogen should be added to the therapy to negate the increased risk of endometrial cancer associated with unopposed estrogen therapy.

- Because progestogens may have significant adverse effects, it is essential to prescribe the minimum effective dose for a given dose of E2.

- The considerations on the hormone dependency of the serum concentration of placental protein 14 lead to the conclusion that the progestogen doses in the present study probably were unnecessarily high, particularly in the smokers.

- The findings are consistent with the changes in serum lipid metabolism during sequentially combined hormone replacement therapy.

- The reduced response among smokers during the E2-only phase and the more pronounced response during the combined E2-progestogen phase may be interpreted as a higher progestogen to E2 ratio in smokers.

Obstetrics and Gynecology:Review 1994-Reproductive Endocrinology References

»Smoking status should be considered an important variable in efforts to find the ideal combination of estrogen and progestogen for the postmenopausal woman.

•One clinical application of serum placental protein 14 may be to establish the optimum progestogen dose for a given E2 dose (i.e., one that adequately opposes the E2 dose) by setting up "titration-curves" for each type of progestogen.

---

6. The spontaneous abortion rate in donor insemination is likely to be highest in those cases where there is

    A. ejaculatory failure.
    B. genetic indication to use a donor.
    C. male infertility.
    *D. male subfertility.
    E. reversed vasectomy.

p. 131 (Amuzu B J, Shapiro S S. Variation in spontaneous abortion rate relates to the indication for therapeutic donor insemination. Obstet Gynecol 1993; 82:128)

6. [F & I: •Background: Therapeutic donor insemination has proven to be a highly effective and well-accepted means to achieve conception, producing an estimated 23,000 pregnancies per year in the United States.

•Unfortunately, patient costs are substantial in terms of time commitment, expenditure of emotional energy, and monetary output.

•It has been estimated that the monetary cost per pregnancy produced by donor insemination is over $6000.

•With recent concern over human immunodeficiency virus transmission, requiring increased donor screening and a change to the exclusive use of frozen, quarantined semen, these costs continue to rise.

•Couples who are contemplating donor insemination frequently ask penetrating questions about the expense and efficacy of the procedure and are given general data obtained from published clinical experience.

•Given the financial and emotional investments required, it is important that therapists be capable of providing specific, individualized estimates of a couple's potential for therapeutic success.

•Women whose husbands are **oligospermic** have **lower** donor insemination fecundity rates than women whose husbands are azoospermic.

•This difference is due to the influence of selective processes that precede the election of therapeutic donor insemination as therapy.

•Oligospermic men whose wives have not attained pregnancy through intercourse are more likely to have partners who are themselves subfertile.

•Objective: To determine whether there might be a difference in pregnancy outcome (frequency of spontaneous abortion) by indication for donor insemination therapy.

•Since the introduction of therapeutic donor insemination into clinical medicine, there has been a widely held assumption that pregnancy outcome from such conceptions mirrors that from the general, non-therapeutic population.

•Most data from donor insemination clinics have been compiled as if those undergoing therapy formed a homogeneous group.

•Fact   °Detail   Page 139   »issue   *answer

- It has become apparent that in terms of fecundity, subsets within this therapeutic cohort may have substantially different experiences.

- Pregnancies conceived from men with significant semen abnormalities produce a higher spontaneous abortion rate, presumably because of **inherent abnormalities in the fertilizing spermatozoa**.

- Recent studies have suggested an increased risk of **preeclampsia** in donor insemination pregnancies, with differences in risk among various subcategories.

  ° The risk increased in oligospermic couples with greater than 3 years of infertility (18.3%), whereas the length of infertility made no difference for azoospermic couples.

- As the frequency and range of indications for therapeutic donor insemination expand, it becomes increasingly important to understand the risks and success rates for individual, specific subcategories of the treatment population.

- Results: A relationship was identified between male partners' semen characteristics leading to donor insemination and resultant abortion rates.

  ° It is likely that this remarkable finding has not been recognized previously because of a lack of effort to determine donor insemination outcomes on the part of most large therapy centers.

- The reason for the relationship between indication for donor insemination and abortion rate is not immediately apparent.

- Several possible mechanisms may be operative:

  ° 1) Exposure to husband's semen may influence pregnancy outcome (41% of respondents admit to having intercourse concurrent with insemination, although the small fraction of pregnancies that might have resulted from the husband's sperm [1-to-2%] would not account for the observed difference);

  ° 2) immunologic properties within oligospermic sperm may induce a response in the partner that increases the frequency of abortion; or

  ° 3) a selection process occurs, similar to that responsible for the diminished fecundity among oligospermic couples participating in donor insemination.

  ° The present data do not allow a distinction to be made between these alternatives or to suggest any other etiologic possibilities.

  ° If the husband's semen interferes directly with the development of donor-conceived pregnancy, a lower abortion rate could be expected among couples who abstain from concurrent intercourse.

  ° If the increase in abortion is due to an immunologic phenomenon, a direct relationship between length of coital exposure and abortion rate should be identifiable.

  ° Should either of these situations be operative, condom use might be beneficial.

- Given data suggesting that exposure to the husband's sperm in the periovulatory period diminishes fecundability rates for donor insemination, there is already reason to advocate condom use for those undergoing therapy because of oligospermia.

- The selection processes that diminish fecundability among oligospermic couples have not been identified or their relative frequencies established with certainty.

- Conditions within the female partner such as endometriosis, luteal phase defects, adhesions, and diminished ovum quality have been proposed.

- Other unrecognized mechanisms may also exist.

• Fact ° Detail »issue *answer

•Most of these could contribute directly or indirectly to the induction of spontaneous abortion and have been suggested as possible etiologic factors in habitual abortion.

»Until more definitive information becomes available, the oligospermic subset may merit a more comprehensive initial evaluation than is ordinarily afforded insemination candidates.

•Increasingly specific information about expected pregnancy rate and outcome can be provided to individual couples during donor insemination counseling.

»To do this, therapists will need to take into account the female partner's age, any superimposed female fertility problems, and the specific male factor that originally led to the prescription of donor insemination therapy.]

---

7. Results to be expected from a 10-day course of naltrexone in obese women with polycystic ovarian syndrome include a **reduction** of serum

    A. androstenedione.
    B. DHEAS.
    C. FSH/LH.
    D. response to GnRH.
*E. testosterone.

---

p.196 (Fulghesu A M, Lanzone A, Cucinelli F, Caruso A, Mancuso S. Long-term naltrexone treatment reduces the exaggerated insulin secretion in patients with polycystic ovary disease. Obstet Gynecol 1993; 82:191)

7. [F & I: •Background: Hyperinsulinemia and obesity are common features in patients affected by polycystic ovary disease.

•The presence of ß-endorphin in the human endocrine pancreas, and the evidence that it may stimulate insulin and glucagon release, suggested the possibility that pancreatic ß-endorphin may influence glycoregulation.

•Plasma immunoreactive ß-endorphin can be elevated in women with polycystic ovary disease compared to control subjects.

•Endogenous opiates are at least partially responsible for hyperinsulinemia and insulin resistance in polycystic ovary disease.

•A relation may exist between high plasma insulin values and elevated circulating androgen levels in these patients.

•A naloxone infusion in a group of hyperinsulinemic women with polycystic ovary disease significantly decreased the insulinemic response to an oral glucose tolerance test (GTT).

•Objectives: To verify the ability of the opioid antagonist naltrexone in long-term treatment to reduce the hyperinsulinemia in patients with polycystic ovary disease.

•To evaluate the endocrine effect of this treatment following the eventual changes of insulin secretion.

•Polycystic ovary disease is characterized by chronic anovulation, elevated serum androgen levels, and an elevated incidence of hyperinsulinism.

°The mechanism of insulin resistance in this disease is partially unexplored.

•Because the circulating levels of ß-endorphin seem to be altered in polycystic ovary disease, a possible effect of opiates on insulin secretion in such patients has been postulated.

- The effectiveness of naloxone infusion on reducing the insulin response to a GTT is related to the hyperinsulinemic status.

  ° The opioid-antagonist treatment reduced the insulin levels in the hyperinsulinemic group, whereas it had no effect in normoinsulinemic subjects with polycystic ovary disease or in controls.

- The use of an oral opioid antagonist allows a longer duration of treatment and presumably a chronic reduction of insulin levels in the hyperinsulinemic woman with polycystic ovary disease.

- Results: Naloxone and naltrexone administration reduced insulin levels after the GTT in the hyperinsulinemic patients with the syndrome; moreover, the degree of such reduction was greater after chronic treatment than after single naloxone administration.

- The glycemic-insulinemic ratio may be considered a marker for insulin resistance.

- After treatment with both narcotic antagonists, the glycemic-insulinemic ratio appeared significantly increased, so that no differences were detectable between the hyper and normoinsulinemic groups.

- As expected from previous data in normoinsulinemic women with polycystic ovary disease, and from the results obtained in normal control subjects, no changes were observed in the normoinsulinemic group for the insulinemic response to the GTT.

- **Overall, these results clearly demonstrate that naltrexone administration could represent a safe and effective method to chronically reduce the hyperinsulinism in women with polycystic ovary disease.**

- The possibility of influencing insulin secretion in these women clarifies some points in the debate about the hyperinsulinism-hyperandrogenism connection in this disease.

- One leading hypothesis is that androgens directly decrease insulin action.

- In studies in which the hormonal environment has been pharmacologically modified, contrasting results have emerged.

  ° Several authors failed to demonstrate any change in insulin resistance in women with polycystic ovary disease after long-term suppression of ovarian steroidogenesis.

- It was also hypothesized that hyperinsulinemia increases androgen production by direct stimulation of ovarian steroidogenesis.

- An in vitro study showed a direct effect of insulin on ovarian steroidogenesis; furthermore, a synergistic effect between insulin and LH in vitro has been proposed.

- No differences were observed in baseline androgen levels between normo and hyperinsulinemic patients with polycystic ovary disease.

- No modification in hormonal indices following the improvement of the metabolic condition in the hyperinsulinemic group was found.

- An inverse relationship was observed between serum sex hormone-binding globulin and insulin in the hyper and normoinsulinemic groups.

- This finding suggests a direct effect of insulin on lowering sex hormone-binding globulin plasma levels.

- The data support these observations, as sex hormone-binding globulin plasma levels were **higher** in normoinsulinemic than in hyperinsulinemic patients, and in patients demonstrating a normalization of insulin levels after naltrexone treatment compared with nonnormalized hyperinsulinemic patients.

•An interesting finding of this study is that in hyperinsulinemic patients with polycystic ovary disease, the decrease of insulin levels after naltrexone treatment was **not** followed by significant changes in hormone levels.

•A normalization of the insulin secretion was reached in eight of 16 hyperinsulinemic patients; a modification of gonadotropin and androgen plasma levels after the therapy was not found.

•On the other hand, it is possible that improvement of androgen secretion needs a longer time of exposure to a normalized insulin secretion.]

---

8. In a population **not** predisposed to abnormal auto-immune function, IgA antibodies against phospholipids and histones are related to

   A. age.
   B. gravidity.
   C. history of fetal loss.
   *D. life-style.
   E. marital status.

---

p.145 (Ober C, Karrision T, Harlow L, Elias S, Gleicher N. Autoantibodies and pregnancy history in a healthy population. Am J Obstet Gynec 1993; 169:143)

8. [F & I: •Background: The function of naturally occurring autoantibodies in healthy individuals is not known.

•They may be beneficial, either by removing damaged or aged tissues, by offering protection against damaging autoimmune responses, or by regulating idiotypic-antiidiotypic networks.

•Polyclonal activation of B cells in the production of autoantibodies may be associated with overt autoimmune disease, such as systemic lupus erythematosus.

•The observation that women have higher levels of natural autoantibodies than men may explain, in part, the increased frequency of autoimmune disease in women compared with men.

•Prevalences of autoantibodies and overt autoimmune disease in females may be augmented by exposure to self-antigens during pregnancy.

•Although there is no direct evidence for this hypothesis, the association between antiphospholipid antibodies and reproductive failure syndromes (i.e., recurrent fetal loss) in otherwise healthy women suggests that pregnancy-induced autoimmunity may occur.

•If the induction of autoimmunity is a consequence of normal pregnancy, then higher levels of autoantibodies should be found in women of higher gravidity than in women of lower gravidity.

•Objectives: To determine whether autoantibodies directed against phospholipids and other cellular components, such as histones and nucleotides, are associated with pregnancy history (gravidity and history of fetal loss) in healthy women.

•To present the results of a population-based survey of the prevalence and distributions of autoantibodies in an unselected, homogeneous white population, the Hutterites.

•Because of their naturally high fertility rates and proscription of contraception, Hutterite family sizes are large (median sibship size 8).

•This population provided a unique opportunity to assess the effects of gravidity on autoantibody levels in healthy subjects.

- The specific goals of this study were to describe natural autoantibody levels in male and female Hutterites and to assess the effects of marriage (exposure to sperm antigens) and pregnancy (exposure to trophoblast antigens) on autoantibody levels in Hutterite women.

- Results: 24% of healthy adults tested positive for at least one autoantibody, similar to prevalences of natural autoantibodies reported for other populations.

- Autoantibody levels were higher in women than in men, in accordance with results of earlier studies in outbred individuals.

- The most common autoantibodies in the Hutterites were IgA antibodies against phospholipids and histones.

- IgA antibody levels were not significantly correlated with age, sex, or marital status or with gravidity or history of fetal loss in women.

- The significance of IgA antibodies is not known.

- This antibody is found in high concentrations in the mucosal secretions of the respiratory and gastrointestinal tract.

- The high prevalence of these antibodies in Hutterites may reflect their farming life-style and chronic exposure to airborne allergens.

- The prevalence of IgG and IgM autoantibodies was 7.0% and 6.0%, respectively, in adult Hutterites.

- Among men, antibody positivity was not associated with age or marital status.

- Among women age was associated with positivity for (1) IgG antibodies, (2) antihistone antibodies, and (3) more than one antibody.

- The association with age in women appears to be primarily because of an increased prevalence of IgG antibodies in women >40 years old.

- In addition, IgM antibodies were decreased in married compared with unmarried females, whereas IgG antibodies were present in married females only.

- The fact that the decrease of IgM antibodies is associated with marriage and not gravidity suggests that exposure to semen, rather than trophoblast, antigens may be associated with a switch from IgM to IgG antibody production.

- Because premarital intercourse and contraception are rare among Hutterites, female subjects are usually first exposed to semen antigens around the time of marriage and to trophoblast antigens within the first year of marriage.

- It is difficult to determine whether exposure to sperm antigens or to trophoblast accounts for the differences observed between unmarried and married women, a trend not observed in men.

- Nonetheless, the increase prevalence of IgG relative to IgM autoantibodies in married women may reflect long-term exposure to antigens, which results in a switch from low-affinity IgM to high-affinity IgG autoantibodies after marriage.

- A history of fetal loss was not associated with antibody positivity in this sample.

- Follow-up information was available for all seven married women who were positive for at least one autoantibody and who had not completed their families at the time of sampling.

- One woman has not yet had a subsequent pregnancy; six women experienced at least one successful pregnancy and none experienced a fetal loss.

•One woman (age 25) who demonstrated positive titers against phosphatidyl serine (IgG), phosphatidyl glycerol (IgG), H2B (IgG), H2A (IgA), and poly(dt) (IgA), has had three untreated pregnancies that resulted in term live births.]

---

9. The major chorionic gonadotrophin component of early pregnancy found in urine is

   *A. beta core.
    B. free α.
    C. free ß.
    D. nicked hCG.
    E. non-nicked hCG.

---

p. 1585 (Cole L A, Seifer D B, Kardana A, Braunstein G D. Selecting human chorionic gonadotropin immunoassays: Consideration of cross-reacting molecules in first-trimester pregnancy serum and urine. Am J Obstet Gynec 1993; 168:1580)

9. [F & I: •Background: Human chorionic gonadotropin (hCC) is a glycoprotein hormone composed of two dissimilar subunits, α and ß, joined noncovalently.

•The hormone (nonnicked hCG) is produced by the trophoblast during pregnancy and is detected by immunoassays in serum and urine.

•The degradation products of hCG, free subunits and fragments of hCG, are also present in serum and urine.

•These include nicked hCG (that cleaved between ß subunit residues 44 and 45 or between 47 and 48), free ß subunit and free a subunit in serum, and ß core fragment (a small peptide one fourth the molecular weight of hCG, composed of ß subunit residues 6 through 40 and 55 through 92) in urine, all of which are inactive or have greatly reduced biologic activities.

•Qualitative urine pregnancy tests, including doctor's office and home pregnancy testing kits, are used to diagnose spontaneous pregnancies 4 or more weeks after the last menses, or in vitro fertilized (IVF) pregnancies 2 or more weeks after embryo transfer.

•Quantitative serum hCG measurements are used to monitor the progress of pregnancy, to assess the date of pregnancy, and to screen for ectopic pregnancy, Down syndrome, and trophoblastic disease.

•Kits, whether for home, office, or laboratory use, rely on a variety of methods to detect hCG.

•These include the classic hCG ß subunit radioimmunoassay or slide or latex test and, in recent years, more sophisticated multiantibody tests.

°The latter include sandwich assays using an anti-a subunit and an anti-ß subunit antibody, antibodies to two sites on the ß subunit, and an anti-hCG α-ß dimer and an anti-ß subunit antibody.

°In these tests one antibody is immobilized and a second labeled with enzyme or radioactivity (laboratory tests) or linked to latex or attached to a colored dye (office and home pregnancy kits).

•Discordance has been reported in hCG assay results, with different kits giving conflicting results for the same serum or urine sample.

•In the past discordance has been attributed to differences in hCG standards, to interference by pituitary luteinizing hormone, or to nonspecific factors.

•Modern immunoassays have little or no cross reactivity with luteinizing hormone and are based on pure hCG standards (first International Reference Preparation for immunoassay and third International Standard).

Obstetrics and Gynecology: Review 1994-Reproductive Endocrinology References

- Classic ß subunit tests and the different multiantibody sandwich assays measure different moieties.

- Although ß subunit tests and certain sandwich assay formats measure hCG-ß or all ß subunit-related molecules (intact and nicked hCG, free ß and ß core fragment), others measure total hCG (nicked + non-nicked hCG) only, total hCG plus free ß or just non-nicked hCG.

- Objective: To examine the levels of total hCG, non-nicked hCG, and hCG-ß in first-trimester pregnancy serum and urine samples.

- To compare the content of samples with the different specificities of pregnancy test kits and show that results from different types of pregnancy testing kits are not necessarily interconvertible and that mismatches in what is present and what is detected causes erroneous or conflicting results.

- Laboratory kits giving conflicting results with the same serum sample and different doctor's office or home pregnancy tests giving either true-positive or false-negative results with a single urine specimen have both been reported.

- Data presented in this study show the occurrence of total and non-nicked hCG, free a and ß subunits in early pregnancy serum samples, and these plus ß core fragment in urine samples.

- From this data levels of hCG-ß (total hCG plus free ß subunit in serum and the same plus ß core fragment in urine) were calculated.

- Significant variation in the levels of total hCG, non-nicked hCG, and hCG-ß are shown in individual serum and individual urine samples.

- A survey of 29 commercial serum and urine hCG assays showed diversity in the specificity of kits.

- One half the kits surveyed were of types detecting total hCG or non-nicked hCG only, and the remaining half were of types detecting hCG-ß.

- The two variables, varying non-nicked, total hCG, and hCG-ß levels, and varying recognition of these by different types of immunoassays together cause mismatches and conflicting hCG results.

- Serum contains non-nicked and nicked hCG molecules and a small but varying amount of free ß subunit.

- Five of the 16 serum hCG assays surveyed used one of three antibody combinations detecting both nicked and non-nicked hCG molecules (or total hCG).

- Two used an antibody to hCG aß dimer detecting only non-nicked hCG molecules.

- The remaining nine used one of three antibody combinations detecting all three molecules (or hCG-ß).

- Although median values for non-nicked hCG were close to or overlapped total hCG values, individual non-nicked hCG values varied widely, from 41% to 163% of total hCG level (because of variation in proportion of nicked hCG molecules).

- As such, a kit detecting non-nicked hCG can give as much as 2.5-fold lower result than a kit measuring total hCG.

- Kits that detect hCG-ß can, in contrast, in the 2 weeks after the missed period when most pregnancy tests are done, give values as much as 45% higher than that measuring only total or only non-nicked hCG.

- Standardization is needed in laboratory hCG kits so that hCG assay results can be repeated at other centers.

- Kits should be labeled as for "total hCG," for "intact" or "non-nicked hCG," or for "hCG-ß."

•Fact   °Detail   »issue   *answer

- Results from clinical laboratories should be referred to in the same way, as should reports in journal articles.

- Pregnancy levels, doubling rates, and cut-off values should be expressed similarly, so that other centers can select the correct type of assay to use and repeat the data.

- **Nonnicked hCG values most closely reflect levels of bioactive hormone.**

- Total hCG values reflect all hCG dimer molecules and, because they include nicked hCG, may be less affected by ongoing nicking of non-nicked hCG.

- hCG-ß tests, in contrast, are preferable for tumor marker applications, where free ß subunit is a major immunoreactivity detected.

- All three types of assays are needed and have specific applications, but their results are not necessarily interconvertible.

- **ß Core fragment is a major component of early pregnancy urine samples.**

- Levels start at a median of 24% of total hCG values at 4 to 5 weeks, exceed total hCG levels at 6 to 7 weeks, and are greater than total hCG levels thereafter (median level 142% of total hCG at 12 to 13 weeks since last menses).

- As such, hCG-ß assays may predominantly detect ß core fragment in urine samples.

- Free ß subunit levels are also higher in pregnancy urines (median 44% to 9.1% of total hCG level).

- Because of the elevated free ß subunit and ß core fragment levels in urine, median hCG-ß values are 1.7- to 3.9-fold higher than total hCG values.

- Wide variation is found in individual hCG-ß and total hCG levels.

- The range of urine hCG-ß values is from 102% to 26,500% of total hCG levels.

- The hCG-ß RIA and the hCG-ß latex tests are common types of assay.

- Because these assays use antibodies raised against ß subunit they generally have preference for binding uncombined ß subunit (free ß subunit and ß core fragment) over hCG.

- This preference can exaggerate the free ß subunit and ß core fragment components of hCG ß values.

- Urine hCG-ß levels are much higher than urine total hCG levels and that values from hCG-ß RIAs and hCG-ß latex tests may be exaggerated further.

- As with serum samples, big variation is observed in individual urine non-nicked hCG and total hCG levels.

- Nonnicked hCG values range from <1.0% to 170% of total hCG levels.

- Considering the extent of individual variation, published urine hCG values may lack meaning unless information is provided about the specificity of the assay used or whether values include nicked hCGß, free ß subunit, and ß core fragment.

- Cut-off values, of the missed period, are assay specific (total hCG, non-nicked hCG or hCG-ß) and become meaningless when used with assays with different specificities.

- Manufacturers should label laboratory and doctor's office urine tests for "intact" or "non-nicked hCG," for "total hCG," and for "hCG-ß."

Obstetrics and Gynecology: Review 1994-Reproductive Endocrinology References

•Values should be referred to in the same way and should not be interconverted.

•Total hCG assays, which detect nicked and non-nicked hCG, appear to be the preferred type for **urine** samples.

°These avoid the complications and variability associated with percent nicking, free ß subunit, and ß core fragment levels.

•hCG-ß tests, which detect total hCG, free ß subunit, and ß core fragment, offer 1.7 to 3.9 times greater sensitivity than total hCG kits.

°They have the potential for the greatest variability, measuring three, versus one, semi-independent antigens.]

---

10. The condition most likely to require laparoscopic (vs transvaginal) oocyte retrieval for in vitro fertilization is

    A. male factor infertility.
    B. mild endometriosis.
*C. pelvic inflammatory disease.
    D. previous tubal ligation.
    E. unexplained fertility.

---

p. 593 (Tureck R W, Garcia C, Blasco L, Mastroianni L Jr. Perioperative complications arising after transvaginal oocyte retrieval. Obstet Gynecol 1993; 81:590)

10. [F & I: •Background: The process for recovery of oocytes for in vitro fertilization-embryo transfer (IVF-ET) and other assisted reproduction technologies is continually evolving.

•Oocytes have been recovered by laparoscopy, laparotomy, or by ultrasound-guided techniques.

•The advantages of sonographically guided oocyte retrieval over laparoscopy or laparotomy include the use of local anesthesia or sedation, rapidity and ease of the procedure, decreased cost to the patient, rapid postoperative recovery, and increased patient acceptance.

•Ultrasonographic ovum capture is accomplished either transvesically or transvaginally

•At first, the majority were performed transvesically.

°As a result of difficulties experienced by patients who underwent the transvesical approach (necessity to distend the bladder, vagal reactions, abdominal-wall hematoma formation, hematuria, and psychological trauma), the transvaginal approach has become a preferred technique.

•Advantages of the transvaginal approach include ease of delineation and improved resolution of the ovaries, minimal discomfort, and psychological acceptance by most patients.

•Injury to structures adjacent to the ovary can occur.

•Oocyte aspiration through a potentially contaminated vaginal route could increase the risk of iatrogenic pelvic infection.

•Objective: To report the perioperative experience of 674 patients undergoing transvaginal retrieval under antibiotic prophylaxis.

•Ovum recovery via transvaginal sonography has been heralded as an important advance for assisted reproduction technologies.

•To date, complications have been limited, posing little concern.

Obstetrics and Gynecology:Review 1994-Reproductive Endocrinology References

•When complications do occur they can be major.

•No infectious complications were reported in 776 patients undergoing laparoscopic ovum retrieval.

»Antibiotic prophylaxis should be used in patients with a history of salpingitis and hydrosalpinges undergoing transvaginal oocyte retrieval.

•Results: 1.5% of patients undergoing assisted reproduction technologies required hospital admission.

•Nine of the ten patients admitted were found to have laboratory and clinical evidence of adnexal infection.

•Admittedly, patients were treated aggressively with IV antibiotics at the first suggestion of adnexal infection.

°Of these nine patients, 67% had a history of salpingitis and/or pelvic adhesions.

•Two patients experienced impressive **vaginal arterial bleeding** after transvaginal oocyte retrieval.

°One patient required a suture to control bleeding.

•No clinically significant intraperitoneal bleeding or collection was noted in any patient undergoing transvaginal oocyte retrieval as assessed by sonography or laparoscopy.

•A laparoscopic approach, despite its many disadvantages, might be used in selected patients to minimize perioperative morbidity.

•If transvaginal oocyte retrieval is not available, laparotomy is necessary to reposition the ovaries for laparoscopic retrieval.

•Another alternative might be transvesical retrieval, which also has its reported problems, including hematuria, hemoperitoneum, urinary tract infections, and **reexacerbation of pelvic inflammatory disease**.

•There were no complications in 38 patients undergoing laparoscopic retrieval.

•The perioperative infections experienced in IVF patients and reported herein may have resulted from the transcervical ET itself.

°Nevertheless, this complication is exceedingly rare, with only one reported case occurring in an agonadal woman after embryo donation.

•Prophylactic antibiotics were routinely used before transvaginal retrieval.

°Their benefit is not clearly proven.]

---

11. The immediate management of a patient undergoing ovulation induction with hMG and hCG who experiences the hyperstimulation syndrome manifested by enlarged ovaries, ascites and evidence of hemoconcentration is

    A. anticoagulation
    B. diuretics
    C. fluid restriction
    *D. paracentesis
    E. salt restriction

p. 110   (Aboulghar M A, Mansour R T, Serour G I, Sattar M A, Amin Y M, Elattar I. Management of severe ovarian hyperstimulation syndrome by ascitic fluid aspiration and intensive intravenous fluid therapy. Obstet Gynecol 1993; 81:108)

•Fact   °Detail   »issue   *answer

11. [F & I: •Background: Ovarian hyperstimulation syndrome is the most serious complication of ovulation induction by gonadotropins.

•The incidence of the severe form of the syndrome varies at 0.6-to-1.8%.

•Severe disease is characterized by ovarian enlargement, ascites, hydrothorax, electrolyte imbalance, hypovolemia, oliguria, and thromboembolism.

•The syndrome is a potentially life-threatening conditions with serious complications including acute renal insufficiency, thromboembolism, adult respiratory distress syndrome, and liver dysfunction.

•Objective: To assess the effect of intensive fluid therapy and immediate complete aspiration of ascitic fluid on the outcome of patients with severe ovarian hyperstimulation syndrome.

•Several methods have been used to reduce the incidence of ovarian hyperstimulation syndrome.

•A combination of serum E2 determination and ultrasonography offers a reasonable chance of predicting the syndrome.

°Complete prevention does not seem possible with the means currently available.

°There is no agreement concerning the E2 level above which hCG should be withheld.

°Even with the most careful and painstaking preventive measures, it seems doubtful that ovarian hyperstimulation syndrome can be eliminated completely because of the narrow margin between ovulation induction dose and hyperstimulation induction dose.

°As assisted conception using ovarian superstimulation becomes more widely available, the occurrence of severe degrees of ovarian hyperstimulation syndrome will probably increase.

•The pathogenesis of ovarian hyperstimulation syndrome is poorly understood, but once the syndrome develops, treatment should aim to prevent serious complications, relieve symptoms, and shorten the hospital stay.

•It is necessary to restore blood volume, correct the hemoconcentration, prevent venous thrombosis, and increase renal perfusion.

•In this series, early intensive infusion of fluids was performed to combat the hemoconcentration in all patients.

•None received diuretics or salt or fluid restriction; on the contrary, they were encouraged to drink as much fluid as they could.

•Plasma was infused in four patients with critically low levels of plasma proteins.

•Transvaginal aspiration of ascitic fluid was found to be safe as well as effective in improving symptoms and shortening the hospital stay.

•Increased intraabdominal hydrostatic pressure in patients with tense ascites acts via the diaphragm to increase intrathoracic pressure and reduce transmural filling pressure in the heart.

•The mean right atrial pressure is increased and venous return is thus impeded.

•Paracentesis should relieve the transabdominal pressure and result in increased venous return and augmented filling of the heart.

•The protein content of the ascitic fluid ranged between 3.1 and 5.4 g/dl, with a mean of 4.6 ± 2.4.

°This level is higher than the protein content of ascitic fluid in cases of liver cirrhosis or congestive heart failure (less than 2.5 g/dl), possibly suggesting a different mechanism of ascites formation in ovarian hyperstimulation syndrome.

•Transvaginal aspiration of ascitic fluid was simple, easy, and done without anesthesia.

•It was performed under **ultrasound guidance,** which eliminated the danger of ovarian injury.

•In all cases, a pocket of ascitic fluid was located below the ovaries, allowing the needle tip to be a reasonable distance from the ovaries.

•The procedure was performed without complications in all patients.

•**Intensive IV fluid** therapy combined with transvaginal aspiration of ascitic fluid resulted in a dramatic increase in renal output, decrease in hematocrit, and marked immediate improvement of symptoms and blood chemistry.

°The only possible drawback is the loss of protein-rich fluid.

•One limitation of this study was the use of a small comparison group (ten subjects).

•The study patients showed marked improvement in symptoms 24 hours after aspiration, whereas symptoms persisted for an average of 9 days in the comparison group.

•The average hospital stay in this series was 3.8 days, which was markedly shorter than that in the comparison group (11 days).]

---

12. A patient who is 10 weeks pregnant presents with a history of pulmonary embolism in her last pregnancy. Heparin prophylaxis is to be considered. The maximum effect of subcutaneous heparin is obtained how many hours after administration?

    A. ½-1
    *B. 2-3
    C. 4
    D. 6
    E. 8

---

p. 79 (Bremma K, Lind H, Blomback M. The effect of prophylactic heparin treatment on enhanced thrombin generation in pregnancy. Obstet Gynecol 1993; 81:78)

12. [F & I: •Background: Pregnancy increases the risk for thromboembolic complications.

•The frequency of these complications in pregnancy is about one in 1000.

•A history of such complications increases the risk to 5-to-12% in a new pregnancy.

•Despite this, there is a reluctance to use prophylactic anticoagulants in high-risk patients because of heparin-induced osteoporosis, a rare but serious complication.

•The effects on osteoporosis are dose and time-related.

•Objective: To detect activation of coagulation, by testing whether the heparin dosage could be kept low without activation of blood coagulation.

•The heparin dose was adjusted by determining the anti-factor-Xa activity because this is the most sensitive current method of heparin analysis.

•In pregnancy, deep venous thrombosis is much more common in the left femoral vein, possibly because of the position of the uterus in the pelvis.

- Results: Show a left-side dominance of thromboembolic complications even in the nonpregnant state.

- In most women without known hereditary blood coagulation defects, a heparin dose of approximately 240 IU per kilogram body weight per 24 hours divided into two doses (generally 7500-to-10,000 IU twice daily) should be sufficient as thrombosis prophylaxis throughout pregnancy.

- After delivery, the dose of subcutaneous heparin was empirically reduced.

- The data, showing that the levels of anti-Xa were too high in most patients but too low in the patient with thromboembolism, imply that the anti-Xa level must be checked postpartum or that oral anticoagulants must be substituted for heparin.

- The marked increase in the protein C level with heparin may indicate that the patients earlier consumed some protein C.

- A small decrease in antithrombin levels was found with prophylactic doses.

- A larger decrease occurred in patients on higher doses of heparin during the treatment of thrombosis.

- Increased levels of fibrinogen and factor VII have been found in subjects prone to cardiovascular complications.

- In the first trimester before heparin administration, the levels of fibrinogen, hemoglobin, and total protein S were already increased compared with those in controls.

- During heparin treatment, not only these factors but also the prothrombin complex (reflecting the sum of prothrombin and factors VII and X) increased more in the study group.

- Little is known about the association between changes in endogenous hormonal and factor VII reactivity in normal women and in women with an increased risk for thromboembolism.

- Compared with the changes in blood coagulation and fibrinolysis variables during the normal menstrual cycle, they seem to be minor.

- A decreased fibrinolytic capacity together with an increase in tissue plasminogen activator inhibitor-1 is the most common finding in young patients with thrombotic disease.

- Near the end of normal pregnancy, an increase in inhibitor-1 and -2 has been shown.

- In the study group, tissue plasminogen activator inhibitor-1 levels were higher 5 weeks postpartum but otherwise were within the levels of the controls.

- Only two women had infants that were small for gestational age, and both were delivered before the last sampling occasion.

  ° A risk of fetal growth restriction was found in these two patients with high titers of **anticardiolipin antibodies**.

- The period of maximum risk for recurrent thromboembolism during any pregnancy is the **puerperium**, and an alternative approach would be to provide treatment only during this period.

  ° Ten subjects had previously developed thrombosis antenatally.

- Early heparin treatment is preferred for patients with previous iliac vein thrombosis or pulmonary embolism.

»Thrombosis-prone women without hereditary thrombophilia should be followed during pregnancy with serial coagulation analyses measuring activation (thrombin formation).

°These assays could be useful in designing optimal therapeutic regimens for decreasing activation of the hemostatic system.

•Enhanced indices of coagulation activation markers were partly reversible by heparin, suggesting that elevated levels result from increased thrombin generation and activity.

•Elevated levels of soluble fibrin are reduced by heparin treatment.

•Conclusion: In early pregnancy, women with previous thrombotic episodes have high plasma levels of biochemical markers of activation of the coagulation cascade.

•This condition persists during antithrombotic treatment, but at a lower level.

•This can be used to predict the need for treatment and, in the future, even to control the treatment.]

---

13. The majority of recurrent pregnancy losses are caused by

   A. anatomical factors
   B. endocrine disorder
   C. immunologic disorders
   D. infection
   *E. none of the above

---

p. 84 (Ecker J L, Laufer M R, Hill J A. Measurement of embryotoxic factors is predictive of pregnancy outcome in women with a history of recurrent abortion. Obstet Gynecol 1993; 81:84)

13. [F & I: •Background: Pregnancy loss before 20 weeks occurs in approximately 15% of clinically recognized gestations.

•Recurrent abortion, classically defined as three or more such losses, has been estimated to affect one in 300 pregnancies.

• Chromosomal defects are found in 3-to-7% of couples with a history of recurrent pregnancy loss and are the only well-established cause of recurrent abortion.

•Other possible associations include anatomical anomalies, endocrine disorders, and infections.

•Even when such potential explanations for recurrent miscarriage are considered, **the majority of cases remain unexplained.**

•Immunologic mechanisms have been suggested as a cause of recurrent abortion.

•Lymphocytes and macrophages from women with a history of recurrent abortion, when stimulated with reproductive antigens (sperm and trophoblast), produced soluble factors that were toxic to developing mouse embryos and human placental cell lines.

•The production of these toxic factors may be involved in reproductive failure.

•It is not known whether these factors are produced during pregnancy, if they vary between successive pregnancies, or whether their production can be altered by therapies such as immunosuppression.

•Objective: To determine whether the embryotoxic factor assay performed at 5 weeks' gestation can be used as a predictor of pregnancy outcome in women with a history of recurrent abortion.

- Methods: Lymphocytes and macrophages from the patients' blood were isolated and maintained in tissue culture in the presence of antigens obtained from a human trophoblast cell line and human sperm.

- Supernatants from these cultures were collected and added to two-cell mouse embryos in culture, with assessment of subsequent blastocyst development.

- A toxic effect was assigned when blastocyst development was less than 50% of control values.

- Human gestation is biologically inefficient, as 50% of pregnancies are lost before the first missed menses and another 10-to-20% end in detectable spontaneous abortion.

- The risk of a subsequent miscarriage after one spontaneous loss is approximately 24%; after two, 26%; after three, 32%; and after four consecutive losses the recurrence risk for a fifth spontaneous abortion is estimated to approach 40%.

- Although the syndrome of recurrent abortion is classically defined as three or more losses before 20 weeks' gestation, many investigators have recommended that this definition be changed to include women with two miscarriages and no term pregnancies.

- Other circumstances warranting earlier evaluation include women older than 35 years having two prior spontaneous abortions and couples having difficulty conceiving or those anxious to initiate an investigation of potential causes for recurrent miscarriage.

- Unfortunately, evaluation often offers no explanation.

- In 1953, Medawar introduced the concept of the fetus as an immunologically privileged tissue, as the mother usually tolerates the intrauterine semi-allograft.

- It was later theorized that pregnancy loss may result from a breakdown of the mechanisms underlying this privileged status.

- The immune systems of many women with a history of recurrent abortion produce factors toxic to mouse embryo development and human trophoblast proliferation when stimulated by exposure to reproductive antigens.

- This response seems unique to many women with recurrent abortion, as women with normal reproductive histories do not produce such factors.

- Results: Women who produce embryotoxic factors when not pregnant do not necessarily produce them in subsequent pregnancies.

- Although the cause of this variation is presently under investigation, the discovery of embryotoxic factors early in gestation may potentially be used to predict the eventual success or failure of that pregnancy.

- The fact that all women found to have embryotoxic factors on their initial evaluation were receiving potentially immunosuppressive doses of progesterone during their subsequent gestations is a confounding variable that needs to be addressed in a double-blind, randomized, placebo-controlled trial before conclusions can be drawn about this form of immunosuppressive therapy.

- In patients with available follow-up data, embryotoxic factor determination in early pregnancy was useful in predicting the ultimate outcome of that pregnancy.

- Among 14 women with two subsequent pregnancies discordant for embryotoxic factors, ten subsequently miscarried during the embryotoxic factor-positive pregnancy and carried to term in the embryotoxic factor-negative pregnancy.

- Neither the positive nor negative predictive value of the embryotoxic factor assay was 100%.

•Many other factors obviously contribute to the eventual success or failure of gestation; measurement of embryotoxic factors may only address one of these.

•Embryotoxic factor activity was reassessed in all women after ultrasound confirmation of fetal cardiac activity.

•In the general obstetric population, the chance of a spontaneous abortion after documenting early fetal cardiac activity was commonly believed to be 2-to-3%.

•Using endovaginal ultrasound, the incidence of spontaneous abortion after documenting fetal cardiac activity at 4 weeks' gestation is 5.8%.

•In this population of women with a history of two or more spontaneous abortions, a 24% chance of aborting a subsequent pregnancy was observed once fetal cardiac activity has been demonstrated.

•In women found to have aberrant cellular immunity to reproductive antigens (sperm and/or trophoblast) as determined by a positive embryotoxic factor finding during evaluation for recurrent abortion, the reassessment of embryotoxic factors during a subsequent pregnancy may be useful in predicting pregnancy outcome.

•Cause-and-effect relationships are difficult to prove from this observational study.

•In women who produce embryotoxic factors, therapies directed at suppressing the maternal immune response warrant further study in randomized, double-blind, placebo-controlled trials.]

---

14. Which of the following is the best predictor of the ability of spermatozoa to bind to zona pellucida?

    A. sperm concentration
    B. sperm linearity
    C. sperm mobility
*D. sperm morphologic pattern
    E. sperm velocity

---

p. 1765   (Oehninger S, Toner J, Muasher S J, Coddington C, Acosta A A, Hodgen G D. Prediction of fertilization in vitro with human gametes: Is there a litmus test? Am J Obstet Gynec 1992; 167:1760)

14. [F & I: •Background: Male-factor infertility remains one of the most challenging barriers to successful (viable) pregnancy in spite of the application of assisted reproductive technologies.

•While some cases of male-related infertility can be suspected on the basis of standard evaluations before in vitro fertilization (IVF) or related techniques are attempted, some are unanticipated and alarming for the couples involved.

•A better way to identify and classify cases of sperm dysfunction would aid in prognostication and allow for a plan before failed or poor fertilization is confirmed.

•Conventionally measured features of semen, according to the World Health Organization (WHO) criteria, including sperm concentration, motility, and morphologic pattern, all affect rates of fertilization in vitro and assisted reproductive technology outcome, as demonstrated in both IVF and gamete intrafallopian transfer (GIFT) techniques.

•The evaluation of sperm morphologic pattern by a more stringent technique (strict criteria) has enhanced objectivity and decreased intraassay and interassay variations while examining this sperm parameter.

•By strict criteria, sperm morphologic pattern has been shown to significantly enhance the prediction of IVF outcome.

- The assessment of sperm motion characteristics by computer-assisted semen analysis has also shown that the amplitude of lateral head displacement, curvilinear velocity, linearity, and straight-line velocity are positively correlated with fertilization rates.

- The hamster zona-free egg-sperm penetration assay constitutes a widely utilized heterologous test to evaluate sperm-oocyte fusion.

- The high incidence of false-negative results and the marked variation in the sperm penetration assay methods from laboratory to laboratory are of concern when the test results are interpreted.

- There is concern about the real clinical relevance of the sperm penetration assay; this bioassay especially in combination with the use of an acrosome reaction-inducing agent, still represents a valuable means by which sperm capacity to undergo the acrosome reaction and oocyte fusion can be indirectly measured.

- Sperm-zona pellucida binding tests have increasingly gained attention in assisted reproductive technology.

- The **hemizona assay** has been introduced and developed as a homologous bioassay to test for tight binding of human sperm to the human zona pellucida.

- This physiologic step may reflect multiple aspects of sperm function and constitutes a critical event leading to fertilization and early preembryo development.

- In the hemizona assay a human oocyte is bisected by surgical micromanipulation, thus allowing for an internally controlled comparison of sperm binding (from a patient versus a fertile control) to matching hemizonae surfaces.

- The assay has been validated by a clear-cut definition of the factors affecting data interpretation (i.e., kinetics of binding, egg variability and maturation status, intraassay variation, influence of sperm morphologic pattern, motility, and acrosome reaction status).

- Initial studies have shown that semen specimens with failed fertilization or poor fertilization rates in IVF had a significantly lower sperm-zona-binding ability than normal samples had.

- The hemizona assay can be used prospectively to identify patients at high risk for fertilization failure.

- Objective: To evaluate sperm parameters (concentration, morphologic pattern, progressive motility, velocity, and linearity of movement) and hemizona binding as predictors of IVF.

- Prediction of the potential of human gametes to achieve fertilization under in vitro conditions has been a major goal of assisted reproductive technology.

- Sperm morphologic pattern (as evaluated by strict criteria) and sperm-zona-binding capacity (as evaluated by the hemizona assay index) are excellent predictors of IVF success or failure.

- Results: Of the classic sperm parameters, **sperm morphologic pattern** was the best predictor of the ability of spermatozoa to bind to the zona pellucida.

- Patients with a poor prognosis pattern (severe teratospermia, <4% normal sperm forms) have an impaired capacity to bind to the zona under hemizona assay conditions, and this finding correlates well with their low IVF rates under standard conditions.

- Increasing the insemination concentration in the hemizona assay enhances binding in teratospermic patients; this corrective measure can be used in IVF to enhance fertilization rates in these patients.

- There is a clear-cut relationship between these two sperm properties.

•Semen samples with a poor prognosis pattern have been found to have significantly poorer velocities and lower recovery rates after swim-up separation of the motile sperm fraction as compared with those of normal semen samples.

•Abnormal sperm morphologic pattern is associated with an impaired capacity to achieve tight binding to the zona pellucida, and dyskinetic deficiencies are also present in these sperm populations.

•Because sperm morphologic pattern is the best predictor of sperm binding to the zona pellucida, the influence of morphologic pattern (as judged by strict criteria) seems to be established in major part through its effect on binding ability to the zona pellucida (possible membrane-receptor deficiencies).

•The ability of sperm to achieve tight binding to the zona pellucida may reflect multiple functions of human spermatozoa, and this may explain why their sperm-zona-binding ratio test (hemizona assay index in this case) was most strongly correlated with IVF results.

•The hemizona assay index was the most measurement of fertilization outcome.

•The discrimination potential of the hemizona assay was maximized by

°(1) attainment of a threshold binding level to the control hemizona pair (fertile control) was required, thereby reassuring a good egg-binding capability and a good control sperm sample and

°(2) only IVF patients having at least two mature, preovulatory oocytes (metaphase I or II at aspiration) were included.

•Motility was the second best predictor.

•These results establish that of the properties analyzed, the ability of sperm to bind to the zona pellucida is fundamental and highly predictive for achieving successful fertilization.

»The relationship between sperm morphologic pattern and IVF results depends on an effect on zona binding.

•Motility adds to the prediction of fertilizaton rate outside the prediction of the hemizona assay.

°Motility, although important to achieve binding, may be more important for cumulus penetration and zona pellucida penetration, factors not directly evaluated in the hemizona assay.

•A model including other sperm motion properties (i.e., hyperactivated motility, the ability of sperm to undergo the acrosome reaction, and sperm-egg fusion) may increase the predictability even more.

•The information gained here may be extremely valuable for counseling patients for IVF (i.e., for a hemizona assay index <35% the chances of poor fertilization are 100%, whereas for a hemizona assay index ≥35% the changes of good fertilization are 81%).

»The analysis of conventional semen parameters with emphasis on sperm morphologic pattern (as judged by strict criteria) and motion characteristics (evaluated by computer-assisted semen analysis) constitutes the first obligatory step for a critical evaluation of male factor patients.

•For the clinician characteristics such as discriminating power and positive and negative predictive power are more meaningful than correlation coefficients.

•Patients in whom fertilization disorders are suspected should be evaluated through bioassays of sperm function of established accuracy.

•The hemizona assay, a bioassay of sperm-zona-binding capacity is here verified to be highly predictive of IVF outcome.

•Ultimately, the biochemical and cellular mechanisms responsible for sperm dysfunctions need to be elucidated.]

15. The addition of the IgG fraction derived from plasma containing antiphospholipid antibodies to normal placental tissue will produce

    A. a decrease in prostacyclin
    B. a decrease in thromboxane
    C. an increase in prostacyclin
  *D. an increase in thromboxane
    E. no change in either prostacyclin or thromboxane because the placental doesn't respond to antiphospholipid antibodies

p. 1546   (Peaceman A M, Rehnberg K A. The immunoglobulin G fraction from plasma containing antiphospholipid antibodies causes increased placental thromboxane production. Am J Obstet Gynec 1992; 167:1543)

15. [F & I: •Background: Antiphospholipid antibodies are circulating immunoglobulins associated with poor obstetric outcomes, including recurrent abortion, maternal thrombosis, fetal death, and early, severe preeclampsia.

    •The clinical findings of thrombosis, thrombocytopenia, or recurrent pregnancy loss in association with the laboratory detection of moderate or high levels of anticardiolipin or lupus anticoagulant is termed the antiphospholipid antibody syndrome.

    •Data from animal models support a causative role for these antibodies in pregnancy complications and justify attempts to suppress antibody activity in affected patients.

    •All proposed treatments are empiric because no controlled trials have been performed to date to document their efficacy in preventing adverse pregnancy outcomes.

    •The choice of appropriate treatments is hampered by the absence of a defined pathophysiology for antiphospholipid antibody-mediated pregnancy loss.

    •Initial studies suggested that lupus anticoagulant, the primary antiphospholipid antibody implicated in recurrent pregnancy loss, affects vascular endothelial cells, resulting in decreased prostacyclin production.

    •The site and mechanism of action for antiphospholipid antibodies remain in doubt.

    •An alternative site in some patients may be on the placenta, with altered prostanoid production at that level being involved in the resulting adverse pregnancy outcome.

    •Objective: To evaluate the hypothesis that the immunoglobulin G (IgG) fraction for plasma containing high levels of antiphospholipid antibody alters the production of prostacyclin or thromboxane when incubated with normal human placental tissue.

    •Results: The addition of the IgG fraction derived from plasma containing antiphospholipid antibodies produced a consistent **increase in thromboxane** production by normal placental tissue over baseline production, whereas IgG from normal nonpregnant patients did not alter thromboxane production.

    •This increase in thromboxane production with antiphospholipid antibody IgG appeared to be dose related.

    •Conversely, no alteration in prostacyclin production by the placenta was seen with the addition of either normal pooled plasma or antiphospholipid antibody IgG at any concentration tested.

    •The placenta is a logical site for the action of antiphospholipid antibodies.

    •Normal pregnancy is thought to be associated with a relative balance between the opposing effects of prostacyclin and thromboxane produced by the placenta.

- Any effect on placental prostanoid production could result in paracrine alteration of the local environment at the maternal-placental interface.

- Decreased prostacyclin and increased thromboxane production are associated with vasoconstriction, platelet aggregation, uterine activity, and decreased uteroplacental blood flow.

- The prostacyclin-to-thromboxane ratio is altered significantly in preeclampsia, a syndrome that shares many pathologic features with the antiphospholipid antibody syndrome.

- It is plausible that antiphospholipid antibodies are active at the maternal-placental interface and alter prostanoid production at that level.

- These data support three hypotheses relating to the pathophysiologic makeup of the antiphospholipid antibody syndrome.

  - First, altered placental thromboxane production rather than a change in prostacyclin production is involved in antiphospholipid antibody-related pregnancy loss.

    - This differs is consistent with the association of increased thromboxane production with abruptio placentae, preeclampsia, and other clinical manifestations of the antiphospholipid antibody syndrome.

  - Second, antiphospholipid antibodies are active at the placental surface.

    - With direct immunofluorescent studies antiphospholipid antibody IgG binds with decidual tissue of treated mice.

    - Alterations in placental production of vasoactive substances may contribute to other pregnancy complications as well.

    - The involvement of the placenta in the pathogenesis of this syndrome is consistent with the finding that most women are primarily symptomatic when pregnant.

  - Last, the adverse effects of antiphospholipid antibodies may be self-contained in the IgG fraction and capable of causing characteristic changes in otherwise normal tissue from unaffected individuals.

    - This concept of an IgG transferable factor has been shown to cause recurrent pregnancy loss in mice and likely pertains to humans as well.

- If a consistent effect on thromboxane production can be confirmed with IgG fractions obtained from other patients with the antiphospholipid antibody syndrome, it might allow development of a bioassay for antiphospholipid antibody activity.

  - Currently, testing for antiphospholipid antibodies, especially anticardiolipin antibody, is not uniform because significant interlaboratory variation exists among testing sites.

  - This variation likely leads to overtreatment of patients with false-positive results and possibly undertreatment of some with false-negative results.

  - Development and validation of a bioassay would allow more accurate identification of affected patients.]

Obstetrics and Gynecology: Review 1994-Reproductive Endocrinology References

Directions: Each set of lettered headings below is followed by a list of numbered words or phrases. For each numbered word or phrase select:

- A. if the item is associated with *(A) only*
- B. if the item is associated with *(B) only*
- C. if item is associated with *both (A) and (B)*
- D. if item is associated with *neither (A) nor (B)*

Items 16-18.

In the treatment of endometriosis:

- A. danazol (800 mg. BID) x 6 months.
- B. leuprolide (3.75 milligrams IM monthly) x 6 months.
- C. both
- D. neither

16. androgenic side effects. — Ans: A

17. increase in serum total cholesterol. — Ans: D

18. skin rash. — Ans: A

---

p. 30 (Wheeler J M, Knittle J D, Miller J D. Depot leuprolide acetate versus danazol in the treatment of women with symptomatic endometriosis: A multicenter, double-blind randomized clinical trial. II. Assessment of safety. Am J Obstet Gynec 1993; 169:26)

16-18. [F & I: •Background: Endometriosis occurs in approximately 10% of all women of reproductive age and is a common cause of pelvic pain and of infertility.

•High recurrence rates within a few years of treatment occur after today's medical and surgical therapy.

•In recent years medical therapy has favored the gonadotropin-releasing hormone (GnRH) agonists, which result in hypoestrogenism and then in atrophy of uterine and ectopic endometrial tissue.

•GnRH agonist side effects are related to the induced hypoestrogenic state, including hot flushes, insomnia, irritability, and bone loss.

•In the United States GnRH agonist administration has required daily injections or inhalations; patient compliance may decline with the requirement of such frequent dosing over months of treatment.

•A depot form of GnRH agonist (leuprolide acetate for depot suspension, or Lupron Depot) provides continuous drug release for 4 weeks after intramuscular injection.

•A depot GnRH agonist may be more acceptable to women with endometriosis and may increase the likelihood of their compliance.

°It can also offer potentially faster, more profound suppression of ovarian estradiol production.

•This randomized clinical trial was conducted to compare the safety and efficacy of leuprolide acetate depot with that of standard danazol therapy in the treatment of women with symptomatic endometriosis.

°This article reports the safety of leuprolide acetate depot as compared with danazol.

•Danazol has been in common use for women with endometriosis since 1973, but its use is often associated with troublesome side effects and high rates of recurrent symptoms.

•Fact   °Detail   »issue   *answer

- GnRH agonists were first used in clinical trials for endometriosis in 1981, and numerous clinical studies document consistent ovarian suppression with reduction of the severity and symptoms of endometriosis.

- Although the majority of patients taking either drug reported significant adverse effects, few women in either group withdrew from the study or otherwise manifested "severe" side effects.

- No patient taking either drug was withdrawn because of a particularly unusual laboratory value.

- Leuprolide acetate depot was associated with more hypoestrogenic symptoms befitting its more complete ovarian suppression, whereas danazol is associated with more androgenic side effects.

- The few changes in serum chemistry and hematologic measurements between the leuprolide and danazol groups were modest and probably of little clinical significance.

- The metabolic effects of these drugs on bone and lipid metabolism are of the greatest concern in terms of long-term toxicity.

- Currently available methods of measuring bone density are imperfect because of inherent variations of ±2% to 5% for repeated measurements, with even greater variation likely between machines.

- Leuprolide acetate depot caused greater bone loss than did danazol.

- Although the bone loss associated with GnRH agonist use in endometriosis is supposed to be reversible, two strategies for minimizing loss may be shorter treatment (e.g., 3 months) or low-dose estrogen or progestin add-back during GnRH agonist treatment.

- Lipid profiles changed according to the anticipated metabolic effects of each drug; changes in patients in the leuprolide group were associated with the symptoms of menopause, and changes in the patients in the danazol group were androgenic in nature.

° Lipid values return to baseline within 60 days after cessation of therapy.

- The clinical significance of these apparently temporary changes in the lipid profile is unknown.]

Items 19-21.

    A. endometrium
    B. breast epithelial cells
    C. both
    D. neither

19. unopposed estrogen enhances development of cancer   Ans: A

20. estrogen receptor declines during the luteal phase   Ans: C

21. progesterone receptor levels content are the same throughout cycle   Ans: B

---

p. 878 (Soderqvist G, Schoultz B, Tani E, Skoog L. Estrogen and progesterone receptor content in breast epithelial cells from healthy women during the menstrual cycle. Am J Obstet Gynec 1993; 168:874)

19-21. [F & I: • Background: Combined estrogen-progestogen therapy is used for contraception and postmenopausal replacement.

- The possibility of an increased cancer risk in target organs has been a matter of debate for several years.

- In the endometrium unopposed estrogen treatment with high doses will enhance proliferation and cancer risk and that the addition of a progestogen will counteract this effect.

- Combined estrogen-progestogen therapy may even reduce the risk to below that of untreated women.

- Whether the breast is affected in a similar manner is unclear and highly controversial.

- Breast cell proliferation in vitro is stimulated by estrogen and inhibited by progestogens.

- Maximal epithelial cell proliferation in breast biopsies has been found during the luteal phase.

- Insight into these processes can be obtained by analysis of the cell content of sex steroid hormone receptors in breast epithelial cells during the menstrual cycle.

- Measurement of the estrogen and progesterone receptors in cytologic smears by use of monoclonal antibodies provides an accurate and reliable technique that can be performed on isolated cells procured through fine-needle aspiration.

- Objective: To evaluate the estrogen receptor and progesterone receptor variations in vivo in normal breast cells from healthy volunteers during the menstrual cycle.

- Most previous studies on the cyclic changes in breast epithelium have been based on tissue specimens obtained from breasts resected for malignancy or biopsy specimens of "normal" breast tissue near fibroadenomas, fibrocystic disease, or breast cancer.

- By using this type of material it is almost impossible to obtain tissue from both the follicular and luteal phase in the same woman.

- The estrogen receptor and progesterone receptor content in normal breast epithelial cells from both the follicular and luteal phase of the menstrual cycle in healthy women was possible by using an immunocytochemical technique for measurement of hormone receptors adapted to cells obtained through fine-needle aspiration biopsy.

- Results: Confirm a **decline** of estrogen receptor detectability during the luteal phase in women with confirmed ovulation.

- In many of the women, but not all, estrogen receptor was **undetectable** in this phase.

- Roughly two thirds of the women had estrogen receptor-positive cells in the follicular phase as compared with one third in the luteal phase.

- In contrast, **progesterone receptor was found to remain constant** throughout the menstrual cycle.

- With respect to estrogen receptor the results suggest a similarity between the epithelial cells in the breast and the endometrium.

    ° In both organs the estrogen receptor declines during the luteal phase.

- The present data indicate a striking difference with respect to progesterone receptor.

    ° In the epithelial cells of the endometrium there is a decline of detectable progesterone receptor during the luteal phase.

    ° This does not occur in breast epithelium.

- These two target organs differ in their hormonal regulation.

- Virtually all endometrial cells proliferate on **low** estradiol levels.

- In the breast the number of proliferating cells is low, amounting to only 1% to 3%.

- Only a fraction of the cells had detectable receptors in the different phases.

- The most likely explanation for this finding is that the technique used, although very sensitive, will not detect low levels of the receptors.

- Thus cells scored as receptor-negative can still show a variation in receptor content that may be of physiologic significance.

- Acinar and ductal cells, which are indistinguishable in fine-needle aspiration smears, may have different physiologic control.

- The variations observed could accordingly also result from different proportions of these two cell types in different aspirates.

- The receptor changes recorded show a basic pattern that seems to be nonrandom.

- The decline of estrogen receptor in the luteal phase may either reflect suppression of receptor-protein synthesis or increased receptor-protein degradation.

- In the endometrium estradiol stimulates and progestogen inhibits proliferation and cancer risk.

- With respect to the breast there is great controversy.

- In the breast nonsteroidal stimulants such as growth factors are relatively more important than in the endometrium.

- The protective effect of progesterone aginst cancer is controversial.

- In contrast to the endometrium there was a marked proliferation of breast epithelium in the luteal phase that was further enhanced by combined and also progestogen-only oral contraceptives.

- Thymidine kinase, an enzyme of the nucleotide synthesis considered to be an important marker of cell growth, is stimulated at physiologic progestogen concentrations.

- Insulin-receptor content and insulin stimulation of cell growth also is enhanced by progestogens in human breast cancer cell lines.

- These data indicate a direct stimulating action of progestogens on the breast.

- Estrogens via estrogen receptor activation are known to stimulate progesterone receptor formation, thus facilitating the action of progesterone in the luteal phase.

- The finding that the progesterone receptor in breast epithelial cells of healthy women was maintained at a constant level during the menstrual cycle indicates important biologic differences as compared with the endometrium.

- The significance of this finding as regards breast cell proliferation, cancer risk, and the effects of exogenous sex steroids remains to be elucidated.]

Directions: For each of the questions or incomplete statements below, ONE or MORE of the answers or completions given is correct. In each case select:

A. if only 1, 2, and 3 are correct
B. if only 1 and 3 are correct
C. if only 2 and 4 are correct
D. if only 4 is correct
E. if all are correct

---

22. True statements about male fertility include

   1. Fertilization can occur in sperm without motility.
   2. Fertilization can occur in a seminal fluid specimen with less than 10% normal forms.
   3. Sperm with abnormal shapes have a normal genetic constitution.
   4. Under zona insemination results in unacceptable rates of polyspermy.

---

p. 332   Ans: A   (Tucker M J, Wiker S R, Wright G, Morton P C, Toledo A A. Treatment of male infertility and idiopathic failure to fertilize in vitro with under zona insemination and direct egg injection. Am J Obstet Gynec 1993; 169:324)

22. [F & I: •Background: The nature of human in vitro fertilization (IVF) therapy has changed since the introduction of micromanipulation for the treatment of male factor infertility.

•Clinical application of single spermatozoon injection into an egg has become feasible.

•This achievement has overturned many previously held beliefs of what constituted a fertile spermatozoon.

•Routine application of the less invasive procedure of under zona insemination has in its own way provided little insight into which spermatozoa are capable of fertilization on a consistent basis.

•This implies that current semen analyses are inadequate, and it is probable that analysis of specific gamete fusogens at the molecular level are needed.

•Clinical practice has run ahead of scientific analysis, allowing treatment of previously untreatable semen samples by means of techniques not yet fully understood.

•In addition to severe male factor infertility where total spermatozoal count is the only apparent limiting factor for treatment, there exists a population of patients undergoing in vitro fertilization who have no apparent reason for what is observed as a consistent failure to fertilize in vitro.

•Such cases of **idiopathic failure to fertilize** represent a true group of patients who provide gametes with no apparent defects on the basis of current analysis; defects can be inferred from their repeated inability to fertilize.

•Such cases can be treated by invasive micromanipulative techniques to enhance the fertilization potential of the gametes, and, although these approaches may seem unwarranted on the basis of spermatozoal count and apparent gamete quality, for many couples these techniques are their only hope for successful fertilization.

•Under zona insemination has enabled a more quantifiable approach to insemination for the treatment of severe male factor infertility and idiopathic failure to fertilize.

•Objective: To report on the first 85 cycles in which the under zona insemination technique has been applied and also report on initial experience with direct egg injection with a single spermatozoon.

•Because of the conflicts of clinical and scientific interests, well controlled comparisons with conventional insemination techniques are not feasible, although results strongly suggest that both under zona insemination and direct egg injection have been of great value to many of the couples reported here.

- IVF may not be an appropriate term for a therapy in which fertilization is either not consistently or never achieved for a specific couple.

- There exist two distinct groups of patients that suffer from a higher chance of fertilization failure during conventional IVF, even using high concentrations of inseminating spermatozoa.

- Those couples in which the male partners have **poor quality semen** clearly are candidates for lower fertilization outcome by virtue of possessing fewer normal viable spermatozoa.

- The second group of couples are those that incur consistent **fertilization failure** in vitro although spermatozoal and egg quality appear normal.

- It is not possible to assess this group of patients prospectively.

- Retrospectively, failed IVF, if consistent, can be thought of as costly diagnosis, albeit rather fruitless therapy.

- From the group of 73 couples (85 cycles) in the current study, it may be thought that certain parameters of seminal quality might be helpful as prognosticators for fertilization failure in IVF, or rather for the need of assisted fertilization.

- In the 20 cycles in which fertilization failed completely with under zona insemination on the day of egg collection, it can be seen that little of significance can be concluded about which seminal parameter may have caused this initial fertilization failure in this relatively small group of patients.

- When fertilization and pregnancy rates are taken where partners spermatozoa were used regardless of the form of insemination and these outcomes are analyzed in terms of either the male factor or idiopathic failure to fertilize groups, **no significant differences** either in fertilization or in viable pregnancy rate occurred between the two groups, in spite of significantly different spermatozoal counts, motilities, and morphologic conditions.

- There is little of prognostic value in these seminal parameters in this group of patients.

- In two of the 73 couples study fertilization was achieved with under zona insemination with samples with **no progressive motility**.

- One of these men had 0% motility as a consequence of testicular exposure to radon, and, as well as achieving fertilization with no motility as has been previously reported from immotile cilia syndrome, this cycle also gave rise to a normal term pregnancy.

- Fertilization and pregnancies were achieved with spermatozoa with a wide spread of normal forms, from 0% to 59% normal forms.

- Seven pregnancies that occurred out of the total group arose using under zona insemination for male factor patients with between 6% and 11% normal forms.

  ° This does not appear to represent a grouping of patients that would more appropriately have been treated with partial zona dissection.

  ° These preliminary data do little to help define those semen samples or couples that require assisted fertilization over conventional insemination.

- Clinical judgment allows embryologists to assess whether complicating factors such as poor ovulatory stimulation, egg quality, or temporarily suppressed seminal quality are at fault in fertilization failure.

- In cases where this is not apparent, criteria such as a minimum of two failed conventional in vitro insemination attempts before the use of assisted fertilization may not be realistic when a couple's economic and emotional situation is considered.

•Whether superfluous or not, if assisted fertilization can deliver greater security of fertilization than conventional insemination, then a couple who have failed fertilization on one previous occasion or who may only suffer from less severe male factor problems may wish to adopt an assisted fertilization approach more readily.

•It is a realistic option to follow up initial fertilization failure subsequent to conventional insemination with reinsemination by either under zona insemination or direct egg injection.

•At least 17 of the severest male factor cases would previously have not been accepted into this clinic's IVF program when only conventional IVF and partial zona dissection approaches were available, although in these cases fertilization was achieved for 15 of them and seven viable pregnancies resulted after the use of under zona insemination and direct egg injection.

•This implies that under zona insemination and direct egg injection may be applicable in virtually all forms of male factor infertility, assuming sufficient viable spermatozoa can be harvested **regardless of motility or normal morphologic conditions**.

•In 14 cases only reinsemination fertilized under zona insemination embryos were available for transfer; although embryonic development was slightly retarded, five viable pregnancies resulted, which is in contrast to the poor outcome when only conventionally reinseminated embryos were available for transfer.

•Although the micromanipulation techniques involved in under zona insemination and direct egg injection are far from simple to master, they are well within the grasp of most clinical embryologists given adequate training.

•The equipment necessary is not prohibitively expensive nor exotic.

•Concerns doubtless will remain for some time relating to the lax and lack of selection of spermatozoa used for under zona insemination and direct egg injection, respectively, which might generate more than acceptable numbers of genetic disorders in the offspring.

•With adequate counseling and thorough prenatal screening, it does seem that there will continue to be many couples who will wish to seek these assisted fertilization techniques as their only chance for pregnancy using their own gametes.]

---

23. Operative in the pathophysiology of infertility caused by *Chlamydia trachomatis*

    1. induction of male antisperm antibodies.
    2. induction of female antisperm antibodies.
    3. inflammation of endometrium.
    4. direct embryotoxic effects.

p. 1461   Ans: E   (Witkin S S, Jeremias J, Grifo J A, Ledger W J. Detection of *Chlamydia trachomatis* in semen by the polymerase chain reaction in male members of infertile couples. Am J Obstet Gynec 1993; 168:1457)

23. [F & I: •Background: *Chlamydia trachomatis* infections of the male and female genital tracts are often asymptomatic.

•Infected persons may not be readily identifiable, and chlamydial infection in men and women may persist for long periods.

•In addition, cytotoxic effects of genital secretions on the cell lines used to culture *C. trachomatis* or loss of *Chlamydia* viability during transport or storage makes it especially difficult to detect this organism in genital tract samples.

Obstetrics and Gynecology: Review 1994-Reproductive Endocrinology References

•A major observable consequence of persistent asymptomatic *C. trachomatis* genital tract infection in women is occlusion of the fallopian tubes and subsequent infertility.

•Women in whom tubal occlusions were first detected at the time of diagnostic laparoscopy for infertility and who were never identified as having a chlamydial infection had a strikingly higher prevalence of antibodies to *C. trachomatis* than did women who did not have tubal infertility:

•*C. trachomatis* can asymptomatically colonize the male urethra and prostate gland.

•If untreated, symptomatic *C. trachomatis* infections of the male urethra often eventually become asymptomatic.

•Objective: To investigate the prevalence of asymptomatic *C. trachomatis* infections in semen from male members of infertile couples was examined by means of polymerase chain reaction.

•Results: More than one third of male partners in couples with unexplained infertility have evidence of a latent chlamydial infection in semen.

•An association between *C. trachomatis* in semen and antisperm antibodies in male and female partners suggests a mechanism whereby an undetected chlamydial infection may contribute to infertility in these couples.

•Although the results were negative for seminal *C. trachomatis* by culture or by DNA probe, more than one third of the 28 male partners in couples with previously undiagnosed infertility had positive test results when tested by the polymerase chain reaction for *C. trachomatis* in semen.

•The most likely explanation for these findings is that these intracellular organisms were present at a concentration below the threshold of these other assays.

•Alternatively, the *Chlamydia* may exist in the male genital tract in a nonculturable, intracellular form.

•The failure of *C. trachomatis* to elicit a systemic humoral immune response in the men with evidence of this organism in semen further indicates that the concentration of organisms is probably very low.

•**In addition, since regions of the male genital tract are inaccessible to the systemic immune system, *C. trachomatis* may persist, as do spermatozoa, in a sequestered state within the tract.**

•Despite the absence of a systemic response, the associations between seminal *C. trachomatis* and both antibodies on the surface of motile ejaculated sperm and poor sperm quality in some of these men suggest that this asymptomatic infection may be capable of inducing an immune response within the male genital tract.

•Antisperm antibodies may be present in semen in the absence of a systemic antibody response, providing a precedent for the occurrence of a male genital tract restricted immune response.

•Both the precise location of *C. trachomatis* within the genital tracts of these men and the predominance of either extracellular elementary bodies or intracellular reticulate bodies remain to be determined.

•The prevalence of asymptomatic male *C. trachomatis* infection may be greater than previously suspected.

•Whether *Chlamydia* detected in semen by the polymerase chain reaction is of clinical significance remains to be definitively established.

•Carriage of *C. trachomatis* in semen is associated with antisperm antibodies on ejaculated sperm and in sera of female partners.

•It has been hypothesized that subclinical chlamydial infections could induce epididymal obstructions that lead to macrophage ingestion of sperm and induction of sperm autoimmunity.

•In male genital tract infections the invading microorganisms can act as immune system adjuvants and induce T lymphocytes to release interferon gamma.

•This enables macrophages to efficiently engulf sperm and present processed sperm antigens to antibody producing cells.

•The current findings add further support to these hypotheses.

•Infertility with evidence of chlamydial infection may have been a result of inactivation of spermatozoa by antisperm antibodies.

•**Alternatively, should conception occur in these couples, repeated exposure to *C. trachomatis* with each act of coitus may eventually induce inflammatory changes in either the cervix, the endometrium, or both, which could impair embryo implantation or development.**

•A subclinical *C. trachomatis* infection may thus be a potential cause of unexplained infertility in some couples.

•It remains to be determined whether antibiotic treatment of infected couples will improve pregnancy outcome.

•The immune sensitization to spermatozoa, once established, would not be affected by elimination of the eliciting microorganism.

»Perhaps a more vigorous screening program to detect *C. trachomatis* in semen from symptom-free, sexually active young men and the prompt treatment of infected persons and their partner(s) would have a greater rate of success in reducing the incidence of unexplained infertility.

•If effective, such screening could also become an integral component of premarital examinations.]

---

24. True statements about the use of GnRH agonists during pregnancy include

  1. There are no known teratogenic effects on humans.
  2. Theoretically it could interfere with placental estrogen synthesis.
  3. GnRH is not found in the embryonic hypothalamus until 10 weeks of gestation.
  4. In the third trimester GnRH is present in high concentration in the placenta.

---

p. 588   Ans: E   (Young D C, Snabes M C. Poindexter A N III. GnRH agonist exposure during the first trimester of pregnancy. Obstet Gynecol 1993; 81:587)

24. [F & I: •Background: Gonadotropin-releasing hormone agonists are analogues of GnRH that are used for the palliative treatment of prostate cancer and endometriosis.

•They are used as adjunctive medication in general gynecology and in the treatment of infertility.

•GnRH agonists are contraindicated in pregnancy because of animal studies showing increased fetal mortality and decreased fetal weight.

•Objective: To analyze the pregnancy outcomes of five infertility patients with unrecognized exposure to leuprolide acetate in the first trimester.

•Gonadotropin-releasing hormone agonists are commonly used in gynecology for the treatment of leiomyomata and endometriosis, and in IVF cycles for pituitary and ovarian suppression before controlled ovarian hyperstimulation with human menopausal gonadotropins.

Obstetrics and Gynecology: Review 1994-Reproductive Endocrinology References

- The patients in this review were in an IVF stimulation protocol that required initiation of GnRH agonist injections on cycle day 21.

- A radioreceptor assay for hCG with a sensitivity of less than 5 mIU/ml performed at this time in a normal menstrual cycle would probably be negative, as hCG is undetectable until 9 days after the mid-cycle peak, which is 8 days after ovulation or 1 day after implantation.

- In other treatment protocols (i.e., endometriosis), patients should begin GnRH agonist administration during menses to avoid possible exposure during pregnancy.

- The potential for fetal morbidity and mortality from exposure to a GnRH agonist in the first trimester is probably related primarily to the drug-induced manipulation of the fetal hypothalamic-pituitary-ovarian axis during the embryonic stage of development.

- **GnRH is not found in the embryonic hypothalamus until 10 weeks.**

- The embryos were probably exposed to the agonist before the appearance of the decapeptide in normally developing embryos.

- In the late stages of pregnancy, the hypothalamic pituitary-ovarian axis is suppressed, probably because of the negative feedback effects of increased ovarian and placental steroids and other factors.

- Pituitary reserve in early pregnancy has not been studied, but based on the initial response observed with GnRH agonist therapy in nonpregnant patients (follicular flare), the length of drug exposure in these patients (14-to-21 days) may have increased maternal serum estrogen or progesterone levels.

- **GnRH agonist exposure during the second or third trimester of pregnancy may not be detrimental because GnRH is present in high concentration in the placenta.**

- Because the precise mechanism of GnRH action in the placenta is not known, it is difficult to speculate on the effect of exposure on early placental function.

- Placental GnRH synthesized in the cytotrophoblast induces an increase in hCG release by the syncytiotrophoblast.

- Because hCG is luteotrophic, it may also regulate steroid production in the fetus, most notably dehydroepiandrosterone sulfate (DHEAS).

- This steroid is important in the placental synthesis of estrogens, primarily estriol, which uses circulating fetal (and maternal) androgens as precursors.

- This synthesis of estrogens is essential for the maintenance of pregnancy.

- In non-human primate studies, GnRH antagonists and agonists have decrease hCG and progesterone production significantly and increase the pregnancy loss rate.

- This decrease in hCG production may possibly affect DHEAS production and estriol synthesis.

- In an unpublished study, a depot suspension of leuprolide acetate on day 6 of pregnancy produced a dose-related increase in major fetal abnormalities in rabbits (dosages of 0.00024, 0.0024, and 0.024 mg/kg), but caused no increase in fetal malformations in rats.

- An increase in fetal mortality and a decrease in fetal weight were observed with the two highest doses of leuprolide acetate in rabbits and the highest dose in rats.

  ° In rats, a dose-related increase in benign pituitary hyperplasia and benign pituitary adenomas was noted at 24 months when leuprolide acetate was administered at high doses (0.6-to-4 mg/kg/day) subcutaneously.

°The equivalent doses in these non-primate studies are, in a 70-kg human, 0.0168-to-280 mg/day, compared to the 0.5-mg/day dose in these patients.

•These studies suggest that the potential for fetal morbidity exists and that pregnant women exposed to GnRH agonists should be observed for potential complications.

•**Pregnancies in these patients should not be terminated based on drug exposure alone.**]

---

25. A patient with hyperandrogenic oligoamenorrhea is thought to have late onset adrenal hyperplasia. She is given a short-term ACTH stimulation test and subsequent 17-hydroxypregnenolone and DHEA levels were found to be twice normal levels. This is most likely due to

   1. increased activity of 17-hydroxylase.
   2. increased activity of 17,20-desmolase.
   3. 21-hydroxylase deficiency.
   4. 3ß-hydroxysteroid dehydrogenase deficiency.

p. 894   Ans: A   (Azziz R, Bradley E L, Potter H D, Boots L R. 3ß-Hydroxysteroid dehydrogenase deficiency in hyperandrogenism. Am J Obstet Gynec 1993; 168:889)

25. [F & I: •Background: Women with mild or partial adrenocortical 3ß-hydroxysteroid dehydrogenase deficiency presumed to represent late-onset adrenal hyperplasia have been identified.

•In contrast to the more severe congenital form of this deficiency, where the defect is often lethal, females with late-onset adrenal hyperplasia usually have hyperandrogenism with hirsutism and acne or primary amenorrhea or oligomenorrhea, although normal ovulatory function has also been described.

•Deficient 3ß-hydroxysteroid dehydrogenase adrenocortical activity has been reported in 5% to 30% of unselected hyperandrogenic women.

•3ß-hydroxysteroid dehydrogenase-deficient late-onset adrenal hyperplasia has been presumed when the enzymatic precursors dehydroepiandrosterone (DHEA) or 17-hydroxypregnenolone increase to above the mean plus **two** standard deviations of normal after adrenal stimulation.

•Alternatively, genetically defined individuals with the more common 21-hydroxylase-deficient late-onset adrenal hyperplasia demonstrate a precursor response to short-term corticotropin (ACTH) stimulation, a response that is at least **three- to sixfold** the upper normal limit.

•Because of these discrepancies in diagnostic criteria, the incidence of 3ß-hydroxysteroid dehydrogenase-deficient late-onset adrenal hyperplasia in hyperandrogenism is unknown, and the value of routinely screening symptomatic patients for this disorder has not been established.

•Adrenal androgens are frequently elevated in women with hyperandrogenism and hypersecretion of adrenal androgens may be secondary to inherited enzymatic deficiencies.

•The role of 3ß-hydroxysteroid dehydrogenase deficiencies in adrenal hyperandrogenism has not been well established.

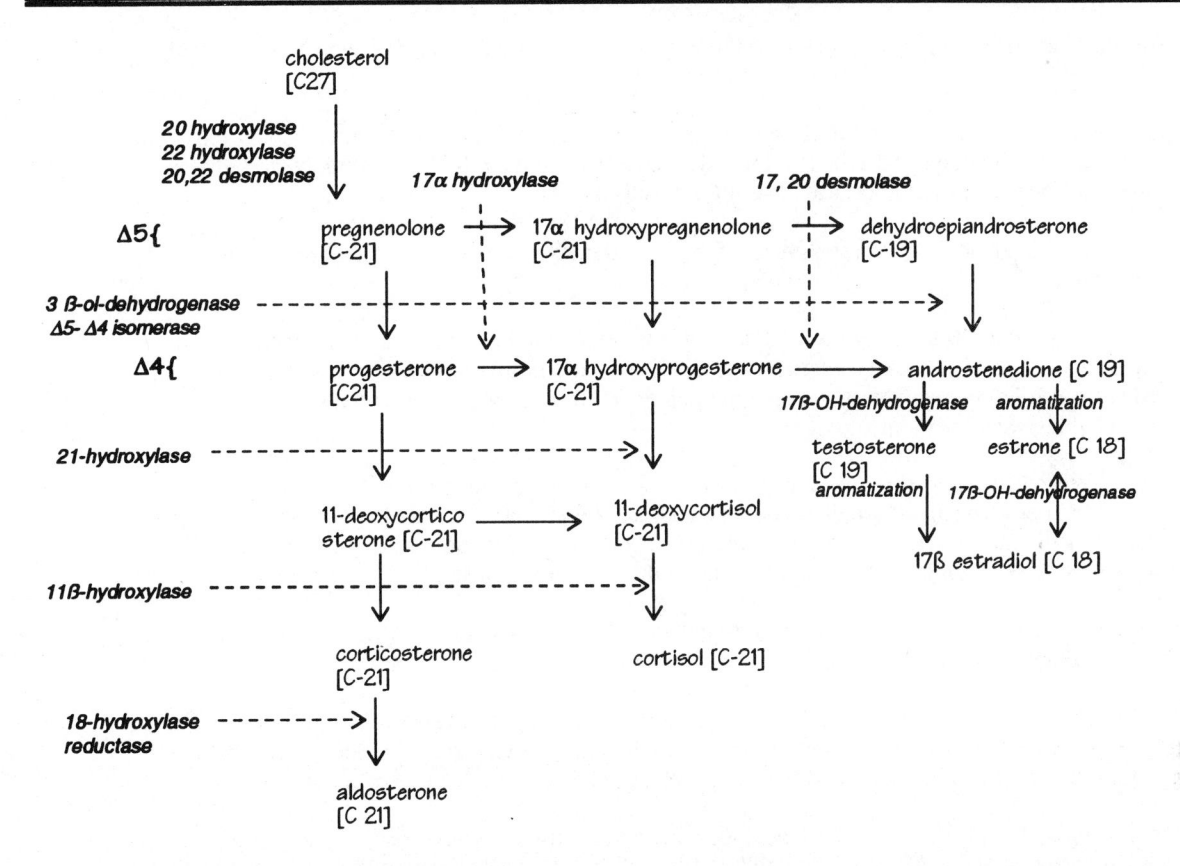

Metabolic Pathways of Ovarian and Adrenal Steroids

- **Objectives:** To determine the incidence of exaggerated 17-hydroxypregnenolone or DHEA responses to short-term ACTH (1-24) stimulation in unselected hyperandrogenic patients, to assess the relationship of these abnormalities with the presence of adrenal androgen excess and to determine the incidence of presumed 3ß-hydroxysteroid dehydrogenase-deficient late-set adrenal hyperplasia.

- The inherited deficiency of 3ß-hydroxysteroid dehydrogenase causes virilization of female fetus and adrenocortical insufficiency in both sexes.

- This deficiency may be seen in the older female, leading to the development of hyperandrogenic symptoms.

- It is presumed that this late presentation is a form of late-onset adrenal hyperplasia.

- Previous studies presume the presence of 3ß-hydroxysteroid dehydrogenase-deficient late-onset adrenal hyperplasia when the poststimulation 17-hydroxypregnenolone or DHEA level, or the 17-hydroxypregnenolone/17-hydroxyprogesterone or 17-hydroxypregnenolone/cortisol ratio, are anywhere above the mean + 2 SD of controls, although no family or genetic studies were available to confirm this criteria.

- Alternatively, individuals with 21-hydroxylase-deficient late-onset adrenal hyperplasia, many of whom the genetic nature of their disorder have been verified by family or molecular genetic studies, have poststimulation levels of the 17-hydroxylated enzymatic precursor at least threefold to sixfold above the upper control limit.

- Although steroid ratios have been proposed for the diagnosis of hydroxysteroid dehydrogenase-deficient late-onset adrenal hyperplasia, these ratios are unnecessary for the diagnosis of 21hydroxylase-deficient late-onset adrenal hyperplasia.

Obstetrics and Gynecology: Review 1994-Reproductive Endocrinology References

- Steroid ratios after short-term adrenal stimulation are much less reproducible than single steroid responses.

- The use of the mean ±2 SD for defining the upper normal limit does not take into account the skewedness in the distribution of hormonal values, skewedness caused by the fact that most steroid assays demonstrate a uniform lower limit because of limited sensitivity.

  ° Defining the upper limit as the 90th or 95th percentile takes into account the shape of this distribution.

  ° If one presumes 3ß-hydroxysteroid dehydrogenase-deficient late-onset adrenal hyperplasia to be present when the 17-hydroxypregnenolone or DHEA poststimulation level is above the mean ±2 SD of control as opposed to above the 95th percentile, the number of individuals presumed to be affected increases markedly.

- For the reasons detailed above, in the absence of appropriate genetic markers the presence of 3ß-hydroxysteroid dehydrogenase-deficient late-onset adrenal hyperplasia was presumed only when the 17-hydroxypregnenolone or DHEA level 1 hour after the short term intravenous administration of ACTH (1-24) was at least threefold the upper 95th percentile of the control response.

- With these criteria not one of 83 hyperandrogenic patients from this general white population could be diagnosed as having this disorder.

- Although approximately 22% and 2% of hyperandrogenic individuals had an exaggerated increment in 17-hydroxypregnenolone and DHEA after adrenal stimulation, respectively, the values were always within twofold the upper 95th percentile of the control response.

- In this report 19 (24%) women demonstrated isolated increases in 17-hydroxypregnenolone, 17-hydroxyprogesterone, DHEA, Δ^5-androstenediol; none of the patients had a response consistent with 3ß-hydroxysteroid dehydrogenase-deficient late-onset adrenal hyperplasia.

- Further evidence that the population of patients studied does not contain individuals with 3ß-hydroxysteroid dehydrogenase-deficient late-onset adrenal hyperplasia is apparent from the distribution of the 17-hydroxypregnenolone poststimulation (17-hydroxypregnenolone$_{60}$) values, where the levels form part of a continuum.

- In contrast, 21-hydroxylase-deficient late-onset adrenal hyperplasia patients are clearly denoted as outliers in the distribution of 17-hydroxyprogesterone values.

- In addition, the response of androstenedione and the 17-hydroxypregnenolone/17hydroxyprogesterone and DHEA/androstenedione ratios after ACTH stimulation were no different between the group of hyperandrogenic patients with and without an exaggerated 17-hydroxypregnenolone or DHEA response to adrenal stimulation.

- These measures of 3ß-hydroxysteroid dehydrogenase activity again suggest that the group of patients with exaggerated 17-hydroxypregnenolone or DHEA levels in response to ACTH do **not** have 3ß-hydroxysteroid dehydrogenase deficiency.

- The rarity of 3ß-hydroxysteroid dehydrogenase-deficient late-onset adrenal hyperplasia in adult hyperandrogenism is not surprising.

- Because inherited defects of this enzyme affect both the adrenals and gonads, a significant defect in the function of this enzyme would impair the production of Δ^4-steroids, including androgens, by the ovaries.

- Androgen production may be hindered, and the disorder could be lethal.

- In fact, boys congenitally affected with this enzymatic deficiency often have incomplete genital development.

•In addition to genetic abnormalities of 3ß-hydroxysteroid dehydrogenase, the activity of this enzyme can be modified by extrinsic factors.

°Some investigators have observed a decrease in 3ß-hydroxysteroid dehydrogenase activity after estrogen administration, whereas others have not observed a change.

°In regard to the effect of extraadrenal androgens on this enzyme, a change in 3ß-hydroxysteroid dehydrogenase activity could not been found, as measured by the DHEA and 17-hydroxypregnenolone response to short-term adrenal stimulation in oophorectomized women treated parentally with testosterone for 3 weeks.

°In the current study hyperandrogenic individuals who had an exaggerated incremental response in either 17-hydroxypregnenolone or DHEA did not have higher mean circulating total or free testosterone or androstenedione levels.

•Patients with an abnormal 17-hydroxypregnenolone or DHEA response had higher mean circulating DHEA sulfate levels than did controls.

°Whether the abnormal adrenocortical response is responsible for or secondary to the elevated levels is unknown.

•Many of the so-called "mild" or "partial" 3ß-hydroxysteroid dehydrogenase deficiencies may not be inherited but are acquired in response to extrinsic factors.

•The adrenal cortex is hyperresponsive to ACTH stimulation in approximately 40% of hyperandrogenic patients, which could also account for the exaggerated response of 17-hydroxypregnenolone and DHEA.

•An exaggerated activity of 17-hydroxylase or 17,20-desmolase may result in hyperandrogenism.

•This dysfunction could, in turn, lead to increased levels of 17-hydroxypregnenolone and DHEA levels after ACTH stimulation.

°Only family or molecular genetic studies of individuals with an exaggerated 17-hydroxypregnenolone or DHEA response to stimulation will determine whether there is a genetic basis for their abnormality.]

---

26. Causes of reproductive failure in patients with mild to moderate endometriosis include

    1. oligo-ovulation
    2. luteal phase defect
    3. luteinized unruptured follicle
    4. aseptic peritonitis

p. 592   Ans: E   (Levia M C, Hasty L A. Pfeifer S, Mastroianni L, Lyttle C R. Increased chemotactic activity of peritoneal fluid in patients with endometriosis. Am J Obstet Gynec 1993; 168:592)

26. [F & I: •Background: The underlying mechanisms indicating an association between minimal to moderate endometriosis and infertility are not clearly understood.

•Recent investigations have focused on the presence of an aseptic inflammation of the peritoneal cavity, resulting in a distortion of the normal function of the pelvic organs, as an important contributory mechanism.

•Other proposed causes for reproductive failure in the less severe cases of endometriosis include oligoanovulation, luteal phase defects, and luteinized unruptured follicle syndrome.

•These suggestions need to be clearly substantiated and each one cannot be considered the sole cause of infertility in patients with endometriosis.

Obstetrics and Gynecology: Review 1994-Reproductive Endocrinology References

•Other factors, which include alterations in the sperm-egg interaction with possible phagocytosis of the sperm or interference with early embryo development, must be taken into consideration when studying the associated infertility of these patients.

•The biochemical modifications that have been described in endometriosis include an increase in the concentration of prostaglandins, cytokines, and complement components in the peritoneal fluid and activation of resident macrophages.

•The activation of leukocytes within the peritoneal cavity is evidenced by cytoskeletal rearrangement of the cells and by changes in the lipid metabolism with activation of protein kinases or release of lysosomal enzymes.

•The role of peritoneal fluid in the physiologic modifications of the peritoneal cavity of patients who otherwise would seem to have a normal pelvic environment has been extensively studied.

•Endometriosis without severe anatomic distortion is associated with an increase in the peritoneal fluid volume, cell number, and concentration of lysosomic enzymes as compared with normal fertile controls.

•The peritoneal fluid arises primarily from two different sources: the plasma as a transudate and the ovary as an exudate; other sources are tubal fluid; retrograde menstruation, and secretions from the macrophages in the cavity.

•The exact source for the biochemical modifications observed in endometriosis is not known.

•Normally the peritoneal fluid contains several types of blood cells, with macrophages and lymphocytes being the most abundant; desquamated endometrial and mesothelial cells are also present.

•This cellular composition is modified in patients with endometriosis.

•Several theories exist regarding the mechanisms responsible for these alterations, one of which is the presence of a chemotactic stimulus that would attract more cells into the peritoneal cavity, or alternatively, activate and induce proliferation of resident macrophages in response to these unknown factors.

•Objective: To further investigate the role of the peritoneal fluid of patients with minimal to moderate endometriosis as a contributor to the inflammatory changes observed in the pelvic cavity of these patients.

•Results: Peritoneal fluid from patients with endometriosis has increased chemotactic activity for neutrophils and macrophages.

•Analysis of the chemotactic fractions gave evidence of the presence of a protein band with an estimated molecular weight of 20 kD only in the endometriosis samples, which is responsible for this activity.

•Patients with medical suppression as treatment for endometriosis have the lowest chemotactic activity.

•The cyclic variations in hormone concentrations are necessary for most of the biochemical modifications observed in the peritoneal fluid in endometriosis.

•This finding suggests that the observation of an increase in chemotactic activity may be hormonally regulated and further that a state of medically induced anovulation suppresses this activity.

•The suppression of chemotaxis to values even lower than those observed for fertile controls lends support to this hypothesis.

• This suppression of chemotactic activity could be considered an indicator of the success of the treatment.

• This would agree with previous reports indicating a reduction in the pelvic inflammation associated with endometriosis after treatment with medroxyprogesterone acetate.

• The chemotactic activity of the fluid is not exclusive for granulocytes because the migration of macrophages is also enhanced.

• Macrophages are the predominant cell type observed in the peritoneal fluid and in the cavity of patients with endometriosis.

• The presence of a chemotactic stimulus that will increase their number may also trigger their activation; this activation would result in the release of cytokines and cytotoxic factors that may be directly responsible for the modifications in the peritoneal environment.

• Endometriosis is a complex disease that involves modifications at the anatomic level with the presence of implants and endometriomas distributed throughout the pelvis; it also produces modifications at the cellular and molecular level, which would explain the findings observed in milder degrees of the disease.

• This is the first report of an increase in chemotactic activity of peritoneal fluid in patients with minimal to moderate endometriosis, which may be one of the many contributing mechanisms for the observed aseptic inflammation in the peritoneal cavity of these patients.]

---

27. Advantages of leuprolide over danazol for the treatment of endometriosis include

   1. more rapid onset
   2. less irregular bleeding
   3. more complete ovarian suppression
   4. decreases the disease process to a greater extent

p. 1370   Ans: A   (Wheeler J M, Knittle J D. Miller J D. Depot leuprolide versus danazol in treatment of women with symptomatic endometriosis. I. Efficacy results. Am J Obstet Gynec 1992; 167:1367)

27. [F & I: •Background: Endometriosis is one of the most common causes of pelvic pain and involuntary infertility in women.

• Treatment of this disease in women desiring future childbearing continues to be disappointing:

• Surgical treatment is associated with high recurrence rates (up to 40% after 5 years), and medical treatment is associated with a high likelihood of side effects and recurrence rates similar to those seen with surgery.

• Three drugs have received Food and Drug Administration (FDA) approval for treatment of women with endometriosis: danazol, depot leuprolide, and intranasal nafarelin.

• Intranasal administration of a gonadotropin-releasing hormone (GnRH) agonist was proved efficacious in treating symptomatic endometriosis by suppressing endogenous estradiol production, with resulting atrophy of uterine and ectopic endometrial tissue.

• Previously, GnRH agonist administration has required multiple daily injections or intranasal inhalations twice daily; concerns with compliance have resulted from these frequent dosing requirements.

• A depot form of GnRH agonist, Lupron Depot 3.75 mg (leuprolide acetate for depot suspension), provides continuous release of drug over a 4-week period when administered as a monthly intramuscular injection.

- For women with endometriosis, the depot formulation promised improved patient acceptability and compliance, as well as potentially faster, more profound suppression of ovarian estradiol production.

- Objective: To compare the safety and efficacy of depot leuprolide and danazol in the treatment of women with endometriosis.

- Danazol has been in common use for women with endometriosis since 1973, but its use is often associated with troublesome side effects and high rates of recurrent symptoms.

- GnRH agonists were first used in clinical trials for treatment of endometriosis in 1981.

- The vast majority of these GnRH agonist studies were uncontrolled cohort studies; there have been only two large multicenter randomized clinical trials comparing a GnRH agonist to danazol.

- Depot forms of GnRH agonist may prove to induce a more rapid suppression of ovarian steroidogenesis than daily injections.

- Daily nasal administration of GnRH agonist suppresses ovarian function less quickly than depot forms but seemingly more quickly than danazol.

- A more rapid induction of ovarian suppression may induce a faster regression of endometriosis implants.

- Depot forms of GnRH agonist may allow shorter courses of medical treatment in the future, thereby decreasing long-term side effects and costs to patients.

- The current study, with its once-monthly administration of GnRH agonist, functionally removes the importance of compliance issues with daily dosage.

- In addition, the depot formulation increases confidence in proper drug administration in this trial, as there is no commonly available serum assay otherwise to assure delivery of GnRH agonist.

- The conclusion that the two drugs are similar in efficacy as measured by the reduction in the revised American Fertility Society score is particularly firm because of the trial's sample size and statistical power, combined with the lack of demonstrable subtle biases that could have swayed the trial toward leuprolide.

- Agreement was found between outcome assessed by total revised American Fertility Society score and that portion of the score contributed by active endometriosis implants without concomitant adhesions.

- Depot leuprolide was proved as effective as danazol in reducing the extent of endometriosis measured by the revised American Fertility Society classification.

- Ovarian suppression by depot leuprolide was more prompt, more complete as judged by estradiol levels, and associated with a slightly greater proportion of rapid onset of amenorrhea without irregular bleeding.

- It seems that depot leuprolide is at least as efficacious as danazol in treating endometriosis.]

GYNECOLOGIC ONCOLOGY

Directions: Each of the questions or incomplete statements below is followed by several suggested answers or completions. Select the BEST answer in each case.

1. A patient has a stage II carcinoma of the fallopian tube treated with platinum and cyclophosphamide subsequent to complete staging and removal of all observably involved tissue. Six weeks after completion of chemotherapy, a negative second look laparotomy was diagnosed. What is the chance that the patient will continue to remain disease free?

   A. 50%
   B. 67%
   C. 75%
   D. 80%
   E. 90%

2. What percentage of women found to have a positive test for HPV DNA using a standard dot-blot hybridization test will eliminate the infection within 18 months?

   A. 5
   B. 10
   C. 15
   D. 20
   E. >25

3. The dose limiting toxicity of Rhenium 186-labeled monoclonal antibody administered intraperitoneally for the treatment of ovarian epithelial cancer is

   A. fever.
   B. gastrointestinal complications.
   C. hepatic toxicity.
   D. myelosuppression.
   E. rash.

4. After fetal lung maturity was assured, a patient with stage IB cervical carcinoma is to have a cesarean hysterectomy. The most common maternal complication to be expected is

   A. deep venous thrombosis.
   B. hemorraghic cystitis.
   C. lymphocyst.
   D. need for blood transfusion.
   E. wound infection.

5. A preoperative distinction between benign and malignant ovarian cysts can be reliably made by

   A. cyst fluid CA 125.
   B. cyst fluid cytology.
   C. serum CA 125.
   D. vaginal ultrasonography with color doppler examination.
   E. none of the above.

6. A patient has a stage IB cervical squamous cell carcinoma with a tumor diameter of four centimeters. Survival can be increased by

   A. chemotherapy followed by radial surgery followed by radiotherapy.
   B. chemotherapy followed by radical surgery.
   C. chemotherapy followed by radiotherapy.
   D. radiotherapy followed by radical surgery.
   E. none of the above.

7. The most cost effective strategy for a patient at low risk (less than 5%) of endometrial cancer who has post-menopausal bleeding is

   A. ambulatory D&C.
   B. hysterectomy.
   C. no further work-up; wait for bleeding to recur, then investigate.
   D. office biopsy.
   E. none of the above

8. The most important feature of a test that evaluates a pelvic mass for possible malignancy is

   A. negative predictive value.
   B. positive predictive value.
   C. sensitivity.
   D. specificity.
   E. All characteristics have the same importance.

9. Associated with improved survival in patients with high risk stage I ovarian cancer

   A. adriamycin.
   B. cisplatinum.
   C. melphalan.
   D. P^{32}.
   E. none of the above.

10. The most powerful predictor of a disease-free interval for patients with stage I ovarian epithelial carcinoma is

    A. ascites.
    B. degree of cellular differentiation.
    C. DNA ploidy.
    D. FIGO substage.
    E. rupture of the capsule during surgery.

11. The most discriminating factor in determining the presence of ovarian cancer in an adnexal mass is

    A. age.
    B. CA 125.
    C. gray scale ultrasound.
    D. pulsatility index.
    E. resistance index.

12. 95% of patients with hydatidiform mole can be expected to have normal hCG levels how many weeks after evacuation?

    A. 6
    B. 7
    C. 11
    D. 19
    E. 25

13. In a closed system, the half-life of CA 125 approximates

    A. 1 day
    B. 5 days
    C. 10 days
    D. 14 days
    E. 21 days

14. A 28-year old patient who had a negative history for cervical neoplasia has a hysterectomy for benign disease. The specimen shows invasive squamous cell carcinoma of the cervix. True statements about this situation include

    A. five-year survival with no further treatment is greater than 50%
    B. reoperation should be immediate
    C. reoperation should include radical parametrectomy, upper vaginectomy, pelvic lymphadenectomy, and bilateral salpingo-oophorectomy
    D. the morbidity from reoperation exceeds its benefit
    E. treatment depends on whether the tumor was cut through

15. A patient with squamous cell carcinoma of the vulva which is 1.5 centimeters in diameter is found to have a positive lymph node metastasis. Using the FIGO surgical classification the cancer is

    A. Stage I
    B. Stage II
    C. Stage III
    D. Stage IV

16. A 180 pound patient is to have a Class III radical hysterectomy and pelvic lymphadenectomy for Stage IB squamous cell cervical cancer. What result can be expected?

    A. increased incidence of bladder dysfunction
    B. increased incidence of blood transfusion
    C. increased incidence of deep pain thrombosis
    D. increased incidence of urinary tract injuries
    E. increased incidence of wound infection

17. Which of the following is the LEAST reliable predictor in cases of stage I invasive squamous cell carcinoma of the cervix?

    A. depth of invasion
    B. flow cytometry analysis
    C. lesion size
    D. lymph node metastasis
    E. penetration of vascular channels

18. True statements about the induction of uterine neoplasms during tamoxifen therapy for cancer of the breast include all of the following EXCEPT

    A. Most cancers are FIGO stage I.
    B. The cancers are only adenocarcinomas and not sarcomas.
    C. The induction is dose-related.
    D. The patients are likely to have symptoms associated with uterine cancer.
    E. The patients are most likely to be postmenopausal.

19. True statements about intraepithelial cervical neoplasia in patients with HIV include all of the following EXCEPT

    A. Cryotherapy is ineffective in treating the CIN.
    B. Patients with CD4 counts below 500 per cubic millimeter are at increased risk of recurrence.
    C. The mode of acquisition of HIV is irrelevant to the recurrent of CIN.
    D. The prevalence rate is related to the degree of immunosuppression.
    E. The recurrence rate is high after standard treatment.

20. The morbidity from selective pelvic and periaortic lymphadenectomy in patients with endometrial carcinoma is related to all of the following EXCEPT

    A. operating time
    B. patient age
    C. patient weight
    D. surgeon
    E. the lymphadenectomy itself

Directions: Each set of lettered headings below is followed by a list of numbered words or phrases. For each numbered word or phrase select:

A. if the item is associated with *(A) only*
B. if the item is associated with *(B) only*
C. if item is associated with *both (A) and (B)*
D. if item is associated with *neither (A) nor (B)*

Items 21-23.

In the treatment of invasive cervical cancer stage IB

    A. Schauta-Amreich vaginal hysterectomy
    B. Wertheim-Meigs abdominal hysterectomy
    C. both
    D. neither

21. complication rate about 5%

22. five-year survival about 80%

23. performed with lymphadenectomy

Items 24-26.

    A. cervical adenocarcinoma in situ
    B. cervical squamous cell carcinoma in situ
    C. both
    D. neither

24. cervical cone biopsy with uninvolved margins and negative ECC is diagnostically accurate

25. cervical cone biopsy is adequate treatment

26. if cone margins are involved expected management is reasonable

Directions: For each of the questions or incomplete statements below, ONE or MORE of the answers or completions given is correct. In each case select:

A. if only 1, 2, and 3 are correct
B. if only 1 and 3 are correct
C. if only 2 and 4 are correct
D. if only 4 is correct
E. if all are correct

27. Survival of patients with epithelial ovarian cancer is affected by

    1. stage of disease.
    2. sensitivity to platinum therapy.
    3. histologic grade.
    4. performance status.

28. Incisions used for the extraperitoneal dissection required for lymphadenectomy in patients with advanced invasive squamous cell carcinoma of the cervix include

    1. bilateral superior groin incision.
    2. unilateral J-shaped incision.
    3. upper abdominal vertical incision.
    4. upper abdominal transverse incision.

29. According to the international classification of cancer of the cervix, characteristics of Stage IB include

    1. must be visible clinically.
    2. the depth of invasion < 5 millimeters.
    3. involvement of the upper third of the vagina only.
    4. horizontal spread greater >7 millimeters.

30. Hypothalamic GnRH is produced by

   1. normal ovary.
   2. placenta.
   3. ovarian epithelial cancer.
   4. dysgerminoma.

31. Patients with invasive endometrial adenocarcinoma should have lymph node sampling if

   1. histology is grade 3.
   2. greater than 50% of myometrium is invaded.
   3. stage II/III disease.
   4. palpably suspicious paraaortic nodes.

32. Tumor markers found in ovarian inclusion cysts include

   1. ß-hCG.
   2. CEA.
   3. CA125.
   4. placental lactogen.

33. Indications for bilateral salpingo-oophorectomy in a premenopausal patient undergoing radical hysterectomy for invasive cervical neoplasia include

   1. 20% of premenopausal patients will experience early gonadal failure.
   2. 5-to-8% will require additional surgery for benign ovarian disease.
   3. 1.4% will develop ovarian carcinoma.
   4. sexual functioning is not adversely affected.

34. Uterine effects of tamoxifen associated with the treatment of breast cancer include increased incidence of

   1. endocervical polyp.
   2. endometrial polyp.
   3. endometrial hyperplasia.
   4. endometrial cancer.

35. Methods used to analyze the zygosity of molar gestations include

   1. protein heteromorphisms.
   2. cytogenetics.
   3. Southern blotting.
   4. polymerase chain reaction.

36. Increased recurrence rates of endometrial carcinoma are associated with

   1. aneuploidy.
   2. increasing percentage of S-phase fraction.
   3. DNA index.
   4. proliferation index.

37. CSF-1 production has been identified with malignancies of

   1. pancreas
   2. ovary
   3. breast
   4. trophoblast

38. True statements about estrogen and progesterone receptors include

   1. there is an inverse relationship between the content of estrogen and progesterone receptors and the stage of endometrial carcinoma
   2. there is an inverse relationship between the content of estrogen and progesterone receptors and grade
   3. adenomatous hyperplasia has relatively high levels of progesterone receptors
   4. receptor rich tumors grow more slowly than receptor poor tumors

39. Factors associated with poor survival in patients with squamous cell carcinoma of the vulva

   1. recurrence within two years
   2. lymph node involvement
   3. tumor grade
   4. initial stage

40. Tumoricidal action of TNF-α against human ovarian cell lines can be increased by

   1. actinomycin D
   2. cycloheximide
   3. emitine
   4. diphtheria toxin

41. Interferon gamma

    1. increases EGF receptor expression
    2. decreases EGF receptor expression
    3. down regulates HER/*neu* levels
    4. increases expression of CEA

42. The E7 oncoprotein associated with HPV 16 promotes

    1. immortalization
    2. growth
    3. altered differentiation
    4. chromosomal abnormalities

43. Histologic variables which significantly increase the risk of other genital primary squamous neoplasms in patients with vulvar carcinoma include

    1. HPV positive VIN
    2. hyperplasia
    3. epithelial-like carcinomas
    4. keratinizing growth pattern

44. Comprehensive surgical staging laparotomy in early ovarian cancer includes

    1. blind biopsies from the anterior and posterior cul-de-sac
    2. omentectomy
    3. cytologic sampling of the right hemidiaphragm
    4. paraaortic lymphadenectomy

GYNECOLOGIC ONCOLOGY REFERENCES

Directions: Each of the questions or incomplete statements below is followed by several suggested answers or completions. Select the BEST answer in each case.

1. A patient has a stage II carcinoma of the fallopian tube treated with platinum and cyclophosphamide subsequent to complete staging and removal of all observably involved tissue. Six weeks after completion of chemotherapy, a negative second look laparotomy was diagnosed. What is the chance that the patient will continue to remain disease free?

   A. 50%.
   B. 67%.
   C. 75%.
   *D. 80%.
   E. 90%.

p. 750 (Barakat R R, Rubin S C, Saigo P E, Lewis, Jr. J L. Jones W B, Curtin J P. Second-look laparotomy in carcinoma of the fallopian tube. Obstet Gynecol 1993; 82:748)

1. [F & I: •Background: Carcinoma of the fallopian tube accounts for 0.31-to-1.11% of all gynecologic cancers.

•Because of the clinical and histologic similarity between tubal and epithelial ovarian carcinoma, most patients are treated in an identical manner with cytoreductive surgery and platinum-based combination chemotherapy.

•There is a 53-to-75% complete response rate to platinum-based combination chemotherapy, with 51% of patients with advanced-stage disease surviving 5 years.

•This result suggests a better response to treatment than that of advanced ovarian cancer.

•Second-look laparotomy, an integral part of management of patients with ovarian cancer, is performed in patients who are clinically free of disease after a prescribed course of chemotherapy.

•The rationale for this procedure is to determine the effectiveness of therapy and to provide information on disease status that cannot be reliably obtained by noninvasive means, thus allowing further treatment if necessary.

•In patients with advanced ovarian cancer, approximately 50% will have disease detected at second-look laparotomy.

•Approximately half of the patients with advanced-stage disease and a negative second-look following platinum-based chemotherapy will eventually have a recurrence.

•Objective: To define more clearly the role of second-look laparotomy in carcinoma of the fallopian tube.

•Tumors were graded by applying the World Health Organization criteria for epithelial ovarian cancer.

•All patients had cytoreductive surgery initially, usually consisting of a total abdominal hysterectomy with bilateral salpingo-oophorectomy as a minimum, and aggressive debulking as indicated.

•In addition to resection of the primary tumor, patients whose disease appeared confined to the pelvis underwent surgical staging including abdominal exploration, peritoneal washings, infracolic omentectomy, and pelvic and/or aortic node sampling.

•Following surgery, all patients were treated with platinum and cyclophosphamide with or without doxorubicin.

Obstetrics and Gynecology:Review 1994-Gynecologic Oncology References

- •Because of the rarity of the disease, most of the currently used treatment strategies for fallopian tube cancer, including surgical debulking and adjuvant chemotherapy, are based on those employed in the management of epithelial ovarian cancer.

- •Disease status at second-look provided important prognostic information.

- •Of the 21 patients with a negative second-look, only four (19%) have had recurrence.

- •This contrasts with advanced stage ovarian carcinoma patients treated with platinum-based chemotherapy, among whom approximately 50% will experience recurrence following a negative second-look procedure, with a median interval of 14 months to recurrence.

- •Excluding the three stage I lesions, only 22% recurred following a negative second-look procedure, with a mean interval of 38 months to recurrence, possibly suggesting a less aggressive biologic behavior of this tumor compared to ovarian cancer.

- •Of concern are two patients who had a recurrence outside of the abdominal cavity after a negative second-look procedure.

- •Based on this experience, second-look laparotomy is recommended in patients with stages II-to-IV tubal cancer.

- •Reexploration provides a more accurate assessment of tumor status so that further treatment can be given if necessary, allows secondary cytoreduction, and provides important prognostic information.

- •Although the numbers are small, patients who have a negative second-look following platinum-based chemotherapy for tubal cancer have approximately an 80% chance of remaining disease-free.

- •Those with persistent disease at second-look can be treated further, and approximately 30% will be expected to survive 5 years.

- •The small number of patients with stage I disease prevents commenting on the usefulness of second-look procedures in this group.]

---

2. What percentage of women found to have a positive test for HPV DNA using a standard dot-blot hybridization test will eliminate the infection within 18 months?

   A. 5
   B. 10
   C. 15
   D. 20
   *E. >25

p. 583 (Moscicki A, Palefsky J, Smith G, Siboshski S, Schoolnik G. Variability of human papillomavirus DNA testing in a longitudinal cohort of young women. Obstet Gynecol 1993; 82:578)

2. [F & I: •Background: Recent advances in DNA diagnostics have found the relationship between human papillomavirus (HPV) infections and human disease.

- •One of the most serious consequences related to HPV infections is cervical precancer or cancer.

- •High-grade precancers and invasive cancers of the cervix are associated with specific HPV types, most commonly HPVs 16 and 18.

- •In studies of the prevalence of HPV infections, women positive for HPV DNA, specifically types 16 and 18, were more likely to have abnormal cytology or histology than women negative for HPV DNA.

- •These studies also found that a significant proportion of women positive for HPV DNA had **no** clinical or cytologic evidence of cervical disease.

- Because these studies were primarily cross-sectional, the long-term implication of these positive HPV DNA tests in "normal" women remains undetermined.

- It has been suggested that all HPV infections result in lifelong carriage of the organism and that the virus may remain "clinically silent" or latent.

- Some HPV DNA-positive women become HPV DNA-negative by dot blot and Southern hybridization techniques when repeated cervical samplings are conducted within a limited period.

- The implication of these repeated negative tests is unknown, as the techniques used in these studies require fairly large copy numbers of viral DNA for detection, and specimens with relatively few DNA copies may give falsely negative test results.

- Few studies have examined the variability in HPV DNA testing over a long period.

- Objectives: To examine the variability in HPV DNA testing of the cervix using a standard RNA-DNA hybridization technique and the more sensitive polymerase chain reaction technique, and to ascertain how these viral DNA detection results compare with the results of repeated cytology determinations in a longitudinal cohort of young women.

- Based on studies showing the existence of HPV DNA in normal tissue, some have hypothesized that HPV infections result in lifelong infection.

- Results: **The data suggest that half of women infected with HPV appear to eradicate the disease**.

- In this longitudinal cohort, 54% of women who were positive for the specific HPV types 6, 11, 16, 18, 31, 33, or 35 at their initial visit appeared to eliminate the original infection, as defined by two or more consecutively negative tests for the specific HPV DNA using RNA-DNA hybridization and polymerase chain reaction.

- When women with other HPV types were included, a similar rate of elimination (52%) occurred.

- The belief that a "true" eradication occurred in this population is supported by the absence of abnormal cytology and by the high sensitivity of the polymerase chain reaction technique, which in principle can detect one virion, but which in practice usually detects 100-to-500 virions.

- Because polymerase chain reaction requires that virus-containing tissue be obtained for analyses, some of the negative tests may have been due to a sampling error, but it is unlikely that this would have occurred repeatedly in the same patient.

- The cervices of patients with repeatedly negative polymerase chain reaction had neither latent nor active HPV cervical infection.

- Age-stratified data for rates of HPV positivity from cross-sectional studies also have suggested that many women clear the infection spontaneously.

- Although these results support the idea that the human host may, in fact, eliminate the viral infection, they do not exclude the possibility of viral latency.

- In comparison with the women who appeared to remain HPV DNA-negative, nearly 50% of the group remained consistently or intermittently positive.

- In contrast to the initial infection with a high viral load, the majority of the persistent infections were low-level ones, defined by tests positive by the polymerase chain reaction only.

- In addition, the majority of these women were intermittently HPV DNA-positive by one or both methods.

- A persistent infection with high viral loads, defined by a consistently positive test by RNA-DNA hybridization, was the exception.

- It is noteworthy that there was no difference in the rates of positivity by either detection method between the first year of follow-up and 24 months or more, suggesting that women who clear the infection do so early on.

- **Taken together, these data seem to indicate that the number of virions decreases over a relatively short period and the infection will be terminated in a subset of women, whereas in another group of women the infection will persist.**

- The persisting infection is predominantly a low-level one with what appears to be an occasional viral activation producing an infection with high viral loads.

- An even smaller subset of this group appears to sustain the infection with relatively high viral numbers.

- These patients warrant further study for the possibility of having developed a true latent HPV infection, for a possibly increased risk of developing cytologic abnormalities, and for consideration of immunologic differences compared to women who successfully terminate the infective process.

- The rates of HPV positivity, regardless of original type, ranged at 20-to-58%, depending on the method and interval.

- This variability is most likely influenced by two factors: the variability of viral replication and the elusive contribution of new infections or re-infections.

- When the women with new HPV types were examined, most reported having acquired a new sexual partner since the last one or two visits from the appearance of the new type.

- The incubation period for HPV (i.e., the period from exposure to a positive test) is unknown.

- The data suggest that the incubation period may be **several months**, as many of the subjects with a new type reported exposure to a new partner over 4 months before the appearance of the new HPV type.

- This period could be substantially shorter, as subjects may have become positive sometime during the 4-month interval.

- The oscillation between positive and negative HPV DNA results by both detection methods in some patients suggests that these "new" types could, in fact, reflect reactivation of previously unrecognized infections.

- These postulates also affect interpretation of the reappearances of the original types, specifically after several months of negative tests.

- Such reappearances may reflect a new infection and not reactivation.

- Unfortunately, this question remains difficult to answer because studies will always be plagued with sampling error, variability in polymerase chain reaction amplification, and unknown partner behavior.

- Although the patterns of positivity and negativity were somewhat perplexing, the preliminary findings suggest a relationship between patterns of HPV DNA testing and the development of cervical disease.

- This relationship was primarily evident for women who eventually became HPV DNA-negative.

- None of these women developed significant cervical disease and all women who appeared to undergo spontaneous regression subsequently became HPV DNA-negative.

- In contrast, the relationship between cervical disease and sustained or intermittent positivity remains ambiguous, most likely because of the small number of subjects who developed significant cervical disease and the relatively short period of follow-up.

•The only woman to develop a high-grade lesion remained HPV DNA-positive by polymerase chain reaction and RNA-DNA hybridization for nearly 3 years.

•Several subjects have been persistently positive for HPV DNA but continue to remain cytologically normal.

•When the results of these two studies are taken together, the presence of a sustained, relatively high level of infection would appear to be necessary, but not sufficient, for the development of CIN or cancer.

•The fact that some persistently infected women are cytologically normal may indicate that cofactors, such as the host immune response, act in the development of cervical disease or that sustained infectivity at a high level may be needed for much longer periods in certain women before CIN ensues.

•Most of the women who remained polymerase chain reaction-positive for a significant length of time but had negative tests using RNA-DNA hybridization did not develop abnormal cytology.

•This implies that women who remain infected with HPV at a low level are at low risk of developing significant disease.]

---

3. The dose limiting toxicity of Rhenium 186-labeled monoclonal antibody administered intraperitoneally for the treatment of ovarian epithelial cancer is

   A. fever.
   B. gastrointestinal complications.
   C. hepatic toxicity.
   *D. myelosuppression.
   E. rash.

p. 590 (Jacobs A J, Fer M, Su F, Breitz H, Thompson, Goodgold H, Cain J, Heaps J, Weiden P. A Phase I Trail of a Rhenium 186-labeled Monoclonal Antibody Administered Intraperitoneally in Ovarian Carcinoma:Toxicity and Response. Obstet Gynecol 1993; 82:586)

3. [F & I: •Background: Ovarian carcinoma is the leading cause of death from gynecologic cancer and the fourth most common cause of cancer mortality among women in the United States.

•The majority of these patients present with metastatic disease, which is usually located in the peritoneal cavity.

•Most such patients die of peritoneal carcinomatosis.

•Optimal treatment of primary metastatic ovarian carcinoma consists of aggressive surgical cytoreduction followed by combination chemotherapy that includes cisplatin or carboplatin.

•Forty to fifty percent of women treated in this manner may demonstrate a complete response at second-look laparotomy, but up to 50% of complete responders experience recurrence.

•Treatment of overt and microscopic peritoneal lesions, although necessary, is not sufficient because a significant minority of patients also harbor extraperitoneal metastases.

•For example, 10-to-20% of women with no extraperitoneal metastases have tumor in the pelvic or aortic nodes.

•Therapeutic strategies must focus on destruction of tumor both in peritoneal and distant sites.

•Intraperitoneal beta-emitting radionuclides have long been used as adjuvant treatment for early ovarian carcinoma, as well as in women with minimal residual disease observed at second-look laparotomy following chemotherapy.

- The most frequently used radionuclide has been colloidal radioactive phosphorus (^{32}P). A large controlled study suggested that intraperitoneal ^{32}P colloid was as effective as oral melphalan in adjuvant postoperative treatment of stage II and high-risk stage I lesions.

- Almost all ^{32}P colloid remains in the peritoneal cavity following administration.

- Beta-emitters penetrate no more than 3 mm into tissues.

- This minimizes enteritis, but makes colloidal ^{32}P ineffective against all but the smallest tumor masses.

- Beta-emitting radionuclides have been complexed with monoclonal antibodies directed against tumor antigens in an attempt to direct the radiation to tumors, thereby allowing treatment of tumor while minimizing exposure of normal tissues to radiation.

- Such complexes are administered in solution, rather than as a colloid, so they are distributed throughout the body.

- The concentration of labeled monoclonal antibody in tumor was demonstrated in 1979 using a labeled antibody against a murine teratocarcinoma.

- Rhenium 186 is an attractive radioisotope for use with monoclonal antibodies.

- Its half-life is shorter than that of ^{131}I or ^{32}P (89.25 hours versus 8.0 and 14.2 days).

- The energy and, consequently, the tissue penetration of the beta emission of ^{186}Re are greater than those of ^{131}I and ^{32}P, Rhenium 186 emits a lower level of gamma radiation than ^{131}I, making it safer to handle, while still permitting the tracking of infused isotope by gamma camera imaging.

- In this study, ^{186}Re was complexed with NR-LU-10, a murine monoclonal immunoglobulin (Ig) reactive with a tumor antigen present on essentially all ovarian cancers.

- This complex was infused intraperitoneally into patients with persistent ovarian epithelial carcinoma in a dose-escalating phase I study.

- Objectives: 1) to determine the maximum tolerated dose and spectrum of toxicity of this preparation,

- 2) to determine whether this complex can effect clinical responses in patients with intraperitoneal metastases of ovarian carcinoma persistent or recurrent after primary treatment with cisplatin-based chemotherapy,

- 3) to measure the radiation distribution to normal structures, and

- 4) to establish the fate of the infused isotope.

- Chemotherapy and, to a lesser extent, whole abdominal external radiation are the standard postoperative adjuvant treatments for ovarian carcinoma.

- They result in a limited number of cures in stages III and IV disease.

- Tumor site-directed therapy represents another strategy with potential promise for treating ovarian cancer.

- In an attempt to control peritoneal disease and enhance overall survival, investigators have administered radioisotopes or cytotoxic drugs directly into the peritoneal cavity.

- Drug distribution after intraperitoneal administration of cytotoxic chemotherapeutic agents show that they are absorbed over the course of a few hours.

- This results in a peritoneal exposure to drugs, as measured by concentration x time, that is 30-to-1000 times greater than can be achieved by IV administration.

- At the same time, systemic concentration x time, as estimated by serial blood drug levels, is comparable to that obtained with IV administration.

- Early results with this form of treatment have shown promise.

- The pharmacologic advantage of intraperitoneal drug administration applies only to the treatment of extremely small lesions, as no drug is likely to diffuse further than 1 mm into solid tumor.

- Intraperitoneal treatment with ^{32}P, a pure beta-emitter given in colloid form, has three potential advantages over cytotoxic drugs.

- First, treatment consists of one administration of isotope and is less time-consuming, inconvenient, and uncomfortable than a course of chemotherapy.

- Second, only 2% of patients should have severe adverse effects consisting of chronic radiation enteritis.

- Finally, few cells are resistant to radiation if the patient has received no previous radiation or chemotherapy.

- Minimal gross disease can be treated adequately provided that the infusate has access to all areas of the peritoneal cavity.

- The disadvantage of such treatment is that essentially all radiation remains confined to the peritoneal cavity and thoracic nodes, leaving untreated any distant disease as well as disease protected by peritoneal adhesions.

- Rhenium 186-NR-LU-10 combines the theoretical advantages of ^{32}P colloid and solutions of cytotoxic drugs.

- It is administered with the same ease as is ^{32}P colloid.

- The peritoneal concentration x time of 186ReNR-LU-10 was 20-to-40 times greater than the comparable serum values.

- This magnitude is similar to that seen with many cytotoxic drugs.

- It is hoped that the monoclonal antibody, which reacts selectively with tumor cells, will enhance the differential radiation exposure between tumor cells and normal peritoneum, providing a greater therapeutic index than might be obtained by administering the isotope without a targeting agent.

- Eventually, this agent must be compared with ^{32}P colloid in a randomized trial to determine whether it offers a therapeutic advantage over the nonspecific colloid.

- The results obtained in this trial are preliminary, but encouraging.

- Rhenium 186-NR-LU-10 can be administered safely in doses capable of producing a clinical response.

- **The dose-limiting toxicity appears to be myelosuppression.**

- Significant myelosuppression was seen when 150 mCi/m^2 of ^{186}Re was infused.

- The maximum safe dose of ^{186}Re-NR-LU-10, given as a single intraperitoneal infusion, appears to be 120-150 mCi/m^2, and the dose-limiting complication is thrombocytopenia.

- In all these patients, previous cytotoxic chemotherapy was a contributing factor in the toxicity of absorbed doses of 110 cGy to marrow.

- Few of the patients in this trial survived long enough to be exposed to chronic radiation enteritis, which has limited the dose of other isotopes given intraperitoneally.

- Final determination of the incidence of enteric complications must await larger trials on women with a longer life expectancy.

- The estimated dose of radiation to both small and large intestine was less than 100 cGy/mCi of isotope injected in any subject, which suggests that enteric complications will not be a major problem.

- The systemic absorption of the isotope provides a rationale for believing that enteric complications will be less likely than after administration of a radionuclide in colloid form.

- The enteric complication rate for ^{32}P has been markedly reduced by insuring good distribution of aqueous intraperitoneal injections before radionuclide infusion, and by eschewing the combination of intraperitoneal radionuclide infusion and external pelvic radiation.

- In this trial, both of these precautions were observed.

- Based on dose escalation studies of IV ^{186}Re-NR-LU10, dosimetric data suggest that patients with adequate renal and hepatic function will **not** develop clinically significant toxicity at doses sufficient to cause myelosuppression.

- Although abnormal liver function tests were observed in most patients, they were readily reversible, and there were no symptoms related to hepatic toxicity.

- In addition, there was no evidence of renal damage.

- In other studies using IV ^{186}Re-NR-LU10, mild fever, elevated liver function tests, and nausea were observed frequently, and were unrelated to the ^{186}Re dose level.

- All patients developed human anti-mouse antibodies.

- This may limit the sequential use of this agent, requiring that it be administered in fractions clustered no more than a week apart.

- This problem most likely can be minimized by use of chimeric or humanized antibodies, or by simultaneous administration of immunosuppressive agents such as cyclosporine A.

- Four of seven women with minimal disease achieved an objective clinical response.

- Most subjects were heavily treated before study entry and had extensive and bulky tumor.

- Clinical responses were limited to those with a relatively small volume of disease and who received only one chemotherapeutic regimen before the radioimmunoconjugate.

- A similar trial using a monoclonal antibody conjugated to yttrium 90 has been performed.

- Myelosuppression was the dose-limiting toxicity.

- Among 14 patients with assessable disease, one experienced tumor regression and one demonstrated palliation of ascites.

- Five to 25 mCi of ^{90}Y activity was used in this study; in contrast, 120 mCi of ^{186}Re as ^{186}Re-NR-LU-10 could be delivered safely.

- When administered complexed to NR-LU-10, ^{186}Re is present in the blood and peritoneal fluid in minimal amounts 4 days after treatment, and is essentially gone a week after treatment.

- This radionuclide does not long survive dissociation from the antibody and is excreted from the body.

•In order for an agent such as ^{186}Re-NR-LU-10 to be clinically useful, it must have advantages over radionuclides in clinical use.

•Such **theoretical** advantages are:

°1) increased therapeutic index, which may be enhanced by selective binding to tumor cells;

°2) efficacy against tumors with diameters too large to treat with radionuclides; and

°3) efficacy against extraperitoneal tumor.

•These advantages remain to be demonstrated.

•Ongoing trials seek to develop a dosage schedule that will maximize the therapeutic index of ^{186}Re-NR-LU-10, anticipating future comparison of this agent with current standard modes of treatment.

---

4. After fetal lung maturity was assured, a patient with stage IB cervical carcinoma is to have a cesarean hysterectomy. The most common maternal complication to be expected is

    A. deep venous thrombosis.
    B. hemorraghic cystitis.
    C. lymphocyst.
*D. need for blood transfusion.
    E. wound infection.

---

p. 600 (Duggan B, Muderspach L I, Roman L D, Curtin J P, d'Ablaing III G, Morrow C P. Cervical cancer in pregnancy: Reporting on planned delay in therapy. Obstet Gynecol 1993; 82:598)

4. [F & I: •Background: Cervical cancer is one of the most frequently encountered malignancies during pregnancy.

•The incidence varies from 1.6-to-10.6 cases of cervical cancer per 10,000 pregnancies, depending upon the inclusion of cases of carcinoma in situ or postpartum patients.

•Diverse findings have been reported regarding the effects of pregnancy and mode of delivery on patient prognosis.

•The treatment schema for the patient with invasive cervical cancer in pregnancy varies with the stage of disease and gestational age at diagnosis.

•Upon diagnosis of invasive carcinoma of the cervix during the first and second trimesters of pregnancy, immediate treatment is recommended without regard to the pregnancy.

•In the late third trimester, delay of therapy is recommended until fetal maturity is documented.

•For the early third trimester, the decision of whether to await fetal maturity or proceed with treatment is less easy.

•There are scant data in the literature regarding the impact of a planned delay in therapy to achieve fetal maturity.

•Objectives: To review experience with invasive carcinoma of the cervix occurring during pregnancy, in order to assess maternal morbidity due to treatment delay and to report maternal and fetal outcome.

•Unlike many malignancies encountered in pregnancy, it is not possible to treat cervical cancer and preserve fetal life.

Obstetrics and Gynecology: Review 1994-Gynecologic Oncology References

- A decision must be made either to initiate therapy without regard to the fetus or to await fetal viability or maturity.

- The incidence of cervical cancer complicating pregnancy in this report is comparatively low.

- This may be due to the exclusion of patients initially diagnosed postpartum and to the inclusion of all pregnancies, not just deliveries.

- It may reflect an absolute decrease in the number of patients diagnosed with invasive cervical cancer during this study period.

- Only a few authors have commented on deliberate delay of therapy in pregnant patients with cervical cancer.

- In this series of eight patients, the deliberate delay of treatment to achieve fetal maturity did **not** appear to adversely affect maternal outcome.

- No progression of disease was documented with delays of 53-to-212 days (7.5-to-30.2 weeks).

- Five patients with stage Ib cervical cancer and three with stage Ia1 cancer who postponed therapy had no evidence of lymph node metastasis at the time of radical surgery.

- All patients are free of disease after a median follow-up of 23 months (range 3-to-124).

- None of the eight patients underwent an unplanned delivery because of adverse sequelae of their cervical cancer.

- Neonatal outcome was uniformly good.

- Combining this series of eight patients with the 43 patients reviewed in the literature, 51 women with cervical cancer complicating pregnancy postponed therapy and awaited fetal viability or maturity before delivery.

- Twenty-six patients with stage Ia cervical cancer are reported to be free of disease and 20 (77%) of these patients have had follow-up of 2 years or more.

- Sixteen of 20 (80%) with stage Ib lesions are disease free; only six (30%) had follow-up of 2 years or more.

- Five patients with stage II lesions had no progression of disease during the pregnancy, but their outcome after treatment is unspecified.

- The results of this retrospective study and literature review suggest no increased maternal risk due to treatment delay for patients with stage Ia and Ib cervical cancers; the number of patients and their duration of follow-up are insufficient to support a definitive conclusion.

- In counseling patients with cervical cancer during pregnancy, many factors must be considered, including the patient's desire for the pregnancy, the stage of disease, the lesion size, and the number of weeks necessary to optimize fetal maturity.

- Any delay of therapy may carry an increased risk of progression of disease; this risk is not easily quantifiable and must be balanced against the benefit of improved fetal outcome.

- At present, the treatment schema recommends delay in treatment for patients greater than 20 weeks' gestational age at diagnosis, for those who have stage Ia or small stage Ib (less than 4 cm) lesions, and for those who desire to continue their pregnancy.

- With close surveillance, a planned delay in therapy to achieve fetal maturity appears to be a reasonable option for patients with microinvasive and early stage Ib cervical cancers.]

•Fact   °Detail   »issue   *answer

Obstetrics and Gynecology: Review 1994 - Gynecologic Oncology References

5. A preoperative distinction between benign and malignant ovarian cysts can be reliably made by

    A. cyst fluid CA 125.
    B. cyst fluid cytology.
    C. serum CA 125.
    D. vaginal ultrasonography with color doppler examination.
 *E. none of the above.

p. 445 (Moran PO, Menczer, Ben-Baruch G, Lipitz S, Goor E. Cytologic examination of ovarian cyst fluid for the distinction between benign and malignant tumors. Obstet Gynecol 1993; 82:444)

5. [F & I: •Background: The preoperative distinction between benign and malignant ovarian cysts could assist in defining two categories of patients.

•Those with a high probability of a malignant neoplasm would obviously undergo appropriate preparation and prompt surgical exploration for definitive diagnostic, therapeutic, and staging purposes.

•In at least some of those with benign asymptomatic cysts, follow-up without any operative intervention could be considered.

•Objective: To assess the feasibility of using cytologic examination of cyst fluid for distinguishing between benign and malignant ovarian tumors.

•Persistent ovarian cysts are often detected accidentally in pre- or postmenopausal women during pelvic examination or ultrasonography, which currently is performed for a variety of reasons.

•These cysts are frequently small and asymptomatic.

•Surgical intervention is usually proposed mainly because of the concern about malignancy.

•Such intervention can be done by operative laparoscopy, a less extensive procedure with lower morbidity and a shorter hospital stay than laparotomy.

•This procedure is not devoid of complications and should not be done unnecessarily.

•Cyst fluid for diagnostic purposes can be obtained safely by ultrasound-guided aspiration.

•This management remains controversial because of the high recurrence rate of the cysts and the uncertainty with regard to malignancy.

•An accurate method of identifying benign cysts could define a group of women in whom any intervention is unnecessary.

•Such a conservative approach can be contemplated because there is no clear evidence that benign cysts eventually undergo malignant transformation or ultimately cause symptoms due to increase in size, rupture, bleeding, or torsion.

•Results: Approximately one-third of the patients with benign cysts had cysts of small diameter, and half were asymptomatic.

•It is reasonable to assume that a considerable proportion of such cysts will remain unchanged indefinitely and not require surgery.

•The preoperative distinction between benign and malignant ovarian cysts is of great clinical significance, and several diagnostic methods have been used for this purpose.

•Vaginal ultrasonography, color Doppler flow examination, and serum CA 125 levels each have limitations.

•The determination of cyst fluid **CA 125** levels for this distinction is **inaccurate** as well.

•Cytologic examination of **aspirated ovarian cyst fluid** is also **not** a reliable method for the distinction between benign and malignant ovarian cysts.

•Although the specificity of the test was 100% (no false positives), the sensitivity for malignancy was very low.

•The number of positive fluid samples was too small for meaningful correlation with stage, histologic category, and grade of differentiation.

°The rate of positive reports was significantly higher in invasive than in borderline tumors.

•The results of studies on cyst fluid cytologic examination are inconsistent.

•In some reports, an accuracy of about 90% was claimed, but another concluded that cytologic examination of ovarian cyst fluid is of doubtful value.

•The reason for the low yield of positive cytologic examination in the fluid from malignant cysts in many of the studies is not known.

• Only a sample of the cyst fluid was examined, which may not have been representative of the entire amount of fluid.

•Because in this series the cytologic slides were not reviewed, misinterpretation also cannot be ruled out.

•The low yield reflects infrequent desquamation of malignant cells.

•The rate of positive cytology may also be low in peritoneal fluid obtained from patients with disseminated ovarian cancer.]

---

6. A patient has a stage IB cervical squamous cell carcinoma with a tumor diameter of four centimeters. Survival can be increased by

   A. chemotherapy followed by radial surgery followed by radiotherapy.
   B. chemotherapy followed by radical surgery.
   C. chemotherapy followed by radiotherapy.
   D. radiotherapy followed by radical surgery.
   *E. none of the above.

---

p. 449 (Zanetta G, Landoni F, Colombo A, Pellegrino A, Maneo A, Leventis C. Three-year results after neoadjuvant chemotherapy, radical surgery, and radiotherapy in locally advanced cervical carcinoma. Obstet Gynecol 1993; 82:447)

6. [F & I: •Background: Surgery and radiotherapy, alone and in combination, represent the treatments of choice for carcinoma confined to the cervix.

•Radiotherapy is the traditional treatment when the tumor has spread to the pericervical tissue and parametria.

•Cure rates of 85-to-90% are attainable in early disease, but they fall with more advanced stages and bulky disease.

•Stage IB cervical carcinoma with tumor diameter of 4 cm or greater has a higher incidence of lymph node metastases, local recurrence, and distant recurrence than do small tumors.

• Lymph node spread represents the main prognostic factor after radical surgery; the presence of four or more metastatic nodes has been related to a reduction in the cure rate of 30-to-50%.

Obstetrics and Gynecology: Review 1994-Gynecologic Oncology References

- •Integrated treatments, adding radiotherapy after surgery, have not significantly improved 5 and 10-year survival rates because of poor control of systemic spread of the tumor.

- • Since the early 1980s, different chemotherapy regimens have been tested for recurrent cervical carcinoma.

- •Regimens containing cisplatin yielded clinical objective responses of 53-to-80%, with complete responses of 8-to-20%, but patient survival did not improve significantly.

- •Responses to chemotherapy may be reduced by a decreased vascular supply to the tumor secondary to previous irradiation or surgery.

- •The use of neoadjuvant chemotherapy as part of multimodality treatment offers some theoretical advantages in advanced disease.

- •Chemotherapy may shrink bulky tumors before surgical and radiation treatment and may also reduce the incidence of lymph node metastases.

- •Following neoadjuvant chemotherapy, radical surgery can remove residual central disease, evaluate lymph node status, and presumably improve cure.

- •Objectives: To report the results of a pilot study with neoadjuvant chemotherapy in locally advanced cervical carcinoma followed by radical surgery with pelvic lymphadenectomy and radiotherapy.

- •To assess the feasibility of this combined treatment and its impact on the survival of patients with locally advanced disease.

- •To assess the effect of preoperative neoadjuvant chemotherapy in decreasing the incidence of lymph node metastases and reducing cervical tumor volume to facilitate surgical excision of locally advanced cervical cancer.

- •The minimum follow-up time of 3 years allows some remarks about the long-term benefits and limits of this relatively new approach to cervical cancer.

- •Results: For patients with locally advanced untreated cervical carcinoma, high clinical response rates can be achieved with platinum-based chemotherapy.

- •Toxicity was mild and the treatment did not complicate the surgical resection; moderate fibrosis of retroperitoneal tissues was observed in chemotreated patients.

- •Radiotherapy was completed in all patients without delays or significant toxicity.

- •Pathologic complete responses were not observed, both patients with complete clinical responses had microscopic residual tumor (one in the lymph nodes, the second in the cervix and lymph nodes).

- •Both of these women are alive with no evidence of disease after 36 and 38 months, respectively.

- •After a minimum follow-up of 36 months, 16 patients had died of disease.

- •This result does **not** seem to represent an improvement in survival compared to the results observed by others or to experience with standard radiotherapy.

- •It seems remarkable that these results were achieved at the cost of a sequence of three "radical" treatments.

- •A limited number of distant recurrences was recorded, possibly reflecting the beneficial effects of systemic treatment on microscopic metastases.

- •In most series examining neoadjuvant treatments for cervical carcinoma, few data were shown on lymph node metastases.

Obstetrics and Gynecology: Review 1994-Gynecologic Oncology References

•In this series, five of eight patients with negative nodes at surgery were alive without evidence of recurrence after 36, 38, 43, 45, and 48 months, respectively.

•Conclusion: Based on these results, neoadjuvant chemotherapy has a potential role in the treatment of locally advanced cervical carcinoma, but the data do **not** seem to confirm the claimed superiority of this multimodal treatment over standard regimens.]

---

7. The most cost effective strategy for a patient at low risk (less than 5%) of endometrial cancer who has post-menopausal bleeding is

   A. ambulatory D&C.
   B. hysterectomy.
   C. no further work-up; wait for bleeding to recur, then investigate.
   *D. office biopsy.

p. 974 (Feldman S, Berkowitz R S, Tosteson A N A, Cost-effectiveness of strategies to evaluate postmenopausal bleeding. Obstet Gynecol 1993; 81:968)

7. [F & I: •Background: Endometrial cancer affects 2-to-3% of American women.

•It usually presents at an early stage and carries a good prognosis.

•Its most common symptom is postmenopausal bleeding.

•Complex hyperplasia, which has been shown to progress to endometrial cancer in 10-to-30% of cases if left untreated, is also associated with postmenopausal bleeding.

•Historically, the standard practice for the evaluation of any amount of postmenopausal bleeding has been D&C.

•This has been questioned because of the cost, morbidity, and accuracy of D&C relative to outpatient office biopsy.

•Nonetheless, there were a total of 379,000 D&Cs performed in the United States in 1987 for a variety of indications, including postmenopausal bleeding.

•The prevalence of endometrial cancer among women who present with postmenopausal bleeding varies from 1.5-to-90%, and textbooks typically report a rate of approximately 20%.

•Recent studies have suggested a prevalence of less than 10%.

•The wide variation in prevalence suggests that the populations studied have different underlying risks (either by virtue of specific patient characteristics or by the duration and amount of bleeding) or that the threshold to evaluate patients differs among groups of physicians.

•Objective: To determine the optimal clinical management strategy for a hypothetical patient who presents for the first time with postmenopausal bleeding, as measured by life expectancy and cost.

•Strategies involved office endometrial biopsy and D&C, and considered patients at 50, 60, 70, and 80 years of age with various underlying risks for cancer and complex hyperplasia.

•Although office biopsy is the least costly of the procedures considered and has a very high reported sensitivity and specificity, there may be some patient groups whose risk for cancer and complex hyperplasia is so low that one should postpone endometrial sampling until further symptoms present.

•There may be groups whose combined risk of cancer and complex hyperplasia is so great that one should forgo endometrial sampling and proceed directly to hysterectomy for simultaneous diagnosis and therapy.

•Fact   °Detail   »issue   *answer

- The analysis questioned whether all patients with postmenopausal bleeding should be evaluated in the same way.

- The life expectancy, costs, and cost-effectiveness of several strategies for evaluating women who present for the first time with postmenopausal bleeding was assessed.

- There was relatively little improvement in life expectancy associated with a more aggressive evaluation strategy, although more aggressive strategies, such as D&C or office biopsy followed by D&C for insufficient tissue, were much more costly than no work-up or office biopsy.

- **Compared with the other procedures, office biopsy was always the most cost-effective way to evaluate an otherwise healthy woman with a normal age-adjusted life expectancy.**

- Office biopsy was the preferred initial strategy even at a cost as high as $2200 or a probability of insufficient tissue as high as 80%.

- A D&C never resulted in an improved life expectancy relative to an office biopsy and was never as cost-effective as office biopsy, regardless of the patient's age, risk for cancer and complex hyperplasia, or the cost of the D&C.

- For patients at low risk for cancer and complex hyperplasia (i.e., 5%) even office biopsy was relatively costly in certain age groups compared with other accepted public health programs (e.g., $30,000-to-$35,000 per useful year of life saved for renal dialysis).

- In particular, for 80-year-old patients the cost per additional year of life saved was $205,000, and for 60-year-olds it was $66,000.

- Close observation with evaluation if or when bleeding recurs may be a reasonable approach in these patients.

- Furthermore, the data suggest a very high sensitivity and specificity for office biopsy.

- If it is assumed that the accuracy of office biopsy may actually be somewhat worse in clinical practice, the evaluation of relatively low-risk patients would become even more costly.

- If insufficient tissue was found after an office biopsy, it was generally more cost-effective to observe the patient closely and to perform a D&C only if postmenopausal bleeding or other relevant symptoms persisted, than to perform a D&C immediately.

- There were some younger patients (age 50-to-60) at moderate to high risk (i.e., greater than 20%) for cancer and complex hyperplasia for whom it was still reasonably cost-effective to proceed directly to D&C following insufficient tissue on an office biopsy.

- The analysis did not consider quality of life.

- Data on quality of life in patients with cancer and complex hyperplasia and quality-of-life decrements associated with office biopsy, D&C, and hysterectomy are required before an adequate analysis of quality-adjusted life-years can be undertaken.

- If one considers quality of life associated with the procedures only, the analysis would favor the option of no work-up or office biopsy to an even greater degree than in the unadjusted analysis.

- One objective of this analysis was to determine whether knowledge of a patient's risk for endometrial cancer or complex hyperplasia should affect her optimal evaluation.

- Although knowledge of a patient's specific risk would be useful, data are not currently available to predict an individual's risk based on her unique characteristics.

- Possible means for determining risk include the development of a clinical prediction rule or the use of a technique such as vaginal probe ultrasound to evaluate the thickness of the endometrium.

- For example, using the data on vaginal probe ultrasound, endometrial thickness of 5 mm may be used to identify a low-risk group (less than 1%) and a high-risk group (33% risk for cancer, 56% combined risk for cancer or complex hyperplasia).

- The model did not address patients who present repeatedly with abnormal bleeding after an initial evaluation or those who have other worrisome signs or symptoms suggestive of cancer, such as a pelvic mass.

- Another potential limitation is that the results depended upon the assumptions that patients who were not initially evaluated remained symptomatic 100% of the time if they had cancer and 50% of the time if they had complex hyperplasia, and that patients with persistent symptoms would promptly undergo a work-up at a future date.

- Because the purpose of the model was to identify the optimal approach to a woman with postmenopausal bleeding, it did not consider the potential litigation costs due to a delay in diagnosis or a complication from a procedure that may have been avoided if evaluation were postponed in some low-risk patients.

- Clinicians may need to consider these potential costs on an individual basis.

- This model looked at many different variables simultaneously, including age, disease prevalence, and aggressiveness of the strategy under a variety of different model assumptions.

- The choice of office biopsy as the preferred initial strategy compared to D&C or hysterectomy was not sensitive to the assumptions, as varying the assumptions gave the same result.

- For any given age group and disease prevalence, because life expectancy remained relatively constant or improved as the evaluation became less aggressive, the decision to postpone a work-up until further symptoms present is unlikely to result in significant harm to the patient.

- Although simple office biopsy is generally cost-effective, in certain low-risk patients (i.e., combined risk of cancer or complex hyperplasia of 5%), initial close observation with evaluation done only if bleeding recurs may be considered an option when a patient presents for the first time with postmenopausal bleeding.]

8. The most important feature of a test that evaluates a pelvic mass for possible malignancy is

   *A. negative predictive value.
   B. positive predictive value.
   C. sensitivity.
   D. specificity.
   E. All characteristics have the same importance.

p. 987 (Schneider V L, Schneider A, Reed K L, Hatch K D. Comparison of doppler with two-dimensional sonography and CA 125 for prediction of malignancy of pelvic masses. Obstet Gynecol 1993; 81:983)

8. [F & I: •Background: High diastolic flow or low resistance is a pathognomonic feature of vessels associated with neoplasms.

- Neovascular vessels lack a muscular intima and form multiple arteriovenous shunts, which result in an increased diastolic flow that is detectable in the Doppler frequency waveform.

- Transvaginal Doppler sonography can be used to detect this specific flow pattern or increased diastolic flow in ovarian cancers.

- Neovascularity is not specific to malignancy; it is shared with benign tumors with high proliferative or inflammatory potential.

- The distinction between benign and malignant adnexal masses using noninvasive diagnostic techniques is a challenge to every clinician.

- Besides pelvic examination, CA 125 serum levels and two-dimensional abdominal or vaginal ultrasonography are accepted diagnostic tools in clinical decision making.

- The validity of these techniques is restricted by their limited sensitivity and specificity.

- Objective: To evaluate the association of abdominal or transvaginal color Doppler sonography to the morphology of adnexal masses and the contribution of this technique to the prediction of malignancy with CA 125 serum levels and two-dimensional sonography.

- Methods: Initially, the adnexal mass was evaluated using transvaginal sonography.

- Malignancy was predicted using sonographic criteria such as size (greater than 5 cm), high echogenicity, multilocular appearance, irregular borders, presence of ascites, and papillary intracystic formations.

- In addition, a sonographic score was calculated applying criteria such as inner-wall structure, wall thickness, septa, and echogenicity.

- Color Doppler sonography was used to identify vessels in the tumor because color mapping is helpful for correct placement of the pulsed Doppler window.

- Vessels in the wall of the tumor were analyzed in case internal vessels were absent.

- A series of at least five similar arterial waveforms was identified, and the resistance index (RI) was calculated using the following formula:

$$\frac{\text{systolic peak} - \text{end diastolic velocity}}{\text{systolic peak}}$$

- The calculation of sensitivity, specificity, and positive and negative predictive values allows accurate evaluation of the validity of a test.

- Additional factors such as prevalence or extent of disease influence the positive predictive value and the sensitivity, respectively.

- Two-dimensional sonography and assessment of CA 125 serum levels are used for the prediction of malignancy in adnexal masses.

- These variables showed a sensitivity of up to 82%, a specificity of up to 93%, and positive predictive values between 31-to-75% with the prevalence of malignancy varying between 15-to-43%.

- Even in these selected patients, at least 18% of malignant tumors are missed by these techniques and up to 7% of benign tumors are considered malignant.

- Two studies used the resistance index with a cutoff of 0.7.

  ° All ovarian cancers (eight) and all benign ovarian cysts (13) were correctly diagnosed.

  ° Applying a cutoff of 0.4, in another study 96.4% of all cancers (n = 56) were recognized and only one out of 624 benign tumors was wrongly diagnosed as malignant.

  ° This latter study showed a positive predictive value of 98.2% for Doppler flow, with a disease prevalence of 8.2%.

- By applying the pulsatility index, two other studies showed similar high sensitivity and specificity of Doppler flow.

- Compared with two-dimensional sonography and CA 125, the pulsatility index proved superior, with a positive predictive value of 94% and a negative predictive value of 97% in a total of 53 patients with a disease prevalence of 32%.

- The findings of the referenced Doppler flow studies were only partly confirmed by these results.

- The resistance index showed the highest sensitivity and the highest negative predictive value compared with two-dimensional sonography and CA 125, but it also showed the lowest specificity and the lowest positive predictive value.

- The high rate of false-positive results was mainly due to endometriosis, leiomyomata, and mucinous cystadenomas.

  ° Two other studies also showed increased diastolic flow in endometriomas and uterine leiomyomata.

- For a more objective interpretation of two-dimensional sonographic findings, a sonographic score was recommended previously, which showed a sensitivity and a negative predictive value of 100% and a specificity of 83%.

- In this study, this scoring system was **not** superior to the two-dimensional assessment, showing lower specificity and predictive values.

- **The negative predictive value is the most important feature of a test that evaluates a pelvic mass because every case identified as benign should be accurate, especially when surgical intervention may be abandoned.**

- The combination of Doppler flow results with two-dimensional data or CA 125 levels resulted in a negative predictive value of 100%.

- In addition, all malignant cases of this series were identified.

- The combination of tests had the disadvantage of lower specificity and lower positive predictive value compared with single tests because malignancy was suspected when only one test was positive.

- The Doppler results showed no advantage compared with established techniques.

- The combination of two-dimensional evaluation and CA 125 resulted in the same sensitivity and negative predictive value but higher specificity (74.4%) and higher positive predictive value (61.6%) than the combination of Doppler flow and two-dimensional sonography or CA 125.

- Doppler sonography can increase the sensitivity and negative predictive value of two-dimensional sonography or CA 125 for the prediction of pelvic malignancy.

- This helps to identify a subset of patients with pelvic masses who need immediate surgical intervention.

- There is a considerable number of false-positive results due to neovascularity of benign tumors.

- In this study with a disease prevalence of 29%, between 52-to-54% of the patients with positive test results had benign findings, and only 51-to-56% of these patients with benign tumors could have been spared surgery.

- These numbers may be helpful when the value of Doppler flow for early detection of ovarian masses is discussed.

- Because the prevalence of disease is much smaller in such settings even when risk groups are screened, the positive predictive value will become smaller and the percentage of operated patients with benign disease higher.

Obstetrics and Gynecology: Review 1994-Gynecologic Oncology References

•In addition, the presence of early-stage cancers will make discrimination between benign and malignant lesions even more difficult.]

---

9. Associated with improved survival in patients with high risk stage I ovarian cancer

    A. adriamycin.
    B. cisplatinum.
    C. melphalan.
    D. P^{32}.
    *E. none of the above.

---

p. 143 (Rubin S C, Wong G Y C, Curtin J P, Barakat R R, Hakes T B, Hoskins W J. Platinum-based chemotherapy of high-risk stage I epithelial ovarian cancer following comprehensive surgical staging. Obstet Gynecol 1993; 82:143)

9. [F & I: •Background: A major advance in the understanding of the natural history of ovarian cancer occurred in the late 1970s and early 1980s with the recognition of the need for comprehensive surgical staging to identify patients with disease limited to one or both ovaries.

•A clinically significant incidence of occult disease metastatic to the peritoneal washings, lymph nodes, omentum, and the diaphragm in patients who appeared clinically to have stage I disease was found.

•The current staging system of the International Federation of Gynecology and Obstetrics (FIGO) incorporates surgical evaluation of these areas into its staging criteria.

•Because most cases of ovarian cancer are found in the advanced stages and because many women with apparent early disease do not undergo appropriate surgical staging, it has been difficult to determine the prognosis and optimum treatment for stage I ovarian cancer.

•Randomized trials of comprehensively staged early ovarian cancer have helped to define low-risk and high-risk groups of patients.

•Patients whose tumors are stage IA or IB, grade 1, are considered to be at low risk for relapse and can be followed without further therapy after definitive surgery.

•Patients whose tumors are stage IC or grade 3 are generally considered to need additional treatment.

•In one series, such patients were randomized to either intraperitoneal ^{32}P or single-agent melphalan, with no difference in outcome in the two arms.

•Although high-risk patients should have adjuvant treatment, the optimum regimen, and the role of platinum-based therapy, will need to be defined by prospective studies.

•In addition, the role of adjuvant treatment in women with grade 2 tumors is unresolved, as the Gynecologic Oncology Group study included only a small number of such patients.

•Objective: To review the outcome of patients with high-risk stage I ovarian cancer treated with platinum-based chemotherapy following comprehensive surgical staging.

•The need for comprehensive surgical staging of apparent early ovarian cancer patients is now well accepted.

•Although the definition of "low risk" has varied somewhat, good survival with no adjuvant therapy in selected patients in the low-risk group has been reported.

•The optimal treatment for patients in the high-risk category has not been defined.

•Among the clinical prognostic factors examined in this study, including substage, cell type, and histologic grade, both **grade and cell type** were significant predictors of recurrence.

•Fact   °Detail   »issue   *answer

•In this patient population, 14 of 15 recurrences (93%) occurred in patients with grade 3 tumors and/or clear-cell histology.

•The nearly 50% rate of recurrence in the patients with grade 3 tumors and the 41% rate of relapse in patients with clear-cell tumors are not encouraging with respect to the ability of systemic platinum to eradicate subclinical residual disease.

•No relapses were noted among 11 patients with stage IA, grade 2 tumors.

•It has not been determined whether such patients should be included in the high-risk category.

•Although the grade 2 patients in the no-treatment arm of the Gynecologic Oncology Group randomized trial did well, only five such patients were included in the study.

•Other authors have suggested that grade 2 patients do require treatment.

•Although there was some variability in the type and duration of platinum-based chemotherapy used in this patient population, no association was found between these factors and the risk of relapse.

•There is evidence that clinical outcome is not related to the duration of platinum-based chemotherapy, the use of adriamycin, or the dose intensity over the commonly used range of doses.

•In this selected patient population, the largest reported to date, an overall disease-free survival of 73% in 62 comprehensively staged stage I ovarian cancer patients treated with adjuvant platinum-based chemotherapy was noted.]

---

10. The most powerful predictor of a disease-free interval for patients with stage I ovarian epithelial carcinoma is

   A. ascites.
   *B. degree of cellular differentiation.
   C. DNA ploidy.
   D. FIGO substage.
   E. rupture of the capsule during surgery.

---

p. 48 (Vergote I B, Kaern J, Abeler V M, Pettersen E O, De Vos L N, Trope C G. Analysis of prognostic factors in stage I epithelial ovarian carcinoma: Importance of degree of differentiation and deoxyribonucleic acid ploidy in predicting relapse. Am J Obstet Gynec 1993; 169:40)

10. [F & I: •Background: Approximately 25% of patients with common epithelial invasive ovarian carcinoma are first seen with disease confined to the ovaries (International Federation of Gynecology and Obstetrics [FIGO] stage I).

•Recently 5-year survival rates of about 70% to 85% were reported for stage I disease.

•The majority of patients with stage I ovarian carcinoma have been treated with either postoperative radiotherapy or cytotoxic agents, yet the curative value of postoperative adjuvant treatment has not been proved.

•Prognostic factors such as degree of differentiation, FIGO substage, histologic type, dense adhesions, large-volume ascites, and patient age have been identified with multivariate analyses as independent prognostic characteristics.

•There is increasing evidence that in a variety of malignancies, including ovarian cancer, the deoxyribonucleic acid (DNA) content is of considerable prognostic value.

•Because of possible interactions between the various prognostic factors, multivariate analysis offers the best approach to assess the value of new prognostic variables.

- Earlier reports on DNA content in ovarian cancer primarily assessed advanced disease, and too few patients with stage I disease were included to permit multivariate analyses in this subgroup of patients.

- Objective: To analyze the prognostic factors and DNA content in a group of 290 patients with invasive epithelial stage I ovarian carcinoma.

- The potential clinical use of **DNA flow cytometry** for prognostic purposes in ovarian cancer has received much attention.

- Most previous reports are limited to stage III or IV malignancies or include fewer than 35 stage I patients.

- Results: A multivariate analysis identified **degree of differentiation** as the most powerful predictor of disease-free survival, followed by DNA ploidy and, finally, FIGO (1986) substage.

- This finding confirms earlier studies suggesting that the degree of differentiation is an important independent prognostic indicator in stage I ovarian cancer.

- Clear cell tumors had a worse prognosis than did the other histologic types.

- It is difficult to grade tumors with clear cell elements because of the great variety of growth patterns.

- The group of clear cell tumors and mixed epithelial tumors with clear cell elements were not graded in the current study and not included in the multivariate analysis of the remaining graded tumors.

- When considering DNA ploidy and FIGO (1986) stage in clear cell tumors and mixed epithelial tumors with clear cell elements, FIGO (1986) stage was an important prognostic variable, whereas DNA ploidy was not significant.

- None of the 77 patients with well-differentiated DNA diploid tumors had a relapse.

- This low-risk group had a significantly better survival than did those with well-differentiated DNA nondiploid tumors and moderately differentiated DNA diploid tumors.

- No significant differences were observed between the other "neighboring" subgroups with graded tumors.

- In the current study dense adhesion was an important prognostic factor in the univariate analysis but was no longer significant in the multivariate analysis.

- Ascites was **not** a prognostic indicator.

  ° Ascites was defined as in the FIGO (1973) classification (i.e., peritoneal effusion that, in the opinion of the surgeon, is pathologic or clearly exceeds normal amounts).

- In the current study only six (2%) received no adjuvant treatment, and no differences in disease-free survival were observed between the different types of adjuvant treatment.

- The efficacy of adjuvant treatment cannot be established on the basis of these studies but only in a large prospective, randomized trial comparing postoperative adjuvant treatment with an untreated observation group.

- Unfortunately, peritoneal washings were not performed routinely in the current study, and the lack of this information prevents comment on its prognostic effect.

- In the 1988 FIGO report the patients treated between 1979 and 1981 were classified retrospectively according to the 1986 classification, although the earlier staging did not require information on cytologic factors.

- The same procedure was followed in this study when reclassifying the patients according to the FIGO (1986) classification.

- In spite of the absence of data on peritoneal cytologic conditions the FIGO (1986) classification was a stronger prognostic indicator than the old FIGO (1973) classification in the univariate analyses and was the third independent prognostic factor in the multivariate analysis.

- In none of the more recent studies performed by multivariate analysis did the state of the tumor capsule have an effect on survival.

- The multivariate analysis in the current study provides evidence for the lack of prognostic significance of rupture and extracapsular growth when analyzed separately.

- But, combining the effects of rupture, extracapsular growth, and ascites in the new FIGO (1986) classification (i.e., FIGO stage Ic) had a significant prognostic effect.

- Recently, extensive surgical staging, including blind biopsies of the pelvic peritoneum, the abdominal gutters, the diaphragm, and paraaortic lymph nodes, has been advocated in early ovarian cancer.

- The extent to which the relapse risk might have been explained by occult peritoneal or nodal spread that would have been detected by meticulous surgical staging could be determined.

- In this group of patients not subjected to this type of surgical staging a subgroup without relapse, which constituted about one third of the patients with graded tumors, could be identified.

- In a recent review of 1300 patients with ovarian cancer (all stages) described in 18 studies, the frequency of DNA nondiploidy was 65%.

- In the current study the frequency of DNA nondiploid tumors is somewhat lower (49%), which is in concordance with previous reports on stage I ovarian cancer.

- This finding supports earlier studies suggesting a relationship between ploidy and FIGO stage.

- In addition, a significant relationship was established between FIGO (1986) stage I substage and ploidy.

- Results of studies evaluating the association between DNA ploidy and grade have been inconsistent.

- In the current study tumors were found to be multiploid in 5%.

- Tetraploid tumors were observed in 16% of the tumors and most often in clear cell tumors.

- No significant differences in disease-free survival were observed between single aneuploid, tetraploid, and multiploid tumors.

- This discrepancy may be because of the different definitions used for tetraploidy and the differences in patient population.

- There was no significant different **disease-free survival** between patients with tumors with a DNA index of 1.1 to 1.3 compared with those with a DNA index of 1.3 to 1.8.

- The DNA index was no longer a prognostic variable after accounting for DNA ploidy in the multivariate analysis.

- The relapse rate was similar in DNA diploid tumors with a coefficient of variation < 8% compared with those with a coefficient of variation >8%.]

11. The most discriminating factor in determining the presence of ovarian cancer in an adnexal mass is

   *A. age.
   B. CA 125.
   C. gray scale ultrasound.
   D. pulsatility index.
   E. resistance index.

p. 910 (Timor-Tritsch I E, Lerner J P. Monteagudo A, Santos R. Transvaginal ultrasonographic characterization of ovarian masses by means of color flow-directed Doppler measurements and a morphologic scoring system. Am J Obstet Gynec 1993; 168:909)

11. [F & I: •Background: Ovarian carcinoma is a disease whose overall survival has not significantly improved in over 20 years and remains approximately 30% for 5-year survival.

•The poor prognosis is attributable to the paucity of signs and symptoms generated by the deeply situated ovaries, leading to late diagnosis.

•The vast majority of these patients are first identified when their cancer has already reached stage III or IV.

•Five-year survival in patients with stage I disease approaches 80% to 85%; if timely identification of early disease can be achieved, a significant improvement in outcome may occur.

•The preliminary studies attempting to screen or identify early-stage ovarian carcinoma, especially in the postmenopausal woman, used transabdominal ultrasonography and was unable to distinguish morphologic characteristics that would identify malignant from benign masses.

•Studies in 1989 were limited by the high numbers of false positives, rendering transabdominal ultrasonography impractical as a screening tool.

•In 1991 a scoring system was devised using traditional gray scale transvaginal ultrasonography to characterize ovarian lesions in the hope of discriminating benign from malignant lesions.

   °This scoring system is based on defining the wall thickness, inner wall structure, characteristics of septae, and echogenicity of the lesion.

   °On the basis of these scores it was possible to characterize the tumors, and benign tumors could be separated from malignancies with reasonable accuracy.

   °The efficacy of a morphologic scoring system alone was hampered by the degree of overlap between malignant and benign-appearing masses.

•Objective: To further refine the characterization of ovarian lesions by including information regarding the presence or absence of low resistance to blood flow.

•The detection of ovarian malignancy by means of color Doppler evaluation of velocity and vessel compliance is based on the fact that fast-growing tumors contain many newly formed blood vessels, and because of this tumor neovascularization these vessels contain little smooth muscle within their walls.

   °**The resistance to blood flow is therefore decreased.**

   °It would be possible to discriminate benign from malignant masses by quantifying this difference.

•Color-coded Doppler flow imaging can be performed which gives semiquantitative definitions and flow measurements by identifying the vessel in question.

•The indexes used in these studies are the pulsatility index and the resistance index, which are widely used in cardiology, neurology, obstetrics, and other specialties in need of flow measurements.

- **Objectives:** To test the feasibility of obtaining color flow Doppler measurements from blood vessels in the wall or the interior of the ovarian or adnexal mass and then once obtained, to determine the optimal cutoff points for the Doppler values obtained, resistance index and pulsatility index, to best differentiate benign from malignant lesions.

- To evaluate the performance of combining the morphologic scoring system with the resistance-to-flow measurements in separating the benign from malignant adnexal masses.

- If performed early enough, during the first and maybe even in the second stage of the development of the malignancy within the ovary, it may actually change 5-year survival rates in the near future.

- It would be overly optimistic to expect perfect discrimination between benign and malignant lesions by means of the velocity and resistance indices alone.

- A combination of morphologic analysis and vessel compliance was analyzed.

- If the scoring system alone would be used, the positive predictive value of correctly diagnosing a malignancy was 60%.

- **Results:** Underscored the validity of measuring indices of resistance to flow in the vessels supplying blood to the ovaries, to detect groups of patients having high and low resistance to flow; this is in addition to the morphologic studies based on the scoring system.

- The cut-off point values of the resistance index and pulsatility index at which the best separation of benign and malignant ovarian lesions occurs were set at 0.40 and 1.00, respectively.

- Most malignancies were found to have measurements below these values.

- The best discriminative cutoff points were 0.46 for the resistance index and 0.62 for the pulsatility index.

- Both indices performed at a relatively high degree of positive predictive value (resistance index 94%, pulsatility index 88%).

- The group of patients in whom a low resistance is observed will contain the patients with ovarian cancer; it will also contain a small number of patients with nonneoplastic disease in which angiogenesis or dilatation of the vessel is present.

- **Inflammatory processes of the adnexa** and highly functional ovarian tissue such as the **corpus luteum** will have to be recognized and separated to lower the false-positive test results.

- The practical aspect of this process is to minimize, as much as possible, the surgical exploration of patients with a nonmalignant lesion.

- The group of simple cysts included two corpora lutea and hemorrhagic cysts in which surgery could have been avoided.

- The combination of the scoring system with the resistance-to-flow indices was better able to discriminate between benign and malignant adnexal lesions.

- This combination correctly identified ovarian cancer in 14 of 16 cases and ruled out the disease in 67 of 67 cases.

- Ten benign masses were identified correctly by flow but scored high.

  ° These benign masses included three fibroma thecomas, three benign teratomas, two simple cysts, one tuboovarian abscess, and one serous cystadenoma.

- The two unidentified cancer cases included one case identified by the flow study but missed by a low score and one case that was identified by the score but missed by the flow study.

»A rigid cutoff point using either resistance index or pulsatility index may **not** be a sole indicator for exploratory surgery, especially in premenopausal women.

»If the results of the flow studies are combined with the transvaginal ultrasonographic characterization of ovarian lesions and preoperative CA 125 levels in those postmenopausal patients, more accurate discrimination of benign from malignant masses is probable.]

---

12. 95% of patients with hydatidiform mole can be expected to have normal hCG levels how many weeks after evacuation?

    A. 6
    B. 7
    C. 11
    D. 19
*E. 25

---

p. 789 (Yedema K A, Verheijen R H, Kenemans P, Schijf C P, Borm G F, Segers M F, Thomas C M. Identification of patients with persistent trophoblastic disease by means of a normal human chorionic gonadotropin regression curve. Am J Obstet Gynec 1993; 168:787)

12. [F & I: •Background: Serial measurement of human chorionic gonadotropin (hCG) serum levels is used to monitor the behavior of residual trophoblastic tissue after evacuation of a hydatidiform mole.

•Postevacuation regression curves allow early identification of patients with persistent trophoblastic disease.

•A persistent rise or plateau in the hCG regression curve identifies those patients requiring chemotherapy.

•In such cases a further spontaneous regression of hCG values is not to be expected because of remaining viable trophoblastic tissue.

•There is no common opinion on the time span required by hCG serum levels to normalize.

•Mean time intervals required for normalization of serum hCG in patients with spontaneous regression range from 49 to 99 days, with maximal disappearance times between 98 and 278 days.

•The wide variation in definitions for abnormal hCG regression explains the variation of persistent trophoblastic disease between 7% and 36% after molar pregnancy.

•Objective: To construct a normal serum hCG regression corridor.

°Data from patients achieving spontaneous regression of a molar pregnancy after evacuation are used in an attempt to provide unequivocal criteria for the identification of persistent trophoblastic disease in patients and for the start of treatment.

•Results: A normal regression corridor was constructed on the basis of hCG regression curves for those patients who achieved uneventful regression of serum hCG without the need for additional chemotherapy after evacuation.

•A biphasic regression pattern was observed comparable to that after abortion or ectopic pregnancy, after delivery, and after intravenous injection of hCG.

•The first phase half-life was 1.8 days.

•The long half-life of 12.8 days in the second phase of regression illustrates the slow hCG regression after molar pregnancies.

•The half-life time of serum hCG was independent of the pretreatment values.

- When the data from patients with persistent trophoblastic disease in this study were retrospectively plotted into the normal regression corridor, it appeared that six patients (8%) had already been treated for persistent trophoblastic disease while their hCG level was still below the 95th percentile.

- Use of a normal regression corridor could possibly have resulted in a more expectant attitude in these cases.

- In addition, one patient with persistent trophoblastic disease deviated to levels above the 95th percentile line, but regressed spontaneously shortly before treatment was started.

- 20 patients with hydatidiform mole (15%) with a temporary hCG plateau or rise, defined as a change <10% or an increase >10% on the basis of at least three consecutive measurements, eventually regressed to normal.

- A previous criterion for persistent trophoblastic disease included failure to regress within 25 weeks from evacuation.

- Because 5% of non-persistent trophoblastic disease patients still had elevated levels at that time, an expectant attitude after this period could be followed if hCG levels continue to decrease.

- **Special caution is merited with those patients with persistent trophoblastic disease after an initial spontaneous regression to normal.**

- Six patients were treated with chemotherapy after initial normalization of hCG serum levels.

  ° All six had complete hydatidiform moles.

  ° Time until normalization ranged from 57 to 316 days.

  ° Reelevated hCG levels were seen in four of six cases within 1 month after initial normalization.

  ° The first samples collected after hCG normalization showed reelevated hCG levels at 138 and 144 days, respectively.

- Follow-up should be continued for at least 1 year after evacuation.

- Ten patients with persistent trophoblastic disease had at review diagnosis partial moles requiring chemotherapy.

  ° Although it can only be presumed that hCG regression in partial moles behaves similarly to hCG regression in complete moles, the data support the opinion that the follow-up of partial moles should be performed in the same way as in the case of complete hydatidiform mole.

- Because most hCG assays vary widely with respect to sensitivity, specificity, and cross reactivity with the free ß-hCG subunits, the current findings only apply to the specific hCG assay at the Dutch Central Registry of Hydatidiform Mole.

- Each individual hCG assay system should be clinically evaluated before applying the test for follow-up of patients with trophoblastic disease.]

---

13. In a closed system, the half-life of CA 125 approximates

    A. 1 day
    *B. 5 days
    C. 10 days
    D. 14 days
    E. 21 days

p. 31 (Brand E, Lodir Y. The decline of CA 125 level after surgery reflects the size of residual ovarian cancer. Obstet Gynecol 1993; 81:29)

13. [F & I: •Background: Primary cytoreduction of ovarian epithelial cancer resulting in "optimal" residual tumor is the single most important therapeutic intervention for survival.

•Residual tumor size is usually estimated by the surgeon and remains somewhat subjective in the presence of "carcinomatosis."

•Most often, there is no reliable way to distinguish postoperatively women having no gross residual cancer, minimal gross residual (less than 0.5 cm), and 1-to-2 cm residual disease.

•The survival of patients with microscopic residual averages 50 months; with 1-to-2 cm residual disease, generally about 24 months; and with lesions over 2 cm, 6-to-16 months.

•Although there is disagreement as to whether 1, 1.5, or 2 cm should be considered "optimal," it seems self-evident that the best residual is no residual.

•Most women with ovarian cancer have suboptimal residual disease.

•Objective: To determine whether CA 125 levels after cytoreductive surgery correlate with the size of residual tumor.

•The rate of decline of CA 125 during chemotherapy correlates with the findings at second-look surgery and with ultimate survival.

•In patients with persistently elevated levels after 60-to-90 days, the likelihood of survival is low.

•Because the absolute level of CA 125 correlates with the stage of ovarian cancer, as well as with the clinical estimate of tumor volume, aggressive cytoreduction should lower CA 125 values in proportion to the amount of residual disease, providing a marker of surgical residual.

•Results: There was a significant difference in surgical half-life among patients with optimal versus bulky residual disease.

•The dynamics of CA 125 half-life are complex.

•In a closed system, **the biologic half-life is 4.8 days**.

•Patients with residual tumor cells continue to produce CA 125 after surgery, and laparotomy alone can elevate levels even when no cancer is present.

•CA 125 ratios were evaluated rather than absolute levels.

•This allowed control for surgical effort despite the initial CA 125 level, which may have no prognostic value.

°This might explain why a woman with a very high CA 125 level who has all visible disease removed and a 90% reduction in CA 125 has a better prognosis than a woman with a low CA 125 level and bulky residual disease yet only a 50% reduction in CA 125, even though the first patient has a much higher pre-and postoperative CA 125 level.

•If these data can be confirmed, one may be able to predict the maximum residual tumor size left after surgery by comparing the level of CA 125 before surgery to the minimum value in the first 2 weeks after surgery.

•In this study, patients with all gross disease resected had a 91% decline in CA 125 postoperatively.

•This was not significantly different than the 85% decline in patients with less than 2 cm residual, but highly significant ($P < .001$) compared with 36% in patients with bulky residual (greater than 2.0 cm).

•Women with a drop of less than 60% postoperatively are likely to have bulky residual disease and may have a very low chance of cure with chemotherapy.

°Such patients should consider re-operation in a center likely to achieve small residual cancer.

°No difference was found in the ability to reduce residual tumor optimally whether the operation was primary or secondary cytoreduction.

•Overall, 81% of the women had optimal residual disease.

°This may be due in part to assisted cytoreductive techniques, ie, the **argon beam coagulator** and **Cavitron ultrasonic surgical aspirator**.

•The goal of surgery was to remove as much cancer as possible in patients who could be reduced to less than 2 cm, and to do minimal surgery if it became apparent that cytoreduction to less than 2.0 cm was not possible.

°It cannot determined whether the volume of tumor removed is as important as the size of residual tumor.

» CA 125 levels in the first 3-to-14 days after surgery may be more useful than late postoperative values obtained after peritoneal inflammation occurs, and more helpful than levels that confound the effects of surgery and chemotherapy.

•The clinical decision to re-operate is a complex one and cannot be based solely on changes in the CA 125 level.

•On the other hand, because the early CA 125 decline may give insight regarding the findings that can be expected at re-operation, this ratio may add to the factors involved in this difficult clinical decision.]

---

14. A 28-year old patient who had a negative history for cervical neoplasia has a hysterectomy for benign disease. The specimen shows invasive squamous cell carcinoma of the cervix. True statements about this situation include

   A. five-year survival with no further treatment is greater than 50%
   B. reoperation should be immediate
   C. reoperation should include radical parametrectomy, upper vaginectomy, pelvic lymphadenectomy, and bilateral salpingo-oophorectomy
   D. the morbidity from reoperation exceeds its benefit
   *E. treatment depends on whether the tumor was cut through

---

p. 933   (Chapman J A, Mannel R S, DiSaia P J, Walker, Berman M L. Surgical treatment of unexpected invasive cervical cancer found at total hysterectomy. Obstet Gynecol 1992; 80:931)

14. [F & I: •Background: Occasionally, postoperative assessment of a uterus removed for a benign indication reveals the surprise finding of invasive cervical cancer.

•Because the recurrence rate following simple hysterectomy done in this situation is approximately 60%, additional treatment is usually given with either radiation therapy or reoperation.

•Survival rates for women treated for cervical cancer by radiation therapy after simple hysterectomy range from 71 to 92% when there is no clinical evidence of residual cancer on pelvic examination.

•Because radiation therapy results in loss of ovarian function and a greater frequency of sexual dysfunction than with operative management, re-operation with removal of the parametria and pelvic lymph nodes is an attractive alternative.

•Most series evaluating radical re-operation grouped women with limited disease with those having extensive residual tumor, thereby precluding an accurate assessment of the treatment efficacy of re-operation.

Obstetrics and Gynecology: Review 1994-Gynecologic Oncology References

- This problem is compounded by a lack of standardization of the operative procedure, which can range from local excision to pelvic exenteration.

- In an effort to standardize surgery for women with limited invasive cervical cancer found after simple hysterectomy, performing a radical parametrectomy, upper vaginectomy, and pelvic lymphadenectomy has been suggested.

  ° In one series, this therapy produced 95% survival at 3 years.

- Objective: To evaluate experience with radical re-operation in 18 women found to have unexpected invasive cervical cancer at simple total hysterectomy.

- Even when routine cervical evaluation is done before hysterectomy for a benign diagnosis, an occasional patient will be found to have invasive cancer on the hysterectomy specimen.

- 27% of the patients with invasive cervical cancer had normal preoperative Papanicolaou smears is consistent with other reports in the literature.

- All patients with abnormal smears underwent colposcopy with biopsies, cervical conization, or both; yet invasive cancer was not diagnosed.

- Thus, even when appropriate steps are taken to rule out invasive cancer preoperatively, there is a small risk that unsuspected invasive cancer will be found at hysterectomy.

- Three patients did not have preoperative Papanicolaou smears which indicates the potential for reduction of unexpected cases.

- Emergency surgery for "uncontrolled hemorrhage" carries a risk of missing a cervical carcinoma.

- Simple hysterectomy is inadequate treatment of invasive cervical cancers.

  ° Survival estimates for women so treated are less than 50% at 5 years of follow-up.

- Radiotherapeutic techniques can cure most patients with unexpected cervical cancer diagnosed at simple hysterectomy.

- If the analysis is limited to radiation therapy in patients fulfilling the criteria of invasive disease with clear margins and no gross residual tumor, the survival rates have been 71 to 92%.

- The actuarial 5-year disease-free survival of 89% in this series confirms the effectiveness of radical parametrectomy, upper vaginectomy, and pelvic lymphadenectomy as an **alternative** to adjuvant radiotherapy in these patients.

- With a median follow-up of 72 months, these patients can achieve cure rates comparable to those in women undergoing primary radical hysterectomy or radiation therapy for stage IB disease.

- Radical re-operation was no more morbid than primary radical hysterectomy when comparing operating room time, estimated blood loss, and hospital stay.

- Re-operation is technically easier if performed at least 4 weeks after the initial surgery; this allowed the inflammation to resolve and appropriate surgical planes to develop.

- A potential disadvantage of radiation after simple hysterectomy is the poor geometry for brachytherapy.

  ° An open implant may be needed, which would require a laparotomy and obviate the major advantage of irradiation.

- The treatment plan is designed specifically for stage IB patients following simple hysterectomy, in whom a radical hysterectomy would have been the standard approach to treatment.

•Fact   °Detail   »issue   *answer

•This is true for younger patients, for whom surgery is often preferred over radiotherapy to avoid the potential side effects of radiation.

•Radiation therapy was avoided in 78% of the patients, and ovarian preservation was effected in all ten women under the age of 40 who underwent ovarian transposition at re-operation.

•Surgery was limited to patients with **no clinical evidence of residual disease**.

•In patients with evidence of tumor cut-through at simple hysterectomy or in those with grossly apparent residual disease, radiation therapy is preferred.]

---

15. A patient with squamous cell carcinoma of the vulva which is 1.5 centimeters in diameter is found to have a positive lymph node metastasis. Using the FIGO surgical classification the cancer is

    A. Stage I
    B. Stage II
    *C. Stage III
    D. Stage IV

---

p. 930 (Shanbour K A, Mannel R S, Morris P C, Yadack A, Walker J L. Comparison of clinical versus surgical staging systems in vulvar cancer. Obstet Gynecol 1992; 80:927)

15.[F & I: •Background: The revised FIGO staging of vulvar cancer has changed from a clinical to a surgical system.

•This change was needed because clinical assessment of inguinal and femoral lymph nodes was often in error.

•Approximately 30% false-positive and 30% false-negative rates in the clinical assessment of inguinal lymph nodes have been reported.

•Because lymph node metastasis is the most critical prognostic factor for vulvar cancer, surgical removal and pathologic assessment of inguinal and femoral lymph nodes are now required before assigning the specific stage.

•Involvement of the perineum is no longer considered in the new staging system.

•Objective: To compare the new surgical staging system with the old clinical staging system for vulvar cancer.

•Results: The new classification system for this disease is a more accurate prognostic indicator of survival than the previous clinical staging system.

•The reason for this appears to be the overriding influence of **nodal metastasis** on survival, along with the poor ability of clinical assessment to determine node status.

•A significant decrease was found in 5-year survival, from 87% in patients with negative nodes to 61% in solitary metastasis and 19% with two or more nodal metastases.

•Clinical assessment of groin lymph node status was associated with 33% false-negative and 36% false-positive rates.

•Overall, 41% of the patients had their stage reassigned after evaluation of nodal status.

•The data support incorporating this surgically determined information into the staging system because it more accurately categorizes patients into appropriate prognostic groups.

•There was a tendency to perform ipsilateral groin node dissection for lateral lesions and superficial inguinal node dissection for lesions of 2 cm or less in diameter with less than 5 mm of invasion.

°Complete bilateral inguinal and femoral lymphadenectomy was done if frozen pathology revealed metastasis.

°Complete node dissection was not performed on all patients.

°The surgical stage would be unlikely to change based on further node dissection because of the rarity of contralateral or deep femoral node involvement in the absence of ipsilateral inguinal node metastasis.

•The new staging system also removes perineal involvement from the stage III category.

°Perineal involvement did not have any adverse influence on survival.

°There was no significant difference in lesion size, lymph node metastases, or survival in patients with perineal lesions compared with the rest of the study group.

°Eleven patients were downstaged based on perineal involvement alone and had no recurrence.

°These data support the removal of perineal involvement from the staging criteria.

•**Tumor size** also correlated well with survival.

°In patients with no nodal metastasis, survival fell from 100% in T1 lesions (2 cm or smaller) to 82% in T2 lesions (larger than 2 cm).

°More important, tumor size appears to be a good predictor of nodal metastasis.

°Although 19% of T1 lesions had nodal metastases, these were all unilateral and solitary and none of these patients had recurrences.

°In contrast, the group of women with lesions larger than 2 cm and nodal metastases accounted for 83% of the recurrences while representing only 36% of the population.

°This is in agreement with the report of the Gynecologic Oncology Group, which considered these patients at high risk for recurrence.

•The stage III category includes patients at low risk for recurrence (ie, tumor measuring 2 cm or less with solitary nodal metastasis) along with a high-risk group of patients (tumor larger than 2 cm with nodal metastasis).

°This information is important when designing treatment protocols for this heterogeneous group of patients.]

---

16. A 180 pound patient is to have a Class III radical hysterectomy and pelvic lymphadenectomy for Stage IB squamous cell cervical cancer. What result can be expected?

   A. increased incidence of bladder dysfunction
   *B. increased incidence of blood transfusion
   C. increased incidence of deep pain thrombosis
   D. increased incidence of urinary tract injuries
   E. increased incidence of wound infection

---

p. 942   (Soisson A P, Soper J T, Berchuck A, Dodge R, Clarke-Pearson D. Radical hysterectomy in obese women. Obstet Gynecol 1992; 80:940)

16. [F & I: •Background: Radiation and radical hysterectomy are equally effective for treating patients with stage IB-IIA cervical cancer.

•The incidence of significant complications for each is essentially the same.

Obstetrics and Gynecology: Review 1994-Gynecologic Oncology References

•The choice of radical hysterectomy or radiation therapy is usually individualized, depending on the patient's age, general medical condition, and body habitus.

•The technical aspects of radical surgery may be more difficult in obese patients.

•The increased incidence of pulmonary complications, thromboembolic disease, and wound infection is directly responsible for the increased morbidity rate associated with radical surgery in overweight women.

•These factors might contribute to a compromise in surgical technique or survival and overshadow the potential advantages of preservation of ovarian and vaginal function usually attributed to radical hysterectomy.

•Blood loss and operative time may also be increased in obese women undergoing radical surgery.

•Radiation therapy is often selected as the primary mode of treatment in obese women with early cervical cancer.

•Objective: To determine both the short and long-term morbidity of radical hysterectomy and pelvic lymphadenectomy in obese women with invasive cancer limited to the cervix and upper vagina.

•Clinicopathologic features, survival, incidence of serious acute and chronic complications, operative time, estimated blood loss, and incidence of perioperative transfusion were analyzed in a large group of women treated with radical hysterectomy and pelvic lymphadenectomy.

•The surgical morbidity and mortality for obese women treated with major gynecologic surgery are increased compared with those for patients with a normal body habitus.

•Of these complications, the increased incidences of anesthetic, pulmonary, thromboembolic, and wound problems in obese women contribute to a relatively high morbidity rate.

•The increased risks of anesthesia due to altered metabolism of anesthetic agents, as well as the technical difficulty of administering anesthesia and maintaining control of the airway, are often significant enough to avoid surgery.

•The perioperative pulmonary complications of atelectasis and pneumonia are estimated to be increased twofold in obese women treated with gynecologic surgery; some complication rates are as high as 56%, especially in patients with pre-existing pulmonary disease.

•Perioperative morbidity in obese women undergoing radical hysterectomy and pelvic lymphadenectomy is not well defined.

•The incidence of deep venous thrombosis is increased in patients treated with radical hysterectomy and is even greater when they are obese.

•Complications of the surgical wound and the incidence of perioperative bleeding are increased in obese women following extensive abdominal surgery.

•Results: There was no difference in wound-related complications in the two groups.

•All women received perioperative antibiotics and had meticulous closure of the abdominal incision in layers to prevent seroma formation.

•Incisional drains or wound irrigation with antibiotic solutions were not used.

•There was a similar incidence of tumor involving the surgical margins, lymphatic metastases, and survival in both groups of women, indicating that the ability to perform an adequate radical hysterectomy was **not** compromised and that clinical staging was not affected by obesity.

•Compromised operative exposure is even more difficult to address, but the increased operative time and greater estimated blood loss indicate that surgery was more difficult in obese women.

Obstetrics and Gynecology:Review 1994-Gynecologic Oncology References

•There was no significant difference in the incidence of major surgical or medical complications compared with women of normal body weight.

•Even though surgery lasts longer and is associated with a statistically significantly greater estimated blood loss and incidence of transfusion, it seems reasonable to consider radical hysterectomy as a treatment option for these patients.

•Strict attention to surgical technique, deep venous thrombosis, and antibiotic prophylaxis should minimize the short-term surgical morbidity in these high-risk patients.

•The technical difficulties and decreased operative exposure can be minimized by using a large abdominal incision and self-retaining retractors.]

---

17. Which of the following is the LEAST reliable predictor in cases of stage I invasive squamous cell carcinoma of the cervix?

    A. depth of invasion
*B. flow cytometry analysis
    C. lesion size
    D. lymph node metastasis
    E. penetration of vascular channels

---

p. 370 (Connor J P, Miller D S, Bauer K D, Murad T M, Rademaker A W, Lurain J R. Flow cytometric evaluation of early invasive cervical cancer. Obstet Gynecol 1993; 81:367)

17. [F & I: •Background: As a result of earlier diagnosis and, to a lesser extent, improved treatment, carcinoma of the uterine cervix is no longer the leading cause of cancer deaths among women in this country as it is in much of the developing world.

°These tumors still account for 4500 deaths annually in the United States.

°Even patients with early cancers confined to the cervix develop recurrence in as many as 20% of cases.

•The use of flow cytometry to measure DNA content and proliferative activity has prognostic significance in terms of risk of recurrence and survival for several human malignancies.

•In invasive cervical cancer, the value of these flow cytometric measurements in terms of predicting biologic behavior and hence patient prognosis has been inconsistent.

•Objective: With these conflicting results in mind, the role of flow cytometry-measured ploidy, DNA index, and S-phase fraction were evaluated as prognostic indicators in 53 women with stage IB malignancies of the uterine cervix who had radical hysterectomy and pelvic lymphadenectomy as primary treatment.

•Multiple specimens were evaluated for each tumor when possible to explore tumor heterogeneity as a potential cause of these conflicting results.

•With the widespread acceptance of the Papanicolaou smear and colposcopy, more cancers of the cervix are being diagnosed at earlier stages and younger ages.

•The proportion of invasive cervical carcinomas in stage I has increased, and now constitutes one-third to one-half of these malignancies.

•With this increased proportion of stage I tumors, authors have attempted to define prognostic factors within this stage to help guide therapeutic decisions.

•Survival has been shown to be inversely related to size of the cervical lesion.

- The depth of tumor invasion as measured histologically predicts survival.

- A negative relationship of survival to lymph and vascular permeation has also been shown.

- The challenge in recent years has been to find a measurable prognosticator that can discern biologically more aggressive cervical tumors in the face of the clinical homogeneity of many stage I patients.

- Determinations of cellular DNA content and proliferative activity have provided just such information in several human malignancies.

- Automated flow cytometry has improved on the Feulgen stains of earlier studies as a more rapid and equally precise measurement of DNA content.

- In addition, it provides histograms from which cell cycle phase distribution can be calculated.

- Concerning tumors of the uterine cervix, a variety of reports on the prognostic significance of ploidy and S-phase fraction have shown conflicting results both between studies and when comparing trends seen in other malignancies.

- When the primary therapy is surgical and the entire tumor is available for analysis, flow cytometry can be done on multiple areas within each tumor, making it possible to address this issue.

- This study reports a group of stage IB patients with similar tumor burden, an overall recurrence rate of 23%, and a mean follow-up of 63 months.

- The use of multiple specimens for each tumor (when available) showed clearly that although heterogeneity between samples was present, the level of variance between samples from different patients was significantly greater than the variance within any single tumor ($P < .0001$).

  ° The level of heterogeneity was greater between patients than within any one tumor.

- Little difference in the statistical correlations was found with recurrence or survival based on the maximum, minimum, or mean values of the flow cytometry data for each subject.

- This indicates that the conflicting results seen in previous studies are not due to tumor heterogeneity.

- If heterogeneity were the cause, the variance within a single tumor would more likely have approached or exceeded the variance between patients, and a different statistical significance between the maximum, minimum, and mean values would have been found.

- Of the prognostic variables evaluated, only depth of invasion predicted recurrence or survival in this patient population.

- Hazard ratios indicated a 30% increase in the risk of both tumor recurrence and death for every 10% increase in the depth of tumor invasion.

- **Of particular interest is the lack of any significant correlation between DNA index or S-phase fraction and recurrence risk or survival.**

- In fact, the mean survival and time to recurrence for aneuploid versus diploid tumors were almost identical.

- The sample size of 53 women with a 23% recurrence rate was sufficient to detect, with 80% power, a difference in death or recurrence of 20 versus 50% between subcategories.

- To be able to detect differences of 20 versus 30%, a sample size of at least 500 subjects would be required.

Obstetrics and Gynecology: Review 1994-Gynecologic Oncology References

•The results clearly indicate that alterations in DNA content (ploidy and DNA index) or proliferative activity (S-phase fraction) in invasive cancers of the uterine cervix do **not** reflect the biologic behavior of surgically treated early-stage malignancies in terms of recurrence or survival.

•Tumor heterogeneity is present in early cancers of the cervix, but this is not of a magnitude to account for the conflicting results seen in the literature.]

---

18. True statements about the induction of uterine neoplasms during tamoxifen therapy for cancer of the breast include all of the following EXCEPT

    A. Most cancers are FIGO stage I.
  *B. The cancers are only adenocarcinomas and not sarcomas.
    C. The induction is dose-related.
    D. The patients are likely to have symptoms associated with uterine cancer.
    E. The patients are most likely to be postmenopausal.

---

p.167 (Seoud A F M, Johnson J, Weed Jr J C. Gynecologic tumors in tamoxifen-treated women with breast cancer. Obstet Gynecol 1993; 82:165)

18. [F & I: •Background: Tamoxifen is a nonsteroidal compound with weak estrogenic activity.

•When given to women who produce estrogen, tamoxifen competes for estrogen receptors and reduces the net estrogenic effect

•In hypoestrogenic women, it has a weak estrogen effect.

•Tamoxifen is widely used to treat estrogen receptor-positive, node-negative carcinoma of the breast.

°It is used for palliation in both premenopausal and postmenopausal women with advanced or recurrent breast cancer and is advocated as long-term adjuvant therapy in node-positive breast cancer patients.

°Breast cancer prophylaxis in high-risk healthy women and treatment of benign gynecologic diseases are other possible uses for this agent

•Tamoxifen has a low incidence of side effects.

•Tamoxifen has been associated with the development of endometrial carcinoma.

•Objective: To review the gynecologic malignancies associated with tamoxifen.

•The literature contains 61 cases of **adenocarcinoma of the endometrium** in tamoxifen-treated breast cancer patients

•There are three cases of uterine **sarcoma** and one sarcoma.

•The total number of gynecologic malignancies reaches 70.

•The mean age for 35 of the patients was 63.9 ± 12.0 years.

•Menopausal status, available for 66 patients, showed that five (7.6%) were premenopausal and 61 (92.4%) were postmenopausal.

•The FIGO stage of the gynecologic tumor, available for 27 of the endometrial adenocarcinomas, was stage I in 25 (92.6%) and stage III in (7.4%).

•The tumor grade, noted in 27 adenocarcinomas of the endometrium, was grade 1 in 11 (40.7%) and grade 2 or 3 in 16 (59.3%).

•Fact   °Detail   »issue   *answer

Obstetrics and Gynecology:Review 1994-Gynecologic Oncology References

- The dose of tamoxifen was 20 mg/day in 15 (23.4%), 30 mg/day in 11(17.2%), and 40 mg or higher in 38 (59.4%).

- Information about the duration of tamoxifen treatment was available for 49 patients; 57% were treated for less than 2 years whereas 43% had used it for more than 2 years.

- Breast cancer is the second leading cause of cancer deaths in women.

- The lifetime risk that any woman will acquire breast cancer is about **one in nine**.

- Certain factors, such as a family history of breast cancer or other malignancies such as ovarian or endometrial cancer, further increase this risk.

- Women with breast cancer also have an increased risk of developing secondary malignancies, especially ovarian, endometrial, and gastrointestinal cancers.

- The breasts, ovaries, and endometrium are especially interesting because of their interrelation with the various sex hormones and because of the possible use of hormonal therapy for tumors in these organs.

- The overall relative risk of endometrial cancer in patients with breast cancer was 1.72

    ° This risk, which was age-dependent, was approximately 1.0 in women younger than 50 years and closer to 2.4 in women 70 years of age or older.

- Tamoxifen has been used with inconsistent results in the treatment of endometrial carcinoma.

- The estrogenic effect of tamoxifen has been implicated in the development of endometrial polyps, endometrial hyperplasia, and uterine leiomyomata in pre and postmenopausal breast cancer patients.

- Whether the increase in the incidence of endometrial adenocarcinoma and, possibly, other gynecologic malignancies in tamoxifen-treated breast cancer patients represents a true increase or an improvement in the rate of detection of very early lesions is unknown

- These patients and most of those in the literature had symptoms (such as bleeding or discharge) for a relatively long time before they were evaluated.

    ° It is important to monitor patients closely and investigate any pertinent complaint promptly.

- The dose level and duration of tamoxifen treatment may be relevant in the development of pelvic malignancies.

- Although doses as high as 60 mg/day were used in some studies, endometrial adenocarcinomas have developed with dosages as low as 20 mg/day.

- The addition of a progestin might alleviate the effect of tamoxifen on the endometrium

- Others have had some reservation, as progestin might negate the beneficial effects of tamoxifen on breast cancer.

- To circumvent this problem, some have advocated regular (annual or semiannual) endometrial biopsies, whereas others have recommended CO_2 hysteroscopy on a yearly basis.

- The majority of reported gynecologic tumors were endometrial adenocarcinomas.

- This is the first well-documented case of mixed mullerian sarcoma of the uterus and fallopian tube carcinoma associated with tamoxifen treatment in breast cancer patients.

- A causal relationship is difficult to establish.

- The rarity of such primary tumors and their unknown potential for estrogen dependency preclude the drawing of any conclusions.

• A potential association between tamoxifen and other cancers, such as **hepatic cancer**, has also been reported.

• Tamoxifen has other side effects such as nausea and vomiting, and occasionally hot flashes.

• Although visual disturbances are usually reported as reversible and minor, long-term use of low-dose tamoxifen (10 mg/day) induced **retinopathy or keratopathy** in four of 63 patients studied prospectively

°Some retinal opacities were irreversible.

• Large-scale trials of tamoxifen for the prevention of breast cancer have begun in England and the United States.

• A full understanding of possible untoward effects must be available to insure informed consent.

• Some researchers object to the use of tamoxifen in healthy women until more information is available

• Tamoxifen is a safe drug with proven value in the treatment of advanced or recurrent breast cancer, as well as in the adjuvant treatment of early breast cancer.

»Rigorous criteria should be used to monitor for cancerous and noncancerous side effects, which include endometrial adenocarcinomas as well as rarer occurrences of hepatic cancer, tubal cancer, mixed mullerian sarcoma, and ocular toxicity.

»The use of tamoxifen for benign breast diseases and other gynecologic conditions should be severely limited until more data are available.

• Experience seems to suggest an association between tamoxifen use and endometrial adenocarcinoma.

»A close follow-up of patients taking tamoxifen and prompt evaluation of all pelvic symptoms should be undertaken.

»Work-up should include a pelvic examination and endometrial biopsy, as well as repeat evaluation every 6 months.

• The efficacy of concomitant ultrasound evaluation of the uterus, endometrium, and adnexa remains to be proven.

• Monitoring for other toxicities, such as ocular toxicity, should also be considered.]

---

19. True statements about intraepithelial cervical neoplasia in patients with HIV include all of the following EXCEPT

    A. Cryotherapy is ineffective in treating the CIN.
    B. Patients with CD4 counts below 500 per cubic millimeter are at increased risk of recurrence.
  *C. The mode of acquisition of HIV is irrelevant to the recurrent of CIN.
    D. The prevalence rate is related to the degree of immunosuppression.
    E. The recurrence rate is high after standard treatment.

---

p. 174 (Maiman M, Fruchter R G, Serur E, Levine P A, Arrastia C D, Sedlis A. Recurrent cervical intraepithelial neoplasia in human immunodeficiency virus-seropositive women. Obstet Gynecol 1993; 82:170)

19. [F & I: • Background: The association between human immunodeficiency virus (HIV) and cervical neoplasia is well established.

Obstetrics and Gynecology: Review 1994-Gynecologic Oncology References

- In populations in which HIV infection is prevalent, patients with cervical neoplasia may have high rates of HIV infection.

- Concomitant HIV infection may alter the natural history of both invasive cervical carcinoma and preinvasive disease.

- Human immunodeficiency virus-positive patients with invasive cervical cancer present with more advanced disease, poorer responses to therapy, and higher recurrence and death rates than HIV-negative women of similar disease status.

- Like renal transplant patients on immunosuppressive drugs, HIV-seropositive women with cervical intraepithelial neoplasia (CIN) have higher-grade lesions with more extensive cervical involvement and multisite lower genital tract involvement with human papillomavirus (HPV)-associated lesions.

- In addition, the presence and severity of cervical dysplasia correlate with both quantitative and qualitative T-cell function.

- Although standard ablative therapy for CIN in immunocompetent women is highly successful with minimal morbidity, there are few data on recurrence rates for preinvasive disease in HIV-positive patients.

- Objective: To compare treatment results after standard therapy for cervical dysplasia in HIV-seropositive and HIV-seronegative women.

- Results: A high rate (39%) of recurrent CIN in HIV-positive women after standard ablative therapy.

- Women positive for HIV are at high risk of developing cervical dysplasia, with frequencies as high as 40%.

- This association can be explained on the basis of both common sexual behavior risks and immunosuppression predisposing to HPV infection and associated neoplasia.

- Intraepithelial neoplasia in such patients may be of higher grade with more extensive cervical involvement and multisite (vaginal, vulval, perianal) involvement with HPV-associated lesions.

- Although the frequency at recurrent CIN is somewhat alarming, it is not unexpected, as higher rates of recurrent neoplasia have been observed in immunosuppressed patients in general and HIV-positive patients in particular.

- Therapy for CIN in immunocompetent patients is usually highly successful, with cure rates between 90-to-96% following ablative techniques such as cryotherapy, laser therapy, and cone biopsy.

- These numbers are consistent with the 9% recurrence rate in the seronegative group.

- Effective treatment of CIN is crucial in HIV-infected women; recent data indicate that untreated CIN is significantly more likely to progress in HIV-positive women than in HIV-negative controls.

- The high recurrence rates observed are of particular concern, and therapeutic strategies that address these treatment failures seem necessary.

- A second major finding was the relationship between immune status and recurrent CIN.

- Patients with CD4 counts **below 500/mm^3** were at extremely **high risk** for the development of recurrent disease, whereas women with counts greater than 500/mm^3 had recurrence rates of only 18%, about twice that of HIV-negative patients.

- Correlations have been established between immune status and many characteristics of cervical dysplasia in HIV-positive women.

- In immunocompetent women, recurrent CIN has been related to increasing grade and lesion size, but in HIV positive women, **degree of immunosuppression** was a more important predictor of recurrence.

- Fact   °Detail   »issue   *answer

•Although HIV-positive patients may represent a high-risk group for many aspects of lower genital tract neoplasia, diagnostic and therapeutic strategies may be stratified based on the degree of immunosuppression.

»Baseline and periodic follow-up CD4 counts should be used in managing CIN in HIV-positive women, with the most aggressive surveillance, treatment, and maintenance regimens reserved for those patients most severely immunosuppressed.

•A third clinically important finding was the **poor outcome after cryotherapy** in HIV-positive patients.

•Because patients with earlier-grade lesions were more likely to be treated with cryotherapy, this trend may be even more important and may explain the excellent results with cryotherapy in the HIV-negative group.

»Although use of cryotherapy in HIV-positive patients may seem attractive because of the absence of bleeding and low risk of iatrogenic transmission of HIV, further studies are needed to define whether cryotherapy is associated with a therapeutic disadvantage in HIV-positive women with CIN.

•Finally, the **mode of HIV acquisition** correlated strongly with recurrent disease.

•**All recurrences** occurred in women who acquired HIV from **heterosexual transmission**, and **none** in those women in whom the etiology was **IV drug abuse**.

•The mode of acquisition of HIV infection affects other aspects of HIV-related disease.

•Theoretical explanations for the varying rates of recurrence of CIN by mode of HIV acquisition include different sexual-behavior patterns, the effect of direct HIV cervical infection, or differences in relative immunosuppression.

•Because of high-frequency, extensive lower genital tract disease and high recurrence rates after standard therapy, complete and definitive management is mandatory.

•5-fluorouracil vaginal cream has been used with some success in the care of immunosuppressed women with lower genital tract neoplasia, and interferon therapy has been used to treat both CIN and other HIV-related diseases.

•Whether these or any other therapies prove to be useful for the management of CIN in HIV-seropositive women remains to be studied.

•Unique therapeutic strategies such as local maintenance therapy, systemic therapy, or optimization of immune function should be developed to address the treatment failures observed.

»Whether standard or extended treatment is used, meticulous post-therapy surveillance with liberal colposcopic biopsy is advised to address recurrent disease and progressive neoplasia.]

---

20. The morbidity from selective pelvic and periaortic lymphadenectomy in patients with endometrial carcinoma is related to all of the following EXCEPT

    A. operating time
    B. patients age
    C. patients weight
    D. surgeon
    *E. the lymphadenectomy itself

---

p. 1230 (Homesley H D, Kadar N, Barrett R J, Lentz S S. Selective pelvic and periaortic lymphadenectomy does not increase morbidity in surgical staging of endometrial carcinoma. Am J Obstet Gynec 1992; 167:1225)

20. [F & I: •Background: The most important component of any treatment plan for early (International Federation of Gynecology and Obstetrics 1970 clinical stages I and II) endometrial carcinoma is hysterectomy, but the indications, timing, and type of radiation therapy have varied widely among different centers.

•The trend is toward primary surgery and omission of the preoperative intracavitary component of adjunctive radiotherapy.

•The only randomized controlled clinical trial reported for radiation therapy failed to show that whole-pelvic radiation therapy improved survival.

•The recent adoption by International Federation of Gynecology and Obstetrics of a new surgical staging system for endometrial carcinoma requires pelvic and periaortic lymphadenectomy because of the lower survival associated with positive pelvic and periaortic nodes.

•Lymphadenectomy is a potentially morbid procedure, which can only be justified in clinical practice if it improves outcome as reflected by either increased survival or decreased morbidity by avoiding radiation.

•Objective: To focus primarily on the morbidity resulting from lymphadenectomy.

•Methods: The selective lymphadenectomy was performed in accordance with the guidelines of the Surgical Manual of the Gynecologic Oncology Group by excising pelvic nodal tissue from the distal one half of the common iliac arteries, anterior and medial external iliac arteries and veins, and the obturator fat pad anterior to the obturator nerve.

•The aortic dissection included excision at the iliac arteries.

•Results: Selective pelvic and periaortic lymphadenectomy was not associated with a significant increase in either surgical morbidity or morbidity from subsequent radiation therapy.

•No radiation cystitis or radiation proctitis was expected because no high-dose vaginal brachytherapy was given.

•The treatment-related mortality was higher for the hysterectomy group (3/104) than for the lymphadenectomy group (1/196), although this was not statistically different.

•Because patients were not randomly assigned to treatment, it is possible that selection bias may have masked real differences in morbidity between the two treatments.

°The fact that patients in the hysterectomy group weighed significantly more than patients in the lymphadenectomy group and that they tended to have higher anesthesia physical status scores would tend to lend credence to this possibility.

°No significant difference in morbidity emerged between the two groups after adjustment for these and other maldistributed covariates.

°Nonetheless, because of the retrospective nature of the study and the low complication rate observed, it is possible that through the operation of subtle selection biases patients in the lymphadenectomy group were at lower risk for complications than those in the hysterectomy group, thus producing increased morbidity associated with hysterectomy.

•Lymphadenectomy did **increase** the operative blood loss significantly, but the increase was minimal, as reflected by the similar transfusion rates for the two treatment groups.

•The amount of blood lost did not affect the frequency of any of the other complications investigated, namely, wound infection, deep venous thrombosis and pulmonary embolus, and aggregate serious morbidity.

- •Serious hemorrhagic complication, especially during periaortic lymphadenectomy, is a hazard and was occasionally encountered, but it did not cause serious or long-term morbidity; excessive blood loss occurred in the hysterectomy group as well.

- •Neither the association of increased blood loss and black race nor the increased operating time could be explained by consideration of other variables such as differences in uterine weights and incidence of pelvic inflammatory disease.

- •Operating time increased with the number of lymph nodes removed, after adjustment for the other variables that affected operating time (weight, race, surgeon, and estimated blood loss).

- •After correction for confounding variables, operating time itself affected the **wound infection** rate but not the frequency of other complications.

- •Patient weight was the only independent risk factor for wound infection after operating time was accounted for.

- •By increasing the operating time, lymphadenectomy may contribute to an increase in the wound infection rate; it was the operating time per se (in addition to patient weight) rather than lymphadenectomy that appeared to be the determinant factor, and this itself was significantly affected by many other variables besides lymphadenectomy.

- •Compared with hysterectomy alone, the lymphadenectomy group had longer operative times, greater blood loss, and a higher transfusion rate.

- •For lymphadenectomy other complications, such as lymphedema, bowel obstruction, and deep venous thrombosis, and mortality rates were also higher, with the conclusion that lymphadenectomy produced significantly more morbidity than did hysterectomy alone.

- •There was a 3.7% (11/300) incidence of thromboembolic complications (nine cases of pulmonary emboli with three deaths and two patients recognized with deep venous thrombosis).

- •Differences in morbidity between the lymphadenectomy and hysterectomy groups were accounted for by factors such as surgeon, weight, race, and age rather than surgical procedure.

- •The current series of patients does indicate that at least four interactive variables (surgeon, age, weight, and race) may decide outcome, and when all of these variables are analyzed with multivariate methods, the addition of selective pelvic and periaortic lymphadenectomy to hysterectomy does **not** have an adverse impact on surgical morbidity in the staging of early endometrial cancer nor does it increase the morbidity associated with subsequent whole-pelvic irradiation.]

Obstetrics and Gynecology: Review 1994 - Gynecologic Oncology References

Directions: Each set of lettered headings below is followed by a list of numbered words or phrases. For each numbered word or phrase select:

- A. if the item is associated with *(A) only*
- B. if the item is associated with *(B) only*
- C. if item is associated with *both (A) and (B)*
- D. if item is associated with *neither (A) nor (B)*

Items 21-23.

In the treatment of invasive cervical cancer stage IB

- A. Schauta-Amreich vaginal hysterectomy
- B. Wertheim-Meigs abdominal hysterectomy
- C. both
- D. neither

21. complication rate about 5% Ans: C

22. five-year survival about 80% Ans: C

23. performed with lymphadenectomy Ans: B

---

p. 933 (Massi G, Savino L, Susini T. Schauta-Amreich vaginal hysterectomy and Wertheim-Meigs abdominal hysterectomy in the treatment of cervical cancer: A retrospective analysis. Am J Obstet Gynec 1993; 168:928)

21-23. [F & I: •Background: Radical vaginal hysterectomy in the treatment of cervical carcinoma was introduced by Schauta at the beginning of this century.

•In 1908 Schauta was able to achieve an eightfold reduction in the mortality rate with equivalent results in terms of survival compared with Wertheim's abdominal hysterectomy, which at the time had a high mortality rate (18.6%).

•In the 1920s Amreich improved Schauta's technique by giving the operation an accurate anatomic support.

•When Meigs combined his radical abdominal hysterectomy with systematic pelvic lymphadenectomy in the 1940s, the goal of a radical surgery procedure seemed to have been reached.

•The role of the Schauta-Amreich vaginal hysterectomy in the treatment of cervical cancer thus appeared to be limited.

•Objectives: (1) to evaluate the results of Schauta-Amreich vaginal hysterectomy in the treatment of carcinoma of the uterine cervix and compare it with the survival rate obtained after the Wertheim-Meigs operation,

•(2) to analyze the differences between these operations in terms of intraoperative and postoperative morbidity and mortality,

•(3) to discuss the role of lymphadenectomy in the treatment of cervical cancer, and

•(4) to investigate the role of surgical adjuvant radiotherapy in patients with nodal metastasis.

•Schauta-Amreich vaginal hysterectomy showed a high rate of cure for cervical cancer, and its use allowed survival rates similar to those of the Wertheim Meigs operation, which is regarded as the gold standard in the surgical treatment of cervical cancer all over the world.

•A statistically significant difference in survival was obtained in stage IB cases.

°This result was not confirmed in patients who underwent surgery only.

•Fact   °Detail   »issue   *answer

°Considering the retrospective approach of the current report, it is not a demonstration of the superiority of the vaginal technique.

•Both procedures were infrequently associated with severe surgical morbidity, whereas mortality, quite low after Meigs operation (0.8%), was zero after the Schauta-Amreich procedure.

•Conclusions: (1) The radical vaginal hysterectomy is as effective as the Wertheim-Meigs operation in the surgical management of stage IB or IIA cervical cancer.

•(2) The therapeutic role of lymphadenectomy is questionable, because the patients who underwent extended vaginal hysterectomy, without any lymphadenectomy, had results similar to those of the patients who had systematic pelvic lymphadenectomy, according to the Meigs abdominal procedure.

•(3) Even the diagnostic role of lymphadenectomy appears to be questionable, because postoperative irradiation in the patients with pelvic lymph nodal metastasis did not yield any improvement in survival.

•Parameters such as grade of lesion and lymphatic involvement were not available from the clinical records, because they were not evaluated at that time.

°It was not possible to control the two groups for these factors.

•In the years 1968 through 1976 the Schauta-Amreich operation was always used except in cases with technical contraindications to the vaginal approach (previous laparotomy, coexistent uteroadnexal abnormality); in the years 1977 through 1983 the Wertheim-Meigs procedure was the standard, and it was performed in all cases except those where patients had contraindications to general anesthesia or to the abdominal approach (obesity).

•The whole series, from 1968 to 1983, was studied and treated by the same group and, especially, all Schauta-Amreich and Wertheim-Meigs operations were carried out by the same surgeon, thus giving a relevant homogeneity to the overall data.

•Considerable doubt persists concerning lymph nodes and their role in antitumor defense, as well as the role of lymphadenectomy.

•Experimental data on the immunologic antitumor response seems to demonstrate a role for local-regional lymph nodes only in the early stages of tumor growth, whereas the possibility that lymph nodes behave as a filter or as barriers against neoplastic spread is not proved once the primary lesion attains considerable size.

•Possibly, in patients who have only lymph node involvement and no systemic disease cure is obtained once the primary lesion is removed.

•There is increasing evidence that biologic features, such as ploidy and fraction of S-phase cells, are strong predictors of survival in many cases of solid tumors and also in cervical cancer.

•The poor results of adjuvant radiotherapy in patients with nodal metastasis are another interesting outcome of the current study.

•Similar results were reported >10 years ago.

•High-dose pelvic irradiation is effective in "sterilizing" neoplastic cells in a certain field, but because immunosupression is also induced, metastatic spread may be enhanced.]

Items 24-26.

A. cervical adenocarcinoma in situ
B. cervical squamous cell carcinoma in situ
C. both
D. neither

24. cervical cone biopsy with uninvolved margins and negative ECC is diagnostically accurate

Ans: C

25. cervical cone biopsy is adequate treatment

Ans: C

26. if cone margins are involved expected management is reasonable

Ans: B

p. 938 (Muntz H G, Bell D A, Lage J M, Goff B A, Feldman S, Rice L W. Adenocarcinoma in situ of the uterine cervix. Obstet Gynecol 1992; 80:935)

24-26. [F & I: •Background: Adenocarcinoma in situ of the uterine cervix was first recognized as a distinct entity in 1953.

•Because adenocarcinoma in situ lacks specific clinical and colposcopic features, study of its natural history was hampered until discovery of criteria for detecting adenocarcinoma in situ on screening cervicovaginal smears.

•Despite improved cytologic detection, the clinical management of women with cervical adenocarcinoma in situ is controversial.

•This is due to the rarity of adenocarcinoma in situ, in contrast to the more common and well-described squamous cell carcinoma in situ (CIS) of the cervix.

•The ratio of cervical adenocarcinoma in situ to squamous cell CIS is estimated at 1:239 ratio.

•Because the incidence of invasive adenocarcinoma of the cervix has been increasing relative to that of squamous cancers, the incidence of adenocarcinoma in situ is most likely increasing as well.

•Objective: To report a clinicopathologic study of cervical adenocarcinoma in situ which evaluated the diagnostic accuracy of cervical conization for women with adenocarcinoma in situ;

•to emphasize the ability to predict residual adenocarcinoma in situ in subsequent hysterectomy specimens and

•to exclude reliably occult invasive adenocarcinoma.

•Cervical conization, assuming uninvolved margins, is adequate for the diagnosis and treatment of squamous cell CIS.

•In contrast, the capability of a cone biopsy to exclude occult invasion and excise all foci of preinvasive disease has been questioned in cases of adenocarcinoma in situ, for which extrafascial hysterectomy is advocated as minimal treatment.

•Early studies of cervical adenocarcinoma in situ emphasized the occasional case of residual disease in hysterectomy specimens following cone biopsies.

•There is a theoretical risk of multifocal disease, deep glandular involvement, and upper endocervical extension leading to occult relapses.

•Although cervical adenocarcinoma in situ lesions can be extensive, most are located at the transformation zone and are unifocal without "skip" lesions.

- Results: Histologic analysis of specimens yielded similar conclusions, with involvement of the endocervical canal almost always occurring in continuity with adenocarcinoma in situ at the transformation zone.

- The pre-conization diagnosis of adenocarcinoma in situ is challenging.

- The diagnosis was suspected before conization in only half of the cases.

- There was also a high frequency (84%) of apparently normal cervicovaginal smears 1 year before the diagnostic conization.

  ° Whether this results from the inherent difficulty in detecting adenocarcinoma in situ, especially in women previously treated for squamous CIN (20% in this series), or from rapid progression from normal glandular epithelium to adenocarcinoma in situ is unknown.

- Despite advances in the cytologic diagnosis of glandular lesions of the cervix, clinicians should expect that many cases of adenocarcinoma in situ will still be recognized only after cervical conization for other indications.

- Involvement of conization margins or ECCs with adenocarcinoma in situ is associated with a significant risk of persistent adenocarcinoma in situ.

- Combined data of several studies yields 84 evaluable cases; 21 of 34 women (62%) with positive cone margins or ECCs had adenocarcinoma in situ detected at hysterectomy, compared with four of 50 women (8%) with uninvolved margins.

- Some women with involved margins were found at hysterectomy to have occult invasive carcinoma not already detected by the preceding conization.

- Conclusion: Women with involved cone margins should at a minimum undergo repeat conization and ECC to assess better the extent of adenocarcinoma in situ and to exclude invasive carcinoma.

- This contrasts with cervical squamous cell CIS, for which expectant management is reasonable for selected women whose cone biopsies have dysplasia at the margins

- A cervical cone biopsy of sufficient size with uninvolved margins and a concomitant normal ECC is diagnostically accurate.

  ° There were no cases of occult invasive carcinoma detected at hysterectomy in the 50 women reported to date.

- The 8% rate of persistent adenocarcinoma in situ in hysterectomy specimens is also low, but the number of women studied is small and post-conization cervicovaginal cytology may not be reliable for detecting persistent or recurrent adenocarcinoma in situ.

- Thus, extrafascial hysterectomy is reasonable in women who have completed their childbearing.

- For women who desire to maintain their fertility, cervical conization alone can be considered adequate treatment for adenocarcinoma in situ, assuming that margins and concomitant ECCs are uninvolved and the patient is closely monitored.

- Whether this approach is as safe for cervical adenocarcinoma in situ as for squamous CIS will require further study.]

Directions: For each of the questions or incomplete statements below, ONE or MORE of the answers or completions given is correct. In each case select:

- A. if only 1, 2, and 3 are correct
- B. if only 1 and 3 are correct
- C. if only 2 and 4 are correct
- D. if only 4 is correct
- E. if all are correct

27. Survival of patients with epithelial ovarian cancer is affected by

 1. stage of disease.
 2. sensitivity to platinum therapy.
 3. histologic grade.
 4. performance status.

---

p. 755   Ans: E   (Carter J, Fowler J, Carlson J, Carson K, Twiggs L B. Borderline and invasive epithelial ovarian tumors in young women. Obstet Gynecol 1993; 82:752)

27. [F & I: •Background: With a median age at diagnosis of 50 years and a peak incidence occurring in the eighth decade, epithelial ovarian cancer is uncommon in young women.

•Young women, defined in this series as less than 40 years of age, represent 3-to-30% of all patients with malignant ovarian tumors.

•Uncertainty exists regarding the occurrence and the etiologic and prognostic factors in this younger subset of patients.

•Objective: To determine the occurrence of borderline and invasive epithelial ovarian tumors and their outcome in women less than 40 years of age.

•Survival of patients with epithelial ovarian cancer is affected by multiple variables, of which the disease stage, grade, and sensitivity to platinum therapy may be the most obvious.

•Age may also influence survival in ovarian cancer in a number of ways.

•Young patients who develop invasive malignancies have more aggressive tumors and poor outcome, whereas older patients with associated multiple medical problems and poorer performance status tend to be less likely to withstand the stress of radical surgery and adjuvant chemotherapy.

•Germ cell ovarian tumors are more common in younger women than their epithelial counterparts.

•Between 3-to-30% of women with epithelial ovarian tumors are less than 35-to-40 years of age.

•Recently, FIGO reported that 8.7 and 31.8% of invasive and borderline tumors, respectively, occurred in women under the age of 40.6.

•The effect of young age on survival in these series is unknown, as cisplatin-based protocols were in their infancy, and many of the series reported the results of simple surgical therapy and adjuvant therapy with external-beam radiation and alkylating agents.

•In a large study of prognostic factors in ovarian cancer, age was not identified as an independent prognostic factor by multivariate analysis, although it was significant by univariate analysis.

•More important than age as a prognostic factor in this series was patient **performance status**, lending further support to the notion that a patient's ability to withstand the effects of therapy is an important prognostic factor regardless of age.

•Similar series have included patients with borderline malignancies, whose survival in early stages approaches 95%.

•Fact   °Detail   »issue   *answer

- Similarly, patients with stage Ia, grade 1 cancers also have a survival greater than 95%.

- Other series have distinguished between borderline and invasive patients, claiming that survival is excellent regardless of stage, but have always qualified this with a statement that widespread disease and death can result from borderline tumors.

- Borderline tumors were included in this analysis as they represent only 15% of the patient population, but borderline and invasive groups were distinguished for statistical analysis.

- Age may influence survival from ovarian cancer in a number of ways.

  ° A study from Germany noted little impact of age on survival after older patients who died within the first 2 months of diagnosis were eliminated from analysis.

  ° If the older patient could survive surgery and the first course of chemotherapy, then the age-adjusted survival was similar for young and old patients.

- **Clinical assessment** is paramount in selecting patients fit enough to undergo aggressive cytoreductive surgery.

- Although the etiology of ovarian cancer remains unknown, there are a number of epidemiologic factors implicated, including low parity, nulliparity, infertility, early menarche, and late menopause.

- These variables all imply that **repetitive and incessant ovulation** leads to stimulation of the ovarian germinal epithelium and subsequent malignant transformation.

- Although the mean parity was 1.0, 32 patients (48%) were nulliparous, the average age at menarche was 13, and 16% gave a history of infertility.

- These facts support the epidemiologic data, but their impact in this young patient population remains uncertain.

- Although the predominant presenting **symptoms** were **pelvic pain and abdominal distention** in 49 and 42%, respectively, nine patients (13%) had no symptoms at all.

- Most patients also had early symptomatology, with 64% having symptoms of less than 6 months in duration.

- Younger women are more likely to have routine gynecologic examinations for birth control and Papanicolaou smears, contributing to the early detection of tumors in this group.

- Prolonged survival of young patients afflicted with epithelial ovarian cancer is associated with earlier stage and lower-grade disease.

- Although ten patients had grade 1 tumors, only 18 (27%) had stage I disease, with the majority (54%) having stage III or IV disease.

- Conservative surgery has been proposed as an alternative to radical surgery in young patients with borderline or grade 1 carcinomas who wish to preserve their fertility.

- Only five patients (7%) had conservative surgery performed.

- The remainder had radical surgery: TAH-BSO, omentectomy, tumor debulking, and node sampling when appropriate.

- As a result of these efforts, 57 patients (85%) were able to be optimally debulked to microscopic or minimal residual disease.

- All but six patients had adjuvant therapy, consisting of either single-agent or cisplatin-based multiagent chemotherapy or radiation therapy.

•The issue of adjuvant therapy in patients with borderline tumors is controversial.

•Patients with advanced-stage disease to treat as if the histology were invasive.

•The median survival of the entire group was 32 months, with a range of 2-to-166 months, and there was a significant difference in survival between the borderline and invasive groups.

•Despite an aggressive surgical approach, the median survival rates of the entire group and borderline and invasive subgroups were less than the optimistic survival rate of 94% in a similar group of patients.

°The rates are still higher than reported for older patients.

•It remains uncertain whether aggressive surgery is warranted in borderline tumors.

•Improved survival in this group may reflect the aggressive surgical approach or a different biologic behavior of borderline tumors, which have a more indolent course and do well regardless of postoperative treatment.]

---

28. Incisions used for the extraperitoneal dissection required for lymphadenectomy in patients with advanced invasive squamous cell carcinoma of the cervix include

    1. bilateral superior groin incision.
    2. unilateral J-shaped incision.
    3. upper abdominal vertical incision.
    4. upper abdominal transverse incision.

---

p. 308   Ans: E   (Gallup D G, King L A, Messing M J, Talledo O E. Para-aortic lymph node sampling by means of an extraperitoneal approach with a supraumbilical transverse "sunrise" incision. Am J Obstet Gynec 1993; 169:307)

28. [F & I: •Background: Since the 1970s, assessment by staging laparotomy procedures on patients with advanced cervical cancer of metastatic disease beyond the usual radiation therapy fields has been performed.

•These earlier surgical studies noted that the incidence of positive paraaortic nodes in clinical stage IIB ranged from 5.2% to 18%; in patients with stage III the incidence ranged from 30% to 38%.

•These data suggested that some diseased nodes would escape being irradiated if only pelvic ports were used.

•Serious bowel complications have occurred in patients with cervical cancer who underwent surgical staging by a transperitoneal approach and later received radiation.

•To avoid these complications, an extraperitoneal approach has been advocated by means of bilateral superior groin incisions, a unilateral J-shaped incision, as described by Berman et al., or an upper abdominal vertical incision as described by Schellhas.

•Because of noted disadvantages of these previously described extraperitoneal approaches (i.e., inability to have adequate access to the nodes around the great vessels on the opposite side of the incision), a midline incision has been used for an extraperitoneal approach.

•Objective: To report on results using a supraumbilical transverse "sunrise" incision to remove paraaortic nodes extraperitoneally in patients undergoing surgical staging for advanced cervical cancer.

•Most phase III studies of advanced cervical cancer from the nation's cancer study groups, such as the Gynecologic Oncology Group, require surgical staging for assessment of paraaortic node metastases before patient entry.

Obstetrics and Gynecology:Review 1994-Gynecologic Oncology References

•These requirements are based on the relatively high incidence of paraaortic node metastases in patients with stage IIB or IIIB carcinoma.

•The extraperitoneal bilateral groin incision approach has the disadvantage of relative inaccessibility to the paraaortic nodes.

•The upper-abdominal vertical incision described by Schellhas has the disadvantage of difficulty in removing the left paraaortic nodes, particularly in obese patients.

•Similarly, the J-shaped incision, described by Berman et al., has the disadvantage of technical difficulty in removing the precaval nodes.

•Easy access to nodes on both sides of the aorta has been noted with the use of a midline approach, but because this midline incision was made in future pelvic irradiation fields, postoperative irradiation was frequently delayed.

•Adequate sampling of paraaortic nodes could be performed with an upper abdominal incision and with few complications, allowing all patients but two to receive pelvic irradiation within 2 weeks of operation.

•The peritoneal surfaces must be carefully inspected after node sampling.

•Any entry to the peritoneum that occurs during its mobilization should be immediately repaired.

•Recent advances in laparoscopic equipment and techniques have led some to remove retroperitoneal nodes with laparoscopes.

•In the hands of experienced laparoscopists, pelvic lymphadenectomy can be performed with minimal morbidity and adequate sampling.

•In patients with advanced cervical cancer, therapists should know the metastatic disease status of the paraaortic nodes, particularly if the patients are candidates for entry to investigational protocols.

•Removing paraaortic nodes through the laparoscope is technically difficult and should be considered experimental until experience and data are accumulated.

•The incisional approach described herein is relatively rapid and extraperitoneal; in addition, the incision can be extended caudad and laterally for removal of unsuspected, bulky pelvic nodes.

•The incision is not in future radiation fields; radiation therapy can be initiated within days of the procedure.]

---

29. According to the international classification of cancer of the cervix, characteristics of Stage IB include

    1. must be visible clinically.
    2. the depth of invasion < 5 millimeters.
    3. involvement of the upper third of the vagina only.
    4. horizontal spread greater >7 millimeters.

p. 599   Ans: D   (Peipert J F, Wells C K, Schwartz P E, Feinstein A R. The impact of symptoms and comorbidity on prognosis in stage IB cervical cancer. Am J Obstet Gynec 1993; 169:598)

29. [F & I:•Background: Cancer has a biologic effect as well as an anatomic form.

•Although both the function of the tumor and its anatomic extensiveness will affect the prognosis, current staging systems rely exclusively on anatomic categories, ignoring the cancer's function and the host-tumor interaction.

- The multiple anatomic or morphologic factors that affect the prognosis include histologic type, tumor volume, vascular or lymphatic space involvement, and depth of stromal invasion, but systematic attention has not been given to factors such as the presence or absence of symptoms, symptom severity, clinical evidence of rate of growth, or the impact of comorbid ailments, in spite of the prognostic importance these factors have shown for diverse other cancers.

- In 1993 in the United States about 13,500 new cases of invasive cervical cancer will be diagnosed, an estimated 4400 deaths will occur as a result of the disease.

- The best method of managing women with localized disease and poor prognostic factors is controversial, and new protocols are evaluating the use of chemotherapy in advanced disease and in patients with "bulky" or extensive localized tumors.

- The choices for treatment of cervical cancer are regularly affected by features of clinical and comorbid severity.

- For example, women who receive radiation are older, generally "sicker," and include more "poor surgical candidates" than women chosen predominantly from groups with a more favorable prognosis who are treated with surgery.

- Because these two groups of patients are not prognostically equal before therapy, a selection bias will distort the results if these factors are ignored in the evaluation of therapeutic efficacy.

- A heterogeneous group of patients exists within each International Federation of Gynecology and Obstetrics (FIGO) stage.

- Careful attention must be paid to clinical variables such as symptom status and the presence of medical comorbidity that can have an impact on survival to control for this heterogeneity.

- Incorporating these variables into estimates of prognosis will provide more accurate and individualized prognostic information for patients and should be useful for prognostic stratification in clinical trials of new forms of therapy.

- Objective: To test the hypothesis that the patient's clinical symptom status and comorbidity would have an impact on prognosis in invasive cervical cancer.

- The specific hypotheses were that survival would be adversely affected by the presence of symptoms (vs no symptoms), the presence of more severe symptoms (vs mild symptoms), and the concomitant presence of severe comorbid conditions.

- The study hypothesis was tested within a single FIGO stage (i.e., stage IB) to control for the effect of morphologic stage on survival.

- If a combination of the symptomatic and comorbid features formed suitable levels of prognostic stratification within FIGO stage IB, impact of clinical variables could later be tested within all FIGO stages.

- **Classification of prognostic information.**

- Each patient's condition immediately before zero time was classified according to conventional anatomic stages and two new clinical axes.

- All classifications were made without prior knowledge of the duration of survival.

- The tumor's anatomic spread, classified according to FIGO guidelines, was listed as axis I.

- Patients had been examined and staged by a gynecologic oncologist, and a radiation oncologist was also involved in staging when radiation therapy was considered for therapy.

- Because the definition of stage IB has changed over time, patients with >3 mm depth of invasion below the basement membrane were considered to have stage IB disease for this study.

- **Classification of symptoms and comorbidity.**

- Clinical manifestations related to the cancer were listed in axis II.

- A "clinical manifestation" was defined as a reported symptom that was attributable or possibly attributable to the cancer.

- To be designated as attributable or possibly attributable, the manifestations had to be consistent with the cancer's anatomic status and customary effects, such as abnormal vaginal bleeding, discharge, pain, or urinary symptoms.

- Primary symptoms included local symptoms such as vaginal bleeding or discharge or possibly regional manifestations such as pain or urinary complaints.

- Systemic symptoms included fatigue or nondeliberate weight loss.

- Patients with profuse bleeding or nondeliberate weight loss of >10 pounds were designated as having severe symptoms.

- Symptom duration was also recorded.

- Within each of the symptomatic and comorbid axes, differential survival rates were noted in the direction hypothesized, but the differences were not statistically significant because of small numbers within each subgroup.

- When symptoms and comorbidity were incorporated into a composite clinical classification system, the clinically important distinctions also became statistically significant.

- The distinctions were retained for patients receiving different modes of therapy.

- The biologic virulence of a cancer can be indicated by its clinical manifestations, which reflect the tumor's functional effects and temporal growth.

- Rapidly growing cancers are particularly likely to produce symptoms rather than no symptoms and severe rather than nonsevere symptoms.

- In prognostic classification primary symptoms can be attributed to the tumor at its site of origin, systemic symptoms occur remote from the cancer's original site but do not imply anatomic dissemination, and metastatic symptoms arise remote from the tumor and imply anatomic dissemination.

- Severe or systemic symptoms are often caused by a more aggressive tumor, and metastatic symptoms indicate a virulent cancer.

- This taxonomy is associated with a "functional" prognostic gradient.

- In asymptomatic patients the tumor has been present for an unknown length of time and might have remained silent for even longer periods of time had the cancer not been accidentally detected.

- In addition, slow-growing "silent" cancers may be detected because of symptoms produced by other gynecologic conditions.

- The duration of symptoms indicate the minimal amount of time a cancer has been present, because the cancer has been present as long as the symptoms.

- For symptoms of short duration no definite conclusions can be drawn about the tumor's rate of growth.

- It may be either growing rapidly or growing slowly with a late appearance of symptoms.

- For symptoms of long duration the cancer is likely to be slow growing, because the tumor has been present for at least as long as its symptoms.

- In addition to patterns of symptoms, the prognostic comorbidity of associated medical conditions adversely affects survival in a variety of chronic diseases.

  ° For example, in endometrial cancer patients without prognostic comorbidity had a 5-year survival rate of 78%, compared with a survival rate of 27% in patients with prognostic comorbidity.

- In a large series of stage I cervical cancer, diabetes mellitus significantly influenced survival in a Cox proportional-hazard model.

  ° Patients with diabetes were generally older and in poorer medical condition.

- Clinical staging systems incorporating patients' initial clinical manifestations have been developed and have shown prognostic gradients for cancers of the lung, larynx, rectum, breast, prostate, and endometrium.

  ° For example, in endometrial cancer patients with primary or local symptoms had a 5-year survival rate of 78%, whereas patients with referred, systemic, or metastatic symptoms had survival rates of 67%, 57%, and 25%, respectively.

  ° The composite symptom-severity staging system produced prognostic distinctions within each FIGO stage of endometrial cancer.

- Current staging systems for cancer identify the anatomic form but not the biologic effect or clinical function of the tumor.

- Although the term "early" is often used to describe anatomic stages such as stage I cervical cancer, it refers to a dimension of time, which is not measured in anatomic systems of staging.

- Although the customary staging systems describe the morphologic appearance and structural damage produced by the tumor, no attention is given to the tumor's duration and rate of growth, which can be manifested as the functional effects of the cancer in structures or systems that may or may not be anatomically invaded.

- Results: Confirm the hypothesis that clinical variables such as symptoms and comorbidity have important prognostic value in stage IB cervical cancer.

- These variables indicate aspects of the cancer's function and rate of growth that are not considered in traditional morphologic staging systems.

- Nevertheless, the morphologic staging systems denote anatomic features of the cancer that cannot be discerned from the clinical variables alone.

- Consequently, both morphologic and clinical features should be considered to produce adequate descriptions of the biologic behavior of a tumor and effective appraisals of prognosis and therapy.

- Numerous investigations in chronic diseases and a variety of malignancies have shown that current methods of classification in cancer staging are incomplete.

- Anatomic and morphologic systems have classified what a cancer *is,* but not what it *does.*

- Because clinical variables such as symptom status and comorbidity influence survival, increase prognostic precision, and improve the evaluation of new therapeutic modalities, these clinical variables should be appraised in gynecologic malignancies.

- Unless the clinical variables are suitably included, prognostic estimates based only on morphologic condition will be imprecise, and therapeutic evaluations may be misleading.]

30. Hypothalamic GnRH is produced by

   1. normal ovary.
   2. placenta.
   3. ovarian epithelial cancer.
   4. dysgerminoma.

p. 609   Ans: A   (Ohno T, Imai A, Furui T, Takahashi K, Tamaya T. Presence of gonadotropin-releasing hormone and its messenger ribonucleic acid in human ovarian epithelial carcinoma. Am J Obstet Gynec 1993; 169:605)

30. [F & I:•Background: In addition to its classic hypophysiotropic action, gonadotropin-releasing hormone (GnRH) may modulate activity in the brain and many peripheral organs, including the ovary.

•GnRH analogs are used in the therapy of breast cancer, prostate cancer, and ovarian cancer.

•Growth of these tumors is inhibited by GnRH analog, and clinical studies have indicated beneficial effects even in the treatment of some metastatic tumors.

•The antitumor action of GnRH analog is presumed to result from a desensitization or down-regulation of GnRH receptors in the pituitary, with a consequent decline in gonadotropin secretion and gonadal hormone production.

•GnRH analog can also suppress the growth of the tumor cells in vitro and the presence of specific binding sites for GnRH is found in the tumors responsive to GnRH analog.

•These findings suggest direct regulatory effects of GnRH on tumor growth.

•Because of the short half-life, GnRH is undetectable or very low in the general circulation.

•It is unlikely that GnRH of hypothalamic origin could reach the peripheral organs in sufficient concentrations to activate its receptors and exert a direct action, although GnRH is supposedly secreted in a pulsatile fashion from the hypothalamus.

•Consideration of these findings lead to the possibility that GnRH might be produced locally within these tumors.

•Objective: To examine human ovarian carcinomas and ovarian carcinoma cell lines for the presence of GnRH and its messenger ribonucleic acid (mRNA).

•Results: Show the mRNA expression of GnRH and the presence of GnRH in human ovarian carcinoma reported to have GnRH binding sites.

•GnRH was detected with immunologic properties indistinguishable from those of authentic GnRH in the acetic acid-ethanol extracts from the human ovarian carcinoma tissue and human ovarian carcinoma cell lines (SK-OV3).

•The possibility that the results could be accounted for by nonspecific immunoreactivity seems highly unlikely because the normal ovary and placenta analyzed in parallel to the ovarian carcinomas were totally negative.

•GnRH found in the ovarian carcinoma was biologically active.

•GnRH and analog are known to bind to GnRH receptor and stimulate phosphoinositide metabolism in granulosa cells and to suppress gonadotropin-induced maturation and steroidogenesis.

•The findings of immunoreactivity and bioactivity clearly indicate the presence of GnRH in the ovarian carcinoma, although the concentration (picogram range per milligram of protein) was much lower than those (nanogram range) in the hypothalamus.

- GnRH-like peptide is present in the normal ovary and placenta.

- Failure to detect immunoreactive GnRH in these tissues might be because of low sensitivity of the assay condition; the tritiated RIA was fivefold less sensitive than the iodine 125 RIA for analysis of GnRH.

- The authenticity of the GnRH and its production by the ovarian carcinoma was further established by the discovery of GnRH mRNA by polymerase chain reaction amplification study in ovarian carcinoma tissues and ovarian carcinoma cell lines.

- The possibility that these results might be accounted for by cross-tissue contamination seemed highly unlikely, because no reverse transcription polymerase chain reaction products were detected when the GnRH primers were used with ovarian nonepithelial tumor dysgerminoma, benign tumor; normal ovary and other cell lines, and because reverse transcription and polymerase chain reaction blanks always remained negative.

- Given these conditions of reverse transcription polymerase chain reaction amplification and direct sequential analysis of the polymerase chain reaction-amplified products, amplified sequences of the cDNA were probably generated from human ovarian carcinoma GnRH mRNA.

- GnRH mRNA was not detected in the human placenta and ovary, the tissues that have the capacity to produce GnRH.

- The most plausible explanation is that the placental or ovarian GnRH gene might differ from that in hypothalamus.

- Previous studies isolated and characterized the human GnRH gene in placental tissue, showing a slight difference from the hypothalamic GnRH cDNA.

- Although the functional role of the receptor in ovarian carcinoma is still obscure, GnRH can stimulate phosphoinositide metabolism through phospholipase C in ovarian carcinoma membrane, in such a way as to permit regulation of tumor growth by GnRH.

- It is unlikely that endogenous hypothalamic GnRH ever reaches concentrations in peripheral blood that are necessary to stimulate ovarian tumor GnRH receptor.

- The current finding that GnRH might be produced locally within the ovarian carcinoma suggests that GnRH receptor could exert an autocrine role on tumor growth.

- The disovery of GnRH production by GnRH-responsive tumor is not without precedent because GnRH has been reported to be expressed in breast carcinoma cells known to have GnRH receptors and to be affected by GnRH analog.

- In the breast carcinoma it is also suggested that GnRH may serve an autocrine regulatory role.

- Last, the current data show that human ovarian epithelial carcinoma can produce GnRH known to have GnRH-binding sites.

- GnRH might act as an autocrine regulator of ovarian carcinoma proliferation, and the relatively high dose of GnRH analog might induce desensitization to GnRH or down-regulation of GnRH receptor with a consequent decline of tumor growth, in an analogous manner to GnRH analog's action on anterior pituitary.

- Thereby it should be interesting to look for a correlation between GnRH response, the histologic condition of the tumors, and the clinical course of the disease.

- This might be part of a possible point of attack for therapeutic approaches with GnRH analog in this malignancy.]

31. Patients with invasive endometrial adenocarcinoma should have lymph node sampling if

1. histology is grade 3.
2. greater than 50% of myometrium is invaded.
3. stage II/III disease.
4. palpably suspicious paraaortic nodes.

p. 176   Ans: E   (Kim Y B, Niloff J M. Endometrial carcinoma: Analysis of recurrence in patients treated with a strategy minimizing lymph node sampling and radiation therapy. Obstet Gynecol 1993; 82:175)

31. [F & I: •Background: Endometrial carcinoma is the most common malignancy of the female genital tract in the United States.

• Surgery and radiation are the most commonly used and effective treatment modalities, but there are significant differences among institutions in how these treatments are selected.

•Recently, primary surgery has been favored because the extent of disease can be accurately defined at the outset of therapy.

•There is no agreement concerning the indications for performing lymph node sampling and administering adjuvant radiation therapy.

•The morbidity of whole pelvic radiation is sufficiently substantial that it should be reserved for patients at significant risk for pelvic lymph node metastases or local recurrence.

•A large Gynecologic Oncology Group study defined several factors that significantly increase the risk of both pelvic and para-aortic lymph node metastases.

°**These factors include high grade, deep myometrial invasion, unfavorable histologic subtype, and surgically defined local spread.**

•Patients with none of these risks have a low risk (less than 6%) of pelvic lymph node metastases.

•Whole pelvic radiation has been limited to patients with at least one of these risk factors.

•Because it is unlikely that lymph node sampling in itself has therapeutic benefit in endometrial carcinoma, lymph node sampling has been limited to patients fulfilling two criteria.

•First, a substantial risk of lymph node metastases should be present.

°This risk can be defined by the criteria described.

•Second, the presence of positive lymph nodes should influence subsequent management.

°The presence of positive pelvic lymph nodes would not change management because any patient with an indication for performing lymph node sampling would receive whole pelvic radiation regardless of pelvic node status.

•Pelvic lymph node sampling has not been routinely performed.

•The effectiveness of para-aortic radiation for patients with positive para-aortic nodes is controversial, but the success reported in small series and the poor performance of historical controls suggest that this modality may be effective in the subset of patients with positive paraaortic nodes.

•Because a positive finding would change management, para-aortic lymph node sampling was performed in patients at risk for such metastases.

•Because patients with no high-risk factors have a low risk of para-aortic lymph node metastases (less than 2%), such sampling was omitted in these patients.

•Fact   °Detail   »issue   *answer

Obstetrics and Gynecology: Review 1994-Gynecologic Oncology References

•Objective: To determine whether using treatment to minimize the use of lymph node sampling and adjuvant radiation therapy compromised outcome in patients with early endometrial carcinoma.

•Experience showed that this was accomplished without compromising either local tumor control or survival.

•Analysis of the patients who developed recurrence following this strategy showed that more aggressive lymph node sampling or radiation therapy would **not** have altered outcome in these patients.

•Lymph node sampling in endometrial carcinoma remains problematic.

•Pelvic and para-aortic lymphadenectomy were routinely performed in a large Gynecologic Oncology Group study to define the pattern of lymph node spread in this disease.

°It is not obvious that this practice should be extended to all patients with endometrial carcinoma.

•Lymph node sampling presents the risk of serious **vascular injury** and results in increased operative blood loss and postoperative ileus.

•Lymph node sampling was performed only in high-risk patients and confined the sampling to the para-aortic lymph nodes.

•Pelvic lymph node sampling is unlikely to benefit a patient who will also receive whole pelvic radiation, which was given to all high-risk patients.

•If a patient had positive para-aortic lymph nodes, an additional portal to the para-aortic nodes was recommended along with whole pelvic radiation.

•Small series have suggested that long-term survival may follow para-aortic radiation.

•These patients have historically done poorly when the para-aortic nodes were not treated.

•The para-aortic nodes were sampled in high risk patients because the decision to add an extended field is based on the status of these nodes.

•Although radiation is widely used as adjuvant therapy for endometrial carcinoma, its limitations should be recognized.

•A survival advantage has not been shown among patients treated with either vaginal cuff radiation or whole pelvic radiation in the adjuvant setting.

•Most studies have documented a decrease in local recurrence but this has not been translated into a difference in survival largely because patients have had distant sites of recurrence.

•This pattern of failure suggests that many patients treated with adjuvant radiation therapy **had distant metastases at the outset of therapy**.

•Although radiation therapy controlled local disease for this subset of patients, recurrence was inevitable because of the lack of systemic therapy.

•The results of this study illustrate this point.

•Of the ten patients suffering recurrence, six had distant sites of recurrence.

•Significantly, four of these patients developed clinically evident lung metastases within 7 months of initial surgery, indicating that they probably had occult lung metastases at the outset of therapy.

•These patients were probably destined to fail regional therapies such as surgery and radiation.

Obstetrics and Gynecology: Review 1994-Gynecologic Oncology References

•Until an adjuvant therapy effective at eradicating distant disease is found, these patients will continue to do poorly despite use of the most aggressive therapies.

•Furthermore, three of the four patients who developed local recurrence had received whole pelvic radiation, and the fourth patient would have received this therapy if not for intercurrent illness.

•The selective approach to lymph node sampling and radiation therapy described in this report did not result in undertreatment of the patients who later developed recurrence.

•This was because every patient who developed recurrence was identified by at least one high-risk factor.

•Six patients had grade 3 tumors, seven had greater than 50% myometrial invasion, and two had papillary serous histology.

•Excluding those patients with significant intercurrent disease, every patient with recurrence received maximal regional therapy, namely, paraaortic node sampling and at least whole pelvic radiation.

•Risks defined by the Gynecologic Oncology Group study are effective in identifying patients at risk for recurrence.

•This is clearly demonstrated by the disease-free survival curves generated while stratifying patients by grade and depth of invasion.

•The survival rates for patients with grade 1 or 2 tumors and less than 50% invasion are excellent, whereas patients with grade 3 disease or greater than 50% invasion clearly do worse despite more aggressive therapy.

•Low-risk patients did extremely well despite the lack of lymph node sampling and whole pelvic radiation therapy.

•The question becomes not whether therapy should be more aggressive, but rather whether more patients in the high-risk group could have been **spared the morbidities of aggressive therapy**.

•This question cannot be answered by this study.

•Two patients with recurrence did not undergo paraaortic node dissection because of inaccurate information.

•Patient no. 4 had deep myometrial invasion which was not recognized intraoperatively.

•Patient no. 10 had poorly differentiated tumor which had been read as grade 1 preoperatively.

•Because patient no. 4 had recurrence distantly in the lung 44 months after diagnosis, it is unlikely that para-aortic node dissection and more aggressive regional therapy would have altered her outcome.

•Patient no. 10 had recurrence in the vagina despite radiation therapy.

°Additional lymph node dissection certainly would not have altered this patient's course.]

---

32. Tumor markers found in ovarian inclusion cysts include

    1. ß-hCG.
    2. CEA.
    3. CA125.
    4. placental lactogen.

p. 185   Ans: E   (Resta L, Russo S, Colucci G A, Prat J. Morphologic precursors of ovarian epithelial tumors. Obstet Gynecol 1993; 82:181)

•Fact   °Detail   »issue   *answer

32. [F & I: •Background: Unlike most neoplasms of the female genital tract, the study of morphologic precursors of the ovarian epithelial tumors is still in its early stage.

•This fact, together with uncertainties as to etiology, pathogenesis, and risk factors, has prevented a full understanding of the early stages of ovarian carcinogenesis.

•Hyperplastic lesions of the ovarian surface epithelium and the related inclusion cysts and their role as substrate for the potential development of ovarian epithelial tumors have been investigated.

•Objective: To correlate the various types of hyperplastic lesions of the ovarian surface epithelium with primary pathology of the female genital tract in order to integrate preceding studies.

•Although the usual normal ovarian epithelium is recognized as being monolayered, flat, cuboidal, or sometimes columnar, a large number of ovaries (39 of 50) from women over 35 years of age have a loss of surface epithelium, which can only be encountered in the lining of the cysts.

•This phenomenon is observed in humans, but not in other mammals.

•Results: A loss of surface epithelium was found more frequently in the group of nonpregnant women without any hyperplastic or neoplastic lesions of the tube, uterus, or vagina than in the other three groups.

•Ultrastructural studies showed continuous destruction of the surface epithelium during ovulation, without reconstruction.

•Such a desquamation was preceded by ultrastructural degenerative changes and might occur regardless of ovulation, suggesting a possible hormonal influence in epithelial trophism and maintenance.

•As a result of this continuous desquamation during a woman's sexual life, the surface epithelium was absent in the postmenopausal ovary.

•In the other three groups, a very different situation was observed: a higher rate of papillomatous hyperplasia and metaplasia both on the surface epithelium and in the inclusion cysts.

•Despite an earlier report in which these changes were considered a generic variant of the ovarian epithelium in postmenopausal women, their expression was quantified in selected groups of women to investigate their significance.

•The high incidence of hyperplastic and mullerian metaplasia on the surface epithelium or in the inclusion cysts in patients with epithelial tumors of the contralateral ovary stresses the potential role of these changes as a substrate for the development of ovarian cancer, which is frequently bilateral.

•Histologically, the changes observed on the surface epithelium and in the inclusion cysts resemble benign cystadenomas, from which they differ only in size; **1 cm** in diameter has been proposed as the dividing criterion.

•The finding, both in the inclusion cysts and on surface papillomas, of markers frequently detected in epithelial ovarian tumors, such as ß-hCG, carcinoembryonic antigen, CA 125, placental lactogen, placental alkaline phosphatase, and clonal antigen MH94, may suggest some confirmation of this hypothesis.

•The occurrence of these changes in most women with **endometrial adenocarcinoma and polycystic ovary disease** suggests that they may be induced by abnormal hormonal stimulation.

°These two diseases have demonstrated an **overproduction of estrogens** of extraovarian origin.

•A sensitivity to steroid hormones has been detected in the surface ovarian epithelium and m the epithelium of the inclusion cysts, as well as in ovarian epithelial tumors.

•Hyperplasia of the surface epithelium has been found in women with polycystic ovary disease.

•They indicated that ovaries with unsuccessful follicle rupture are always covered by an intact epithelium.

•Considering the low frequency of ovulation in polycystic ovaries and the normal desquamation of the ovarian epithelium with or without ovulation, hyperplasia and metaplasia of the ovarian epithelium and inclusion cysts are probably not related to ovulatory trauma but to hormonal stimulation.

•The preventive effect of oral contraceptives on epithelial ovarian tumors may be unrelated to the inhibition of ovulation.

•Similar to what has been postulated for endometrial and breast duct epithelium, the progestins in oral contraceptives might have a stabilizing effect on the ovarian epithelium.

•The inclusion cysts, which are thought to be secondary to reparation of the surface epithelium after ovulation, may simply result from **hormonal stimulation** of the epithelium at the bottom of the invaginations.

•Two types of inclusion cysts can be distinguished: fetal inclusion cysts, produced during fetal life because of the absence of the basal membrane; and acquired inclusion cysts, probably produced by hormonal stimuli.

»The observations on the different changes in the ovarian surface epithelium and in the related inclusion cysts in normal women and in those with ovarian or endometrial cancer and polycystic ovary disease further support a hormonal role in the development of epithelial ovarian tumors, possibly through an intermediate phase characterized by hyperplastic, papillomatous, and mullerian metaplastic changes.

•These changes are histologically more similar to the benign than to the malignant epithelial tumors.

»On the other hand, neither "premalignant" lesions nor transition from papillomatosis, hyperplasia, metaplasia, and inclusions cysts to ovarian neoplasia has been described in ovarian tumors, the premalignant phase is probably fast and difficult to observe.]

---

33. Indications for bilateral salpingo-oophorectomy in a premenopausal patient undergoing radical hysterectomy for invasive cervical neoplasia include

   1. 20% of premenopausal patients will experience early gonadal failure.
   2. 5-to-8% will require additional surgery for benign ovarian disease.
   3. 1.4% will develop ovarian carcinoma.
   4. sexual functioning is not adversely affected.

---

p. 189   Ans: E   (Parker M, Bosscher J, Barnhill D, Park R. Ovarian management during radical hysterectomy in the premenopausal patient. Obstet Gynecol 1993; 82:187)

33. [F & I: •Background: The decision to remove or retain grossly normal ovaries in premenopausal patients at radical hysterectomy for early-stage cervical carcinoma involves several competing factors.

•Variables to consider include the woman's age, suspicion of ovarian metastasis, potential for premature ovarian failure postoperatively, risk of surgery for subsequent primary benign or malignant adnexal disease, compliance with hormone replacement therapy, psychological impact of surgical castration, expense of hormone supplementation, and expense of treating future ovarian disease.

•Objectives: To provide follow-up information on premenopausal women who had radical hysterectomies without adjuvant therapy for stage I cervical carcinoma.

•To examine the advantages and disadvantages of ovarian conservation.

•The average age at natural menopause in the United States is approximately 51 years.

Obstetrics and Gynecology: Review 1994-Gynecologic Oncology References

- The decision to preserve ovarian tissue in a premenopausal woman undergoing radical hysterectomy for cervical carcinoma is, in part, based on an expectation of continued normal hormonal function postoperatively.

- This study reveals an **early gonadal failure rate** of at least 20% among the 30 women with retained ovaries who were premenopausal at the time of their radical hysterectomies.

- Although no patient has developed ovarian cancer in a preserved ovary, recent data have estimated that 1.4% of all American women will develop ovarian cancer during their lifetime.

- Younger women reported a higher rate of compliance with hormone replacement therapy.

- The postoperative intervals of the younger and older patients were compared to determine whether this could explain the unequal compliance rates, but no significant difference was found.

- The psychological impact of castration on a premenopausal woman can only be estimated.

- Castration did not have an adverse impact on sexual function.

- The level of sexual satisfaction was not related significantly to use of hormone replacement therapy.

- The expense of hormone replacement therapy for castrated women can be compared to the costs of treatment for ovarian disease and hormone medication for premature ovarian failure in those with ovarian retention.

- Using this data for all premenopausal patients, the mean age at radical hysterectomy was 37 years, the mean age at detection of early ovarian failure was 41 years, and subsequent oophorectomies were required on average at age 40 years.

- A rough estimate of the difference in hormone costs between the BSO and retention groups can be made, assuming equal compliance rates.

- At today's prices, the lifetime cost of daily estrogen replacement therapy for 150 castrated patients would be approximately: 150 x $120/year for estrogen therapy x 42 years (79 years average life expectancy 37 years for average age at radical hysterectomy) = $756,000.

- Among 150 women with retained gonads, 110 would be expected to undergo menopause at approximately 51 years, and their subsequent hormonal expense would be 110 x $120/ year x 28 years (79 years average life expectancy 51 years for average age at menopause) = $369,600.

- Thirty in the retention group would experience premature ovarian failure, and ten would require oophorectomies for benign disease.

- These 40 women would incur a medication expense as follows: 40 patients x $120/year x 38 years (79 years average life expectancy 41 years for average age at early ovarian failure or oophorectomy) = $182,400.

- The difference in hormone replacement therapy costs for the BSO and the retention groups would be approximately $204,000.

- Assuming that 1.4% of the women with retained ovaries will develop ovarian cancer, in addition to the ten patients needing subsequent oophorectomies for benign disease, two women in the retention group would require an exploratory laparotomy with an ovarian staging or debulking procedure, and possibly postoperative chemotherapy, second-look laparotomy, and terminal supportive care for ovarian carcinoma.

    » It is possible that the costs of treating these 12 women would exceed the difference in hormonal expense between those with removed versus preserved gonads, making it more expensive overall to preserve the ovaries than to remove them.

- Recommendation: Elective BSO for most premenopausal women undergoing radical hysterectomies for cervical carcinoma because of the following:

°At least 20% of those with retained ovaries will experience early gonadal failure,

°5-to-8% will require additional surgery for benign ovarian disease, and

°1.4% may develop ovarian carcinoma;

°compliance with hormone replacement therapy in the young patient appears to be high;

°sexual function is not adversely affected; and

°the cost of preserving the ovaries may exceed that of removing them.]

34. Uterine effects of tamoxifen associated with the treatment of breast cancer include increased incidence of

1. endocervical polyp.
2. endometrial polyp.
3. endometrial hyperplasia.
4. endometrial cancer.

p. 660   Ans: E   (Lahti E, Blanco G, Lauppila A, Apaja-Sarkkinen M, Taskinen P J, Laatikainen T. Endometrial changes in postmenopausal breast cancer patients receiving Tamoxifen. Obstet Gynecol 1993; 81:660)

34. [F & I: •Background: The beneficial effect of tamoxifen for the treatment of breast cancer is attributable to its antiestrogen effect.

•Tamoxifen has an estrogenic effecton the vaginal epithelium.

•Longterm tamoxifen treatment increases the occurrence of endometrial polyps, hyperplasia, and cancer.

•An increased risk of endometrial cancer also occurs in breast cancer patients who have not received tamoxifen, and this also may be true of benign endometrial diseases.

•Objective: To compare endometrial findings in breast cancer patients with or without tamoxifen treatment.

•Results: Larger uterine size and thicker endometrium was found in postmenopausal breast cancer patients receiving tamoxifen than in similar breast cancer patients without hormonal therapy.

•Factors that may affect endogenous estrogen production and uterine size, such as parity, age, menopausal age, and BMI, did not differ between the groups.

•Hysteroscopy is a reliable method for evaluating endometrial atrophy, which was found in 87% of the controls but only 28% of those receiving tamoxifen.

•Tamoxifen has an estrogenic effect on the vaginal epithelium in breast cancer patients, and the findings extend this estrogenic effect to the corpus and the endometrium of the uterus.

•**Transvaginal sonography** is an effective and practical screening method to detect pathologic changes in the endometrium, uterus, and ovaries.

•A thin endometrium (less than 5 mm) accompanies endometrial atrophy without any pathologic findings in curettage.

°Curettage may not be suitable for clarifying transvaginal sonography findings in post menopausal women, because polyps are often missed and the endometrial samples are often insufficient to confirm atrophy.

•Fact   °Detail   »issue   *answer

•Curettage was combined with hysteroscopy in this study.

•All the pathologic findings, including polyps, three cases of endometrial adenocarcinoma, and two endometrial hyperplasias, involved an endometrial thickness of **more than 5 mm** at sonography.

•If transvaginal sonography were used as a screening method with a cutoff limit of 5 mm, further examinations such as hysteroscopy and curettage would be warranted in 20% of breast cancer patients without hormonal treatment and in 84% of those receiving tamoxifen.

•Endocervical polyps were twice as common and endometrial polyps three times as common in the tamoxifen group than in the control group.

•Decidual reaction of stromal cells was not found in the endometrial polyps in the tamoxifen group.

•Although fewer cases of endometrial polyps were found in the breast cancer patients without hormonal therapy, two large polyps with adenomatous hyperplasia were found in this group.

•A thick endometrium during ultrasonography (greater than 5 mm) without the presence of polyps was detected in 26 patients in the tamoxifen group.

°This appeared as a well-defined, highly reflective layer, which is a typical finding described as being associated with various forms of endometrial hyperplasia in postmenopausal women.

°Unexpectedly, one case of adenomatous and one case of atypical hyperplasia was found in these patients.

°An estrogenic effect was detected in 19 of them, but the changes were rather slight.

•The present series of 103 breast cancer patients was too small to evaluate the risk of endometrial cancer; the detection of three cases was more than could be expected in asymptomatic post-menopausal women, for whom the prevalence is 6.96 per 1000.

•As only one atypical hyperplasia was found in the tamoxifen group, the present investigation failed to demonstrate any increased occurrence of precancerous lesions in association with tamoxifen treatment.]

---

35. Methods used to analyze the zygosity of molar gestations include

    1. protein heteromorphisms.
    2. cytogenetics.
    3. Southern blotting.
    4. polymerase chain reaction.

---

p. 1549   Ans: E   (Mutter G L, Pomponio R J, Berkowitz R S, Genest D R. Sex chromosome composition of complete hydatidiform moles: Relationship to metastasis. Am J Obstet Gynec 1993; 168:1547)

35. [F & I: •Background: Complete hydatidiform moles are associated with a substantial risk of developing persistent gestational trophoblastic tumor.

•An outstanding question is whether there is any feature of the mole itself that will predict which fraction of cases will persist or progress to metastasis.

•Histologic grading has been claimed to have such predictive value, but this has been disputed.

•Complete hydatidiform mole variables, especially genetic markers, that predict clinical outcome might be useful in patient management.

•The maternal genome is excluded during creation of a complete mole, enabling the paternal genome to disproportionately influence postfertilization development.

Obstetrics and Gynecology: Review 1994-Gynecologic Oncology References

- The genetic composition of complete moles varies according to the number of sperm that successfully fertilize the egg.

  ° Approximately 75% to 85% are the products of **monospermy** with endoreduplication of the haploid product to generate a 46,XX genotype.

  ° Most of the remainder are created by **dispermy**, producing a diploid stem cell that could have a 46,XX, 46,XY, or 46,YY genotype.

  ° Moles with a 46,YY genotype have not been described, probably because such a conceptus, whether created by monospermy or dispermy, is not viable.

- Dispermic moles can be recognized by heterozygous genetic autosomal markers in 46,XX cases or by sex chromosome genotype in 46,XY cases.

- Previous attempts to define any relationship between molar dispermy and monospermy and natural history have been complicated by rarity of the lesions of interest, imprecise genetic analysis, maternal contamination of the molar tissue studied, and controversial definition of clinical outcome.

- Criteria for defining persistent trophoblastic disease vary among centers in frequency, timing, and interpretation of human chorionic gonadotropin (hCG) follow-up.

- The identification of metastatic disease is more standardized, requiring demonstration of a physical extrauterine lesion in a patient with high hCG levels.

- Objective: To compile a series of complete hydatidiform moles with unequivocal and different clinical outcomes, either nonmetastatic (spontaneous remission or nonmetastatic gestational trophoblastic tumor) or metastatic gestational trophoblastic tumor (all treated by chemotherapy and diagnosed at time of persistence).

- Results: The prevalence of Y chromosome-containing complete moles was 7.7% for the metastatic and 9.1% for the nonmetastatic groups, not a statistically significant difference.

- This corresponds closely to the overall rate of Y chromosome-containing complete moles estimated by others as 4% to 15%.

- Rejection of the null hypothesis that the two outcome groups have equivalent Y-chromosome frequencies would be very difficult in such a small sample in which a low-frequency event is the subject of study.

- If the actual frequencies of Y chromosome moles for the two groups is at the observed level of 7.7% and 9.1%, this sample size would be unable to confirm them as different (power = 0.13).

- A threefold difference in Y chromosome-positive moles between metastatic and nonmetastatic groups would have been detectable (at a power of 0.7) in these experiments, assuming a 10% nonmetastatic mole rate of Y-chromatin positivity.

- In some series complete moles with a heterozygous genotype have a higher risk of progression than do homozygous moles.

- One study reported a persistence rate of 50% after heterozygous complete moles, contrasting with 4% for homozygous moles.

- This suggests a 12 to 24-fold increased risk associated with heterozygosity. This has not been confirmed by several later studies that show equivalent risk.

- The current report, confined to analysis of heterozygotes that are Y chromosome positive, has not shown an increased risk for metastasis in Y chromosome-positive versus Y chromosome-negative moles.

•Fact   °Detail   »issue   *answer

- Direct examination of the genotype of metastatic or persistent lesional tissues might define the high-risk genotypes of antecedent normal and abnormal gestations.

- Too few of these lesions have been studied to reach any conclusions.

- Furthermore, it is incorrect to assume that the aggressive lesion has biologic continuity with the immediately preceding gestation making it difficult to identify which antecedent gestation was the precursor lesion.

- Methods used to analyze the zygosity of molar gestations are numerous, including "F-body" scoring, protein heteromorphisms, cytogenetics, Southern blotting, and polymerase chain reaction.

- **F-body scoring** for identification of the Y chromosome is very subjective, with sensitivity and specificity highly dependent on the protocol used and on the tissue condition.

- Karyotypic analysis requires fresh tissue and can be complicated by sampling bias incurred during culture.

- Newer methods of chromosome identification by **fluorescent in situ hybridization** have tremendous potential for extracting cytogenetic information from frozen tissues and will no doubt be increasingly used in the future, although application to paraffin-embedded tissues is less reliable than to frozen tissues.

- **Protein heteromorphisms** may be analyzed on fresh or frozen tissue but are tedious to perform and provide limited information.

- **Southern blotting** is time consuming and difficult to apply to paraffin-embedded tissues.

- Autosomal marker systems are necessary to differentiate heterozygous from homozygous 46,XX moles.

- **Polymerase chain reaction-based** methods capable of scoring informative autosomal zygosity markers are available, but application to archival paraffin-embedded material is difficult because

    ° (1) accurate interpretation of maternal contamination requires marker studies on normal maternal and paternal tissues and

    ° (2) the DNA quantity and quality from paraffin sections require high cycle numbers to detect a strong signal, a process that with repetitive sequences may induce artifactual bands subject to misinterpretation.

- Polymerase chain reaction identification of Y chromosome-containing tissues by means of primers that only amplify Y-chromosome sequences is subject to two significant errors:

    ° (1) a false-negative result, caused by failure to amplify degraded Y-chromosome sequences, and

    ° (2) a false-positive result, caused by amplification of contaminating DNA.

- Genetic features of complete hydatidiform moles that predict persistent or metastatic gestational trophoblastic tumor have not yet been identified.

- The current study uses objective and reproducible molecular methods to identify Y chromosome-containing moles and shows **no correlation of this parameter with clinical aggressiveness as defined by metastatic disease.**]

36. Increased recurrence rates of endometrial carcinoma are associated with

   1. aneuploidy.
   2. increasing percentage of S-phase fraction.
   3. DNA index.
   4. proliferation index.

p. 1207   Ans: E   (Podratz K C, Wilson T O, Gaffey T A, Cha S S, Katzmann J A. Deoxyribonucleic acid analysis facilitates the pretreatment identification of high-risk endometrial cancer patients. Am J Obstet Gynec 1993; 168:1206)

36. [F & I: •Background: Endometrial carcinoma is the most common cancer (45%) of the female genitalia in the United States.

•According to 1992 estimates 32,000 new cases and 5600 deaths are anticipated from this neoplastic process during this calendar year.

•This represents an increase of >90% (from 2900) in the estimated number of deaths since 1987, an interval during which the estimated annual number of new cases of corpus cancer was essentially unchanged (decrease over 5 years of 8% to 9%).

•The estimated number of annual deaths attributable to cancer of the endometrium surpassed cancer of the cervix in 1991 and presumably will account for approximately 23% of all cancer-related deaths of the female genital organs this year.

•The major therapeutic prognostic determinants include stage, histologic grade, and depth of myometrial invasion.

•The limitations associated with development of treatment are readily apparent in the lack of precision associated with clinical staging and with histologic grading and subtyping of sampled endometrial specimens.

•Neither the depth of myometrial invasion nor the surgical stage is ascertainable before commencement of definitive therapy.

•The ability to triage and appropriately refer to the gynecologic oncologist those patients at high risk for advanced primary disease or subsequent recurrences continues to be significantly compromised.

•The ability to identify patients at low risk for advanced disease or recurrence, thereby avoiding excessive therapeutic manipulations and their associated costs and morbidity, is equally important.

•The deoxyribonucleic acid (DNA) content in patients with endometrial carcinoma is strongly correlated with patient prognosis.

•Increased recurrence or decreased survival rates (or both) were correlated with aneuploidy and increasing percent of S-phase fraction, DNA index, and proliferative index.

•These more quantifiable molecular variables may better identify certain tumor types that predispose to such virulent courses as reflected by early dissemination, early recurrence, treatment refractoriness, and compromised survival.

•Ideally, the assessment of such therapeutic determinants before initiation of therapy would facilitate treatment dispositions and translate into enhanced salvage rates.

•Objective: To examine DNA content in curettage specimens containing endometrial carcinoma obtained immediately before definitive surgical staging and cytoreduction.

°DNA ploidy, S-phase fraction, and proliferative index were independently assessed as a function of surgical stage and progression-free survival to determine the proficiency of each factor for stratifying patients accurately according to risk for advanced disease (surgical stage III or IV) and the development of recurrent disease.

- A flow cytometer was used to generate DNA histograms.

- The cell cycle distribution was determined by analyzing ungated data from 10,000 nuclei in a rectangular S-phase computer model.

- Tumors with only one G0/G1 peak were designated as diploid (2n), whereas tumors with histograms suggesting more than one G0/G1 population were categorized as aneuploid.

° Tumor samples with 29% of nuclei associated with the 4n peak were considered tetraploid.

- The DNA index was calculated as the ratio of the mean channel of the aneuploid G0/G1 population compared with the diploid G0/G1 channel.

° Diploid tumors possessed a DNA index of 1.0, tetraploid 2.0, and aneuploid >1.0, with the most prominent population in multiploid tumors used to assign a DNA index.

- The current mechanisms for assignment of surgical stage and myometrial invasion require surgical intervention and pathologic evaluation.

- The prognostic value derivable from only the histologic assessment of a curettage specimen without knowledge of other prognostic variables is limited.

- In addition, clinical stages III and IV reliably incorporate only those patients with obvious extrauterine spread, whereas patients with clinically occult extrauterine spread are masked within clinical stage I or II.

- The progression-free survival for clinical stage I patients paralleled the survival for the entire population, suggesting that a significant percentage of patients with advanced disease were included with clinical stage I patients.

- Simultaneous alignment of surgical and clinical stages demonstrated incorrect clinical designations in 24% of the patients, reconfirming similar disconcordance rates observed by other investigators.

- The clinical identification of only five of 26 patients (sensitivity of 19%) with advanced disease further attests to the limited role of clinical staging.

- Because patients with surgically documented advanced disease accounted for only 19% of the sample population but 63% of the observed recurrences, preoperative identification of these high-risk patients would facilitate the triage processes for definitive treatment.

- An analysis of cellular DNA content was initiated to examine the applicability of cytometric variables in identifying patients with advanced disease or patients at high risk for recurrence (or both).

- Nondiploid patterns, increased S-phase fraction, abnormal DNA index, and increased proliferative index are associated with an increased frequency of post-treatment recurrences and cancer-related deaths.

- The frequency of ploidy, DNA index, S-phase fraction, and proliferative index aberrations correlate with increasing levels of tissue dedifferentiation.

° Stratification of well and moderately differentiated tumors into diploid and nondiploid groups identified two distinctly different risk subsets.

- The correlation between cytometric variables and the depth of myometrial invasion and the stage of disease remains to be defined.

- Results: DNA ploidy, percent of S phase, and the proliferative index were analyzed in sections from paraffin-embedded blocks of curettage specimens containing endometrial carcinoma obtained before definitive staging and cytoreduction.

•In the study population that received definitive primary surgical management and adjunctive therapy on the basis of surgical and pathologic findings, the recurrences and cancer-related deaths were correlated with nondiploid DNA patterns (29% of population, 50% of recurrences, 54% of deaths), an S-phase fraction 29% (41% of population, 67% of recurrences, 75% of cancer-related deaths), and a proliferative index ≥14% (45% of population, 73% of recurrences, 79% of deaths).

•Aneuploid tumors with a DNA index >1.5 had significantly higher recurrence and death rates than lesions with a DNA index <1.5, suggesting the probability of further risk stratification.

•These observations confirm a less favorable prognosis for patients with malignancies characterized by aneuploidy, increased-phase fraction, and higher DNA indexes.

•Because of the strong correlation between aberrant cytometric variables noted in curettage specimens, the recurrence frequency, and the limited information in the literature suggesting that patients with metastatic disease more frequently harbor aneuploid tumors, an assessment of the distribution of ploidy, S-phase fraction, and proliferative index in patients at risk for advanced disease was initiated.

•Aneuploidy, S-phase fraction 29%, and proliferative index >14% were used as discriminators in an attempt to stratify patients with advanced disease.

•Although aneuploid tumors represented 23% of the sampled population, 46% of patients in surgical stages III and IV harbored aneuploid tumors.

•Curettage specimens containing carcinoma with S-phase fraction ≥9% or proliferative index ≥14% were detected in 41% and 45% of the entire population, respectively.

°Both subsets identified 69% of the patients with advanced disease.

•These data suggest that the information derived from cytometric DNA analysis of the pretreatment curettage specimen identifies a significant number of patients at high risk for advanced disease and recurrences or cancer-related deaths.

•This information should favorably influence treatment-planning processes.

•Although the deaths attributable to endometrial cancer increased during the past 5 years, this disease remains relatively amenable to therapy.

•The identification of one or more quantifiable molecular variables that directly or indirectly assess tumor biology would assist the clinician in profiling patients' risk status and selecting treatment options.

•The DNA ploidy and cell kinetic data derived from pretreatment curettage specimens in the current study identified a significant proportion of patients at risk for extrauterine spread and compromised longevity.

•High-risk patients can be readily afforded access to individuals and institutions with special expertise in managing advanced or recurrent endometrial carcinoma.

°This approach would facilitate the evaluation and application of new or modified therapeutic modalities.]

37. CSF-1 production has been identified with malignancies of

   1. pancreas
   2. ovary
   3. breast
   4. trophoblast

p. 526   Ans: E   (Price F V, Chambers S K, Chambers J T, Carcangui M L. Schwartz P E, Kohorn E I, Stanley E R, Kacinski B M. Colony-stimulating factor-1 in primary ascites of ovarian cancer is a significant predictor of survival. Am J Obstet Gynec 1993; 168:520)

37. [F & I: •Background: Expression of the genes encoding the glycoprotein cytokine colony-stimulating factor (CSF-1) and its receptor, the *c-fms* protooncogene, has been found in hematologic and epithelial neoplasms and tumor-derived cell lines by a variety of immunochemical and molecular biologic techniques.

•In normal tissues CSF-1 and its receptor function in the terminal phases of macrophage differentiation and in placental implantation.

•CSF-1 is a reliable circulating marker of neoplastic disease activity in patients with hematologic, endometrial, and ovarian cancer.

•In ovarian and endometrial cancers high levels of *c-fms* transcripts correlate strongly with high histologic grade and advanced stage, both of which are strongly prognostic of poor clinical outcomes.

•The presence of malignant cells in peritoneal washings and ascites is a recognized prognostic factor in ovarian carcinoma, and in the International Federation of Gynecology and Obstetrics (FIGO) staging system malignant cells in peritoneal fluid advances the stage of early ovarian tumors.

•Tumor markers in ascites, peritoneal washings, and peritoneal fluid have been analyzed because these body fluids are in direct contact with disseminated ovarian cancer cells.

•Ascites fluid from patients with ovarian carcinoma contains a variety of growth factors which facilitate the growth of some cell lines.

•Objectives: To determine whether a relationship exists between CSF-1 concentration in the ascites of patients with ovarian carcinoma and their prognosis and to compare the concentration of CSF-1 in ascites with other accepted indicators of clinical behavior.

•CSF-1 levels in ascites of advanced ovarian cancer may be a significant independent predictor of survival.

•The hematopoietic growth factor CSF-1 is a mitogen, chemoattractant, and phenotypic activator for nonneoplastic macrophages and monocytes.

•Circulating levels are elevated during pregnancy, and locally produced CSF-1 may regulate the differentiation and replication of trophoblasts, which proliferate and invade the uterine, much as cancer cells do during dissemination from their organ of origin.

•CSF-1 is produced in pancreatic, breast, lung, endometrial, choriocarcinoma, and ovarian carcinoma cell lines.

•Levels of CSF-1 receptor measured by quantitative in situ hybridization or immunohistochemistry correlate with histologic grade and advanced stage of ovarian and endometrial carcinomas at presentation.

•Serum CSF-1 levels follow changes in clinical disease status of patients with tumors that produce CSF-1, including patients with certain hematologic malignancies and gynecologic adenocarcinomas.

•It is not surprising that the levels of CSF-1 in the ascites that bathes ovarian carcinoma are elevated and that ascites CSF-1 concentration has implications for prognosis.

•The presence of growth factors such as CSF-1 in high concentrations in and around carcinoma cells may, in part, explain the proliferative and invasive characteristics of these tumors.

°They may modify host immune antitumor responses.

•Although the inappropriate activation of the CSF-1 gene in *c-fms* bearing neoplastic hematopoietic cells leading to an autocrine state has been implicated as a secondary event in tumor progression in the mouse, it is still unknown whether derangements in the local and systemic concentrations of growth factors such as CSF-1 in humans arise as a result of their production by tumor cells, as a response of the host to an invasive cancer, or as a combination of both.

•Ascitic fluid CSF-1 concentrations were measured in patients who had ascites associated with ovarian cancer at the time of their initial staging laparotomy.

•In 37 of 44 patients (84%), disease was advanced (FIGO stage III and IV) at the time of diagnosis.

•Long-term follow-up of these patients allowed ascites CSF-1 concentration at presentation to be analyzed retrospectively as an indicator of prognosis.

•Patients with low levels of CSF-1 in ascites were found to have longer survival compared with patients with higher levels of CSF-1.

•These differences were more significant than for any other prognostic indicator, except for zero residual disease after cytoreductive surgery.

•High CSF-1 concentrations in serum and overexpression of the *fms* oncogene in tumor specimens have been shown to correlate with high grade and advanced stage, indexes already known to influence clinical behavior.

•The advantage of ascites fluid analysis is that it is readily accessible by paracentesis.

•If ovarian carcinoma were clinically or radiographically suspected, ascites could be aspirated and a prediction could be made about the likelihood of successful surgical debulking.

•Patients with high ascites CSF-1 levels, in whom a poor survival from diagnosis may be predicted, may be candidates for neoadjuvant chemotherapy or other nonstandard approaches, particularly if the trend observed in prediction of the feasibility of optimal surgical cytoreduction is borne out in future studies with larger numbers of patients.]

38. True statements about estrogen and progesterone receptors include

   1. there is an inverse relationship between the content of estrogen and progesterone receptors and the stage of endometrial carcinoma
   2. there is an inverse relationship between the content of estrogen and progesterone receptors and grade
   3. adenomatous hyperplasia has relatively high levels of progesterone receptors
   4. receptor rich tumors grow more slowly than receptor poor tumors

p. 1340   Ans: E   (Nyholm H C J, Nielsen A L, Lyndrup J, Norup P, Thorpe S M. Biochemical and immunohistochemical estrogen and progesterone receptors in adenomatous hyperplasia and endometrial carcinoma: Correlations with stage and other clinicopathologic features. Am J Obstet Gynec 1992; 167:1334)

38. [F & I: •Background: Endometrial carcinoma is generally accepted to be an endocrine-related neoplasm.

•Like normal endometrium, many endometrial carcinomas contain estrogen and progesterone receptors.

•The receptor content appears to correlate with several histopathologic features, in particular with tumor differentiation.

•Potential precancerous lesions of the endometrium, such as adenomatous hyperplasia with or without nuclear atypia, may contain levels of estrogen and progesterone receptors distinct from carcinoma.

•In determining estrogen and progesterone receptor levels, biochemical and immunohistochemical analysis can be applied.

•The biochemical methods determine the receptors in whole-tissue homogenates and cannot discriminate between receptors in malignant tissue versus nonmalignant tissue that may be intermingled in the carcinoma.

•Immunohistochemical analysis of the receptors directly on tissue sections yields a semiquantitative estimation of the receptor content at the cellular level, and the distribution of receptors between malignant and nonmalignant cells can be studied.

•Objective: To examine the correlation between estrogen and progesterone receptors, determined both biochemically and immunohistochemically, and tumor histologic type, stage, patient age, years since menopause, and previous use of estrogens in endometrial carcinoma.

•Results: A close inverse relationship between tumor grade and the content of estrogen and progesterone receptor, determined both biochemically and immunohistochemically.

•The receptor content, and the histologic grade and the carcinoma tissue percentage are very uniform in samples from the same tumor, suggesting that one single specimen is representative for the overall tumor histopathologic type and content of receptors.

•The correlations between total immunohistochemical histologic score and grade and between cancer immunohistochemical histologic score and grade were similar, probably reflecting the finding that the malignant tissue component predominated in the majority of samples.

•It is uncertain whether the cancer score is of greater relevance than the total score in characterizing endometrial carcinoma.

•The overall agreement between the biochemical and the immunohistochemical method was good.

•The immunohistochemical methods detect receptor epitopes that are distinct from the ligand binding sites of the receptors.

•The fixative of the tissue may alter the antigenic site of the receptor protein, which could lead to negative immunohistochemical analysis in dextran-coated charcoal-positive tumors.

•The preparation technique applied in immunohistochemical analysis may affect estrogen and progesterone receptors differently, and this might be one reason for the divergent sensitivities of the estrogen and progesterone receptor immunohistochemical analysis.

•This study is the first in which the receptor content is related to the revised 1988 FIGO grading system, which includes nuclear atypia that, if inappropriate for the architectural grade, raises the grade by one.

•In more than 20 studies published since 1980 an inverse correlation between biochemical receptor presence and grade has been shown, i.e., poorly differentiated endometrioid adenocarcinomas are more often receptor negative or display lower amounts of receptors than do well-differentiated and moderately differentiated lesions, differences between the latter two often being less pronounced.

•The frequency of estrogen receptor-positive tumors ranges from 77% to 94% in FIGO grade 1 to 27% to 56% in grade 3 and of progesterone receptor-positive tumors from 70% to 93% in grade 1 to 22% to 44% in grade 3 (frequencies for grade 2 tumors resemble those for grade 1).

•There are several possible reasons for the discrepancies between various studies: divergent receptor analysis methods, analysis threshold levels, and chosen cutoff values.

•Differences in histopathologic evaluations may also account for discordant results.

•By means of a multiple regression model, a significant decrease of estrogen and progesterone receptor content with stage, independent of histologic grade, was found.

• The observation that the clinical stage correlates better with the receptor content than with the postsurgical stage may simply be a consequence of more subgroup classes in the postsurgical classification.

Obstetrics and Gynecology:Review 1994-Gynecologic Oncology References

•A number of studies analyzing single variables have examined correlations between clinical stage and biochemical receptor status (positive/negative) with varying results, ranging from no correlation to correlations between only estrogen receptor, progesterone receptor only, or both receptors and stage.

•The finding of an independent relationship between the estrogen and progesterone receptor contents and the stage of tumor is interesting, because it may reflect the biologic behavior of the tumor.

•The inverse relationship suggests that "receptor-rich" tumors may grow more slowly than do "receptor-poor" tumors and vice versa or alternatively that the receptors, as the tumor grows, may gradually be lost or undergo degenerative changes and thereby escape detection.

•The latter theory would be in accordance with the demonstration of reduced receptor levels in recurrent endometrial carcinoma and metastases, similar to findings in breast carcinoma.

•Myometrial invasion did not correlate with receptor content when correcting for histologic grade or stage.

•Progesterone receptors were relatively high in adenomatous hyperplasia.

°This may support the theory that adenomatous hyperplasia is associated with increased estrogen influence, because one cellular effect of this is known to be stimulated progesterone receptor synthesis.

•This study establishes a significant, inverse correlation between the content of estrogen and progesterone receptors and the stage of endometrial carcinoma independent of tumor grade and furthermore shows that the content of estrogen and progesterone receptors is distinctively associated with the histologic grade of the tumor.

°The immunohistochemical analysis cancer score was closely related to the total score, probably reflecting the finding that the malignant tissue component predominated in the majority of biopsies.]

---

39. Factors associated with poor survival in patients with squamous cell carcinoma of the vulva

    1. recurrence within two years
    2. lymph node involvement
    3. tumor grade
    4. initial stage

---

p. 1387   Ans: E   (Tilmans A S, Sutton G P, Look K Y, Stehman F B, Ehrlich C E, Hornback N B. Recurrent squamous carcinoma of the vulva. Am J Obstet Gynec 1992; 167:1383)

39. [F & I: •Background: Radical vulvectomy with bilateral inguinal lymphadenectomy is the accepted primary management for squamous carcinoma of the vulva.

•Conservative resection rather than more extensive procedures has been recently advocated for some subsets of patients.

•Many have attempted to define reliable prognostic variables that allow a more limited resection.

•The overall 5-year survival for all stages is approximately 75%.

•Patients with recurrent disease have a poor prognosis, especially with regional or distant failure.

•Objectives: To evaluate the clinical aspects of recurrence and to optimize management, particularly emphasizing therapy, prognosis, and special problems unique to vulvar cancer.

•The recurrence rate for vulvar carcinoma after surgery is 20% to 30%.

•The prognosis for patients with recurrent cancer has historically been poor.

Obstetrics and Gynecology:Review 1994-Gynecologic Oncology References

- FIGO stage, nodal status, and tumor site may be of prognostic significance in patients at high risk for recurrence.

- In addition, lymph vascular space invasion, depth and pattern of invasion, and grade and surgical margin may also help predict those patients whose tumors are likely to recur after initial therapy.

- Efforts to control recurrence will probably fail in at least 50% of cases.

- With disease outside the pelvis, no curative therapy is available.

- The site of recurrence, interval to recurrence, and tumor grade were prognostically significant for both overall survival and survival after retreatment.

- Initial FIGO stage was also predictive of overall survival.

- The interval between primary therapy and recurrence tends to be long.

- 44% of patients in this series had disease recurrence within 1 year, and only 63% had recurrences within two years.

- The patients who had recurrences within 16 months of initial therapy had poorer outcomes than did those who had recurrences later.

- The site of recurrence significantly influences the survival after retreatment.

- Lymph node involvement or distant metastases were ominous signs.

- Of the recurrences in the current series, 43% were located in the vulva with no evidence of regional or distant metastases.

- Other series report that 66% to 71% of recurrences are confined to the vulva.

- Retreatment for local recurrence was primarily surgical, although four patients were treated with radiotherapy alone.

- Historically, irridiation of the vulva and perineum has produced significant morbidity.

- Moist skin desquamation requiring frequent treatment interruptions, radiation fibrosis, lymphedema (particularly after groin node dissection), skin ulceration, and other severe morbidity were not uncommon.

- The compromised blood and lymphatic drainage of the perineal tissue also was thought to contribute to radiation therapy's limitations.

- Factors thtat may be responsible for the success of radiotherapy include the size and depth of the recurrence, groin node size, perineal skin involvement, and the degree of tumor tissue necrosis.

  ° Radiation doses of 5500 to 8500 cGy were required and external beam therapy was integrated with brachytherapy.

- Vulvar carcinoma is radioresponsive and that those with recurrent tumors can occasionally be salvaged with radiotherapy.

- Patients with groin recurrences may benefit from a more aggressive retreatment strategy.

- In anal carcinoma the addition of 5-fluorouracil and mitomycin C is more beneficial than radiation or surgery alone for primary tumor control.

  ° This regimen appears to be cytotoxic for microscopic distant disease, as well as local disease.

  ° Also, a synergistic effect of 5-fluorouracil is evident when it is combined with radiotherapy.

Obstetrics and Gynecology: Review 1994 - Gynecologic Oncology References

°The combination of cisplatin and 5-fluorouracil has confirmed activity against cervical cancer.

•Patients with vulvar carcinoma require long-term follow-up.

•Most recurrences are vulvar surface lesions that can easily be detected.

•Although the majority of recurrences are seen within 2 years, a significant number are found later.

•Patients should undergo careful restaging.

•Recurrence site, interval to recurrence, and grade were significant predictors of survival after retreatment.

•Retreatment tended primarily to involve surgery, with postoperative radiotherapy reserved for the treatment of regional disease.

°Radiotherapy does provide significant palliation.

•The poor prognosis for patients with groin node involvement warrants additional evaluation.

°These patients may benefit from chemoradiotherapy as an adjunct to surgery.

°They generally tolerate aggressive retreatment with acceptable morbidity, in spite of their advanced ages.

°In others with poor performance status, judicious second-line therapy is appropriate.]

---

40. Tumoricidal action of TNF-α against human ovarian cell lines can be increased by

 1. actinomycin D
 2. cycloheximide
 3. emetine
 4. diphtheria toxin

(Two references.)
p. 1868   Ans: E   (Quantitation of tumor necrosis factor-α, interleukin 1ß, and interleukin-6 in the effusions of ovarian epithelial neoplasms. Am J Obstet Gynec 1992; 167:1870)

40. [F & I: •Background: Ovarian carcinoma is the fifth leading cause of cancer death in women and the leading cause of cancer death from gynecologic malignancies.

•More than 12,000 women die annually of this type of cancer.

•In spite of extensive chemotherapy, radiotherapy, and surgery, the age-adjusted cancer death rate for cancer of the ovary has continued to increase since 1930, with a current rate of 10 deaths per 100,000 female population.

•The survival of neoplastic cells was thought to be dependent on the escape from recognition and eventual destruction by the host immune system.

•The human female host is able to recognize ovarian tumor cells as foreign and to initiate an immune response containing specific antibody molecules.

•Autologous antibodies have shown cytotoxic potential in vitro against human ovarian neoplastic cell lines.

•Attention has been focused on the direct and indirect actions of multifunctional cytokines on human ovarian tumor cells after the report that interleukin-1ß (IL-1ß) and interleukin-6 (IL-6) were produced by tumor-associated macrophages from human ovarian carcinoma.

- The presence of tumor necrosis factor-α (TNF-α) in the peripheral blood of patients with ovarian cancer is also of interest.

- The use of multifunctional cytokines alone or in combination with current chemotherapeutic protocols for the treatment of human ovarian cancer has also been suggested.

- The culture of human ovarian cancer cells with TNF-α alone has resulted in both tumor cell cytotoxicity and tumor cell proliferation.

- In vitro studies have found both proliferative and antiproliferative effects on human ovarian carcinoma cells cultured with TNF-α in combination with interferon.

- Objective: To determine if the host might respond to ovarian neoplasia with the production of multifunctional cytokines.

- Methods: Cyst and ascitic fluids were obtained from 35 patients with ovarian neoplasms, and the concentrations of TNF-α, IL-1ß, and IL-6 were determined by sensitive immunoassay.

- Thirty-five different samples of effusions from human ovarian epithelial neoplasms were quantitatively analyzed for TNF-α, IL 1ß, and IL-6.

- The possibility that the amounts of the multifunctional cytokines present varied with histopathologic type of tumors was investigated.

- Results: When compared with IL-1ß and TNF-α, IL-6 was found in the largest quantities in all fluid samples studied.

- It is possible that these cytokines were produced by the immune cells of the host in response to the tumor.

- Peritoneal macrophages obtained from women with benign gynecologic diseases produce TNF-α and IL-1ß in vitro.

- Human ovarian carcinoma cells produce TNF-α in vivo and IL-Iß in vitro.

- TNF-α, IL-Iß, and IL-6 are produced by monocytes, macrophages, and lymphocytes, as well as by cells of other types.

- These cytokines display growth-stimulatory and growth-inhibitory actions, depending on various culture conditions, cell types, and cytokine concentrations.

- Detectable levels of all three cytokines in fluid from patients with different histopathologic types of tumors were found.

- Although it is possible that the cytokines detected were produced by the tumor cells, it is likely that they were produced by the T lymphocytes and macrophages that infiltrate the tumors and surround the tumors in ascites.

- TNF-α, IL-1ß, and IL-6 have been measured in the peritoneal fluid of individuals with nonmalignant conditions.

- IL-6 levels in papillary serous cystadenocarcinoma and papillary adenocarcinoma that were tenfold higher than those of the peritoneal dialysates.

- Significant differences were not detected in the levels of TNF-α in any diagnostic groups of ovarian cancer fluid when compared with benign cyst fluid.

- The interactions between the immune system and tumor cells are complex.

Obstetrics and Gynecology: Review 1994-Gynecologic Oncology References

•The tumoricidal action of the macrophage cytokine TNF-α against human ovarian cell lines was increased in the presence of the protein synthesis inhibitors actinomycin D, cycloheximide, emetine, and diphtheria toxin.

•The resistance to killing of the SKOV-3 ovarian carcinoma line in the presence of TNF-α was converted to sensitivity with the addition of cycloheximide.

•These effects were independent of differences in the expression of the TNF-α receptors.

•It is likely that the **protein synthesis inhibitors are blocking the production** of a factor that can neutralize the action of TNF-α.

•The serum ultrafiltrate of human cancer contains a **blocking factor** that inhibits the cytotoxic activity of TNF-α in vitro.

°A similar blocking factor has been isolated from the ascites of patients with ovarian cancer.

°This 28 kD protein is derived from the TNF-α cell membrane receptor.

•The presence of a TNF-α-blocking factor in the ascites of patients with ovarian cancer may explain the relatively lower levels of TNF-α detected by ELISA, in comparison with those of IL-6.

•It also provides an explanation for the escape from host control of ovarian tumor.

•The expression of HER2/Neu oncogenes in human ovarian tumor cells confers a proliferative advantage because of the induction of resistance to several host cytotoxic mechanisms.

•This tumor resistance to host control was significantly reversed with the addition of protein synthesis inhibitors.

•Conclusion: Ovarian cancer is recognized by the immune system, as evidenced by the production of specific antibodies and perhaps also multifunctional cytokines.

•The administration or activation of these biologic response modifiers, alone or in combination with other chemotherapeutic modalities, may offer significant advances in the care of ovarian cancer patients.]

(Second reference.)

p. 1870   (Williams S, Mutch D G, Xu L, Collins J L. Divergent effects of taxol on tumor necrosis factor-α -mediated cytolysis of ovarian carcinoma cells. Am J Obstet Gynec 1992; 167:1864)

J-12-1864 [F & I: •Background: Ovarian carcinoma is the leading cause of death from gynecologic malignancy.

•Treatment for this disease is aimed at decreasing tumor burden, generally through surgery followed by chemotherapy.

•Cisplatin-based chemotherapy has resulted in an increase in the frequency of response but little increase in the overall cure rate.

•Significant problems remain with cisplatin-based therapy because of continued low survival, dose-limiting toxicities, and development of drug resistance.

•The age-adjusted death rate for women with ovarian carcinoma has remained constant for 35 years.

•Taxol, a plant-derived antimitotic agent, is a potential new drug in the treatment of epithelial ovarian cancer.

•Taxol is derived from extracts of the bark of the western yew tree (Taxus *brevifolia);* its complex taxane ring structure has so far eluded attempts at complete synthesis.

•Fact   °Detail   »issue   *answer

Obstetrics and Gynecology: Review 1994-Gynecologic Oncology References

- Although other antimitotic chemotherapeutic agents disrupt microtubules, the unique antimitotic activity of taxol arises from its ability to stabilize microtubules, preventing their disassembly.

- Phase II clinical trials of taxol in patients with drug-refractory epithelial ovarian cancer have response rates of 30% to 37%.

- Phase III trials are presently ongoing.

- Tumor necrosis factor-α (TNF-α) may be involved in host protective mechanisms, either as a macrophage-secreted product capable of mediating cytolysis directly or as a membrane-bound effector molecule associated with cytotoxic cells.

- Patients with ovarian carcinomas (and carcinomas of other tissues) have significantly elevated serum levels of TNF-α, suggesting that this is a response to these cancers.

- Because taxol is capable of increasing the release of TNF-α from macrophages, as well as decreasing the number of TNF-α receptors on some cancer cells.

- Objective: To investigate the effect of taxol on TNF-α-mediated cytolysis of human ovarian carcinoma cells in vitro.

- Results: Taxol increased the TNF-α-mediated cytolysis of Caov-3 and A2780 while decreasing the TNF-α-mediated cytolysis of OVCAR-3, SK-OV-3, and L929.

- Possible explanations for these results include:

    ° The mechanism by which taxol diminished TNF-α cytolysis in L929, OVCAR-3, and SK-OV-3 could be that it **decreased the number of TNF-α receptors** on the cell surface.

    ° This would result in decreased internalization of TNF-α and thereby diminished activation of the cytolytic mechanism.

    ° If taxol decreased TNF-α receptors in these cell lines and if the decrease was responsible for the decrease in TNF-α-mediated cytolysis, then exposing these cells to TNF-α before their exposure to taxol should at least reduce the level of inhibition of TNF-α-mediated cytolysis by taxol.

    ° The fact that taxol was equally inhibitory whether it was added 2 hours before or 2 hours after TNF-α suggests that taxol does not decrease the TNF-α-mediated cytolysis of these cells by decreasing TNF-α receptors.

- Taxol caused an increase in TNF-α-mediated cytolysis in Caov-3 and A2780.

    ° The results seen in these cell lines cannot be due to a decline in either the number or the function of TNF-α receptors.

    ° Because TNF-α-mediated cytolysis in Caov-3 is increased by taxol in the absence of protein synthesis inhibitors, the possibility exists that taxol might be acting as a **protein synthesis inhibitor**.

    ° When protein synthesis was measured, it was at equivalent levels of TNF-α-mediated cytolysis in the presence of taxol or emetine, the levels of protein synthesis inhibition differed markedly (i.e., it was necessary to inhibit protein synthesis to a greater extent with emetine than with taxol to achieve similar levels of TNF-α-mediated cytolysis.

- Circulating levels of TNF-α are increased in the sera of patients with epithelial ovarian cancer.

- TNF-α messenger ribonucleic acid has been detected in situ in ovarian cancer.

- If TNF-α is involved in the surveillance of ovarian cancer, treatment with taxol could cause an alteration in the host response by acting synergistically or antagonistically with TNF-α, resulting in divergent effects on TNF-α-mediated cytolysis.

- Fact   ° Detail   »issue   *answer

•In those patients responsive to the combined effects treatment strategy may include administration of both taxol and TNF-α.]

41. Interferon gamma

   1. increases EGF receptor expression
   2. decreases EGF receptor expression
   3. down regulates HER/*neu* levels
   4. increases expression of CEA

p. 1877   Ans: E   (Boente M P, Berchuck A, Rodriguez G C, Davidoff A, Whitake R, Xu F J, Marks J, Clarke-Pearson D L, Bast R C. The effect of interferon gamma on epidermal growth factor receptor expression in normal and malignant ovarian epithelial cells. Am J Obstet Gynec 1992; 167:1877)

41. [F & I: •Background: The epidermal growth factor (EGF) receptor is a membrane-spanning glycoprotein that includes an extracellular ligand binding domain, a hydrophobic membrane-spanning region, and an intracellular tyrosine kinase domain.

•Binding of EGF or transforming growth factor-α to the extracellular domain results in activation of the tyrosine kinase, which is involved in transmitting the mitogenic signal to the nucleus.

•In addition, the receptor-ligand complex subsequently is internalized, which results in down-regulation of cell surface EGF receptor levels.

•Because the EGF receptor and its ligands can stimulate proliferation of many cells, their role in growth regulation and transformation of human ovarian epithelial cells has been investigated.

°Normal ovarian epithelial cells express EGF receptors (10^4 to 10^5 receptors per cell) and that EGF acts to stimulate proliferation of these cells (two- to fivefold).

°Ovarian cancer cell lines express similar numbers of high-affinity EGF receptors, but most of these cells lines were relatively resistant to the growth-stimulatory effect of EGF.

°Expression of EGF receptor and overexpression of HER-2/neu, a closely related receptor-tyrosine kinase, are associated with **poor** survival in breast and ovarian cancer.

•Like EGF, the interferons affect growth of a wide range of cell types.

•In general, proliferation of cancer cell lines is inhibited by interferons, but in some cases interferons can stimulate proliferation.

•Although the mechanisms of action remain largely unknown, interferons can modulate expression of cell surface molecules.

•Interferon gamma (IFN-γ) can increase expression of both major histocompatibility complex antigens and tumor-associated antigens such as carcinoembryonic antigen and tumor-associated glycoprotein-72.

• IFN-γ **down-regulates** HER-2/neu levels in cells that overexpress this receptor.

•IFN-γ can either increase or decrease EGF receptor expression, depending on the cell line studied.

•Objective: To examine the effect of IFN-γ on proliferation and EGF receptor expression in normal and malignant ovarian cells.

•The interferons are a heterogeneous family of molecules that were first discovered because of their ability to induce cellular resistance to viral infection.

- Interferons also influence cellular proliferation and differentiation and have immunomodulatory properties.

- The interferon α/ß superfamily encompasses a large group of structurally related genes, whereas IFN-γ is encoded by a single gene on chromosome 12 that is structurally unrelated to members of the α/ß family.

- In humans activated T lymphocytes are the predominant cellular source of IFN-γ, and this lymphokine is active in the immune response to viruses and other antigenic stimuli.

- In addition to immune functions, interferons act to decrease proliferation of a wide range of cells in culture, but in some cells modest growth stimulation has been observed.

- IFN-γ also has antitumor activity against human ovarian cancer xenografts in nude mice.

- Interferons have modest antitumor activity in clinical trials when they were used both alone and in combination with conventional cytotoxic chemotherapy to treat ovarian cancer.

- Mechanisms of interferon action are not well understood, but they can alter expression of receptor tyrosine kinases (EGF receptor, HER-2/neu), which are important in transmitting growth-regulatory signals.

- There is not a consistent relationship between the effect of interferons on proliferation and receptor expression.

- IFN-α **decreases** EGF receptor synthesis in renal carcinomas that are growth inhibited by IFN-α, whereas there is no effect on receptor levels in renal cancers that are unresponsive to IFN-α.

- IFN-α **up-regulates** EGF receptor levels in two squamous carcinoma cell lines (A43 1, KB) that also are growth inhibited by interferons.

- Interferons **down-regulate** HER-2/neu expression in breast and ovarian cancer cell lines that overexpress this putative growth factor receptor.

- Results: Similar to the prior studies in which IFN-γ decreased proliferation of several ovarian cancer cell lines, IFN-γ inhibited proliferation of three ovarian cancer cell lines (OVCA 429, OVCA 432, OVCA 433).

- In all three cell lines and in SKOv3 cells IFN-γ treatment increased EGF receptor expression.

- The most striking evidence of receptor up-regulation was seen at the cell surface; total cellular EGF receptor content also was increased by 1.4- to 4.2-fold.

- In contrast, IFN-γ treatment of normal ovarian epithelial cells had no effect on EGF receptor expression.

- Potential mechanisms that could contribute to increased EGF receptor expression in ovarian cancer cell lines after IFN-γ treatment include:

    ° Increased production of EGF receptor because of higher rates of transcription or translation of the EGF receptor gene or messenger ribonucleic acid, respectively.

    ° Increases in EGF receptor synthesis occur in other types of cells in which interferons up-regulate EGF receptor expression.

    ° A greater portion of total cellular EGF receptor protein is present on the cell surface after interferon treatment.

    ° Newly synthesized EGF receptor normally is inserted into the cell membrane.

°When a ligand (EGF, transforming growth factor-α, monoclonal antibody) binds to the EGF receptor, the receptor-ligand complex is internalized into the cytoplasm by clatherin-coated pits.

°Receptor may then be recycled back into the cell membrane or alternatively routed to lysosomes for degradation.

°Thus up-regulation of cell surface EGF receptor levels by interferon may be caused by increased recycling and decreased degradation of receptor and by increased production.

•It is unknown whether interferon-induced up-regulation of EGF receptor levels have an impact on cellular growth regulation or is an unrelated phenomenon.

•Because the EGF receptor is overexpressed in some squamous cancers, often because of gene amplification, this cell surface molecule might be an effective target for immunotherapy and imaging with monoclonal antibodies conjugated to cytotoxins or radioisotopes

•Growth factor receptors are appropriate targets for immunotoxins, because internalization of the receptor-immunoconjugate complex facilitates delivery of the toxin to the interior of the cell.

•Anti-EGF receptor-ricin A-chain immunoconjugates can inhibit in vitro and in vivo growth of epidermoid cancer cell lines that express high EGF receptor levels.

•Although overexpression of EGF receptor is not observed in ovarian cancers, most of these cancers express detectable levels of EGF receptor.

•Interferon treatment represents a potential method of increasing EGF receptor levels in ovarian cancer cells.

•This is particularly appealing in view of the finding that up-regulation occurs preferentially in cancer cells relative to normal cells.

•Finally, regulation of growth factor receptors has the potential to affect proliferation of ovarian cancer cells.

•Although it has been assumed that this is because of the direct antiproliferative effect of interferons, regulation of growth factor receptors, either up or down, could lead to interference with autocrine or paracrine growth regulatory pathways involving EGF or other factors.]

---

42. The E7 oncoprotein associated with HPV 16 promotes

   1. immortalization
   2. growth
   3. altered differentiation
   4. chromosomal abnormalities

---

p. 11 Ans: E   (Mittal R, Tsutsumi K, Pater A, Pater M M. Human papillomavirus type 16 expression in cervical keratinocytes: Role of progesterone and glucocorticoid hormones. Obstet Gynecol   1993; 81:5)

42. [F & I: •Background: Human papillomaviruses (HPVs) may be involved in the etiology of cervical malignancies.

•Of the more than 60 types identified, **HPV 16** is the prevalent "high-risk" HPV and is strongly associated with high-grade cervical intraepithelial neoplasia (CIN) and invasive cervical carcinomas.

•Lesions containing HPV 16 DNA also have a strong tendency to progress through successively higher grades of CIN.

•The DNA of HPV 16 is **episomal** in benign and low-grade CIN lesions, whereas in most cervical tumors and all cervical tumor-derived cell lines it is integrated into the host genome.

Obstetrics and Gynecology: Review 1994 - Gynecologic Oncology References

- The **integration event** causes oncogenic changes in viral and cellular gene expression.

- HPV infection is not likely to be sufficient to produce a fully malignant state, as cancer is usually observed decades after infection and progression from low-grade dysplasia to invasive carcinoma appears to depend on the cumulative effect of a number of cellular genetic changes.

- Steroid hormones may be involved in the etiology of cervical carcinoma.

   ° There are many reports of a correlation between the duration of oral contraceptive use and the presence and grade of CIN.

   ° Steroid hormones might act by **increasing the susceptibility** of cervical cells to HPV infection.

   ° Hormones could have a promoting effect in **inducing expression of the viral oncoproteins**.

- Progesterone/glucocorticoid response elements are found within the regulatory regions of several HPVs associated with genital lesions, and these regulatory regions respond to steroid hormones.

- These observations suggest a direct role for steroid hormones in the life cycle of anogenital HPVs.

- Dexamethasone and progesterone can increase markedly the efficiency and frequency of transformation of primary rodent cells by HPV 16.

- Glucocorticoids enhance the efficiency of HPV 16 in **immortalizing** primary human foreskin keratinocytes and enhancing transformation of such immortalized cells by the ras oncogene in a dose-dependent manner.

- Objective: To examine the role of these hormones in the episomal expression of HPV 16 in primary human cervical keratinocytes.

- Cultured human epithelial cells were used from the ectocervix as a model system for early events in HPV 16 infection; expression of HPV 16 required either progesterone or glucocorticoid hormones.

- The effectiveness of the anti-progestin RU 486 showed that this response was mediated by the hormone receptor, because RU 486 is known to block hormones from complexing with the progesterone or glucocorticoid receptors.

- Hormones may promote cervical cancer through enhanced HPV expression in the target cells due to the cells' release from growth arrest by hormones.

- The Ki67 result suggests that this does not apply in this in vitro system, but does not exclude the possibility that a block in cell cycling in vivo is overcome by hormonally induced HPV 16 expression.

- Hormones might first modulate the expression of specific cellular genes, which then modulate HPV gene expression.

   ° The greatly enhanced induction observed when the HPV 16 hormone response element was mutated to the consensus sequence suggests a **direct hormone action**.

- The direct induction of viral expression was confirmed, as there was no hormone response when the three HPV hormone response elements were mutated.

- This model system has clearly showed that all three hormone response elements are independently functional and that the function of one or more is sufficient for steroid hormone-dependent expression of HPV 16 in human ectocervical keratinocytes.

- Primary human ectocervical cells are the natural target for hormones and are permissive for expression of HPV 16, which is highly associated with high-grade CIN and invasive cervical carcinoma.

- The transfected HPV 16 DNA remains episomal and is intact; thus, it can regulate with its own control region the expression of all viral products seen in HPV-associated early cervical lesions.

• Fact   ° Detail   »issue   *answer

- Progression to cervical carcinoma involves **integration** of the viral DNA into the host chromosomes.

- Integration can eliminate hormone induction of expression of the viral DNA because of the regulatory influences of an adjacent cellular sequence.

- Because HPV-infected benign/premalignant lesions contain viral DNA in an episomal form, as do the epithelial cells in this model system, steroid hormones may have an important role in the early stages of oncogenesis.

- For HPV 16-associated lesions, the progression to cervical malignancy occurs in approximately half of the cases and rates of progression increase with disease severity, suggesting that early-stage events are pivotal for progression.

- For a number of cervical carcinoma cell lines, growth was linked to the expression levels of E6-E7 oncogenes of HPV.

- The tumorigenicity of cells from a carcinoma cell line could be strongly inhibited by reducing E6-E7 expression levels.

- The transforming activity of HPV 16 has been mapped to the E6 and E7 oncogenes in epithelial cells from the human genitalia.

- The E6 and E7 oncoproteins produce growth promotion, immortalization, and altered differentiation.

- HPV 16 E7 oncogene induced genetic instability, as evidenced by chromosomal abnormalities in mouse and human keratinocytes.

- E7 has the potential to induce the various chromosomal deletions, translocations, duplications, and aneuploidy typically observed in cervical carcinomas.

- Considering these properties of the HPV oncogenes and the present results showing the role of steroid hormones in the induction of high levels of expression of these genes in human cervical cells, high induced levels of expression of the viral oncogenes in preneoplastic cervical cells may initiate the dynamic chromosomal instability that follows.

- This HPV-induced instability could facilitate the integration of viral DNA into the host genome.

- Some of these random integration events would then deregulate expression of viral and/or cellular genes and promote progression into malignancy.

- Another important consideration is that RU 486 abolished steroid hormone-dependent expression of HPV 16 genes in ectocervical cells.

  ° This raises the issue of whether RU 486 or other anti-progestins could be useful for prophylaxis and treatment of HPV-induced lesions.

  ° These lesions might be subject to the effects of oral contraceptives.

  ° Naturally circulating glucocorticoids and progesterone might cause critical and recurrent increases in HPV gene expression during the normal ovulatory cycle or during pregnancy.

» The development of new and safe anti-progestins could provide a treatment modality for early cervical lesions induced by HPVs.]

Obstetrics and Gynecology: Review 1994-Gynecologic Oncology References

43. Histologic variables which significantly increase the risk of other genital primary squamous neoplasms in patients with vulvar carcinoma include

   1. HPV positive VIN
   2. hyperplasia
   3. epithelial-like carcinomas
   4. keratinizing growth pattern

p. 17 Ans: B   (Mitchell M F, Presad C J, Silva E G, Rutledge F N, McArthur M C, Crum C P. Second genital primary squamous neoplasms in vulvar carcinoma: Viral and histopathologic correlates. Obstet Gynecol 1993; 81:13)

43. [F & I: •Background: Cancer of the vulva, an uncommon disease with an incidence of approximately 1.8 per 100,000, principally afflicts women in their seventh and eighth decades of life and is rare in women under age 30.

   •Risks for vulvar cancer include other genital carcinomas, chronic vulvar inflammatory disorders, vulvar carcinoma in situ (vulvar intraepithelial neoplasia [VIN]), smoking, and prior history of genital warts.

   •Squamous cancers and pre-cancers of the cervix are associated with human genital papillomaviruses (HPVs), and the role of HPV in the genesis of vulvar carcinoma is yet to be determined.

   •Up to 90% of VIN lesions contain HPV 16 or other "high-risk" HPV types.

   •HPV nucleic acids have been detected in only 28-to-45% of invasive vulvar carcinoma.

   •Invasive vulvar carcinomas most likely to harbor HPV include those variants classified as condylomatous or "warty" carcinomas, those associated with VIN, and those that are less differentiated and/or exhibit intraepithelial-like or basaloid growth patterns resembling VIN.

   •In contrast to the more differentiated keratinized tumors, intraepithelial-like carcinomas infiltrate in broader, well-demarcated epithelial sheets or nests, with cells arranged perpendicular to the epithelial stromal interface.

   °Because the epithelial organization resembles VIN, the pattern is termed "intraepithelial-like."

   °This pattern must be observed within the invasive component.

   •Objective: To determine whether patients whose vulvar carcinomas exhibited both histopathologic and viral characteristics distinguish subsets of vulvar carcinoma, were at greater risk for other genital primary squamous neoplasms.

   °A second genital primary may reflect a "field effect," and may link these neoplasms to a sexually transmitted disease agent.

   °Its presence (or absence) may distinguish tumors of different etiologies.

   •A substantial proportion of women with vulvar cancer have other squamous primary lesions in the genital tract, and the relative risk of a second genital primary neoplasm is estimated to be as high as 29.8%.

   •About 20% of vulvar cancers are associated with a current, previous, or subsequent second primary lesion of the cervix or vagina.

   •The precise relationship of this risk of a second genital primary to the presence of HPV nucleic acids, or to morphologic features that identify cases at risk for associated HPV nucleic acids, has not been studied in detail.

   •Both VIN and invasive carcinoma are associated with additional primaries.

•Fact   °Detail   »issue   *answer

- Although this may be evidence that second primaries were preferentially related to HPV-related precursors (ie, VIN), it does not address the concept that invasive carcinomas associated with VIN would be more likely to have second primary neoplasms.

- Results: The presence of VIN served as a marker for an increased risk of a second primary neoplasm.

- A second variable, intraepithelial-like growth patterns in the tumor itself, correlated strongly with the presence of VIN and, although of borderline significance, tended to indicate a second primary.

- These data suggest that certain histologic variables significantly increase the risk of other genital primary squamous neoplasms.

- In contrast, other variables did not, such as non-neoplastic epithelial alterations (hyperplasias) or other growth patterns of squamous cell carcinoma.

- The direct demonstration of HPV nucleic acids in the tissues appeared to influence the risk for additional genital primary neoplasms, although this characteristic could not be separated from some of the morphologic variables themselves.

- Both intraepithelial-like growth pattern in the tumor and associated VIN were strongly related to one another and to HPV nucleic acids.

- Although the HPV-positive VIN or intraepithelial-like carcinomas were more likely to be associated with multifocal disease than were their HPV-negative counterparts, the association was not significant.

- When HPV-positive tumors containing these morphologic variables were compared with tumors lacking both these variables and HPV, the associations were statistically significant.

- Epithelial hyperplasias coexisting with HPV-positive tumors were significantly associated with multifocal disease; in these cases, one of the other growth patterns associated with HPV was often present.

- By themselves, both epithelial hyperplasias and keratinizing growth patterns were negatively associated with the presence of HPV and not significantly associated with multifocal disease.

- HPV DNA analysis, specifically DNA-DNA in situ hybridization, is less sensitive than other detection methods (i.e., Southern blot hybridization).

  ° Thus, it was not possible to determine the precise proportion of cancers associated with VIN or an intraepithelial growth pattern that contained HPV nucleic acids.

- Because VIN and intraepithelial growth patterns are not always associated with HPV nucleic acids suggests that within each morphologic group there exist both HPV-positive and -negative subsets.

  ° This could contribute to the lower frequency of HPV nucleic acids.]

---

44. Comprehensive surgical staging laparotomy in early ovarian cancer includes

    1. blind biopsies from the anterior and posterior cul-de-sac
    2. omentectomy
    3. cytologic sampling of the right hemidiaphragm
    4. paraaortic lymphadenectomy

p. 952   Ans: E   (Soper J T, Johnson P, Johnson V, Berchuck A, Clarke-Pearson D L. Comprehensive restaging laparotomy in women with apparent early ovarian carcinoma. Obstet Gynecol 1992; 80:949)

44. [F & I: • Background: Although epithelial ovarian carcinomas are the second most prevalent gynecologic malignancy, they have the highest death-to-case ratio, accounting for almost half of all deaths

- from gynecologic malignancies and ranking as the fourth most frequent cause of cancer-related death in women.

- Mortality is high in part because the majority of patients have an advanced stage at the time of diagnosis, for which the likelihood of cure is small.

- Survival in "early-stage" ovarian carcinomas remains poor, with only 55-to-75% and 45% 5-year survival rates for women with stages I and II epithelial ovarian carcinomas, respectively.

- Many patients with apparent early ovarian epithelial carcinomas have more advanced disease, detected only with comprehensive surgical staging.

- The majority of women with ovarian carcinoma undergo exploration by obstetrician-gynecologists or surgeons, who often omit critical steps of the staging procedure for ovarian carcinoma.

- Women with low-risk early ovarian carcinoma defined by strict staging laparotomy do not benefit from additional therapy, and women with higher-risk factors have comparable survival after treatment with intraperitoneal radiopharmaceuticals or simple chemotherapy.

- Given an incompletely evaluated patient with apparent early ovarian carcinoma who has a substantial risk of having more advanced disease, the morbidity of a second restaging laparotomy must be weighed against the toxicity of systemic chemotherapy for presumed advanced-stage disease.

- Objective: To review experience with comprehensive restaging laparotomies in women with apparent early ovarian carcinoma who were referred for evaluation after incomplete initial surgery.

- Results: Positive findings occurred in all peritoneal sites and in both pelvic and paraaortic lymph nodes.

- Despite knowledge for over 15 years that even apparent early ovarian carcinoma has the potential for occult intraperitoneal and retroperitoneal metastases, women continue to be referred for definitive therapy after incomplete initial staging procedures.

- Even with a preoperative or intraoperative suspicion of ovarian carcinoma, a simple visual inspection of the abdominal wall clearly indicated the inadequacy of the primary exploration as a staging procedure for ovarian carcinoma.

- Forty percent of patients had Pfannenstiel and 43% had other subumbilical incisions.

- Basic staging procedures (omentectomy and peritoneal washings for cytology) were performed in a minority of patients.

- Patients who were reexplored had positive findings from a variety of sites.

    ° Only one-third of these had grossly apparent disease which stresses the need to perform biopsies of any adhesions and to obtain random biopsies from multiple pelvic and upper abdominal peritoneal sites.

    ° The finding of positive pelvic and para-aortic nodes in different patients emphasizes the need for sampling lymph nodes from both sites even when these are not grossly enlarged.

- A model for the comprehensive surgical staging laparotomy in early ovarian carcinoma is described in the Gynecologic Oncology Group studies.

- The procedure requires systematic performance of multiple washings for cytology; blind biopsies from the anterior and posterior cul-de-sac, pelvic sidewalls, bilateral pericolic gutters, and mesentery or serosa of the small intestine; performance of omentectomy; and biopsy or cytologic sampling of the right hemidiaphragm.

- •In addition, these studies included removal of lymph nodes from the external iliac, obturator, common iliac, and paraaortic chains bilaterally if the patients had no gross evidence of intraperitoneal metastasis.

- •Although advanced histologic grade and papillary serous histology were predictors of positive findings at restaging laparotomy, the small numbers of patients with non-papillary histologies, particularly the clear-cell subtype, limit the reliability of histologic subtype as a predictor.

- •Only four patients with grade 1 lesions were reexplored but 20% of patients with grade 2 lesions had positive findings, emphasizing the need for restaging even these patients or treating them as if they have advanced disease.

- •The initial assessment of stage did not correlate with the final stage established by restaging laparotomy.

- •Perhaps other markers of biologic differentiation might prove to be better predictors of occult metastasis than are simple histopathologic features of early ovarian carcinoma.

- •Tumor ploidy, phase fraction, and expression of certain oncogenes correlate with prognosis in ovarian carcinoma but the utility for predicting occult disease spread will have to be confirmed in prospective studies.

- •The cost and morbidity of a second procedure to establish reliably the stage of presumed early ovarian carcinoma are considerable.

- •Although most of the morbidity observed was modest, representing transfusions and wound separations, others have reported substantial morbidity comparable to that of primary staging procedures with tumor resection.

- •This is probably related to the postoperative adhesions or retroperitoneal reaction and induration observed in the majority of patients.

- •The cost and morbidity of a second procedure must be weighed against the cost and morbidity of treating all patients with presumed early disease but incomplete surgical staging with aggressive cytotoxic chemotherapy for the possibility of advanced disease.

- •Noninvasive techniques using serum tumor markers and vaginal probe ultrasound may aid in increasing the preoperative suspicion for ovarian carcinoma before performing primary surgery.

- •Elevated serum levels of antigen CA 125 have greater than 80% sensitivity and specificity for discriminating malignant from benign pelvic masses in postmenopausal women.

- °The sensitivity drops to only approximately 50% in women with stage I disease.

- •Criteria indicating an increased risk of malignancy based on characteristics of adnexal masses using vaginal probe ultrasound or more sophisticated Doppler color flow studies also may increase the level of suspicion preoperatively.

- •Patients with a high index of suspicion should be explored in a clinical setting where intraoperative consultation is available to perform a comprehensive staging laparotomy for early ovarian carcinoma if this is found at laparotomy.

- •The performance of comprehensive surgical staging as part of the initial pre-therapy laparotomy for early ovarian carcinoma allows selection of appropriate postoperative therapy for individual patients.

- •Those with low-risk early-stage disease may not require any further therapy, whereas patients with high-risk early disease may be treated with either cytotoxic chemotherapy or intraperitoneal radiopharmaceuticals.

- •Patients with occult extrapelvic metastases could be spared the toxicity of inappropriate or ineffective therapy and be treated initially with appropriate cytotoxic therapy for advanced disease.]

OBSTETRICS

Directions: Each of the questions or incomplete statements below is followed by several suggested answers or completions. Select the BEST answer in each case.

1. Early onset intrauterine growth retardation is most likely to be found in

   A. Klinefelter XXY
   B. trisomy 13
   C. trisomy 21
   D. Turner XO
   E. XYY syndrome

2. A patient has a blood pressure of 150/90. What is her mean arterial pressure?

   A. 80
   B. 90
   C. 110
   D. 120
   E. 140

3. A patient who is 16 weeks pregnant complains of severe abdominal pain unresponsive to over the counter analgesics. On pelvic examination a firm parauterine mass which is exquisitely tender is palpated. Ultrasound examination is suggestive of either an ovarian mass or a leiomyoma. The next best step in her management is

   A. begin a trial of ketorolac.
   B. do an exploratory laparotomy.
   C. obtain a serum CA125.
   D. obtain a serum LDH.
   E. order an MRI of the pelvis.

4. Gravidas who are seropositive for HIV

   A. are at greater risk for infectious complications.
   B. have a decreased incidence of risk behaviors while pregnant.
   C. have acceleration of their disease.
   D. have an increased risk for delivery of fetuses with birth defects.
   E. have an increased risk for intrapartum complications.

5. Signs or symptoms highly suggestive of the onset of HELLP syndrome include

   A. chest pain.
   B. diarrhea.
   C. pedal edema.
   D. polyuria.
   E. right upper quadrant pain.

6. Which of the following treatments will increase fetal lung maturity in an otherwise normal patient who has spontaneous premature rupture of the membranes at 26 weeks gestation?

   A. Antibiotics.
   B. Corticosteroids.
   C. Observation.
   D. Tocolysis.
   E. None of the above.

7. Of predictive value in patients with catastrophic uterine rupture during an attempted vaginal delivery following previous cesarean section:

   A. increased vaginal bleeding during labor.
   B. maternal age.
   C. maternal parity.
   D. number of previous VBACs.
   E. previous cesarean section disproportion.

8. At 31 weeks a patient has confirmed spontaneous premature rupture of the membranes. The best predictor of microbial invasion of the amniotic cavity is amniotic fluid

   A. glucose.
   B. Gram stain.
   C. IL-6 determination.
   D. leukocyte esterase activity.
   E. white blood count.

9. What should be the serum glucose threshold value after a one hour 50 gram glucose challenge screening test done at 20 weeks?

   A. 130 mg/dl.
   B. 135 mg/dl.
   C. 140 mg/dl.
   D. 145 mg/dl.
   E. 150 mg/dl.

10. In a term vertex presentation, failure of descent of the fetal vertex after transabdominal fundal pressure is applied (The Mueller-Hillis maneuver) is predictive of

    A. increased need for oxytocin.
    B. increased risk for abdominal delivery.
    C. increased risk for forceps delivery.
    D. increased risk prolonged second stage.
    E. none of the above.

11. Diagnostic of severe maternal CMV infection during pregnancy

    A. fetal hyperechogenic masses in the abdomen.
    B. maternal serum ALT.
    C. maternal serum AST.
    D. maternal serum GGT.
    E. none of the above.

12. The fetal bladder should always be visualized on ultrasound by what gestational week?

    A. 7
    B. 9
    C. 10
    D. 11
    E. 13

13. What is the earliest time during gestation that the constrictive effect of indomethacin can be found in the fetal ductus arteriosus?

    A. 23 weeks.
    B. 24 weeks.
    C. 25 weeks.
    D. 26 weeks.
    E. 27 weeks.

14. The most important risk for Chlamydia infection during pregnancy is

    A. low socioeconomic status.
    B. nulliparity.
    C. race.
    D. tobacco use.
    E. young age.

15. The drug of choice for treating bacterial vaginosis during pregnancy is

    A. ceftriaxone intramuscularly.
    B. clindamycin vaginal gel.
    C. oral ampicillin.
    D. oral metronidazole.
    E. sulfonamide vaginal cream.

16. Which of the following is increased in lactation as compared to a nonlactating puerpera?

    A. Estrogen.
    B. High-density lipoproteins.
    C. Progesterone.
    D. Triglycerides.
    E. Two-hour blood sugar after a glucose tolerance test.

17. Significant deviations from singleton growth do not occur in twin gestations until how many weeks?

    A. 24.
    B. 28.
    C. 30.
    D. 32.
    E. 34.

18. Advantages of expectant management of labor in class B diabetics include

    A. decreased incidence of larger gestational age infants.
    B. decreased incidence of shoulder dystocia.
    C. increased incidence of successful VBACs.
    D. reduction in incidence of cesarean section.
    E. none of the above.

19. Which of the following accurately describes the action of cocaine on myometrium?

    A. Increases α-adrenergic receptor binding.
    B. Increases ß-adrenergic receptor binding.
    C. Inhibits α-adrenergic receptor binding.
    D. Inhibits ß-adrenergic receptor binding.
    E. None of the above.

20. The greatest risk to the fetus of the patient with clinically significant aortic stenosis is

    A. congenital heart disease.
    B. depression at birth from general anesthesia.
    C. fetal growth retardation.
    D. preterm delivery.
    E. teratogenic effects of cardiac glycosides.

21. Near term, the maximal oxytocin concentration in maternal blood occurs about

    A. 2:00 a.m.
    B. 8:00 a.m.
    C. 4:00 p.m.
    D. 10:00 p.m.
    E. midnight.

22. Which of the following is the best predictor of neonatal survival in extremely low birth weight infants?

    A. Biparietal diameter.
    B. Birth weight.
    C. Estimated fetal weight.
    D. Femur length.
    E. Pediatric estimate of gestational age.

23. Factors predictive of successful external cephalic version near term include

    A. breech at station -1.
    B. maternal weight greater than 200 pounds.
    C. parity greater than 2.
    D. tocolytic therapy.
    E. type of breech.

24. In managing a gestational diabetic patient if all fasting glucose levels are normal, the 2-hour post-prandial blood sugar in is predictive of

    A. larger for gestational age fetus.
    B. macrosomia.
    C. need for cesarean section.
    D. shoulder dystocia.
    E. none of the above.

25. Of the following the procedure which best predicts abruptio placentae **early** on is

    A. D-dimer slide test.
    B. determination of low amplitude-high frequency contractions by tocodynamometer.
    C. determination of partial thromboplastin time.
    D. doppler color flow studies of placental bed.
    E. ultrasonic imaging.

26. Complications from the use of uterine packing to control postpartum hemorrhage include

    A. concealed hemorrhage.
    B. delayed hemorrhage.
    C. infertility.
    D. sepsis.
    E. none of the above.

27. At five weeks following a term normal spontaneous vaginal delivery, a patient has a curettage for delayed post-partum hemorrhage. The most likely interpretation of the tissue retrieved by that procedure is

    A. decidua.
    B. endometritis.
    C. involution of the placental bed.
    D. normal endometrium.
    E. retained placental tissue.

28. Post-cesarean endometritis can be effectively prevented if

    A. there is a special skin prep with parachlorometaxylenol and saline lavage of the pelvic and subcutaneous tissue.
    B. there is a special skin prep with parachlorometaxylenol and no pelvic or subcutaneous irrigation.
    C. there is a standard skin preparation with povidone iodine and the normal saline lavage of the pelvic and subcutaneous tissue.
    D. there is standard skin preparation and cefazolin irrigation of the pelvic and subcutaneous tissues.
    E. There is no evidence to show that either skin prep or pelvic lavage is effective in preventing endometritis.

29. In mothers on methadone maintenance, neonatal plasma methadone levels are lower than maternal levels because

   A. extensive biotransformation takes place in the placenta.
   B. fetal enzymes rapidly metabolize methadone.
   C. methadone levels are about the same in maternal and neonatal tissues.
   D. placentally transferred methadone is rapidly stored in fetal tissues.
   E. plasma protein-bound methadone is increased in pregnancy.

30. The major handicap associated with surviving neonates delivered at 24 weeks is

   A. blindness.
   B. bronchopulmonary dysplasia.
   C. cerebral palsy.
   D. deafness.
   E. mental retardation.

31. The correct order of restitutive maneuvers for the optimal management of shoulder dystocia is

   A. fundal pressure, McRoberts maneuver, release of posterior arm, Zavanelli maneuver.
   B. suprapubic pressure, McRoberts maneuver, release of posterior arm, Zavanelli maneuver.
   C. rotate the shoulders to the oblique, McRoberts maneuver, release of posterior arm, Zavanelli maneuver.
   D. suprapubic pressure, release of posterior arm, Zavanelli maneuver.
   E. none of the above.

32. Effects of elective amniotomy at term in an otherwise uncomplicated pregnancy include increased incidence of

   A. cesarean section.
   B. meconium passage.
   C. neonatal depression.
   D. prolonged decelerations.
   E. none of the above.

33. Magnesium sulfate inhibits uterine contractions by

   A. decreasing extracellular calcium.
   B. down regulating oxytocin receptors.
   C. elevating intracellular free magnesium.
   D. inactivating calmodulin.
   E. suppressing lysosomal metabolism.

34. Routine weekly cervical examinations in twin gestations after 20 weeks is likely to result in

   A. increased incidence of post-partum infections.
   B. increased incidence of preterm labor.
   C. increased incidence of ruptured membranes.
   D. increased incidence of neonatal sepsis.
   E. none of the above.

35. Spontaneous version of a twin pregnancy is influenced by

   A. amniotic fluid volume.
   B. birth weight discordancy.
   C. gestational age.
   D. parity.
   E. placental location.

36. Of the following the most common cause of preterm labor is

   A. cervical incompetence.
   B. faulty placentation.
   C. fetal anomalies.
   D. immunologic factors.
   E. intrauterine infection.

37. Which of the following are **fetal** effects of maternal ingestion of low-dose aspirin prophylactically?

   A. Decreased amniotic fluid.
   B. Myocardial dysfunction.
   C. Premature closure of the ductus.
   D. Thrombocytopenia.
   E. None of the above.

38. The use of indomethacin in the treatment of preterm labor should be limited to those fetuses that are how many weeks old?

   A. 28
   B. 29
   C. 30
   D. 31
   E. 32

39. Which of the following increase the risk of uterine rupture during attempted vaginal delivery after cesarean section?

    A. Epidural anesthesia.
    B. History of cesarean section previously for CPD.
    C. Macrosomia.
    D. Two or more previous cesarean sections.
    E. Unknown uterine scar from previous cesarean section

40. Which of the following in the most rapid and reliable test for the detection of group B streptococci which have colonized the reproductive tract of pregnant patients?

    A. DNA probe.
    B. Enzyme immunoassay.
    C. Gram stain.
    D. Latex agglutination test.
    E. Todd-Hewitt broth culture.

41. Approximately, what percentage of fetuses with trisomy 18 have congenital heart disease?

    A. 50
    B. 67
    C. 75
    D. 85
    E. 99

42. Which of the following carries the highest risk for premature labor?

    A. Chorioamnionitis
    B. Cigarette smoking
    C. Multiple gestation
    D. Previous preterm labor
    E. Uterine anomalies

43. At 36 weeks a patient presents with a blood pressure of 180/110, backache, blurred vision, and abdominal pain. Urinalysis is negative for protein, sugar and leukocyte esterase. Within 45 minutes her blood pressure is 110/70 with supportive treatment. The diagnosis is

    A. anxiety neurosis.
    B. chronic hypertension.
    C. cocaine intoxication.
    D. pheochromocytoma.
    E. preeclampsia.

44. The minimum dose of aspirin to effectively reduce the incidence of preeclampsia is

    A. 80 mg.
    B. 100 mg.
    C. 160 mg.
    D. 250 mg.
    E. 500 mg.

45. The antibiotic to which *M. hominis* is sensitive and *U. urealyticum* is resistant is

    A. chloramphenicol
    B. clindamycin
    C. erythromycin
    D. quinolones
    E. tetracycline

46. Which of the following **single** oral GTT plasma glucose levels is associated with LGA infants?

    A. elevated fasting blood sugar
    B. elevated 1 hour blood sugar
    C. elevated 2 hour blood sugar
    D. elevated 3 hour blood sugar
    E. All are associated with large for gestational age infants.

47. Associated with hypothyroidism in pregnancy

    A. gestational hypertension
    B. macrosomia
    C. maternal anemia
    D. post-date pregnancy
    E. postpartum hemorrhage

48. Preeclampsia is associated with an increase in the effect of which substance on placental arteries?

    A. Angiotensin II.
    B. Endothelin.
    C. PGF2α.
    D. Prostacyclin.
    E. None of the above.

49. Umbilical vessel oxytocin administration for retained placenta is to be undertaken. Which technique is likely to deliver the most oxytocin to the placental capillary bed?

    A. Allow the cord to bleed, clamp, inject 20 ml of saline with 20 units of oxytocin into the umbilical vein.
    B. Do not allow the cord to drain, clamp the cord, inject 20 ml with 20 units of oxytocin into the umbilical vein.
    C. Do not allow the cord to drain, clamp the cord, inject 30 ml into the umbilical vein and milk the cord toward the placenta.
    D. Do not allow the cord to drain, clamp the cord, inject 30 ml with 20 units of oxytocin into the umbilical vein.
    E. Do not the allow the cord to drain, clamp the cord, inject 30 ml into the umbilical artery.

50. Following amniocentesis for genetic anomalies, a fetus is discovered to have a balanced translocation. What is the empiric risk for the fetus to have anomalies or develop mental delay?

    A. 0%
    B. .5%
    C. 1%
    D. 5
    E. 10%

51. Which of the following antibiotics does NOT disrupt bacterial cell walls?

    A. ampicillin
    B. bacitracin
    C. cephalosporin
    D. gentamicin
    E. vancomycin

52. Clinically useful in discriminating true labor from false labor in the early third trimester

    A. bed rest
    B. cervicovaginal levels of oncofetal fibronectin
    C. hydration
    D. morphine sedation
    E. observation of fetal breathing movements on ultrasound

53. The drug of choice for post-partum endometritis caused by enterococcus is

    A. ampicillin
    B. cephalexin
    C. clindamycin
    D. gentamicin
    E. none of the above

54. The approximate number of Down Syndrome cases that can be detected by prenatal testing using advanced maternal age (greater than 35 years) as a criterion is

    A. 20
    B. 25
    C. 33
    D. 50
    E. 57

55. During pregnancy the terbutaline induced glucose intolerance is caused by

    A. decreased levels of C peptide.
    B. decreased levels of insulin.
    C. increased insulin resistance.
    D. increased levels of pancreatic peptide.
    E. Terbutaline does not cause glucose intolerance in pregnancy.

56. Magnesium sulfate causes plasma endothelin-1 levels in preeclamptic pregnancies to decrease because of

    A. decreased production of angiotensin converting enzymes
    B. direct suppression of Et-1 production
    C. increased production of nitric oxide
    D. increased vasodilatation and release of prostacyclin
    E. none of the above

57. In late pregnancy the increased uterine activity seen between midnight and 2:00 a.m. is secondary to

    A. decreased maternal progesterone
    B. increased maternal catecholamines
    C. increased maternal estrogen
    D. increased maternal oxytocin
    E. increased maternal prostaglandins

58. What percentage of functioning nephron mass is lost when serum creatinine is 0.8 mg/dl during gestation?

    A. 15
    B. 20
    C. 25
    D. 33
    E. >50

59. The greatest sensitivity in predicting subsequent clinical infection in patients with premature rupture of the membranes is

    A. amniotic fluid glucose level
    B. Gram stain
    C. leukocyte esterase estimation
    D. limulus amebocyte lysate assay
    E. white blood count

60. Predictive of learning deficits in the older child (9 to 11 years)

    A. fetal asphyxia
    B. intrauterine growth retardation
    C. newborn encephalopathy
    D. newborn infections
    E. newborn respiratory complications

61. A patient is admitted at term with a vertex presentation. Active management of labor is to be undertaken. Success in achieving vaginal delivery includes all of the following EXCEPT

    A. development of chorioamnionitis.
    B. maternal height.
    C. need for oxytocin augmentation.
    D. the station of the vertex on admission.
    E. use of epidural anesthesia.

62. True statements about the standing position in pregnancy at term include all of the following EXCEPT

    A. a decrease in maternal cardiac output.
    B. a decrease in fetal heart rate accelerations.
    C. an increase in fetal vessel resistance.
    D. an increased incidence of inferior vena cava compression with the vertex engaged.
    E. diminished venous return.

63. Increased physiologic effects in preeclampsia all of the following EXCEPT

    A. calcitonin gene-related peptide.
    B. endothelin.
    C. plasma fibronectin.
    D. thromboxane.
    E. total plasma activator inhibitors.

64. Predictors of severe meconium aspiration syndrome (i.e. prolonged ventilation) include all of the following EXCEPT

    A. delivery by cesarean section.
    B. fetal heart rate abnormality.
    C. intubation in the delivery suite for resuscitation.
    D. low Apgar score.
    E. presence of meconium below the cords.

65. Factors predisposing to preeclampsia all of the following EXCEPT

    A. advanced maternal age.
    B. cigarette smoking.
    C. family history of hypertension.
    D. high body mass.
    E. multiparity.

66. All of the following drugs may be safely prescribed in pharmacologic doses upon indication for a breast-feeding mother EXCEPT

    A. diclofenac.
    B. flurbiprofen.
    C. ibuprofen.
    D. mefenamic acid.
    E. naproxen.

67. All of the following affect the maternal homeostatic response to hypermagnesemia EXCEPT

    A. 1α,25-dihydroxycalciferol.
    B. calcitonin.
    C. dietary intake of fortified cow's milk.
    D. exposure to sunlight.
    E. parathyroid hormone.

68. The rapid eye test used in the screening of substance abuse includes all of the following EXCEPT

   A. evaluation of pupil size
   B. testing for corneal reflexes
   C. testing for frequency of blinking
   D. testing for nystagmus
   E. testing reaction of pupil to light

69. The Doppler indices of placental function are affected by all of the following EXCEPT

   A. diabetes mellitus
   B. erythroblastosis fetalis
   C. intrauterine growth retardation
   D. preeclampsia

70. Associated with a decreased length of pregnancy predicted by Naegele's rule all of the following EXCEPT

   A. age less than 19
   B. alcohol
   C. coffee consumption greater than 5 cups per day
   D. low educational achievement
   E. multiparity

71. Infants who develop major neurological deficits are likely to have all of the following EXCEPT

   A. hypercarbia
   B. infection
   C. late decelerations
   D. metabolic acidemia
   E. oligohydramnios

72. Using decreased amniotic fluid glucose as marker for intraamniotic infection, all of the following can be responsible for false positive tests EXCEPT

   A. advanced gestational age
   B. fetal growth retardation
   C. placental insufficiency
   D. preeclampsia
   E. ureaplasma colonization of amniotic cavity

OBSTETRICS REFERENCES

Directions: Each of the questions or incomplete statements below is followed by several suggested answers or completions. Select the BEST answer in each case.

---

1. Early onset intrauterine growth retardation is most likely to be found in

   A. Klinefelter XXY
   *B. trisomy 13
   C. trisomy 21
   D. Turner XO
   E. XYY syndrome

p.1527 (Drugan A, Johnson M P, Isada N B, Holzgreve W, Zador I E, Dombrowski M P, Sokol R J, Hallak M, Evans M I. The smaller than expected first-trimester fetus is at increased risk for chromosome anomalies. Am J Obstet Gynec 1992; 167:1525)

1. [F & I: •Background: The diagnosis of symmetric IUGR in the second trimester indicates the need for further invasive diagnostic testing (e.g., amniocentesis, late chorionic villlus sampling, cordocentesis) to exclude fetal anomalies.

•Up to 25% of fetuses with severe early onset IUGR are aneuploid, and such a diagnosis has a major impact on pregnancy management and fetal prognosis.

•Studies of fetal hematologic and liver function and blood gases imply that growth-retarded aneuploid fetuses have a pattern of laboratory value alterations consistent with fetuses having IUGR with **placental insufficiency**.

•The aneuploid placenta provides inadequate respiratory and nutritional support for the developing fetus.

•IUGR in aneuploid gestations is often observed on ultrasonography in the late second trimester, somewhat earlier than seen with chronic placental insufficiency.

•The clinical impression is that the impact of aneuploidy on fetal growth is evident much earlier; the aneuploid fetus may appear smaller than dates on ultrasonography even in the first trimester, probably because of an inherent effect of aneuploidy on cell growth and proliferation.

•In the first trimester measurement of the crown-rump length is the most useful parameter for pregnancy dating, with a 95% confidence interval of plus or minus 5 to 7 days.

•Errors in crown-rump length estimation may arise from flexion of the embryo or from inadvertent inclusion of the yolk sac in the measurement.

•In diabetics a crown-rump length significantly smaller than normal in early pregnancy is associated with a significant risk of fetal malformations.

•Objective: To investigate the association between a smaller-than-expected crown-rump length and fetal aneuploidy in patients referred for first-trimester prenatal diagnosis by chorionic villus sampling.

°The majority of these patients were ≥35 years of age, and extrapolation to younger patients must be made cautiously.

•IUGR has been commonly classified into two types.

•Fact   °Detail   Page 275   »issue   *answer

°Type I (or symmetric IUGR) refers to decreased growth potential caused by intrinsic factors in the fetus (i.e., chromosome anomalies) or extrinsic factors affecting the fetus and placenta from early stages of development, e.g., congenital infections and some teratogenic drug effects.

°In type I IUGR (about 20% of cases) the effect on fetal growth is predominantly on cellular hyperplasia; there is a fairly uniform decrease in body size without selective sparing of any organs.

°Data on trisomy 18 suggest that even with aneuploidy some organs may be differentially spared at different stages of gestation.

°What has been previously called symmetric IUGR appears to be an asymmetric pattern that is dynamic in nature and may change through the course of gestation.

•Asymmetric (type II, brain-sparing) IUGR is often associated with placental insufficiency, which is commonly manifested only in the third trimester.

•The cordocentesis data in aneuploid pregnancies imply that in these cases IUGR may also be mediated through dysfunction of the **chromosomally abnormal placenta**.

•In the chorionic villus sampling population, a crown rump length smaller than expected by dates with a viable fetus is found in 8.6% of pregnancies scanned.

°In these pregnancies the risk of aneuploidy was 2.5 times higher than that encountered in gestations with appropriate-for-age fetal size.

°The size-dates discrepancy of aneuploid pregnancies in the first trimester appears to be dependent on the type of aberration involved and is more accentuated with severe or lethal chromosome anomalies than with trisomy 21 or sex chromosome aneuploidy.

•Aneuploid gestations with low viability potential had gestational age discrepancies significantly greater than those in pregnancies affected by chromosome anomalies with moderate viability potential;

°The more severe the chromosome anomaly, the larger the impact on fetal growth and pregnancy development.

•In term deliveries infants with trisomy 13 or 18 have severe IUGR, whereas newborns affected by trisomy 21 or sex chromosome aneuploidy are usually appropriate for gestational age.

•The effect of aneuploidy on fetal growth is not age dependent but is evident at all gestational ages, modulated primarily by the **type of aneuploidy involved**.

•The yearly increase in rate of chromosome anomalies diagnosed by chorionic villus sampling has been observed.

°An obvious explanatory phenomenon (a change toward more advanced maternal age) could not be documented.

°It is tempting to speculate on environmental factors (pollution, cosmic ionizing radiation, etc.) causing a change in population risk for these disorders, but much larger studies over a longer period of time would be needed to substantiate such a theory.]

2. A patient has a blood pressure of 150/90. What is her mean arterial pressure?

   A. 80
   B. 90
   *C. 110
   D. 120
   E. 140

p. 803 (Combs C A, Rosenn B, Kitzmiller J L, Khoury J C, Wheeler B C, Miodovnik M. Early-pregnancy proteinuria in diabetes related to preeclampsia. Obstet Gynecol 1993; 82:802)

2. [F & I: •Background: Preeclampsia is a serious complication affecting 10-to-20% of pregnancies in women with diabetes.

•Hypertensive disorders may be responsible for as many as one-third of preterm deliveries among diabetic women and half of deliveries before 32 weeks' gestation.

•Diabetic nephropathy is a major risk factor for preeclampsia.

•Overt nephropathy is defined by persistent dipstick-positive proteinuria, by urinary albumin excretion greater than 300 mg/day, or by urinary total protein excretion of more than 500 mg/day.

•Overt nephropathy is preceded by a 5-to-10-year phase of subclinical or "incipient" nephropathy characterized by lesser degrees of proteinuria.

•Because incipient nephropathy is an early manifestation of diabetic microvascular disease, women with incipient nephropathy, like women with overt nephropathy, are at high risk of preeclampsia.

•Objective: To test the hypothesis that the risk of preeclampsia in diabetic mothers could be related to the amount of proteinuria in early pregnancy.

•Results: The risk of preeclampsia rose dramatically with early pregnancy protein excretion rates above 190 mg/day.

•The 40% overall rate of preeclampsia in women with proteinuria of 190-to-499 mg/day was not significantly different than the 47% rate with overt diabetic nephropathy (proteinuria of 500 mg/day or more).

•By logistic regression, the risk of preeclampsia attributable to baseline proteinuria persisted after controlling for the effects of nulliparity, chronic hypertension, retinopathy, and glycemic control.

•There is difficulty in distinguishing "true" preeclampsia from a transient worsening of chronic hypertension and proteinuria in women with overt diabetic nephropathy.

•In the presence of baseline proteinuria, the definition of preeclampsia is arbitrary.

°The distinction may be irrelevant to the obstetrician.

•With worsening hypertension and proteinuria, the only practical management options are either to deliver the infant or admit the mother for hospital bed rest and close observation, with possible antihypertensive therapy.

•Which alternative is preferred depends on the severity of the maternal condition and on assessment of fetal maturity and well-being.

°Preterm delivery is often necessary.

•Elevated glycohemoglobin is associated with preeclampsia, that is, gestational hypertension with proteinuria.

•The association persists after controlling for early-pregnancy proteinuria, nulliparity, and chronic hypertension.

•Poor glycemic control in the late second trimester might interfere with the second wave of trophoblast invasion and thereby predispose to preeclampsia.

•Glucose may have some direct effect on the vascular endothelium that could predispose to hypertensive disorders.

»Women with baseline proteinuria of 190-to-499 mg/day have incipient diabetic nephropathy.

•This early phase in the natural history of nephropathy is characterized by normal creatinine clearance and by protein excretion rates too low to be reliably detected with standard dipstick testing.

•In nonpregnant diabetic subjects, sensitive assays for albumin have been used to define incipient nephropathy as albumin excretion rates of 25-to-300 mg/day.

•Patients with so-called "microalbuminuria" in this range almost always progress to overt nephropathy within 10 years, whereas those with lower albumin excretion rates rarely do.

•In pregnancy, baseline protein excretion rates increase; thus, no standards exist for the definition of incipient nephropathy during pregnancy.

•By the end of the first trimester, the excretion rates of all proteins increase by 50-to-100% over pre-pregnancy values.

•The upper limit of normal urinary total protein in early pregnancy in nondiabetic subjects is about 200 mg/day, nearly identical to the 190 mg/day found with an increasing risk of preeclampsia in diabetic subjects.

•Long-term follow-up studies are needed to demonstrate conclusively whether early pregnancy proteinuria greater than 190 mg/day is a marker of incipient nephropathy.

•It has been recommended that diabetic patients undergo annual assessment of the albumin excretion rate to detect possible incipient diabetic nephropathy.

»Assessment of protein excretion after pregnancy is of particular importance for women with a history of preeclampsia and for those whose early-pregnancy protein excretion exceeds 190 mg/day.

•Early detection of incipient nephropathy allows interventions, such as strict glycemic control and antihypertensive therapy, that may slow the progression to overt nephropathy and end-stage renal disease.]

---

3. A patient who is 16 weeks pregnant complains of severe abdominal pain unresponsive to over the counter analgesics. On pelvic examination a firm parauterine mass which is exquisitely tender is palpated. Ultrasound examination is suggestive of either an ovarian mass or a leiomyoma. The next best step in her management is

   A. begin a trial of ketorolac.
   B. do an exploratory laparotomy.
   C. obtain a serum CA125.
   D. obtain a serum LDH.
   *E. order an MRI of the pelvis.

p. 836 (Curtis M, Hopkins M P, Zarlingo T, Martino C, Graciansky-Lengyl M, Jenison E L. Magnetic resonance imaging to avoid laparotomy in pregnancy. Obstet Gynecol 1993; 82:833)

3. [F & I: •Background: The diagnosis of an adnexal mass during pregnancy will usually lead to laparotomy, preferably in the second trimester.

•The incidence of adnexal mass in pregnancy is somewhere between one in 200 to one in 1000.

•Although there have not been a large number of series reported, most found that a small proportion of patients underwent laparotomy for leiomyoma.

•In pregnancy, the usual management of the leiomyoma found at laparotomy is conservative, with removal performed after delivery unless the leiomyoma is pedunculated and producing symptoms.

•If a more definitive diagnosis of leiomyoma could be made without laparotomy, it would be preferable because of the risk of miscarriage associated with laparotomy in pregnancy.

•Unfortunately, there is no definitive preoperative test to distinguish leiomyoma from a solid adnexal tumor.

•Objective: To determine whether magnetic resonance imaging (MRI) would be a useful diagnostic test in the differential diagnosis of an adnexal mass in pregnancy.

•Magnetic resonance imaging has become a valuable imaging modality over the past decade.

•It provides excellent tissue contrast, allows unlimited planes of view, eliminates artifact from bone and air, and avoids the use of ionizing radiation.

•Magnetic resonance imaging permits visualization of the more lateral and posterior areas of the true and false pelvis, which may be obscured by gas or bony fetal structures during ultrasound examination.

•Normal ovaries not found on ultrasound may be identified separate from the mass, allowing exclusion of ovarian malignancy on MRI.

•Because of its relatively recent development, the use of MRI in obstetric patients has been limited.

•To date, there is a **lack of evidence of fetal risk** due to MRI, and its use in pregnant patients has slowly but steadily increased.

•This modality has also been used to evaluate gynecologic malignancy.

•When pelvic masses are discovered during pregnancy, MRI can be a valuable complement to sonography.

•Magnetic resonance imaging has been reported to be a safe and effective method to evaluate various pelvic structures, both in the pregnant and nonpregnant state.

•It appears to have excellent resolution in distinguishing ovarian from uterine tissue.

•Leiomyomas contain signals that are more consistent with uterine tissue, allowing a more definitive diagnosis in pregnancy.

•The use of high-resolution ultrasound has also contributed to the management of pelvic masses.

•In three of these patients, ultrasound was highly suggestive of a leiomyoma.

•The MRI scan contributed to the diagnosis by giving further information and reassurance that the visualized structures on ultrasound were in fact uterine in nature.

•Magnetic resonance imaging cannot distinguish a leiomyosarcoma from a benign leiomyoma, but this should be a rare occurrence in the pregnant population.

•Fact   °Detail   Page 279   »issue   *answer

•In addition, during pregnancy, leiomyomas are usually not removed at laparotomy and are merely followed expectantly.

•Ultrasound can be used during the remainder of the pregnancy to ensure stability in the size of the leiomyoma once the diagnosis is firmly established.

•MRI can be useful in the differential diagnosis of the adnexal mass in pregnancy.

•It allows expectant management in a percentage of women.

•Although it may not avoid cesarean delivery at term for obstetric reasons, it will help to avoid laparotomy in the second trimester, when very little should be done for myomas involving the pregnant uterus.

•Because more women are delaying childbearing and because the incidence of leiomyoma increases with age, one can expect that this will be a problem of increasing magnitude.

•In this report, the four patients with leiomyoma were nulliparous and at least 35 years old.

•Sonography remains the primary diagnostic imaging tool in obstetric patients who present with pelvic masses.

•When ultrasound results are equivocal, the addition of MRI may provide valuable information and obviate surgery.]

---

4. Gravidas who are seropositive for HIV

   A. are at greater risk for infectious complications.
   *B. have a decreased incidence of risk behaviors while pregnant.
   C. have acceleration of their disease.
   D. have an increased risk for delivery of fetuses with birth defects.
   E. have an increased risk for intrapartum complications.

---

p. 787 (Alger L S, Farley J J, Robinson B A, Hines S E, Berchin J M, Johnson J P. Interactions of human immunodeficiency virus infection and pregnancy. Obstet Gynecol 1993; 82:787)

4. [F & I:•Background: Seropositivity rates for HIV in women delivering in large-city, municipal hospitals along the entire eastern seaboard lie in the 1-to-5% range.

•Although infection is less prevalent in other parts of the country, the biggest percentage increases in seropositivity rates are occurring in cities with populations of less than 100,000.

•To counsel these patients appropriately, the natural history of HIV infection in pregnant women and its effect on pregnancy outcome must be determined.

•Both HIV infection and pregnancy exert **immunosuppressive** effects independently.

•During pregnancy, the T-cell helper-suppressor ratio falls and cell-mediated immunity is somewhat diminished.

•Pregnancy and HIV infection might operate synergistically to depress maternal immune function.

•Early reports suggested that disease progression from asymptomatic to symptomatic expression and to frank AIDS and death was more likely to occur in association with pregnancy.

•Several types of viral infections are associated with fetal malformation and adverse pregnancy outcome.

- On this basis, infected women have been counseled that proceeding with pregnancy may involve risks in addition to that of vertical transmission.

- Most previous studies have been conducted in symptomatic populations with relatively advanced disease, have not had all appropriate control group, or have been limited to intravenous (IV) drug users.

- Information regarding populations other than those of New York and Miami has been limited.

- In Baltimore, consistent with national figures, it was estimated that approximately 50% of seropositive women are, or have been, IV drug users.

- Heterosexual contact has become a major route of acquisition, reflecting a nationwide trend.

- Objectives: To investigate the validity of earlier findings in a group of largely asymptomatic women who had risks not limited to drug use and hence were more representative of the majority of seropositive American women presenting for prenatal care.

  ° This population would allow assessment of the interactions of HIV infection itself with pregnancy, rather than the effects of the many other serious disorders that can be associated with AIDS.

- To determine whether HIV infection has an adverse effect on pregnancy outcome and whether pregnancy negatively affects the short-term course of HIV disease.

- Initial reports on the interaction of maternal HIV infection and pregnancy suggested an adverse effect on both mother and infant.

- Infected gravidas appeared to have more rapid progression of their disease, and infected infants were more likely to be delivered prematurely, have low birth weight, and exhibit abnormal physical characteristics.

- Seropositive women are generally asymptomatic, disproportionately black, current or former IV drug users, or the sexual partners of IV drug users, in keeping with the national profile of HIV-infected gravidas.

- To assess the validity of earlier studies, the study population was selected from a group of women of unknown antibody status who shared similar demographic and socioeconomic characteristics and who identified risks for HIV acquisition at the initial prenatal visit.

- Except for a small group of known seropositive women, subjects were enrolled before their HIV test results were obtained.

- To further differentiate between the effects of HIV infection on pregnancy outcome and those of socioeconomic or life-style factors associated with at-risk behavior, both groups were compared to the general obstetric population delivering over 1 year.

- Women at risk for HIV acquisition were older and more frequently single than the general obstetric population, in keeping with the substantial number of IV drug users in both groups.

- Associated with an increase in maternal age was a proportionate increase in parity.

- There was no evidence of impaired fertility in either group.

- **As expected, the most common risk for participants was injection drug use.**

  ° Over half of the patients had risks associated with heterosexual contact.

Obstetrics and Gynecology: Review 1994-Obstetrics References

- Because many of the patients had multiple risks, it was often impossible to determine the route of HIV acquisition.

- One in eight infected women denied any risks even after extensive discussion.

- The current partners of some of these women were seronegative.

- Some women, who do not consider themselves to be at risk, are acquiring the disease from partners they believe to be at low risk.

- This supports the current practice of screening all prenatal patients after obtaining informed consent.

- **Women in both groups were less likely to report high-risk behaviors during pregnancy than before conception.**

- The present study design did not permit a determination whether this reduction was related to counseling by staff or more directly to the patient's pregnancy.

- None of the uninfected women seroconverted during pregnancy.

  ° A single seronegative woman delivered a child who was subsequently determined to be HIV-infected, suggesting recent maternal infection with delivery before seroconversion.

- Based upon this large, prospectively followed population of asymptomatic women, the findings failed to find any evidence of accelerated HIV disease during pregnancy.

- Infected women were more likely to have a history or physical evidence of condylomata, and there was a trend toward a greater likelihood of genital candidal infections at enrollment, but the clinical status of these women changed little over the duration of prenatal care.

- Seropositive women were more likely to complain of at least one HIV-related symptom (e.g., oral thrush, recurrent fever, night sweats, weight loss), but **no single complaint increased during pregnancy.**

- Seropositive women were **not** at greater risk for antepartum **medical or infectious complications**, such as asymptomatic bacteriuria or pyelonephritis.

- **None** of the 16 patients with CD4 counts less than 200/μl developed serious infections antenatally, although the patient with the lowest count did so postpartum.

- This finding differs from a previous report and highlights the need for further perinatal study of women with low CD4 counts before definitive conclusions can be drawn.

- Both groups of women studied were **more likely** to have historical, physical, or laboratory evidence of **STD** than the general population.

- This was particularly true for seropositive women, who had significantly higher rates than their seronegative counterparts and tended to develop **a new STD** more often during the antenatal course.

- Although seropositive women were affected in greater numbers for all infectious diseases investigated, the only infectious agent significantly associated with seropositivity was genital **human papillomavirus (HPV).**

- **Heterosexual contact** appears to be an important route of HIV acquisition.

- A trend toward an increased frequency of abnormal Papanicolaou smears is in keeping with a previous report of an association between HIV infection, HPV infection, and abnormal cervical cytology.

- During the first 6 weeks postpartum, seropositive women were more likely to develop an infection and to require antibiotics.

- Perhaps related to this use of antibiotics, only HIV-positive women complained of genital candidal infection in the postpartum period.

- **Neither antepartum nor intrapartum complications were associated with HIV infection.**

- Although there were no increases in chorioamnionitis, systemic infections, or intrapartum temperature elevations above 100.4°F, seropositive women were more likely to receive antibiotics.

- Because seropositive women did present to the delivery suite with higher temperatures on average, the increased use of antibiotics may represent a lowering of the therapeutic threshold for clinicians; it appears that there was greater willingness to treat seropositive patients who exhibited even slight temperature elevations.

- As anticipated, multiple **hematologic indices** were altered in seropositive women.

- For patients with paired data, no significant changes in CD4 or CD8 percentages were noted between prenatal and delivery measurements.

- There are conflicting reports on the effect of pregnancy on CD4 lymphocyte counts in the general population, and the influence of HIV infection is uncertain.

- An increase in absolute lymphocyte counts was found in infected women between enrollment and delivery, resulting in an increase in both the CD4 and CD8 counts but no change in the CD4-CD8 ratio.

  ° Despite this increase, the mean CD4 count remained substantially below the mean for uninfected women.

- Antibody status had little influence on pregnancy outcome.

- Because of the subjects' delay in seeking prenatal care, it could not be determined whether HIV infection predisposed to spontaneous abortions, but abortion rates were low for both groups.

- Seropositive women were **not** at increased risk for **preterm labor, tocolysis, premature rupture of membranes, or preterm delivery.**

- Even the subgroup of patients with CD4 counts less than 200/µl had favorable outcomes, although the infants of these women are at risk for developing HIV disease.

- **Maternal weight gain, infant birth weight, and placental weight were not associated with maternal antibody status.**

- **Fetal distress and low 5-minute Apgar scores** were seen **no more frequently** in either group than in the entire population.

- Failure to control for maternal drug use may account for much of the discrepancy in findings between these various investigators.

- The majority of subjects did not use drugs during pregnancy, but equivalent numbers of IV drug users were present in both groups.

- No increase in anomalies or other somatic differences in the offspring of infected women were found, even in women who were current drug users and despite a 30% vertical transmission rate.

  ° The subgroup of **infants** who do acquire HIV infection in utero may have **poorer outcomes** at birth than those who remain uninfected.

- The policy for all patients is to perform a cesarean only when vaginal delivery is not an option.

- It is not surprising that there was no reduction in operative delivery for seropositive women.

- At the same time, the performance of an **episiotomy** is often discretionary.

  ○ The significant decrease in the use of episiotomy at vaginal delivery in seropositive women most likely represents recognition that an episiotomy repair can result in a needlestick injury to the surgeon and also expose the infant to a greater amount of blood at delivery.

  ○ Episiotomies were also performed less frequently in the seronegative group as compared to the general population.

  ○ Obstetricians consider women from high-risk groups to represent a possible infection risk despite a negative HIV test result.

- Similarly, use of an **electrode** to monitor the fetus during labor is frequently elective.

  ○ Any break in the fetal integument increases the risk of intrapartum HIV transmission.

  ○ Hence, there was significantly less use of fetal scalp electrodes in seropositive women.

  ○ Because there are known maternal risks associated with performing an unnecessary cesarean, and the fetal risk of scalp electrode use is hypothetical, scalp electrodes were still used in one-quarter of the deliveries of seropositive women.

- The majority of HIV-infected women are in the reproductive age group.

- These findings support a growing body of information indicating that for women who are asymptomatic at enrollment for prenatal care, pregnancy has no discernible effect on the early progression of maternal HIV disease.

- In addition, seropositivity does not influence maternal or neonatal outcome.

- In industrialized countries where there is access to adequate food and health care, such women are likely to have a favorable outcome even with significant reductions in the CD4 count.

- Although longitudinal studies with follow-up for several years will be necessary to assess the influence of pregnancy on long-term prognosis, at present the risk of vertical transmission appears to be the greatest threat associated with pregnancy.]

---

5. Signs or symptoms highly suggestive of the onset of HELLP syndrome include

   A. chest pain.
   B. diarrhea.
   C. pedal edema.
   D. polyuria.
   *E. right upper quadrant pain.

p. 1004 (Sibai B M, Ramadan M K, Usta I, Salama M, Mercer B M, Friedman S A. Maternal morbidity and mortality in 442 pregnancies with hemolysis, elevated liver enzymes, and low platelets (HELLP syndrome. Am J Obstet Gynec 1993; 169:1000)

5. [F & I: Background: HELLP syndrome has become the subject of considerable controversy because of the lack of standardized diagnostic criteria used to diagnose it.

- Another reason for the controversy is the failure to distinguish between patients whose onset of HELLP syndrome occurred before or after delivery.

- There are few studies with an adequate sample size to describe incidences of important maternal outcomes in HELLP syndrome.

- There is little or no information regarding the influence of the time of onset of HELLP syndrome (antepartum or postpartum) on maternal morbidity.

- Objectives: To describe a 15-year experience with the management of 442 cases of HELLP syndrome to

  ° (1) describe incidences of serious maternal morbidities associated with HELLP syndrome;

  ° (2) detect potential clinical or therapeutic factors that may affect maternal morbidity, and

  ° (3) compare maternal morbidity between patients in whom HELLP syndrome develops before and after delivery.

- Diagnosis of HELLP syndrome was based on the clinical diagnosis of preeclampsia and all the following laboratory abnormalities: characteristic peripheral blood smear, serum lactic dehydrogenase >600 U/l (or total bilirubin >1.2 mg/dl), serum aspartate aminotransferase >70 U/l, and platelet count <100,000/mm^3.

- Routine laboratory evaluation included serial measurements of liver function tests, complete blood cell count, coagulation profile, and renal function tests.

- Disseminated intravascular coagulation was defined as the presence of low platelets (<100,000/mm^3), low fibrinogen (<300 mg/dl), positive fibrin split products (≥40 ug/dl), and prolonged prothrombin (≥14 seconds) and partial thromboplastin times (≥40 seconds).

- Acute renal failure was diagnosed in the presence of oliguria-anuria in association with severe reduction in renal function (creatinine clearance of ≤20 ml/min).

- The diagnosis of pulmonary edema was made on the basis of clinical and chest x-ray findings.

- Severe ascites was defined as the presence of ascitic fluid estimated at >1000 ml at either cesarean section, laparotomy, ultrasonography, or computed tomographic scanning of the abdomen.

- Abdominal computed tomographic scanning was performed in 26 of these women.

- Patients with HELLP syndrome routinely received intravenous magnesium sulfate to prevent and control convulsions.

- Bolus doses of hydralazine or nifedipine or a continuous infusion of sodium nitroprusside were administered to control severe hypertension.

- Blood and blood products were used to correct coagulation abnormalities and anemia as needed.

- Laparotomy was performed when necessary to control major intraabdominal bleeding.

- In addition, all patients received close monitoring of fluid intake and output, and dialysis was performed for severe azotemia or hyperkalemia.

- The patients represent the largest well defined group of patients with the HELLP syndrome in the medical literature.

- All patients met the strict criteria for HELLP syndrome.

- The incidence among patients with severe preeclampsia-eclampsia in this study was 18.9%.

- This high incidence is because of the high percentage of complicated cases referred from five different states in the region.

- Indeed, 55% of the patients studied in this report were referred or transported.

- Interestingly, the incidence of HELLP syndrome in women with eclampsia was only 10%.

- In addition, the incidence of eclampsia was similar in patients having HELLP syndrome before and after delivery.

- In the past severe preeclampsia had been defined as the presence of elevated blood pressure (systolic ≥160 mm Hg or diastolic ≥110 mm Hg) in association with either generalized edema, proteinuria, or both.

- **In some women with HELLP syndrome, hypertension and proteinuria may be absent or slight.**

  ° These women may have a variety of signs and symptoms, none of which are diagnostic of classic severe preeclampsia.

- A large percentage of the referred patients had clinical symptoms that might have presaged the onset of HELLP syndrome.

- Some of these symptoms may be nonspecific, especially in the absence of diagnostic hypertension or proteinuria, and may be missed by the nurse or physician during routine antepartum care.

- » It is imperative that all health professionals caring for pregnant women be familiar with the clinical signs and symptoms that might herald the onset of HELLP syndrome.

- HELLP syndrome is associated with increased maternal morbidity and mortality.

- This high incidence of maternal complications reflects the high-risk population of this perinatal center.

- Many patients were referred because of significant complications before or after delivery.

- It is also possible that patients with "mild" presentations of HELLP syndrome and those with uncomplicated preeclampsia-eclampsia were not referred to this center.

- These factors may explain the differences in the incidence of maternal morbidity in HELLP syndrome between this study and those reported by others.

- The role of disseminated intravascular coagulation in the pathogenesis of HELLP syndrome is controversial.

- In clinical practice disseminated intravascular coagulation is diagnosed in the presence of thrombocytopenia, prolonged prothrombin and partial thromboplastin times, and low fibrinogen concentration.

- With these criteria Weinstein found disseminated intravascular coagulation in only one (4%) of 26 patients with HELLP syndrome.

- Some authors have suggested that all patients with HELLP syndrome will have evidence of disseminated intravascular coagulation if sensitive laboratory tests are used.

- Laboratory evidence of disseminated intravascular coagulation was found in 92 patients with HELLP syndrome (21%).

- The majority of these cases occurred in women who had antecedent abruptio placentae or peripartum hemorrhage and in all four women who had subcapsular liver hematomas.

- If these cases are excluded from the analysis, then the incidence of disseminated intravascular coagulation developing de novo in HELLP syndrome was < 5%.

- The presence of disseminated intravascular coagulation was associated with an increased frequency of renal and pulmonary complications.

- Indeed, 33 patients had acute renal failure, of whom 10 requires dialysis.

- Abruptio placentae, disseminated intravascular coagulation, and hemorrhagic complications leading to hypotensive shock were responsible for the majority of cases of acute renal failure.

- This complication underscores the need for aggressive blood and volume replacement.

- Subcapsular liver hematoma is a life-threatening, but fortunately rare, complication of the HELLP syndrome.

- In most instances rupture involved the right lobe and was preceded by the development of a parenchymal hematoma.

- Ruptured subcapsular liver hematoma resulting in shock is an indication for massive transfusion of blood, fresh-frozen plasma, and platelets and for immediate laparotomy.

- Four patients suffered this complication: all required massive transfusions and laparotomy for control of hemorrhage, and three survived without long-term morbidity.

- Thirty percent (133) patients developed the manifestations of HELLP syndrome for the first time during the postpartum period.

- Importantly, 20% of these 133 patients had no evidence of preeclampsia before delivery.

- In addition, many of these patients had HELLP syndrome after being discharged from the recovery area or from the hospital.

- These patients were more likely to have pulmonary edema and renal failure than those who had HELLP syndrome before delivery.

- Because it is currently routine practice to discharge women with uncomplicated deliveries during the first 24 to 48 hours postpartum it is important to counsel all postpartum patients about the prodromal symptoms of HELLP syndrome.

- This counseling should be routinely undertaken before discharge, because this entity occurs in both normotensive uncomplicated postpartum women and preeclamptic women.

- In such women the diagnosis of HELLP syndrome should be suspected on the basis of patient symptoms (nausea, vomiting, **upper gastric pain,** or bleeding) and should be subsequently confirmed by complete blood cell count and liver enzyme evaluation.

» All such women be evaluated by a complete blood cell count that includes a platelet count.

- If the platelet count is <100,000 mm^3, then liver enzymes should be examined.

- Patients with delayed resolution of HELLP syndrome, particularly those with progressive deterioration in laboratory findings, represent a management dilemma.

- Exchange plasmapheresis with fresh-frozen plasma has been advocated as a treatment by some authors, whereas prostacyclin treatment has been recommended by others.

•Management of these women consisted of close observation of fluid intake and output, transfusions as needed, and supportive care.

•Dialysis was used as indicated.

•Virtually all such patients will have spontaneous resolution of the microangiopathy with supportive care alone.

•Because exchange plasmapheresis is an invasive and expensive procedure that carries a high risk of plasma-transmitted infection, its routine use for this indication should await the results of a randomized trial.]

---

6. Which of the following treatments will increase fetal lung maturity in an otherwise normal patient who has spontaneous premature rupture of the membranes at 26 weeks gestation?

    A. Antibiotics.
    B. Corticosteroids.
    C. Observation.
    D. Tocolysis.
*E. None of the above.

---

p. 1047 (Hallak M, Bottoms S F. Accelerated pulmonary maturation from preterm premature rupture of membranes: A myth. Am J Obstet Gynec 1993; 169:1045)

6. [F & I: Background: Preterm premature rupture of the membranes is an important cause of preterm delivery and is dangerous for both the fetus and the mother.

•Although prematurity and its inherent problem of pulmonary immaturity are a threat to survival and to the quality of life of the neonate, amnionitis may endanger both the mother and the fetus.

•Survival rates of preterm infants are between 0% to 10% at 23 weeks' gestation to between 78% and 91% at 28 weeks with of the survivors having long-term disability.

•The main hazard to the life of the small live-born infant is respiratory distress syndrome (RDS).

•The obstetrician who is engaged in managing a case of premature rupture of membranes often tries to gain time for the fetus in utero if there are no signs of amnionitis.

•It is widely believed that pulmonary maturation continues as a function of lengthening the time that the fetus stays inside the uterus and that premature rupture of the membranes by itself has an important effect on the acceleration of fetal pulmonary maturity.

•Objectives: To determine both whether fetal pulmonary maturation is accelerated after premature rupture of the membranes and the duration of premature rupture of the membranes required to achieve this effect.

•The management of preterm premature rupture of the membranes is controversial.

•Previous studies have provided information concerning the risks and benefits of conservative, expectant management of preterm premature rupture of the membranes.

•Of 70 patients with premature rupture of the membranes before 26 weeks' gestation, amnionitis developed in 43%, 52% of the neonates had RDS, and the overall perinatal survival rate was 63%.

•Of the survivors, 68% had normal neurologic and physical development after the first year of life.

- Tocolysis, prophylactic antibiotic, and corticosteroid treatment were not found to be more beneficial than expectant management alone.

- It is widely believed that premature rupture of the membranes accelerates fetal pulmonary maturity.

- A number of authors have reported that prolonged premature rupture of the membranes is associated with a decreased incidence of RDS.

- All but one of these studies have a common flaw: they controlled for gestational age and time of premature rupture of the membranes rather than for gestational age at delivery.

- It would be expected that the 35-day increase in the mean gestational age at delivery seen in the data would decrease the frequency of RDS irrespective of premature rupture of the membranes.

- The evidence suggesting that premature rupture of the membranes does not accelerate fetal pulmonary maturation is strong.

- This study is by far the largest study that controlled for gestational age at delivery.

- The National Natality Survey data failed to suggest accelerated fetal pulmonary maturation in association with premature rupture of the membranes and actually indicated that **premature rupture of the membranes increases the risk of RDS**.

- The possibility of error in assessing gestational age by controlling for birth weight was considered and comparable results were found.

- A "dose-effect" relationship was looked for by considering the duration of premature rupture of the membranes and again evidence was found to indicate that premature rupture of the membranes may increase the risk of RDS.

- The analyses of duration of premature rupture of the membranes excluded most cases with other medical or obstetric indications for delivery that might have accelerated pulmonary maturation.

- Another potent bias was that 30% of patients with intact membranes before 32 weeks received steroid therapy.

- Again, the analysis of duration of premature rupture of the membranes excluded these cases.

- Finally, when controlled for numerous factors related to RDS in a multivariate model, the duration of premature rupture of the membranes was positively correlated with the incidence of RDS.

- Conclusion: Pulmonary maturation continues but is not accelerated after premature rupture of the membranes.

- In fact, there is a strong suggestion that premature rupture of the membranes actually increases the risk of RDS at a given gestational age.

- The practice of delaying delivery for only 48 hours after preterm premature rupture of the membranes is more likely to result in chorioamnionitis than accelerated pulmonary maturation.

- Significant maturation with premature rupture of the membranes requires a longer period of expectant management.

7. Of predictive value in patients with catastrophic uterine rupture during an attempted vaginal delivery following previous cesarean section:

   *A. increased vaginal bleeding during labor.
   B. maternal age.
   C. maternal parity.
   D. number of previous VBACs.
   E. previous cesarean section disproportion.

p. 950 (Leung A S, Leung E K, Paul R H. Uterine rupture after previous cesarean delivery: Maternal and fetal consequences. Am J Obstet Gynec 1993; 169:945)

7. [F & I: Background: The rate of cesarean delivery in the United States peaked at 24.7% in 1988.

   •It was thus the most common major surgical procedure in the United States, with slightly more than 30% being repeat operations.

   •This high incidence has led to active advocacy of attempting vaginal birth after cesarean section to reduce this rate.

   •The high success rate and relative safety of trial of labor has been well documented.

   •A residual concern is the small but finite risk of 0.3% to 1.7% of uterine rupture.

   •Rupture of the gravid uterus is an unexpected and potentially devastating complication.

   •Limited and conflicting information is available to counsel patients regarding the maternal and neonatal outcome in cases of uterine rupture during a trial of labor after a previous cesarean section.

   •The differences among studies may be partly attributed to the many variations in the definition of uterine rupture.

   •Uterine scar **separation** includes a spectrum of problems varying from asymptomatic scar dehiscence to overt uterine rupture with complete fetal extrusion from the uterus into the maternal abdomen.

   •The latter condition would likely qualify as a "catastrophic rupture," which is noted as "rare" in the guidelines of The American College of Obstetricians and Gynecologists.

   •Another obvious factor affecting outcome is the elapsed time between diagnosis of uterine rupture and delivery.

   •Objectives: To identify the risks associated with overt, catastrophic uterine rupture, including fetal extrusion, and to report the maternal and neonatal outcome.

   •In addition, the fetal heart rate (FHR)-uterine contraction patterns were analyzed, and the elapsed time for delivery of an uncompromised neonate in cases of uterine rupture was investigated.

   •Both the charts and the FHR uterine contraction monitor strips from cases of uterine rupture were studied.

   •For the purpose of this study uterine rupture was defined as symptomatic uterine scar separation that required emergency laparotomy.

   •Indications for laparotomy included acute fetal distress, maternal bleeding with hypotension or shock, and repair of a urinary tract or peritoneal defect after vaginal delivery.

   •Asymptomatic uterine scar dehiscences were excluded.

- The study results were from in an indigent, urban, Hispanic population.

- This study probably presents the most severe spectrum of uterine rupture because most patients (90%) undergoing a trial of labor had unknown uterine scars.

- In a more stable population knowledge of previous incision and patient history would probably reduce some of the complications that were found.

- It is encouraging to note that the overall incidence of uterine rupture in patients undergoing a trial of labor was only 0.87%.

- A major concern for those managing a trial of labor is the rare catastrophic uterine rupture with its attendant maternal and neonatal complications.

- Uterine rupture that occurred before an observed trial of labor complicated 13 of the 99 cases of uterine rupture.

- Of note, nine of these 13 subjects had either a previous classic or three or more prior cesarean sections.

- If these facts had been known, most would have undergone an elective repeat cesarean.

- Only three uterine ruptures could have been prevented by elective cesarean section in those patients with uterine rupture near term and a history of unknown uterine scar.

- Performing elective repeat cesarean section in patients with prior unknown uterine scars to prevent uterine rupture and its attendant untoward neonatal outcome is **not** supported.

- Of significance, all 13 patients had some symptoms of abdominal pain, vaginal bleeding, or uterine contractions for few hours before arrival at the hospital.

- **It is thus prudent to advise the patients who desire a trial of labor that symptoms of new onset of uterine contractions, abdominal pain, or vaginal bleeding require evaluation as soon as possible.**

- The remaining 86 (86%) cases of uterine rupture occurred in hospitalized patients who were undergoing a trial of labor.

- Complete fetal extrusion complicated approximately one third of the cases.

- Except for a **higher** incidence of **intrapartum vaginal bleeding**, other variables such as maternal characteristics, prior obstetric history, or intrapartum events were of no predictive value to the impending catastrophic extent of uterine rupture.

- Decrease of uterine tone or cessation of uterine contractions at the time of uterine rupture was **not** observed.

- **Fetal distress was the most common signal of uterine rupture.**

- Fetal distress secondary to uterine rupture was manifested by prolonged, late, or variable decelerations.

- Prolonged decelerations in cases with complete or partial extrusion of the fetus were most devastating and required immediate intervention.

- The American College of Obstetricians and Gynecologists guidelines for vaginal birth after cesarean section of 30 minutes from the diagnosis of fetal distress to the beginning of the surgical procedure does not provide the best outcome of the fetuses that were extruded through the ruptured uterus into the abdomen.

•Significant neonatal morbidity was encountered when ≥**18 minutes** elapsed between the onset of prolonged deceleration and delivery.

•Patients who had severe, repetitive late decelerations should also undergo prompt delivery.

•Fetuses appeared to tolerate a shorter length of prolonged decelerations when it was preceded by severe late decelerations.

•A reasonably low perinatal morbidity and mortality rate was achieved with prompt operative intervention in neonates completely or partially extruded into the abdomen.

•The most common maternal morbidity associated with rupture of the uterus was the need for **blood transfusion**.

•Other morbidities such as bladder rupture (six of 11,405; 0.05%) and hysterectomy secondary to unrepairable rupture of the uterus (13/11405; 0.1%) were uncommon.]

---

8. At 31 weeks a patient has confirmed spontaneous premature rupture of the membranes. The best predictor of microbial invasion of the amniotic cavity is amniotic fluid

   A. glucose.
   B. Gram stain.
   *C. IL-6 determination.
   D. leukocyte esterase activity.
   E. white blood count.

---

p. 850 (Romero R, Yoon B H, Mazor M, Gomez R, Gonzalez R, Diamond M P, Baumann P, Araneda H, Kenney J S, Cotton D B, Sehgal P. A comparative study of the diagnostic performance of amniotic fluid glucose, white blood cell count, interleukin-6, and Gram stain in the detection of microbial invasion in patients with preterm premature rupture of membranes. Am J Obstet Gynec 1993; 169:839)

8. [F & I: Background: Microbial invasion of the amniotic cavity is present in approximately one third of patients with preterm premature rupture of membranes.

•An early diagnosis of this condition is important because neonates born to mothers with microbial invasion are at high risk for infection-related and non-infection-related complications.

•Clinical chorioamnionitis occurs late during the course of this disease and the results of the microbial cultures are often not available in time for important patient management decisions.

•Rapid tests for the diagnosis of microbial invasion of the amniotic cavity by analysis of amniotic fluid include Gram stain white blood cell count, glucose concentrations, leukocyte esterase activity, leukoattractants, and interleukin-6 (IL-6) concentrations.

•The value of these tests has been examined in patients with preterm labor and intact membranes and in patients with preterm premature rupture of membranes.

•There is little data about the comparative diagnostic and prognostic value of these tests in patients with preterm premature rupture of membranes.

•Objectives: To compare the diagnostic performance of these tests in the detection of microbial invasion of the amniotic cavity and in the prediction of the duration of pregnancy and neonatal outcome in patients with preterm premature rupture of membranes.

•To compare the diagnostic performance of these tests in patients with preterm labor with intact membranes and preterm premature rupture of membranes.

- Results: Patients with preterm premature rupture of membranes and a positive amniotic fluid culture have a **shorter** amniocentesis-to-delivery interval than patients with a negative amniotic fluid culture.

- The rate of neonatal complications was higher in patients with microbial invasion of the amniotic cavity than in those without it.

- Collectively these data provide strong evidence about the importance of microbial invasion of the amniotic cavity as a risk factor for adverse pregnancy and neonatal outcome.

- The **most common** microorganisms isolated from the amniotic fluid were **mycoplasmas**.

- Patients with preterm premature rupture of membranes have a higher rate of microbial invasion exclusively by mycoplasmas than do patients with preterm labor with intact membranes.

- Although mycoplasmas are extremely frequent facultative microorganisms in the lower genital tract, it is unlikely that their mere presence is the explanation for the observation because other prevalent microorganisms (e.g., *Lactobacillus sp.*) were not found as often in the amniotic cavity of patients.

- Microbial invasion of the amniotic cavity with mycoplasmas is capable of eliciting a host response because patients with positive cultures for mycoplasmas had a higher amniotic fluid IL-6 and white blood cell count than did patients with a negative amniotic fluid culture.

- No difference was found in the median amniotic fluid IL-6 and white blood cell count between patients with microbial invasion exclusively by mycoplasmas and that by other aerobic and anaerobic bacteria.

- Inoculum size is an important factor in determining the changes in amniotic fluid glucose, white blood cell count, and IL-6 concentrations.

- Patients with more than 10^5 colony-forming units per milliliter had significantly higher amniotic fluid IL-6 and white blood cell count and lower glucose concentrations than did patients with $<10^5$ colony forming units per milliliter.

- A limitation of this study is that this hypothesis was not tested in the context of microbial invasion with mycoplasmas because quantitative cultures for these microorganisms were not performed.

- The results clearly show that **amniotic fluid IL-6 determinations are better predictors of amniotic fluid culture results, the duration of the admission-to-delivery interval, and neonatal morbidity and mortality than are Gram stain, amniotic fluid white blood cell count, and amniotic fluid glucose.**

- An amniotic fluid IL-6 concentration above 7.9 ng/ml had a sensitivity of 80.9% in the detection of a positive culture but a specificity of 75%.

- The false-positive rate of 25% is more apparent than real as virtually all patients delivered within 72 hours and had neonatal complications and histologic chorioamnionitis.

- Gram stain of amniotic fluid had an extremely low sensitivity (23%) in the detection of microbial invasion of the amniotic cavity.

- The most likely explanation for this is that **mycoplasmas**, the most common isolates in this study, **are not visible on a Gram stain examination.**

- There was only one positive Gram stain in patients with positive amniotic fluid culture with mycoplasmas.

- This case may represent either a false-positive Gram stain or a false-negative culture for other bacteria.

- All rapid tests for the detection of microbial invasion of the amniotic cavity performed significantly better in patients with preterm labor and intact membranes than in patients with preterm premature rupture of membranes.

- Amniotic fluid glucose, white blood cell count, and IL-6 concentrations largely reflect host responses to microbial invasion; the data was interpreted as indicating that there are differences in the biologic characteristics of microbial invasion in preterm labor with intact membranes and in preterm premature rupture of membranes.

- Microbial invasion of recent onset, such as the one that probably occurs after rupture of membranes may be sufficient to lead to a positive culture but not to a robust host response.

- In contrast, microbial invasion of the amniotic cavity that occurs in patients with intact membranes is of longer duration and thus allows a more robust host response.

- Evidence to support this contention comes from previous studies in which the amniotic fluid concentrations of tumor necrosis factor and interleukin-1α, interleukin-1ß, and IL-6 were significantly higher in patients with preterm labor and intact membranes than in patients with preterm premature rupture of membranes (both with microbial invasion of the amniotic cavity.

- Amniotic fluid IL-6 concentration was an independent explanatory variable of admission-to-delivery interval and the occurrence of neonatal complications.

- Amniotic fluid IL-6 concentrations added significantly to gestational age when modeling the occurrence of neonatal morbidity and mortality.

  ° Measurements of amniotic fluid IL-6 would add new and significant information to the clinician.

- A practical consideration is whether assays for IL-6 are clinically available and practical.

  ° Several biotechnology companies offer immunoassays for the determination of IL-6 in the tissue culture media and biologic fluids.

- IL-6 is a group of differentially phosphorylated glycoproteins.

- It is extremely important that assays are carefully and extensively validated for the biologic fluid of interest.

- Insofar as the speed of the assay, immunoassays can be configured to produce very quick results.

- It is possible to develop a dip-stick test for immediate results in the antepartum and labor and delivery ward.

- These formats shall narrow the distance between research and clinical application.

- It is clear that these tests do not perform as well as IL-6 in the prediction of interval to delivery and neonatal complications.]

9. What should be the serum glucose threshold value after a one hour 50 gram glucose challenge screening test done at 20 weeks?

   A. 130 mg/dl.
   B. 135 mg/dl.
   *C. 140 mg/dl.
   D. 145 mg/dl.
   E. 150 mg/dl.

---

p. 517 (Monteros A, Parra A, Carino N, Ramirez A. The reproducibility of the 50-g, 1-h glucose screen for diabetes in pregnancy. Obstet Gynecol 1993; 82:515)

9. [F & I: •Background: The measurement of blood glucose performed 1 hour after a 50-g oral glucose load has been used since 1959 for detecting a "prediabetic" state during pregnancy.

•This test is usually recommended for screening for gestational diabetes mellitus, and has a 79% sensitivity and 87% specificity.

•Although this test was originally applied at any gestational age, now it is used mainly between 24 and 28 weeks' gestation.

•There are certain circumstances in clinical practice in which it would be convenient to perform this test as soon as possible.

•The Third International Workshop-Conference on Gestational Diabetes Mellitus reported: "The recommendation for universal 50-g 1-h glucose challenge testing at 24-to-28 week gestation should not preclude earlier testing depending on the circumstances."

°In some studies, a good sensitivity and specificity were reported as early as 10 weeks, but others suggested that routine screening is not warranted in a low-risk population before 20 weeks.

•For several years this screening test has remained unchallenged, but two studies have questioned whether the accepted threshold of 140 mg/dl should be changed based on current techniques for glucose determination and use of the fasting or fed condition before the test.

•Objective: To analyze the day-to-day variability of the 1-h glucose screening test, performed in the morning under an identical or opposite sequence of fed and fasting conditions on 2 consecutive days, in women at less than 24 weeks and at 24-to-28 weeks of pregnancy.

•Consequently, the only aim of the study was to explore the reproducibility of this screening test in the same women under identical fasting or fed conditions (fast-fast and fed-fed) or with an opposite sequence of fasting and fed states before the test (fast-fed and fed-fast) on 2 consecutive days.

•Both before and after the 24th week of pregnancy, a significant day-to-day variability was observed in mean serum glucose values, when comparing fasting both days and for the subgroups fast-fed and fed-fast.

•The mean values were lower on the second than on the first day in both fast-fast subgroups, and on the fed day in the subgroups fast-fed and fed-fast.

•These findings might suggest that in both fast-fast subgroups, stress could be inducing higher glucose levels on the first day of the study, whereas its effect was considerably diminished on the second day, when the pregnant woman was acquainted with the procedure.

•These findings suggested that the fed state may dampen the usual insulin resistance observed in fasting pregnant women.

- They also could indicate that the pancreatic beta-cell is already primed by a previous breakfast and thus can respond better to the subsequent oral challenge.

- The stress influence, if present, may then be overcome.

- The results in the fed-fed subgroups, showing no significant differences between days, lend further support to this hypothesis.

- The percentage of samples with a paired variability in serum glucose values of less than 10% on both days was below 50%, regardless of the group or subgroup analyzed.

- These results agree with the previous assessment of the screening test as "moderately reproducible."

- Among women before 24 weeks of pregnancy, the finding of nearly a 50% possibility that a first-day serum glucose value above any given threshold would be observed again the next day agrees with previous reports supporting either a good or poor sensitivity and specificity at these gestational ages.

- At 24-to-28 weeks' gestation, the probability of reproducing a high serum glucose concentration on the second day was more than 83%.

- The results also suggest that, up to 28 weeks' gestation, if a first-day glucose concentration is below a given threshold, there is a 90% probability that it will also be below that threshold on the second day, although this may deteriorate as pregnancy progresses.

- It is possible that only those women with a-screen value higher than 140 mg/dl at 12-to-23.6 weeks of pregnancy are truly at risk for gestational diabetes.

- Serial tests are needed to identify those women who really fail the 1-h, 50-g oral glucose test.

- The results support the current recommendation that the screening test can be performed in either the fasting or fed condition, although the use of different thresholds seems warranted.

- There may be better reproducibility if the test is done in the fed condition.]

---

10. In a term vertex presentation, failure of descent of the fetal vertex after transabdominal fundal pressure is applied (The Mueller-Hillis maneuver) is predictive of

   A. increased need for oxytocin.
   B. increased risk for abdominal delivery.
   C. increased risk for forceps delivery.
   D. increased risk prolonged second stage.
   *E. none of the above.

---

p. 521 (Thorp Jr. J M, Pahel-Short L, Bowes W A. The Müeller-Hillis maneuver: Can it be used to predict dystocia? Obstet Gynecol 1993; 82:519)

10. [F & I: •Background: An intrapartum screening test for dystocia would be a valuable addition to obstetric practice.

- In 1886, Mueller described an antepartum test in which an assistant applies fundal pressure and a second examiner determines descent of the presenting part.

- Descent implied that vaginal delivery was likely.

- The Mueller maneuver was modified in 1930 by Hillis.

- The modification consisted of a single operator applying fundal pressure and assessing descent.

- Such a test is now labeled the **Mueller-Hillis maneuver**.

- Modern obstetricians have endorsed the Mueller-Hillis maneuver as an intrapartum test for dystocia.

- Objectives: To describe the results of this test in a normal population of laboring women and to determine its utility in predicting dystocia.

- Methods: The examination was performed using the modification of the Mueller maneuver first described by Hillis.

- With the patient in the lithotomy position in a hospital bed, the examining fingers were inserted into the vagina and the ischial spines and infant skull were identified.

- Pressure was then applied transabdominally with the opposite hand on the breech.

- The pressure was begun gradually and then slowly released.

- The descent of the head with reference to the interspinous line was evaluated.

- The interspinous line was considered to be zero station, with centimeters above it labeled -1, -2, and -3 and centimeters below labeled +1, +2, and +3.

- Examinations were not performed during uterine contractions.

- Neither Mueller nor Hillis presented any data with their articles; each only described the technique and how they used it in practice.

- Results: **This work refutes the belief that the Mueller-Hillis maneuver can predict dystocia.**

- Women with no descent were as likely as women with descent to need abdominal delivery, operative vaginal delivery, and oxytocin augmentation.

- Similarly, women with no descent were no more likely than women with descent to have prolonged second stages (greater than 2 hours) or abnormalities detected by the blinded review of their labor curves.

- One can always argue that if more patients had been studied, significant differences between groups may have been detected.

- Perusal of the RR estimates and their 95% CIs indicates that there were no clinically important differences between the groups.

- In fact, many of the outcome variables tended to be less common (RR estimates less than 1.0) in patients without descent, which is the reverse of the finding one would expect if the test were useful.

- Likewise, one could speculate that performing the maneuver in women with abnormal labors would increase the prevalence of various outcomes and thus increase the predictive value.

- Fortunately, the RR estimates should remain the same in groups with either a low or high prevalence of various outcomes.

- The principal shortcomings of this study include an inability to quantitate the variables affecting maneuver outcome, lack of a precise inception cohort, failure to control for observer variation, and failure to account for the use of regional anesthesia.

- The force applied, resistance of the maternal abdomen, cervical resistance, and station, position, and flexion of the vertex, all of which might affect descent were **not** quantified.

- Entering the subjects throughout the active stage of labor rather than at a more clearly defined point may have biased the outcomes.

•Having a single examiner do only a single examination precludes evaluation of inter- and intra-observer variation.

•If there were a large degree of such variation, the maneuver would be of no value to the clinician for that reason alone.

•Finally, if epidural anesthesia can cause labor abnormalities, as suggested by some, then the failure to account for this variable could have influenced the results.]

---

11. Diagnostic of severe maternal CMV infection during pregnancy

    A. fetal hyperechogenic masses in the abdomen.
    B. maternal serum ALT.
    C. maternal serum AST.
    D. maternal serum GGT.
*E. none of the above.

---

p. 485 (Donner C, Liesnard C, Content J, Busine A, Aderca J, Rodesch F. Prenatal diagnosis of 52 pregnancies at risk for congenital cytomegalovirus infection. Obstet Gynecol 1993; 82:481)

11. [F & I: •Background: Cytomegalovirus (CMV) is the most common cause of intrauterine infection.

•The incidence of congenital CMV infection is 0.2-to-2% of live births.

•In Europe, 55% of pregnant women are seronegative at the beginning of pregnancy, and primary infection occurs in about 1-to-2% of pregnant women.

•After primary infection, the rate of transmission to the fetus is about 40%; 10% of infected fetuses are clinically affected at birth and a further 10-to-15% will develop symptoms later in life such as hearing loss or intellectual function impairment.

•Among symptomatic children at birth, mortality can be as high as 30%, and late complications almost invariably develop among the survivors.

•Transmission may occur at any stage of pregnancy and infection may be severe in early or late pregnancy.

°Primary CMV infection in the first half of pregnancy may have more severe sequelae.

•CMV can be diagnosed prenatally.

•Cytomegalovirus can be isolated in the amniotic fluid (AF) and in fetal blood samples, and specific immunoglobulin (Ig) M antibodies can be identified.

•Objective: To report results obtained prospectively in 52 pregnancies at risk for congenital CMV infection.

•Methods: Forty cases were referred because of abnormal results obtained on CMV screening; 12 other cases were referred after serologic investigation because of a symptomatic maternal infection.

•The women were divided into two groups.

•In group A (32 cases), maternal primary infection was defined by either the appearance of specific IgG and IgM antibodies in a patient who had been seronegative in the year before the pregnancy (28 cases), or a significant rise in titer of IgG in the presence of IgM (three cases), or the association of clinical symptoms and biologic alterations in the presence of IgM without evolution of IgG (one case).

- Group B contained 20 other patients, in whom the first serum obtained between 6 and 20 weeks' gestation and later sera showed IgM and IgG without IgG augmentation, and without symptoms or biologic alterations.

  ° In these cases, it was not possible to differentiate with certainty a primary from a recurrent infection or to determine the exact time of onset of the infection, as anti-CMV IgM antibodies can be detected in primary and recurrent infections and as the immune status of these women before pregnancy was not known.

- The pregnant women were also divided into three groups based on gestational age when the first positive serology was detected: Group 1 had infection early in pregnancy or in the periconception period (before 6 weeks); group 2 had infection between 6 and 20 weeks' gestation; and group 3 was infected after 20 weeks' gestation.

- The diagnostic procedure applied differed according to the gestational age at the time of referral.

- Nine women had only one amniocentesis, 29 had one procedure for both fetal blood and AF sampling, and 14 women referred early in pregnancy underwent AF sampling at 16 weeks' gestation and both fetal blood and AF sampling at about 22 weeks.

- Ultrasound examination was performed every 4 weeks from the time of referral to the end of the pregnancy.

- In group A cases with demonstrated primary CMV infection, transmission occurred in 12 of 32 cases (37%).

- In group B with positive IgM, four of 20 fetuses were infected (20%).

- The difference in fetal infection rates between group A and group B could be explained in that group B probably included an unknown number of primary infections that took place months before pregnancy, as well as recent primary infections and recurrent infections.

- This problem of diagnosis should be solved by routine serologic testing of women of childbearing age to determine their immune status with respect to CMV.

- The sensitivity of prenatal diagnosis was 81%.

- Cytomegalovirus culture and polymerase chain reaction in AF allowed the diagnosis in 12 of 13 cases, showing as in other studies that **amniocentesis is the best diagnostic test**.

- The sensitivity for CMV IgM antibody detection in fetal blood was 69%; this rate has varied at 20-to-75% in previous series.

- The best results seem to be obtained in studies using capture ELISA.

- Repetitive testing late in the second trimester should increase the accuracy of the diagnostic procedure and would give some information on the natural history of congenital CMV infection.

- The risk of sampling AF and fetal blood seems reasonable; no complications occurred after funipuncture in 255 pregnancies at risk for congenital infection including CMV and toxoplasmosis.

- The sensitivity of virologic investigations in AF before 21 weeks' gestation is unknown and seems to be moderate; five amniocenteses of eight performed before 21 weeks were negative in congenitally infected fetuses.

  ° In the three other cases, a positive diagnosis was obtained before 21 weeks, allowing early decisions concerning pregnancy management.

  ° This advantage could balance the relatively low sensitivity of early amniocentesis.

•Eight of the 12 terminated pregnancies were studied and showed clear evidence of CMV infection.

°Among the four uninvestigated aborted fetuses, two had **hydrocephalus** on ultrasound and one showed CMV inclusions in the placenta, suggesting viral infection in these fetuses.

°In three of these uninvestigated fetuses, evidence of CMV infection in the AF was established by two different procedures (culture and polymerase chain reaction), essentially excluding the possibility of a false-positive result.

•The detection of the virus in AF and the presence of IgM in fetal blood are evidence of fetal infection, but neither has prognostic value for the development of serious disease or severe sequelae.

•Fetal blood analysis could provide additional information about the fetal condition.

•Elevated alanine aminotransferase and thrombocytopenia are the most frequent laboratory abnormalities in symptomatic newborns, each seen in 80% of cases.

•Gamma-glutamyl transferase determination did not aid the diagnosis of infection.

•This finding contradicts published data in which gamma-glutamyl transferase was elevated in six infected fetuses.

•Alanine aminotransferase and aspartate aminotransferase have some role in the diagnosis of fetal infection.

•It remains to be seen whether signs of reticuloendothelial involvement such as thrombocytopenia and hepatic abnormalities in the fetus can be correlated with symptomatic disease at birth.

•Ultrasonographic abnormalities (cerebral ventriculomegaly, FGR) were present in five cases and were probably associated with severe disease.

•A fetal abdominal echogenic mass was present in one case; together with three other cases reported in the literature, it underlines the association between hyperechogenic areas in the fetal abdomen and the presence of fetal CMV infection.]

---

12. The fetal bladder should always be visualized on ultrasound by what gestational week?

   A. 7
   B. 9
   C. 10
   D. 11
   *E. 13

---

p. 490 (Bronshtein M. Bar-hava I, Blumenfeld Z. Differential diagnosis of the nonvisualized fetal urinary bladder by transvaginal sonography in the early second trimester. Obstet Gynecol 1993; 82:490)

12. [F & I: •Background: The urinary bladder on transvaginal sonographic examination can be seen as a midline hypoechoic cystic structure in the lower fetal abdomen.

•**The bladder is visible beginning at 10-to-12 weeks and should always be visualized by the 13th week of gestation.**

•The bladder normally fills and empties repetitively in cycles of 30-to-155 min, and this also should be visualized by 13 weeks' gestation.

•This cyclical change in bladder volume over time is helpful in its differentiation from other cystic structures, such as potential cystic lesions in the fetal lower abdomen and pelvis.

- The fetal bladder must be identified in the early second trimester within 30 minutes of examination.

- The combination of a nonvisualized bladder with a normal amount of amniotic fluid (AF) and normal-appearing kidneys on sonographic examination should raise the suspicion of bladder exstrophy, especially if an anterior protruding mass is demonstrated at the lower fetal abdominal wall.

- Objective: To report preliminary experience with seven cases in which persistent and repeated sonographic scans failed to visualize the fetal urinary bladder.

- The introduction of high-resolution transvaginal sonography allows detailed visualization of different stages in fetal embryogenesis and provides an opportunity to identify and follow dynamic processes in the development of fetal malformations.

- Whereas in late pregnancy severe oligohydramnios serves as a major sonographic marker of a nonfunctioning urinary system, in early gestation there are additional contributors to AF production.

- Severe renal malformations can coexist with a normal amount of AF.

- Approximately 90% of dysplastic kidneys result from urinary tract obstruction during nephrogenesis, and probably a lag in time is necessary for the insult to become sonographically detectable.

- Identification of a normal-appearing bladder in early pregnancy does not guarantee a normal functioning urinary system in late gestation.

- Multicystic kidney dysplasia is a bilateral disease in 20% of cases.

- Multicystic kidney dysplasia in the first-trimester has been diagnosed.

- The only clue to pathology of the urinary system was the persistent nonvisualization of the urinary bladder.

- Two other possibilities for persistent nonvisualized urinary bladder are bladder exstrophy and bilateral renal agenesis.

- Bladder exstrophy occurs in one of 25,000-to-40,000 births.

- This malformation is the end result of a persistent cloacal membrane, which prevents the normal process of midline mesoderm fusion.

- When the cloacal membrane eventually ruptures, the result is a ventrally exposed urinary bladder.

- Prenatal diagnosis of bladder exstrophy in advanced pregnancy has been described.

- The main aspect of the diagnosis of bladder exstrophy was **persistent nonvisualization of the fetal bladder during examination periods of 30 min or longer**, while concomitantly finding normal kidneys and a normal amount of AF.

- Another clue to the diagnosis of bladder exstrophy was the small **mass that protruded anteriorly from the lower abdominal wall**.

  ° This mass may represent herniation of the posterior bladder wall and bowel loops.

  ° On postabortal examination, this mass could not be identified; instead a shallow crater was observed in the same place.

- The different dynamic appearance might be explained by different intrauterine intraabdominal pressure during early pregnancy.

•Another possible sonographic sign for the diagnosis of bladder exstrophy, i.e., **a more caudal insertion of the fetal umbilical cord into the lower abdomen.**

•Because the average length of the entire fetal abdomen at the 14th week of gestation is approximately 3-to-4 cm, this sign has not been clearly found.

•The diagnosis of Potter syndrome in late pregnancy usually consists of nonvisualization of the urinary bladder and kidneys.

»In early pregnancy, the bladder can be identified despite the absence of urine production, probably because of retrograde filling.

•An alternative explanation may be the visualization of a **urachal cyst** and its misinterpretation as the urinary bladder.

•Only in four of eight cases of Potter syndrome has the urinary bladder been undetectable by early second-trimester transvaginal sonography.

•In the other four, the urinary bladder visualized at 14-to-15 weeks' gestation gradually disappeared during the following month.

•Persistent nonvisualization of the bladder (on repeated examinations, each longer than 30 min) concomitant with a normal amount of AF in the early second trimester is an indication for a careful examination of the fetal kidneys.

•One should bear in mind that some of the urinary system malformations develop relatively late, after the period of organogenesis; a normal-appearing fetal urinary tract on early ultrasound examination does not rule out urinary malformations.

•If the kidneys appear morphologically normal concomitant with an absent bladder, the differential diagnosis is bladder exstrophy or late-onset multicystic kidney dysplasia.

•When the kidneys are large and hyperechoic, late-onset infantile-type polycystic kidney disease should be suspected.

•One should be aware of the possible misinterpretation of the fetal adrenals (which are hypoechoic and lack a pelvis) as kidneys in cases of Potter syndrome.

•In both Potter syndrome and late-onset infantile-type polycystic kidney disease, the urinary bladder can be identified until 14 or 15 weeks of gestation.]

---

13. What is the earliest time during gestation that the constrictive effect of indomethacin can be found in the fetal ductus arteriosus?

    A. 23 weeks.
    B. 24 weeks.
    C. 25 weeks.
    D. 26 weeks.
*E. 27 weeks.

---

p. 500 (Van den Veyver I B, Moise Jr, K J, Ou C, Carpenter Jr R J. The effect of gestational age and fetal indomethacin levels on the incidence of constriction of the fetal ductus arteriosus. Obstet Gynecol 1993; 82:500)

13. [F & I: •Background: Indomethacin can effectively inhibit uterine contractility.

•Premature constriction of the fetal ductus arteriosus after the use of indomethacin for treatment of preterm labor is a well-known side effect.

- Initially it was believed that this complication of maternal indomethacin ingestion occurred only after 34 weeks' gestation.
  ° This complication can be detected with Doppler ultrasound and can occur before 34 weeks.
- Transplacental transfer of indomethacin from the maternal to the fetal circulation was first found in cord blood samples obtained at delivery in patients who received indomethacin before the onset of labor.
- Indomethacin crosses the placenta easily and prenatal transplacental transfer is unrelated to gestational age in the human fetus (maternal fetal serum ratio 0.97 ± 0.07).
- Objective: To evaluate the relationship between gestational age and ductus arteriosus constriction to determine the threshold time in pregnancy when the ductus becomes sensitive to the effects of indomethacin.
- The fetal circulation is dependent on a patent ductus arteriosus.
- Prostaglandins (PGs) (PGE2 and prostacyclin) are the most important mediators of vasodilation of the ductus arteriosus during fetal life.
- Maternal ingestion of PG synthetase inhibitors during the third trimester of pregnancy is associated with intrauterine closure of the fetal ductus arteriosus, leading to fetal and neonatal pulmonary hypertension and the syndrome of persistent fetal circulation.
- Although a large series of neonates exposed to indomethacin antenatally failed to show any adverse side effects, constriction of the ductus arteriosus after maternal indomethacin ingestion can be detected with Doppler flow ultrasound.
- Normal values of peak systolic and peak diastolic flow velocities through the ductus arteriosus are 50-to-140 and 6-to-30 cm/second, respectively, between 20 and 39 weeks' gestation.
- Constriction of the ductus arteriosus was seen with a peak systolic velocity of greater than 140 cm/second and/or a peak diastolic velocity greater than 35 cm/second.
- Only the value of the peak diastolic velocity was used to define constriction, because it is much less influenced by high-output states than is the peak systolic velocity.
- Constriction of the ductus arteriosus as early as 26.5 weeks' gestation was observed.
- This finding contrasts with earlier recommendations that indomethacin can be safely used before 34 weeks.
- Results: Using a peak diastolic flow velocity of greater than 35 cm/second as the cutoff value to diagnose ductal constriction before 27 weeks' gestation, the effect on the fetal ductus arteriosus is minimal.
- After 30 weeks, this seems to be an important side effect, with a mean diastolic flow of 39 cm/second.
- The gestational age when the majority of fetuses will begin to show constriction of the ductus arteriosus is 27-to-30 weeks.
- These data were obtained in fetuses with a pathologic condition (Rh disease), which theoretically could affect extrapolation of the results to a healthy population.
- By eliminating anemic fetuses, an attempt was made to correct for the most important confounding factor that could affect results.

•This study did not evaluate other side effects of indomethacin such as a decrease in fetal urinary output causing oligohydramnios.

•There are no good data on the relationship of this phenomenon to gestational age, but it has been found early in the second trimester.

•Even though the drug seems to be relatively safe from a cardiovascular standpoint before 27 weeks, one should be attentive to these other side effects in all patients.

•The lack of a relationship between fetal serum indomethacin levels and ductal constriction was not a surprising finding in this study.

°The efficient and equal placental transfer of indomethacin occurs in humans at all gestational ages and there is no difference between patients.

•The significant correlation found with gestational age in this multiple regression analysis is consistent with the results of the first part of the study, which showed an increased sensitivity of the ductus with increasing gestational age.]

---

14. The most important risk for *Chlamydia* infection during pregnancy is

    A. low socioeconomic status.
    B. nulliparity.
    C. race.
    D. tobacco use.
    *E. young age.

p. 401 (Alary M, Joly J R, Moutquin, Labrecque M. Strategy for screening pregnant women for chlamydial infection in a low-prevalence area. Obstet Gynecol 1993; 82:399)

14. [F & I: •Background: *Chlamydia trachomatis* is a major cause of cervicitis and pelvic inflammatory disease in women, and urethritis and epididymitis in men.

•In pregnancy, vertical transmission during vaginal delivery occurs in 50-to-70% of infants, causing neonatal conjunctivitis or chlamydial pneumonia.

•Most studies performed in the United States in the late 1970s or early 1980s found prevalence rates of chlamydial infection in pregnant women of 7-to-13%.

•The prevalence rate was only 2% among private obstetric patients, but well over 20% among younger women receiving care at public clinics.

•It is currently estimated that 155,000 infants in the United States are exposed to this organism each year during the birth process and that approximately 100,000 become infected.

•In addition, maternal infection per se may have severe consequences for the mother.

•Erythromycin or tetracycline ophthalmic ointments are used to prevent neonatal conjunctivitis, but they provide incomplete protection and do not prevent neonatal pneumonia.

•Treatment of infected pregnant women is effective in preventing transmission of *C trachomatis*.

• Because of this, screening of pregnant women is currently recommended by Canadian authorities and the Centers for Disease Control.

•Screening pregnant women for chlamydial infection using direct antigen testing is cost-effective only if the prevalence exceeds 6%.

- If culture is used for screening, the prevalence threshold for cost-effectiveness reaches almost 15%.

- Objectives: To determine the prevalence of genital chlamydial infection in pregnant women, to assess risk factors associated with this infection, and to identify criteria for the implementation of a screening program.

- Because culture techniques for the detection of *C. trachomatis* are considered highly specific but not perfectly sensitive (estimated sensitivity of 82% in pregnant women), the prevalence figure of 1.9% for genital chlamydial infection in pregnant women probably reflects a slight underestimation of the true prevalence.

- It does not explain the large differences between the results of this study and those reported previously or even a more conservative estimate of 5%.

- This discrepancy could be related to several possibilities.

  ° First, the sensitivity of the culture technique used in this study could be lower than previously reported.

  ° This is unlikely because all samples underwent a blind passage, a procedure that is known to increase the sensitivity of culture.

  ° Assuming a sensitivity of 81% and a specificity of 97% for ELISA as compared to culture, this figure would be comparable to a prevalence rate of 1.6% if culture had been used.

  ° Second, the most important risk for chlamydial infection was **young age**.

  ° This age group represented only 15.1% (1080 of 7150) of all subjects.

  ° Adjusting data on this previous age structure (57% under 24 and 43% 24 and older) would yield a prevalence of 3.2%, a figure much closer to the estimated prevalence of 5% in the United States.

  ° Finally, black pregnant women and those of low socioeconomic status are at higher risk of infection with *C. trachomatis*.

- Although related to young age, **a new sexual partner and nulliparity** remained significantly associated with chlamydial infection in the logistic regression model.

- These two factors generally reflect a relatively short period since the beginning of a stable sexual relationship.

- Women with one or more of these three risk factors may be at increased risk because of their past sexual behavior or that of their partners.

- The numbers of sexual partners and previous STDs over the last year were **not** associated with chlamydial infection in this study.

  ° Few women reported these conditions, which may be accurate but could also reflect underreporting because of the difficulty of admitting past behavior or disease, especially at the beginning of a pregnancy, when the stability of a relationship is of paramount value.

- The results of the case-control study contained in this prevalence survey suggest strongly that the application of simple pre-screening criteria could improve the use of diagnostic tests for *C. trachomatis*.

- According to this simple model, restricting culture to pregnant women who are younger than 25, those who have had a new sexual partner in the last year, or those who are nulliparous would lead to the detection of over 80% of the culture-positive women while screening only 40% of the whole population of pregnant women.

•Criteria to perform selective screening of chlamydial infection have been proposed for nonpregnant women, but these models have generally been derived from populations with prevalences of more than 9%.

•Although related to chlamydial infection, **mucopurulent cervicitis** was identified in less than 30% of infected women in several studies.

•The usefulness of cervical examination in identifying chlamydial infection in pregnant women is not well established.

•In a low-prevalence population, the application of prescreening criteria is attractive because it may increase cost-effectiveness.

•In this study, application of these criteria would increase prevalence to 3.7% in the screened population.

•Such a low prevalence is under the suggested cutoff value for cost-effectiveness of screening with an antigen detection test.

•In addition, assuming a sensitivity of 81% and a specificity of 97% with an ELISA test, the positive predictive value of screening in this population would be only 51%.

•The use of new direct tests with specificities of 99% may improve the positive predictive value.

•If data suggesting an association between chlamydial infection and adverse pregnancy outcome are confirmed, the minimum prevalence required for a screening program to be cost-effective could be greatly reduced.

•Screening all pregnant women for *C. trachomatis* without taking into account the local epidemiology of this infection may involve costs that are not worthy of the program's benefits.

•Before implementation, any screening program for *C. trachomatis* infection in pregnant women should be evaluated in the setting in which it will be applied.]

---

15. The drug of choice for treating bacterial vaginosis during pregnancy is

   A. ceftriaxone intramuscularly.
   *B. clindamycin vaginal gel.
   C. oral ampicillin.
   D. oral metronidazole.
   E. sulfonamide vaginal cream.

---

p. 409 (Fischbach F, Petersen E E, Weissenbacher E, Martius J, Hosmann J, Mayer H. Efficacy of clindamycin vaginal cream versus oral metronidazole in the treatment of bacterial vaginosis. Obstet Gynecol 1993; 82:405)

15. [F & I: •Background: Bacterial vaginosis is a common complaint among those who seek treatment at gynecology clinics, sexually transmitted disease clinics, prenatal clinics, and doctors' offices.

•Approximately 45% of all symptomatic abnormal vaginal discharges are due to this clinically mild disease, the most common and constant symptom of which is a fishy-smelling vaginal discharge.

•Clinically, bacterial vaginosis is characterized by a vaginal discharge that is thin and homogeneous, has a pH greater than 4.5, gives off a fishy-amine odor when mixed with a 10% potassium hydroxide solution, and contains clue cells on microscopic examination.

•The etiology of bacterial vaginosis is unknown, although current evidence suggests that it is a polymicrobial infection involving *Gardnerella vaginalis,* anaerobic bacteria including *Bacteroides* species (other than *B. fragilis), Mobiluncus* species, *Mycoplasma hominis,* and anaerobic cocci.

- Bacterial vaginosis occurs when vaginal concentrations of anaerobic bacteria reach 100 to 100,000 times that in the normal vagina, in association with suppression of some components of the normal vaginal flora such as *Lactobacillus* species.

- The factors that trigger the overgrowth of bacteria leading to bacterial vaginosis are unknown, but the frequency with which bacterial vaginosis occurs in sexually active women suggests that it may be sexually transmitted.

- Oral metronidazole 250-to-500 mg twice daily for 7 days has a reported cure rate of approximately 61-to-96%, and is currently the treatment of choice for bacterial vaginosis.

- Metronidazole has potential toxicities and, because of this teratogenic potential, is not recommended for use during early pregnancy.

- There is a need to develop effective, safer treatments for bacterial vaginosis that can be used by both nonpregnant and pregnant women.

- Susceptibility testing has indicated that the organisms isolated from patients with bacterial vaginosis are susceptible in vitro to clindamycin.

- Intravaginal clindamycin has response rates of 61-to-94% 4 weeks post-therapy.

- Objective: To compare the efficacy and safety of clindamycin phosphate vaginal cream and oral metronidazole for the treatment of bacterial vaginosis.

- Numerous antimicrobial therapies have been recommended for the treatment of bacterial vaginosis, including intravaginal sulfonamide creams, tetracyclines, ampicillin, and amoxicillin.

- The efficacy of many of these regimens has been disappointing or questionable.

- In recent years, oral metronidazole has been suggested to be the preferred treatment for bacterial vaginosis.

- Systemic metronidazole is associated with a number of side effects such as nausea, a bitter taste in the mouth, a disulfiram-like effect with alcohol ingestion, and, rarely, a peripheral neuropathy.

- Metronidazole use during the first trimester of pregnancy is contraindicated because of possible risks of teratogenicity and mutagenicity.

- In this large, multicenter, double-blind study, clindamycin vaginal cream and oral metronidazole again had comparable efficacy for the treatment of bacterial vaginosis in nonpregnant women.

- Results: Cure or improvement rates at the first follow-up were 85% in the clindamycin group versus 87% in the metronidazole group.

- One month after therapy, the cure or improvement rates were 83 and 78%, respectively.

- Bacterial vaginosis is a clinical syndrome without a specific etiologic agent.

- Although *G. vaginalis* is not the etiologic agent causing bacterial vaginosis, it appears to be a marker for the disease when it is present in large quantities.

- Over 40% of normal women carry *G. vaginalis*, but usually in a much lower concentration than in women with bacterial vaginosis.

- The higher cure rate in the metronidazole group (61%) compared to the clindamycin group (45%) at the first follow-up visit appeared to be mainly due to a more rapid decrease in vaginal fluid pH.

• Clindamycin is bactericidal to resident *Lactobacilli*, whereas metronidazole has **no** effect on vaginal *Lactobacilli*.

• This probably explains the difference in vaginal pH immediately after treatment.

• For this study, strict criteria to diagnose bacterial vaginosis—the presence of the three most objective clinical findings (**pH, odor, and clue cells**) plus a Gram stain compatible with bacterial vaginosis were used.

• The same three clinical criteria were used for the efficacy evaluation.

• Both clindamycin vaginal cream and oral metronidazole were well tolerated.

• Topical therapy has the potential advantage of fewer side effects because of a lower dosage and low systemic absorption of clindamycin cream.

• The most common medical event was vaginitis due to *C. albicans*, reported in 8.5% of the clindamycin patients and 4.7% of the metronidazole patients.

• The specific relationship of this disease to the study drugs is unknown but is consistent with suppression of vaginal bacteria, allowing overgrowth of *Candida* species.

• Other medical events, mainly diarrhea, nausea, and vomiting, were mild and comparable between the treatment groups.]

---

16. Which of the following is increased in lactation as compared to a nonlactating puerpera?

   A. Estrogen.
   *B. High-density lipoproteins.
   C. Progesterone.
   D. Triglycerides.
   E. Two-hour blood sugar after a glucose tolerance test.

---

p. 453 (Kjos S L, Henry O, Lee R M, Buchanan T A, Mishell Jr D R. The effect of lactation on glucose and lipid metabolism in women with recent gestational diabetes. Obstet Gynecol 1993; 82:451)

16. [F & I: • Background: The puerperium is a period of intense hormonal and metabolic changes.

• Placental steroid and peptide hormone blood levels, elevated ten to 100-fold during pregnancy, drop to virtually nil.

• Insulin resistance, increased two to threefold during pregnancy, returns to normal; lipoprotein levels elevated during pregnancy return to pre-pregnancy levels.

• Lactation adds another dimension to this period of dynamic metabolic change.

• Serum prolactin (PRL) levels remain elevated while estrogen and progesterone levels remain suppressed compared to levels in nonlactating women.

• Lactation may result in a more rapid return to prepregnancy weight as the extra body fat stored during pregnancy is used for milk production.

• Objective: To evaluate glucose and lipid metabolism after approximately 6 weeks of lactation in women who had exhibited during pregnancy the metabolic abnormalities associated with gestational diabetes.

• Many women with previous gestational diabetes continue to exhibit persistent abnormal glucose tolerance and associated adverse lipid changes in the puerperium.

- The hypothesis was that lactation, which has been associated with beneficial effects on carbohydrate and lipid metabolism in the early puerperium in healthy women, should similarly affect women with recent gestational diabetes.

- Lactating women had improved glucose metabolism as indicated by significantly lower area under the glucose curve, with lower fasting and 2-h glucose levels compared to nonlactating women.

- Lactating women also were found to have **higher fasting HDL** cholesterol levels.

- Lactation requires the interaction of several hormones, but these hormones, singularly or in concert, may have an opposite effect in other target tissues.

- In a study of healthy lactating women 8 weeks after delivery, fasting serum estradiol, insulin, and glucose levels were found to be lower, whereas PRL levels were higher compared to nonlactating women.

- No differences were seen in fasting serum progesterone, FSH, LH, and glucagon levels.

- Abnormally high levels of PRL in women with pituitary tumors decrease glucose tolerance and elevate serum insulin levels.

- Basal PRL levels in women nursing for 2-to-12 weeks postpartum remain slightly elevated, with 10- to 20-fold increases following a period of nursing.

- This physiologic elevation of PRL in lactating women has not been associated with a deterioration in oral glucose tolerance, but rather with significantly lower mean fasting glucose and insulin levels 8 weeks postpartum.

- Results: Significantly lower fasting and 2-h glucose levels and decreased total area under the glucose tolerance curve after controlling for age, BMI, and insulin use in pregnancy was found.

- The severity of glucose intolerance in gestational diabetes is only broadly defined by ACOG as either class A1 or A2.

- To investigate whether improved glucose tolerance in the lactating group was a result of nonrandom selection of women with less severe gestational diabetes, the study population was stratified into those who achieved fasting euglycemia by diet control during pregnancy and those who had persistent fasting hyperglycemia requiring insulin therapy.

- This division resulted in significantly different populations, with the insulin-treated group being older and heavier, with higher blood pressure and parity and more compromised glucose and lipid metabolism compared with the diet group.

- When the analysis was repeated separately in both the diet and insulin-treated groups while controlling statistically for age, BMI, and MAP, the findings in both groups were similar to the overall analysis: **The mean fasting serum glucose remained significantly lower and mean HDL cholesterol was significantly higher in lactating women compared to nonlactating women.**

- The intriguing finding of a twofold reduction in the development of diabetes mellitus in the lactating group compared to the nonlactating group invites further exploration into alterations in insulin sensitivity during lactation.

- Lactation may increase insulin sensitivity, thereby explaining increased metabolic efficiency in response to noradrenaline infusion in healthy women during lactation.

- Milk production requires approximately 500 extra calories per day, with approximately half of these calories existing in the form of triglycerides.

•Healthy lactating women have higher levels of HDL cholesterol, phospholipid, and apoprotein A-I and A-II at 6 weeks postpartum compared to nonlactating women.

•The substantial demand for triglycerides in healthy lactating mothers is met by enhanced VLDL catabolism and generation of increased HDL components via the transfer of surface remnants.

•An increase in HDL cholesterol was found in lactating mothers who had recent gestational diabetes.

•The increased HDL cholesterol levels in women who are at high risk for diabetes and its sequelae should be particularly desirable.

•Mild adverse changes in lipid profiles appear to precede the development of diabetes in these women.

•In a recent study, significantly lower HDL cholesterol levels were found during the puerperium in gestationally diabetic women who developed diabetes mellitus within the following 3 years compared with a similar cohort who did not develop diabetes.

•Analysis of the effect of lactation on metabolism is complicated by many factors.

°First, a woman's decision to nurse probably involves cultural, educational, and health biases.

°Women treated with insulin during pregnancy chose to nurse less often (44%) compared to those treated with diet (52%).

°This may reflect a lower cesarean delivery rate in the diet group, allowing earlier recovery from physical limitations to breastfeeding and possibly a patient's perception of better health.

°Second, lactation may result in earlier return to prepregnancy weight.

°Without increased caloric intake, catabolism of fat stores supplies the additional energy requirement of nursing.

°Lactation-associated lipid catabolism appears to favor specific tissue sites.

°Basal rates of fat breakdown have been found to be higher in femoral compared to abdominal adipose tissue in lactating women compared to nonlactating women.

°This may be explained by the lower levels of adenosine reported in the femoral tissues of lactating women.

°Adenosine is a local-acting, insulin-like effector, which in lower quantities would preferentially allow local lipid mobilization.]

---

17. Significant deviations from singleton growth do not occur in twin gestations until how many weeks?

   A. 24.
   B. 28.
   C. 30.
   D. 32.
   *E. 34.

p. 595 (Luke B, Minogue J, Witter F R, Keith L G, Johnson T R B. The ideal twin pregnancy: Patterns of weight gain, discordancy, and length of gestation. Am J Obstet Gynec 1993; 169:588)

17. [F & I: •Background: During the 1980s twin births in the United States increased at twice the rate of singleton births.

- By 1989, the 92,916 twin births in this country set an all-time high.

- Twin births currently account for approximately 2.2% of all live births but contribute disproportionately to perinatal morbidity and mortality.

- Compared with singletons, infants of a twin gestation have relative risks of 9.6 of being born with very low birth weight (<1500 g), 10.3 of being born with low birth weight (<2500 g), 6.6 of dying in the first year of life, and, among survivors, 1.4 of having a postnatal handicap.

- Studies of perinatal outcomes in twin pregnancies pose special clinical and methodological challenges.

- Definitions that are used and accepted in singletons, such as low birth weight and preterm birth, may not have the same implications when applied to twin infants.

- Research of twin births are complicated by the unique variable of discordancy and by the challenge of characterizing the growth of each twin individually and both twins as a pair.

- In addition, studies have indicated that maternal anthropometric factors such as pregravid weight and weight gain, which are strongly associated with singleton birth weight, also exert a therapeutic influence in twin gestations.

- Other measures such as rates and patterns of weight gain that are associated with birth weight and length of gestation in singletons have not yet been evaluated in twin pregnancies.

- Objectives: To evaluate those factors that influence the intrauterine growth of twins and to identify specific factors and combinations of factors associated with the best intrauterine growth and lowest morbidity ("ideal twin pregnancy").

- Because of the considerations cited above, a series of unique variables were formulated for this study.

- These variables incorporate specific aspects of those factors that influence perinatal outcome in singletons and at the same time consider the special situation of twins.

- This study builds on a previous analysis of the same data set, which evaluated the association between maternal weight gain and the average birth weight of twin pairs.

- This current study extends the previous analysis by characterizing the birth weight of each twin infant in several ways and by formulating an optimal, or "ideal," twin model.

- Results: The best intrauterine growth and lowest morbidity is achieved **earlier** for twins than for singletons.

- The maturation process is accelerated in twin gestations, resulting in more rapid aging of the twin placental and earlier attainment of a mature lecithin/sphingomyelin ratio.

- Because of these differences, that which is defined as "term" for singletons may actually be "postterm" for twins.

- The "ideal" window of gestation for twins should be that period associated with the best intrauterine growth for gestational age and the lowest morbidity.

- Using length of stay and growth retardation criteria (model 1), nearly 70% of ideal twin pregnancies were deliveries between 35 and 38 weeks' gestation.

- In contrast, late term birth (39 to 41 weeks' gestation) was negatively associated with the sum of twin birth weight ratios (indicating greater deviation from singleton growth curves) and a fivefold increased risk of intrauterine growth retardation (IUGR) of the smaller of the twin pair (odds ratio 5.23, 95%

confidence interval 1.4, 19.0) and an eightfold increased risk for IUGR of the larger of the twin pair (odds ratio 7.96, 95% confidence interval 2.7, 23.8).

•**The findings that significant deviations from singleton growth do not occur until after 34 weeks' gestation confirm previous investigations.**

•The intrauterine growth of singletons and twins begins to diverge at about 30 weeks, and differences become significant by 35 weeks.

•The peak growth rate in weight for singletons is about 250 g/week at 33 weeks compared with 175 g/wk at 31 weeks for twins.

•After 31 weeks twin birth weight falls progressively behind that of singletons so that by 38 weeks the singleton 10th percentile is equivalent to the twin 50th percentile, and the singleton 50th percentile is equivalent to the twin 90th percentile.

•In this study gestations of ≥39 weeks were associated with significant deviation from singleton growth (birth weight ratio) for the larger of the twin pair and substantial increased risk of growth retardation (birth weight ≤10th percentile) for both the smaller and larger of the twin pair.

•**Discordancy**, both in magnitude and period of gestation when it occurs, was associated with adverse outcomes in this study.

•Because discordancy of ≥15%, ≥20%, and 25% had all been shown to be significantly associated with subsequent neonatal or postneonatal morbidity and mortality, all three definitions were evaluated in this study.

•Discordancy of ≥15% was negatively associated with birth weight and birth weight ratio of the smaller of the twin pair.

•Discordancy was also associated with IUGR of the smaller twin; this risk paralleled increasing discordancy (odds ratio 4.16, 95% confidence interval 1.0, 17.6 for >15% discordancy and odds ratio 5.35, 95% confidence interval 1.2, 23/7 for ≥20% discordancy).

•In model 1 of the ideal twin pregnancy, discordancy of both ≥15% and ≥20% were associated with substantially increased risks of morbidity and growth retardation.

•When the additional limitation of 35 to 38 weeks' gestation was added (model 2 of ideal twin pregnancy), only discordancy of ≥20 was associated with increased risk.

•The findings suggest that a substantial portion of neonatal morbidity in newborn twins is a secondary result of IUGR.

•The pattern of **maternal weight gain** of low early and low late was negatively associated with all measures of intrauterine growth and with an increased risk for IUGR that was greater for the smaller versus the larger of the twin pair.

•In both models of ideal twin pregnancy this pattern of weight gain was associated with increased risk of a nonideal outcome.

•Additionally, in model 2 the pattern of low early and high late was associated with a decreased risk of a nonideal outcome.

•Among singletons, inadequate early weight gain (<9.5 pounds by 24 weeks) is associated with an increased risk of IUGR.

•**Maternal body weight** (including body fat), alone or in combination with gestational weight gain, may exert its effect on birth weight through the presence (or absence) of energy reserves and by influencing the hormonal response to pregnancy.

- Body fat is a significant extragonadal source of estrogen and a storage site for steroid hormones.

- Increases in body fat during pregnancy, reflected in the pattern of weight gain, may influence the complex hormonal mechanisms mediating intrauterine growth.

- The hormonally induced expansion of the plasma volume and the placental hormone production secondary to placental size and metabolism are also important components in the overall hormonal milieu influencing fetal growth.

- The only factor contributing to the hormonal regulation of fetal growth that can potentially be augmented is **gestational weight gain.**

- Inadequate weight gain may limit the full hormonal response to twin pregnancy and result in poor intrauterine growth.

- The relationship between poor patterns of weight gain and growth retardation, as inadequate gain before 24 weeks or between 28 and 32 weeks, may be an indirect reflection of the hormonal role of body fat on birth weight.

- In studies of singleton pregnancies, skinfold changes, estimating the accretion and use of body fat, correlate with better birth weights and longer gestations.

- In the current study, low gain before 24 weeks' gestation was adversely associated with all measures of intrauterine growth and with increased risks of nonideal outcomes in both models 1 and 2.

- Subsequent high gain after 24 weeks for pregnancies of 35 to 38 weeks was associated with a decreased risk of a nonideal outcome (model 2).

- The retrospective nature of this study limits the variables that could be evaluated.

- Ideally, the intrauterine growth of twins should be studied prospectively, with serial evaluations of maternal body fat (by means of skinfold measurements or ultrasonography), hormonal assessments, and tests of placental function and (at delivery) placental size and structure.

- Although length of stay >8 days as a measure of morbidity for twins was appropriate in this study because of the obstetric practices during the decade under study, different criteria need to be developed to make this factor more universally applicable.

- In spite of these limitations, this study adds to the mounting body of evidence that "term" for twins is achieved earlier than for singletons and that "postterm" (39 to 41 weeks) is associated with greatly increased risks of IUGR and morbidity.

- Weight gain, as patterns of gain, were significantly associated with all measures of intrauterine growth and both models of ideal twin pregnancy.

- **These results suggest that weight gain may be potentially beneficial in improving perinatal outcome in twin gestations.**]

18. Advantages of expectant management of labor in class B diabetics include

   A. decreased incidence of larger gestational age infants.
   B. decreased incidence of shoulder dystocia.
   C. increased incidence of successful VBACs.
   D. reduction in incidence of cesarean section.
   *E. none of the above.

p.614 (Kjos S L, Henry O A, Montoro M, Buchanan T A, Mestman J H. Insulin-requiring diabetes in pregnancy: A randomized trial of active induction of labor and expectant management. Am J Obstet Gynec 1993; 169:611)

18. [F & I:•Background: The infant of the diabetic mother and the infant of the mother with untreated gestational diabetes are at increased risk of perinatal death.

•Until recently the risk of fetal death in term infants of diabetic mothers prompted elective delivery at 38 completed weeks of gestation, after documentation of fetal lung maturity.

•In insulin-requiring diabetic pregnancies, this practice of active induction may have contributed to an increased cesarean delivery rate, which in some studies ranges up to 71%.

•In the Los Angeles County University of Southern California Women's Hospital, 45% of women with insulin-requiring gestational diabetes, and non-insulin-dependent diabetes before pregnancy requiring insulin treatment during pregnancy, and class B insulin-dependent diabetes were delivered by cesarean section in 1987 through 1990.

•In Ireland a low cesarean section rate of 20% was achieved by allowing all uncomplicated pregnancies of insulin-dependent diabetic mothers to continue through 40 weeks.

•Objective: To assess whether the cesarean delivery rate could be safely reduced by expectant management as opposed to active induction of labor at 38 weeks.

•**Active induction of labor management.**

•Amniocentesis was performed to assess fetal lung maturity in pregnancies where the gestational age could not be determined with accuracy (i.e., first physical examination after 20 weeks or first ultrasonographic scan after 26 weeks).

•Induction of labor was scheduled within 5 days for those mothers with (1) accurate estimation of fetal age or (2) with evidence of fetal lung maturity, a lecithin sphingomyelin ratio ≥2.0.

•If fetal lung maturity was not confirmed, amniocentesis was repeated 1 week later, while patients continued twice weekly antepartum surveillance (nonstress test and amniotic fluid volume index) and home insulin therapy.

•Labor was induced with intravenous oxytocin in accordance with standard protocol.

•In women with favorable Bishop scores (<4), unscarred uteri, and normal amniotic fluid indexes (>5.0 cm), up to three applications of vaginal prostaglandin (3 mg) were used for cervical ripening before oxytocin treatment.

•**Expectant management.**

•Expectant management consisted of daily split-dose insulin therapy and home blood glucose monitoring, weekly antenatal clinic visits, and twice-weekly antepartum testing.

•Induction of labor was undertaken only if any of the following developed: (1) suspected fetal distress as indicated by decelerations or unreactive nonstress testing or low volume of amniotic fluid, (2) preeclampsia, (3) maternal hyperglycemia exceeding the thresholds stated above or ketonuria, (4) estimated fetal weight ≥4200 g, or (5) 42 weeks' (294 days') gestation.

- Otherwise spontaneous labor was awaited.

- Maternal age was determined at delivery.

- Gestational age was calculated from the first day of the last menstrual period, adjusted if ultrasonographic estimation (before 22 weeks) differed from the menstrual age by ≥10 days.

- Birth weight for gestational age was assessed by reference to data published for California.

- Infants whose birth weights were ≥90th percentile were classified as large for gestational age (LGA).

- After delivery the infants were fed early, capillary blood glucose was monitored for hypoglycemia, and physical examination was performed by a neonatologist.

- Both pregestational insulin-dependent diabetes mellitus and gestational diabetes are associated with increased perinatal mortality.

- Early elective delivery was introduced to reduce such deaths.

- Most American obstetricians and fetal medicine specialists electively deliver at least 70% of mothers with insulin-dependent diabetes mellitus.

- Induction of labor after the thirty-eighth week of pregnancy is widely advocated and is standard practice for all mothers with insulin-dependent or non-insulin-dependent diabetes mellitus or gestational diabetes who require insulin therapy during pregnancy.

- The practice of active induction of labor may have contributed to the high cesarean delivery rate in diabetic women.

- In the United States the 1986 cesarean section rate was 53% in women with diabetes mellitus and 34% in those with "abnormal glucose tolerance."

- The former incidence was approximately double the overall cesarean section rate of 24% in the United States for that year.

- Obstetric intervention in diabetic mothers can be minimized by intensive control of diabetes and postponement of delivery until 40 weeks' gestation.

- In this study of a selected group of women with uncomplicated, insulin-requiring diabetes, the cesarean section rate was not reduced by expectant management of pregnancy (31%) compared with active induction of labor (25%).

- Women with previous cesarean sections were routinely offered a trial of vaginal delivery.

- Against this background, it was decided not to exclude such women from the current study.

- The incidence of cesarean section was not significantly different in the expectant management and induction of labor groups, either when all women were included or when those who had a prior cesarean section were excluded.

- The high rate of induction of labor in the expectant management group (49%) and of cesarean delivery in both groups may reflect a low threshold for interventions that exists in the management of pregnancies with complications such as diabetes.

Obstetrics and Gynecology: Review 1994 - Obstetrics References

•Diabetes, both gestational and non-insulin-dependent diabetes mellitus, occurs more frequently in older mothers, in women with higher parity, and in those with a previous large infant, all of whom are at risk of having bigger babies and hence cesarean sections.

•Infants of mothers managed expectantly had significantly more infants with larger birth weights and more LGA infants than those managed by active induction of labor.

•Birth weight is affected not only by diabetes but also by gestational age and maternal weight.

•In spite of correcting for maternal age, maternal weight before delivery, and gestational age at delivery, there was still a higher prevalence of LGA infants in the expectant management group compared with the active induction of labor group.

•This finding suggests that the rate of growth is greater than among the reference California population used in assessing LGA.

•Prolonging the gestation in diabetic pregnancies appears to be associated with an absolute increase in size and an increase in size corrected for gestational age.

•In this study of expectant management and active induction of labor, there were few intrapartum or postpartum problems.

•The three cases of mild shoulder dystocia all occurred in the expectant management group and there were no permanent sequelae.

•Conclusion: Expectant management of pregnancy in women with insulin-treated gestational diabetes or class B pregestational diabetes failed to decrease the cesarean section rate compared with active induction of labor.

•In the expectant management group more cases of **shoulder dystocia** occurred, and there was a significant increase in LGA infants.

•In view of the accelerated growth of some infants of diabetic mothers at term, any advantage of expectant management must be weighed against the risk of macrosomia.

•**There appears to be no advantage in delaying delivery in women with insulin requiring diabetes past 38 to 39 weeks' gestation.**

•If delivery is postponed, careful monitoring of fetal size and growth must be performed.]

---

19. Which of the following accurately describes the action of cocaine on myometrium?

    A. Increases α-adrenergic receptor binding.
    B. Increases ß-adrenergic receptor binding.
    C. Inhibits α-adrenergic receptor binding.
    *D. Inhibits ß-adrenergic receptor binding.
    E. None of the above.

---

p. 644 (Hurd W W, Gauvin J M, Dombrowski M P, Hayash R H. Cocaine selective inhibits ß-adrenergic receptor binding in pregnant human myometrium. Am J Obstet Gynec 1993; 169:644)

19. [F & I: •Background: In some urban areas as many as 17% of women abuse cocaine during pregnancy.

•The premature delivery rate among cocaine users of 17% to 25%, is approximately double the normal rate.

•Because prematurity is a major cause of perinatal morbidity and mortality, understanding the relationship between cocaine use and premature labor is of clear clinical significance.

- The mechanism by which cocaine abuse is linked to premature labor is unknown.

- The increase in circulating catecholamines associated with cocaine abuse may increase uterine contractility and thus increase the risk of premature delivery.

- Increases in catecholamines associated with stress correlates with prolonged labor, suggesting that increased levels of circulating catecholamines may actually inhibit uterine contractility.

- Because α-adrenergic receptor stimulation increases uterine contractility and ß-adrenergic receptor stimulation inhibits contractility, the association of prolonged labor with stress suggests that increased circulating catecholamines may have a predominantly ß-adrenergic effect in vitro.

- In addition to systemic effects, cocaine also directly augments the adrenergic response of some tissues.

- This effect may be caused by the ability of cocaine to increase α-adrenergic receptor affinity for catecholamines.

- Alternatively, cocaine could augment contractility by interfering with ß-adrenergic receptors.

- If cocaine either selectively increases α-adrenergic receptor binding or blocks ß-adrenergic receptor binding, the net effect would be an increase in uterine contractility.

- The effect of cocaine on adrenergic receptor binding has not been reported.

- Objective: To determine if cocaine alters binding to either the α– or ß-adrenergic receptors of pregnant human myometrium.

- In vitro receptor-binding assays were performed in the presence and absence of cocaine, using human myometrium obtained at cesarean section from women not in labor.

- Results: Cocaine selectively and competitively **inhibits** ß-adrenergic receptor binding in the pregnant human myometrium (inhibition constant 132 µmol/l).

- Although cocaine also had an effect on α-adrenergic receptor binding, inhibition was seen only at much higher concentrations (inhibition constant 1.63 mmol/l).

- This situation is similar to that for most adrenergic compounds, which usually have different affinities for α– and ß-adrenergic receptors.

- In light of the limited structural analogies between cocaine and catecholamines, the ability of cocaine to competitively inhibit adrenergic receptor binding was unexpected.

- Cocaine may have a direct effect on α-adrenergic receptors, which increases receptor binding efficacy, perhaps by inducing conformational changes in α-adrenergic receptors.

- In the pregnant human uterus cocaine has little effect on α-adrenergic binding affinity.

- At extremely high concentrations (1 mmol/l) cocaine actually inhibited receptor binding.

- This finding probably has little clinical significance because this level of cocaine is approximately 300 times higher than serum concentrations associated with smoking alkaloidal "crack" cocaine, one of the most potent forms of the drug.

- In contrast to α-adrenergic receptors, an effect of cocaine on ß-adrenergic receptor binding has not been previously suggested.

- Cocaine increases the adrenergic response of various types of smooth muscle when both α- and β-adrenergic receptors are stimulated but has no effect on the adrenergic response when β-adrenergic receptors are blocked with propranolol.

- These observations, together with the findings in the current study, suggest that cocaine augments the adrenergic response by interfering with β-adrenergic receptor function in some systems.

- The lowest concentration of cocaine at which inhibition of β-adrenergic receptor binding could be shown was 30 μmol/l, which is 10 times the serum concentrations found after smoking "crack" cocaine (3 μmol/l).

- In spite of the insensitivity of the assay at this low concentration, even small changes in receptor binding may have clinical implications because of the pattern of repeated and prolonged abuse associated with cocaine.

- Although this study indicates that cocaine is a competitive inhibitor of β-adrenergic receptor binding, it does not address the question of whether cocaine is an adrenergic agonist or antagonist.

- In general, cocaine is not an adrenergic agonist in other systems and does not have catecholamine-like properties.

- Competitive inhibition of β-adrenergic binding by cocaine may result in an antagonist effect at the receptor.

- Could selective inhibition of β-adrenergic receptor binding by cocaine result in an increased incidence of premature delivery?

  ° Before labor the uterus remains in a senescent state in spite of stimulation of both α- and β-adrenergic receptors by circulating catecholamines.

- With cocaine abuse circulating catecholamines are increased twofold to threefold, which presumably increases the adrenergic stimulation of the uterus.

- Local catecholamine concentrations at the uterine receptors may be further increased by cocaine's ability to block uptake and metabolism of catecholamines by both the endometrium and myometrium.

- It is questionable if these factors alone would increase uterine contactility, because increased serum levels of catecholamines resulting from stress in labor are associated with a **prolongation** of labor.

  ° If cocaine selectively blocks the relaxant effect of β-adrenergic receptor stimulation, this may shift the balance so that catecholamine stimulation results in increased uterine contractility.

- Another consideration is the effects of **repeated exposure** to cocaine, because a common pattern of cocaine abuse appears to be repeated episodes of use throughout pregnancy.

- Although patients report that cocaine use "speeds up labor" and has been associated with precipitous labor, it may be that chronic recurrent uterine exposure to cocaine rather than acute exposure is more important as a cause of premature delivery.

- In either case, how cocaine use leads to premature delivery can only by surmised because the mechanism of the onset of labor remains uncertain.

- Although cocaine may also have the various central and systemic effects that contribute to the association of cocaine abuse with premature delivery, the results of this study suggest that direct effects of cocaine on myometrial receptors may play an important role.]

20. The greatest risk to the fetus of the patient with clinically significant aortic stenosis is

   *A. congenital heart disease.
   B. depression at birth from general anesthesia.
   C. fetal growth retardation.
   D. preterm delivery.
   E. teratogenic effects of cardiac glycosides.

p. 544 (Lao T T, Sermer M, MaGee L, Farine D, Colman J M. Congenital aortic stenosis and pregnancy-A reappraisal. Am J Obstet Gynec 1993; 169:540)

20. [F & I: •Background: Congenital valvular aortic stenosis has been a contraindication to pregnancy, because maternal and perinatal mortalities, reported more than two decades ago and often quoted since, is 17% and 32%, respectively.

•An earlier series, reviewing patients with congenital heart disease delivered between 1975 and August 1986, did not substantiate the high maternal and perinatal mortality rates reported earlier.

•Objective: To review the maternal and perinatal outcome of pregnancies complicated by maternal congenital aortic stenosis.

•Experience with pregnancy in patients with congenital aortic stenosis is rare, because it is more commonly found in men, and severe stenosis is unusual in women of childbearing age as it is a progressive cardiac lesion with average age at clinical presentation of about 48 years.

•The literature quotes a maternal mortality of 17%, a figure based on data published in 1978.

•There was no clear recommendation on the advisability of pregnancy in this condition, but pregnancies have been discouraged or terminated because of the high maternal mortality rate.

•Results: No maternal mortality in 25 pregnancies in 13 patients, including the five pregnancies that underwent therapeutic abortion.

•The data lend support to the more optimistic opinion that these patients should have a favorable outcome.

•Differences in maternal mortality may have been related to reporting bias, because most of the patients in 1978 had symptoms and had more severe disease (average survival after onset of symptoms in aortic stenosis is <5 years).

•Recent case reports of congenital aortic stenosis in pregnancy also tended to focus on patients with severe disease, especially those requiring cardiac intervention and having adverse maternal outcome.

•The current series, reflecting total experience since 1986 in patients with congenital aortic valvular stenosis, may be more representative of the spectrum of this condition as seen in clinical practice today.

•As for perinatal loss, the often-quoted figure of 32% included abortions.

•Once abortions were excluded, the fetal loss was 0% in the current series.

•The incidence of preterm birth among all the reported pregnancies was 5% (4/82).

•**For the fetus the greatest risk is probably congenital heart disease.**

•The 5% to 26% risk of congenital heart disease justifies a fetal echocardiogram performed before 20 weeks' gestation to search for significant fetal cardiac anomalies.

•The presence of other congenital heart lesions in the mother can be a significant additional risk.

- The association of aortic stenosis with coarctation of the aorta has not been discussed in the obstetric literature.

  ° Coarctation of the aorta is commonly associated with bicuspid aortic valves; it was found in 31% of these patients.

- Although a history of aortic coarctation is not predictive of severity of aortic stenosis, it does suggest increased risk because correction of the coarctation does not necessarily prevent associated complications such as dissection of the aorta or rupture of cerebral aneurysms

- The major maternal concern in patients with congenital aortic stenosis is deterioration in their cardiac status.

- Three of 11 patients (27%) in class I had deterioration during pregnancy; in one of these patients deterioration occurred once during a multiple gestation and once after successful completion of a singleton pregnancy.

- Also, both patients who required therapeutic abortion for cardiac indications had deterioration very early in gestation.

- Early monitoring of cardiac status in pregnancies complicated by aortic stenosis is essential, especially in patients with severe stenosis.

- **Antepartum functional classification should not be the sole predictor of cardiac deterioration.**

- **Echocardiographic assessment**, which correlates well with cardiac catheterization assessment, which in turn correlates well with cardiac catheterization studies, should be used in all patients.

- In general, and especially in pregnancy, echocardiographically calculated valve area is a better index of severity than is pressure gradient estimation alone, because the latter can be exaggerated by the high-flow state of pregnancy and by combined aortic stenosis and regurgitation, yielding a so-called "pseudocritical stenosis."

- In patients with aortic stenosis, **pulmonary congestion** may occur secondary to left ventricular failure, which can be made manifest or exacerbated by the hypervolemia of pregnancy.

- Evidence of pulmonary congestion should be treated promptly.

- Also, a **decrease in venous return** because of hypovolemia, vasodilatation, or inferior vena caval obstruction, especially in the peripartum period, can lead to low cardiac output and sudden death.

- These causes of decreased venous return must be prevented and rapidly corrected should they occur.

- An invasive cardiac intervention may be required for patients whose cardiac status deteriorates during pregnancy.

- **Balloon valvuloplasty**, used successfully in severe mitral stenosis in pregnancy and in aortic stenosis in nonpregnant patients at high risk for aortic valve replacement, has been reported previously in two patients with aortic stenosis in pregnancy.

- In an additional report "valvuloplasty" (type not specified) performed at 30 weeks' gestation was associated with preterm labor 2 weeks later with delivery of a healthy infant.

- Because balloon valvuloplasty is appropriate only in patients without significant aortic regurgitation and whose valves are not heavily calcified, open surgical valvuloplasty or valvular replacement may be necessary in other patients.

•In two reports there were no maternal deaths in 11 patients with aortic valve replacement although the overall maternal mortality related to cardiac surgery with cardiopulmonary bypass was 1.5%.

•In contrast, the overall fetal mortality with open heart surgery varied between 16% (11/68) and 20% (9/45) and was as low as 10% in cases performed after 1969.

•Aortic valve replacement in particular seems to be associated with exceptionally high fetal loss, 40% (4/10) in the whole group and 57% (4/7) in patients with aortic stenosis.

•Thus open heart surgery during pregnancy for aortic stenosis is probably a last resort.

•These results indicate that, although deterioration in functional cardiac status may occur in patients with congenital aortic stenosis, the maternal and perinatal outcome is much less dismal than previously reported, if proper maternal monitoring is available and intervention is provided when necessary.

•In indicated patients therapeutic abortion appears to be a safe option.

•Fetal echocardiography is indicated in all patients with continued pregnancies because of the increased risk of congenital heart disease in the offspring.]

---

21. Near term, the maximal oxytocin concentration in maternal blood occurs about

    A. 2:00 a.m.
    B. 8:00 a.m.
    C. 4:00 p.m.
    D. 10:00 p.m.
    *E. midnight.

---

p. 419 (Hirst J J, Haluska G J, Cook M J, Novy M J. Plasma oxytocin and nocturnal uterine activity: Maternal but not fetal concentrations increased progressively during later pregnancy and delivery in rhesus monkeys. Am J Obstet Gynec 1993; 169:415)

21. [F & I: •Background: Pregnant rhesus monkeys and women with normal pregnancies have 24-h rhythms in uterine activity with episodes of increased uterine activity during the hours of darkness.

•Episodes of nocturnal uterine activity are correlated with elevated concentrations of oxytocin in the maternal plasma and were abolished by oxytocin antagonist infusions.

•Elevated oxytocin levels in the maternal circulation are responsible for the generation of these episodes in rhesus monkeys.

•Nocturnal uterine activity episodes are most pronounced on the several nights preceding the spontaneous onset of labor; it is possible this activity contributes to the initiation of labor at night, which is typical for rhesus monkeys.

•The sensitivity of the myometrium to oxytocin increases progressively during late gestation; the contribution of maternal or fetal nocturnal oxytocin secretion to changing patterns in nocturnal uterine activity has not been investigated at multiple time points during late gestation.

•Whether oxytocin crosses the placenta during late gestation remains controversial, and the role of fetal oxytocin in stimulating uterine activity in primates or women is unknown, since previous studies were based on maternal and fetal comparisons only at delivery or at cesarean section.

•Because there are rapid changes in oxytocin concentrations at delivery, erroneous conclusions may be drawn from a comparison of maternal and fetal oxytocin levels on the basis of cord blood sampling.

•The action of fetal oxytocin in the control of uterine activity has not previously been investigated in primates that are unanesthetized and chronically catheterized.

- **Objective:** To elucidate the roles of maternal and fetal oxytocin in the development of nocturnal uterine activity episodes during late pregnancy.

- The possibility that fetal oxytocin concentrations display circadian variation or contribute to maternal levels was also addressed.

- The maternal plasma oxytocin concentrations observed during daylight hours were similar to those previously reported for pregnant rhesus monkeys and for women in late pregnancy not in labor.

- The maximal oxytocin concentrations, observed around **midnight**, are also consistent with levels previously reported for catheterized rhesus monkeys.

- There is little evidence of pulsatile variations in oxytocin concentrations.

- Nocturnal uterine activity episodes are closely correlated with elevated concentrations of oxytocin, suggesting that these episodes are driven by oxytocin in the maternal plasma.

- The pivotal role of oxytocin in the generation of nocturnal uterine activity is supported by the observation that these episodes are abolished by oxytocin antagonist treatment in rhesus monkeys.

- The proportion of animals that display a nocturnal peak in uterine activity increases steadily during late gestation, particularly during the 10 days immediately before spontaneous labor.

- The current finding of a parallel progressive rise in nocturnal uterine activity and oxytocin concentrations with advancing gestation indicates that the increasing levels of uterine activity result in part from rising nocturnal oxytocin concentrations in the maternal plasma as term approaches.

- The finding that there was no increase in daytime oxytocin concentrations with advancing gestation is in agreement with previous studies in rhesus monkeys and pregnant women.

- Although both the levels of uterine activity and oxytocin rise in parallel at night during late gestation, there is some divergence from complete parallelism in this relationship at term.

- In spite of markedly higher levels of nocturnal uterine activity near parturition, there was no further increase in nocturnal oxytocin concentrations on the night before vaginal delivery or in the 1- to 3-h period before delivery compared with the levels attained between 150 to 156 days of gestation (about 1 week before delivery).

- These observations suggest that the overall **myometrial oxytocin sensitivity also increases** substantially during the days immediately before delivery.

- Uterine responsiveness to oxytocin also exhibits a 24-h rhythm that coincides with the nocturnal rhythm in uterine activity.

- An increased responsiveness of term myometrium may also result from interactions with **prostaglandins**, which in turn depend on the development of an appropriate concentration of oxytocin receptors in the decidua.

- Oxytocin stimulates uterine prostaglandin $F_{2\alpha}$ production, particularly by the decidua, and an adequate prostaglandin response appears to be essential for the successful induction of labor with oxytocin.

- The combined effects of elevated nocturnal oxytocin secretion and enhanced myometrial sensitivity to oxytocin result in a crescendo of uterine activity on the nights immediately before the spontaneous initiation of labor.

- The increased magnitude of nocturnal oxytocin secretion near term in the rhesus monkey may represent the maternal drive to initiate labor at night.

- All animals were delivered during the hours of darkness, which is typical for rhesus monkeys.

- The possibility that increased nocturnal oxytocin secretion contributes to the timing of the initiation of spontaneous labor must also be considered in women.

- The observations that maternal oxytocin concentrations rose during the late second stage of labor are consistent with previous studies in women.

- The high levels of oxytocin attained during expulsion of the fetus probably resulted from the additive effects of nocturnal oxytocin secretion and the stimulation of further oxytocin secretion by the **Ferguson reflex**.

- Stimulation of estrogen production by the fetoplacental unit leads to the enhancement of nocturnal uterine activity, whereas the experimental suppression of estrogen production has been found to abolish episodes of nocturnal uterine activity.

- Rising estrogen concentrations during late pregnancy play a support nocturnal uterine activity.

- Because estrogens promote the development of **myometrial oxytocin receptors**, estrogens likely support nocturnal uterine activity by inducing a heightened myometrial sensitivity.

- Estrogens also have a stimulatory effect at the level of the hypothalamus and pituitary, resulting in increased oxytocin synthesis and release into the circulation.

- No change was found in fetal plasma oxytocin concentration during the hours of darkness, indicating that, unlike the mother, the fetus does **not** display cyclic changes in oxytocin levels.

- The absence of a rise in fetal oxytocin concentrations during episodes of nocturnal uterine activity or during labor also indicates that oxytocin secretion by the fetus is unlikely to contribute to the generation of nocturnal uterine activity or to the initiation and maintenance of labor.

- Graded infusions of oxytocin into the fetal circulation raised fetal plasma levels more than fifty-fold had no effect on maternal oxytocin concentrations or on uterine activity, suggesting that fetal oxytocin does **not** cross the primate placenta during late gestation.

- The current results do not exclude the remote possibility that during delivery some oxytocin escapes from the fetal circulation and may influence uterine activity.

- Human studies have suggested the ability of pharmacologic doses given by intraumbilical injection to aid in placental expulsion, but the results have been highly variable.

- The findings with graded oxytocin infusions in chronically catheterized animals indicate that even supranormal levels of oxytocin in the fetal circulation do not elicit uterine contractions during late gestation and suggest that fetal oxytocin does not contribute to processes leading to the initiation of labor.

- The rising nocturnal plasma concentration may be a key maternal influence leading to the initiation of labor at night in primates.]

22. Which of the following is the best predictor of neonatal survival in extremely low birth weight infants?

   *A. Biparietal diameter.
   B. Birth weight.
   C. Estimated fetal weight.
   D. Femur length.
   E. Pediatric estimate of gestational age.

p. 490 (Smith R S, Bottoms S F. Ultrasonographic prediction of neonatal survival in extremely low-birth-weight infants. Am J Obstet Gynec 1993; 169:490)

22. [F & I: •Background: Fewer than 1% of infants have birth weights <1000 g but up to 50% of mortality among structurally normal infants occurs in this group.

•Approximately 30% of the survivors have a significant permanent handicap requiring expensive financial support.

•Parents' expectations, the opinions of other medical professionals, and medicolegal considerations may encourage active intervention even when the prospects for intact survival are minimal.

•The chances for survival of infants weighing <1000 g have greatly improved.

•Approximately 60% survive, ranging from <10% weighing below 500 g to 80% weighing from 900 to 1000 g.

•Although maturity is more important for survival than birth weight, inconsistencies and current limitations in methods, such as the known inaccuracy of the Ballard examination before 28 weeks, have made survival rates that are based on gestational age subject to great variation.

•Consequently, the obstetrician frequently relies on survival rates that are based on birth weight.

•Clinical estimates of fetal weight are often inaccurate, and ultrasonographic fetal weight determination is associated with a mean error of at least 10% to 15% among fetuses weighing <1000 g.

•Underestimating fetal weight influences obstetric management and is associated with higher perinatal mortality rates.

•Correlating ultrasonographic biometry directly to neonatal survival might improve the accuracy of neonatal prognosis by avoiding some of the error inherent in estimating fetal weight.

•Objectives: To evaluate ultrasonographic measurements as predictors of neonatal survival and to compare them with estimated fetal weight, actual birth weight, and pediatric assessment of maturity.

•Results: Using BPD to determine neonatal prognosis is significantly more reliable than the current practice of using estimated fetal weight.

•The BPD is surprisingly accurate in predicting survival.

•It performed as well as actual birth weight and better than pediatric assessment of gestational age.

•This finding was consistent throughout the analysis.

•Using receiver-operator characteristic curves, controlling for the method of delivery, or comparing critical cut points all yielded the same conclusion.

•Comparing the predicted numbers of nonsurvivors was particularly convincing.

- Estimating prognosis on the basis of estimated fetal weight from survival tables that are based on actual birth weight is a two-step process.

- The error inherent in calculating estimated fetal weight can only compound the uncertainty of basing prognosis on actual birth weight.

- This does not explain why estimated fetal weight was less accurate than BPD in this study, because estimated fetal weight was correlated directly with neonatal survival.

- A better explanation is that **survival is more closely related to maturity than to size.**

- The smallest survivors frequently have fetal growth retardation, a condition in which growth of the head is often spared.

- Estimated fetal weight emphasizes abdominal circumference, the measurement most susceptible to alterations in growth and least well correlated with gestational age.

- BPD is also measured more accurately than estimated fetal weight; this could have important clinical implications.

  ° For example, with a mean error of 10% in estimated fetal weight, errors of ≥20% are encountered in some cases.

  ° A 20% underestimation of fetal weight in a 600 g infant would result in an estimated fetal weight of 480 g, and possibly there would be little or no intervention on the basis of fetal indications.

  ° An infant of this size would probably have a BPD of about 60 mm.

- The 95% confidence interval for BPD measurement has been estimated to average ±5 mm throughout pregnancy, with lesser degrees of error in early gestation.

- A 20% (12 mm) error in measuring BPD would be extremely unlikely.

- It is important to appreciate the limitations of applying these results to clinical practice.

- Extreme dolicocephaly or brachycephaly might be expected to decrease the accuracy of prognosis on the basis of BPD, although these conditions were not excluded.

- Early pregnancy dating and medical or obstetric complications were not considered in this analysis.

- With major advances such as surfactant replacement there is continued improvement in neonatal prognosis.

- Hopefully, current thresholds for neonatal survival will be obsolete within a few years.]

---

23. Factors predictive of successful external cephalic version near term include

    A. breech at station -1.
    B. maternal weight greater than 200 pounds.
    *C. parity greater than 2.
    D. tocolytic therapy.
    E. type of breech.

p. 247 (Newman R B, Peacock B S, VanDorsten J P, Hunt H H. Predicting success of external cephalic version. Am J Obstet Gynec 1993; 169:245)

23. [F & I: •Background: External cephalic version is described in the writings of Hippocrates and was commonly performed earlier in this century.

•It fell from favor because of unacceptably high complication rates and failure to improve on the relatively high spontaneous version rate.

•During the last decade external cephalic version at term was resurrected with success rates of 60% to 70% with parallel reductions in the incidence of breech presentation in labor and subsequent cesarean delivery.

•Objective: To review external cephalic versions between 1984 and 1986 to identify maternal and fetal variables that influence the outcome of this procedure.

•This retrospective analysis was used to develop a prognostic scoring system, which was then prospectively tested on the women admitted for external cephalic version between October 1986 and October 1992.

•Methods: Patients admitted to labor and delivery underwent a real-time ultrasonographic examination, a nonstress test, and a pelvic examination.

•The ultrasonographic examination was to confirm a nonvertex presentation, the adequacy of the amniotic fluid volume (pocket ≥2 cm in vertical diameter), fetal measurements consistent with a term gestation, and estimated fetal weight.

•Ultrasonography was also used to confirm the absence of any gross fetal anomalies and to identify placental location.

•Placental location was described as being anterior, posterior, fundal, or lateral.

•After obtaining a reactive nonstress test or negative contraction stress test, an intravenous line was established for infusion of ritodrine hydrochloride at 100 µg/min.

•In the latter years of the investigation a 250 µg subcutaneous injection of terbutaline sulfate was substituted for the intravenous ritodrine hydrochloride.

•In five patients with insulin-requiring diabetes magnesium sulfate was used intravenously for tocolysis.

•After 20 min the external cephalic version was attempted by two operators.

•The "forward roll" technique was usually attempted if the fetal head crossed the maternal midline.

•The "back flip" was used if the initial method failed or occasionally as the initial technique if the fetus did not cross the midline.

•Version attempts were discontinued for excessive patient discomfort, for a persistently abnormal fetal heart rate tracing, or after multiple failed attempts.

•Real-time ultrasonography confirmed version outcome before discontinuation of tocolytic therapy.

•For Rh-negative, unsensitized patients Rh immune globulin was administered after version.

•After the procedure fetal heart rate monitoring was continued until a reactive nonstress test was obtained.

•Anesthesia and immediate operative facilities were available throughout the external cephalic version.

- There were few absolute contraindications to external cephalic version, but these included abruptio placentae, placenta previa, premature rupture of the membranes, or evidence of fetal compromise during preliminary fetal heart rate monitoring.

- Transverse lie, prior uterine scar, or maternal weight ≥200 pounds were not considered contraindications to external cephalic version.

- On the basis of experience and previous reports in the literature, 10 potentially influential maternal and fetal variables were selected for analysis as prognostic factors: these factors were

    ° (1) maternal weight,

    ° (2) parity,

    ° (3) gestational age,

    ° (4) type of breech (frank, complete, incomplete, or transverse lie),

    ° (5) amniotic fluid volume (oligohydramnios, average, or polyhydramnios),

    ° (6) placental location (anterior, posterior, lateral, or fundal),

    ° (7) cervical dilatation,

    ° (8) cervical effacement,

    ° (9) station of presenting part, and

    ° (10) the estimated fetal weight at the time of the external cephalic version.

- By means of these 10 variables, an initial stepwise linear regression analysis was performed on the 108 women who had undergone external cephalic version to determine those variables correlating best with procedure success.

- Increasing fetal weight is associated with greater success, presumably because of an improved ability to manipulate the fetus.

- Estimation of **fetal weight** will be the most difficult variable to determine in the scoring system.

    ° With the increasing use of ultrasonography an acceptable margin of error should be achieved, especially considering the wide birth weight categories.

- A patient who would not be a candidate for vaginal delivery because of gross **macrosomia** may need to be reconsidered as a version candidate.

- The effect of placental location on the success of external cephalic version has probably been the most controversial.

- Posterior, lateral, and fundal placentas were more frequently associated with success than were anterior placentas.

    ° Cornual implantations would be considered as either fundal or lateral depending on the predominant location.

- There were no successes in cases where descent of the breech into the pelvis reached a -1 station or lower.

- The great controversy in the literature regarding prognostic factors suggests that no one variable will optimally predict procedure success.

•In fact, when the individual components of the external cephalic version scoring system and other clinical factors not included in the scoring system were evaluated in the 266 breech presentations tested prospectively, no single factor really stood out other than **deep descent of the breech into the pelvis and maternal parity of two or more.**

•The proposed scoring system is not all inclusive; rather, it addresses clinical variables that can be easily evaluated on every external cephalic version candidate.

•The predictive accuracy of any scoring system will be best for those patients from which it was derived.

•Much like the confirmation of the Zatuchni-Andros score in predicting the likelihood of successful vaginal breech delivery at term, the true value of any scoring system is found in its prospective application.

•The performance of this predictive scoring system was acceptable when it was applied prospectively to the next 266 women with breech presentations undergoing external cephalic version.

•There was a positive relationship between a rising version score and the likelihood of procedure success.

•There were no successful versions with a score ≤2, and all breech versions were successful with a score of 9 or 10.

•Approximately 35% of the women in the prospective trial had a version score of ≤4 or ≥8 where the likelihood of success was either significantly worse or better than for the remainder of the study group.

•The women with transverse lies were excluded because the retrospective evaluation was specifically designed to predict the success of external breech version and because the **overall success rate for external version of the transverse lie is generally higher, ranging from 80% to 90%.**

°In this investigation 90% of the transverse lies undergoing external cephalic version were successful.

•On the basis of the prospective of evaluation of this external cephalic version scoring system, the women scoring ≤4 may simply not be candidates for external cephalic version.

•Appropriate delivery plans should be made and a costly and futile attempt at version avoided.

•Alternatively, those women with favorable scores of ≥8 would appear to be optimal candidates, with success rates significantly greater than those generally quoted.

•This scoring system is an easily applicable and quantifiable tool that can improve both physician selection of version candidates and patient informed consent in over one third of breech presentations undergoing external cephalic version.]

---

24. In managing a gestational diabetic patient if all fasting glucose levels are normal, the 2-h postprandial blood sugar in is predictive of

    A. larger for gestational age fetus.
    B. macrosomia.
    C. need for cesarean section.
    D. shoulder dystocia.
    *E. none of the above.

---

p. 262 (Huddleston J F, Cramer M K, Vroon D H. A rationale for omitting two-hour postprandial glucose determinations in gestational diabetes. Am J Obstet Gynec 1993; 169:257)

Obstetrics and Gynecology: Review 1994-Obstetrics References

24. [F & I: •Background: Gestational diabetes is a state of deranged carbohydrate metabolism first discovered during pregnancy.

•Maternal gestational adaptations include many hormonal changes that promote insulin resistance.

•Pregnancy is diabetogenic.

•Carbohydrate metabolism is increasingly stressed during the second half of pregnancy.

•Most pregnant women are able to produce insulin in amounts adequate to overcome this stress, but 2% to 3% of pregnant women cannot do so and become functionally, and usually temporarily, glucose intolerant.

•The fetus is subjected to an environment that contains excessive concentrations of glucose and amino acids, those metabolic fuels normally controlled by maternal insulin.

•The usual fetal response to these excesses is an exaggerated output of insulin, a major fetal growth hormone.

•Uncontrolled gestational diabetes mellitus can increase perinatal morbidity and, rarely, mortality.

•Risks to the neonate include macrosomia, birth trauma, hypoglycemia, hypocalcemia, polycythemia, and hyperbilirubinemia.

•Obstetric complications include hydramnios, preeclampsia, cesarean delivery, and preterm labor, which is made more serious in gestational diabetes mellitus by the tendency to delayed lung maturity.

•Many of the perinatal complications are attributable to fetal hyperglycemia and its consequent hyperinsulinemia.

• Better understanding of gestational diabetes mellitus has resulted in standardized management protocols that have reduced the risk of perinatal mortality to the level found in pregnancies without this complication.

•Currently accepted management is based on strict attention to glycemic control, which in most cases can be achieved by following an appropriate American Diabetes Association diet.

•Patients typically are monitored with fasting and 2-hour postprandial plasma glucose values, and those who do not achieve or maintain adequate control with diet alone are placed on insulin.

•Fasting plasma glucose conditions are reasonably easy to define and control.

•The 2-h postprandial glucose test is subject to variations in composition of the breakfast and in timing of the venipuncture.

•The current protocol recommended by The American College of Obstetricians and Gynecologists suggests a fasting plasma glucose level of 105 mg/dl and a 2-h postprandial glucose of 120 mg/dl as threshold values for consideration of insulin therapy.

•Objectives: To answer three questions: (1) How well does the fasting plasma glucose predict the 2-h postprandial level, especially if the fasting value is normal?

•(2) For patients with all normal tasting plasma glucose values, are there outcome differences between those with normal and those with elevated 2-h postprandial glucose values?

•(3) Is the 2-h postprandial glucose test really necessary?

•Fact   °Detail   »issue   *answer

•If some or all 2-h postprandial testing could be safely omitted, patients with gestational diabetes mellitus would avoid the discomfort, expense, and inconvenience associated with the additional venipunctures.

•Control of gestational diabetes mellitus is believed to be important in avoiding complications.

•The ideal management scheme and appropriate threshold glucose values for beginning insulin have yet to be firmly established.

•Some protocols suggest prophylactic insulin for many or all patients, some managing patients with fasting plasma glucose alone, others with the 2-h postprandial glucose alone, and several suggesting even tighter glycemic control than the current American College of Obstetricians and Gynecologists suggestions.

•Suggested glucose monitoring has ranged from one value taken at a weekly or biweekly visit to seven values per day by means of home monitoring.

•Results: Only 5% of 2-h postprandial glucose results after a normal (<105 mg/dl) fasting plasma glucose will be ≥140 mg/dl.

•The uncertainty of breakfast composition and timing may further discourage reliance on 2-h postprandial data.

•Because patients with 2-h postprandial glucose elevations alone are typically not placed on insulin, these values are of minimal diagnostic help, so that the cost and inconvenience to the patient are probably unwarranted.

•Similarly, of those with a fasting plasma glucose value ≥110 mg/dl, 73% will also have an elevated 2-hour postprandial value but would have insulin therapy initiated on the basis of the fasting value alone.

•The lack of any significant difference among the tested outcome measures suggests that, **if the fasting plasma glucose level is persistently normal and the result is available while the patient is still in the clinic or office, the 2-h postprandial glucose test can be safely eliminated from the management protocol.**

•In this study a cost savings of nearly $10,000 could have been realized and directed toward other clinical needs.

•This change in testing scheme would result in no apparent compromise of the ability to correctly identify those gestational diabetics requiring insulin and with no apparent increased risk of poor outcome.]

---

25. Of the following the procedure which best predicts abruptio placentae **early** on is

   *A. D-dimer slide test.
   B. determination of low amplitude-high frequency contractions by tocodynamometer.
   C. determination of partial thromboplastin time.
   D. doppler color flow studies of placental bed.
   E. ultrasonic imaging.

p. 267 (Nolan T E, Smith R P, Devoe L D. A rapid test for abruptio placentae: Evaluation of a D-dimer latex agglutination slide test. Am J Obstet Gynec 1993; 169:265)

25. [F & I: •Background: Early diagnosis of abruptio placentae can be difficult because its typical signs and symptoms, such as vaginal bleeding, increased uterine tone and tenderness, and fetal distress, are often late manifestations.

•Early symptoms of abruptio placentae may be confused with preterm or prodromal term labor.

- Ultrasonography and standard laboratory measures of coagulation factors rarely clarify the diagnosis of abruptio placentae until the process is well advanced.

- As abruptio placentae progresses, there is increasing placental site hemorrhage and local consumption of factors responsible for clot formation, stabilization, and lysis.

- In this process, fibrinogen is converted to fibrin; fibrin complexes are formed and then cleaved, which results in the generation of D-dimer.

- The detection of D-dimer may be an early marker for abruptio placentae.

- Objective: To evaluate a recently developed rapid latex agglutination slide test for the detection of D-dimer and its use as a potential screening method for abruptio placentae.

- This investigation was performed in groups of patients who were without complications, who had abruptio placentae, or who had conditions that could be associated with possible coagulation factor abnormalities such as preeclampsia and preterm labor.

- The management of abruptio placentae is best served by early diagnosis and treatment, which may be impeded because its clinical signs mimic more common benign conditions such as bloody show and early labor.

- By the time vaginal bleeding, uterine tenderness, or uterine hypertonus has appeared, fetal hypoxia or asphyxia may have occurred already, thereby resulting in brain damage or death.

- Laboratory tests have limited value in early diagnosis of abruptio placentae.

- It was anticipated that ultrasonographic imaging would aid in the diagnosis of abruptio placentae.

- Available case reports suggest that this has proved difficult because of wide variation in the manifestations of abruptio placentae.

- Marginal placental detachments have been correctly diagnosed in as many as 60% of cases, but these are usually accompanied by vaginal bleeding.

- **Ultrasonographic diagnosis** of abruptio placentae is difficult when a retroplacental hematoma is present because its echogenic image is similar to that of normal placental tissue.

- This technique was shown to have a sensitivity of only 29% in a large series.

- The addition of **Doppler color flow** studies of the placental bed may be of value.

   ° This application is yet unproved and requires special expertise that is not usually available during labor and delivery.

- **Electronic fetal monitoring** measures important variables that may be affected by abruptio placentae.

   ° Fetal heart rate and uterine pressure tracings reflect uteroplacental blood flow and fetal well-being.

- Abruptio placentae can be characterized by **certain uterine contraction** patterns such as low-amplitude, high-frequency contractions, high-frequency, high-amplitude contractions ("irritable uterus"), and increased uterine tone.

- None of these findings is either sensitive to or pathognomonic for abruptio placentae.

- Abruptio placentae is a major cause of obstetric disseminated intravascular coagulation.

- The degree of placental separation or the amount of retroplacental bleeding is usually directly related to consumption of coagulation factors.

- Thrombocytopenia, hypofibrinogenemia, and consumption of clotting factors measured indirectly with prolonged prothrombin and partial thromboplastin time give indirect evidence of disseminated intravascular coagulation.

- Unfortunately, no prior studies have indicated that any of these tests are particularly accurate; or are they considered early indicators of abruptio placentae.

- The role of fibrinogen in the coagulation cascade has been well described.

- Fibrinogen, activated in the presence of platelets or tissue phospholipids, is converted to fibrin, which occludes defects in vessel walls or disrupted tissue.

- In the presence of fibrin stabilizing factor, fibrin crosslinks are formed, and the clot stabilizes.

- When fibrin is digested during clot lysis, a breakdown product, D-dimer, is released.

- D-dimer fragments arc cross-linked at set intervals, which allows for their quantification distinct from other released fragments.

- Consequently, D-dimer is increasingly being used as a test to determine the presence of fibrinogen breakdown in consumptive coagulation syndromes.

- Although the D-dimer test results were positive in only 67% of the cases with abruptio placentae, this performance level was clearly superior to that provided by the other standard tests.

- In at least eight (53%) of these cases the degree of abruptio placentae was relatively slight (~10%).

- Although these results were encouraging, the fact remains that one third of the cases with clinically confirmed abruptio placentae were associated with negative results.

- Four of the five patients in this group had a 10% abruptio placentae, and the fifth had a 20% abruptio placentae.

- Another possible explanation for the false-negative results is that the abruptio placentae was proceeding so rapidly at the time of blood sampling that clot lysis had not yet occurred to a significant degree and minimal amounts of D-dimer had been formed.

- This preliminary study is encouraging because the D-dimer test is quite simple and rapid to perform.

- It appears to offer a potential method to evaluate patients in whom abruptio placentae must be distinguished from other clinical conditions.

- Clearly, these data need to be confirmed by larger studies.

- The findings of positive D-dimer test results in patients with preeclampsia is consistent with earlier reports.

- It is also intriguing that approximately one fifth of the patients in preterm labor had positive results.

- This suggests the possibility that this condition may be triggered occasionally by subclinical abruptio placentae which may be an investigative avenue worth pursuing.]

26. Complications from the use of uterine packing to control postpartum hemorrhage include

   A. concealed hemorrhage.
   B. delayed hemorrhage.
   C. infertility.
   D. sepsis.
   *E. none of the above.

---

p. 320 (Control of postpartum hemorrhage with uterine packing. (Maier R C.. Am J Obstet Gynec 1993; 169:317)

26. [F & I: •Background: Postpartum hemorrhage is a sudden, potentially life threatening event.

•Unusual and frequently unpredictable in its occurrence, expedient and thorough management is essential.

•After passage of the placenta and lacerations of the genital tract have been excluded, the physician's management is directed at methods to increase uterine muscular tone (contraction) to stop the hemorrhage.

•Objective: To present nine patients with postpartum uterine hemorrhage treated with uterine packing.

•Because of the clinical situation, postpartum uterine hemorrhage will be difficult to investigate in a randomized study.

•In a matter of minutes the clinical condition can evolve into a state of urgency.

•These nine patients and reports from the past medical literature permit some contemporary thought on the procedure.

•Historically, the practice of uterine packing for postpartum hemorrhage was endorsed by many standard textbooks of the 1930s and 1940s.

•The practice fell out of widespread use from the 1960s to the 1980s.

•Reports of its successful use continued to appear.

•Since the mid-1980s most articles in the obstetric literature have made no specific reference to uterine packing, while promoting several medical and surgical therapies.

•A recent American College of Obstetricians and Gynecologists Technical Bulletin briefly referred to uterine packing in control of postpartum hemorrhage as a technique that is being "abandoned."

•The variation in these opinions has been proposed to be best explained by differences in technique.

•If DeLee and Greenhill in the 1940s could identify 398 cases of postpartum hemorrhage successfully treated by uterine packing out of a total of 400, the procedure must have merit.

•The technique of uterine packing has been explained by these authors as a careful attempt to pack all areas of the uterine cavity in a uniform, consistent manner.

•Aside from not being physiologic, historic objections to the postpartum uterus being packed have been the fear of infection and concealed hemorrhage.

•In the nine patients in this paper and in the references provided, the procedure has been rarely associated with concealed hemorrhage when properly performed.

- In the successful cases provided in this study the patient's bleeding ceased, clotting disorders (if present) resolved, and once the patient was stabilized no further clinical deterioration occurred.

- With removal of the pack, which was invariably deeply stained with serosanguinous fluid, there was no further bleeding and no expressible clots.

- In contrast to the fear of concealed hemorrhage, on review of the medical records of these patients a poorly controlled clinical dilemma on the brink of a major abdominal surgery resolved in instances where the bleeding was controlled by uterine packing.

- If the procedure was not successful, it was clinically apparent during the immediate time after the procedure was completed.

- There are no examples in these nine cases, and rarely in the reviewed literature, of concealed hemorrhage.

- In theory, uterine packing would seem to be a predisposition for uterine infection.

- The presence of a foreign body in the uterine cavity could be proposed as a nidus for bacterial proliferation.

- In the older literature efforts were made to use medically treated gauze, probably out of fear of infection.

- In the nine cases in this report and those from recent literature no antiseptic solutions were used on the packing material, but antibiotics were administered parenterally during and after the procedure.

- There have been no incidences of serious infections.

- This favorable condition is likely because of the packing being removed in a short period of time or the use of antibiotics.

- The knowledge that patients observed for weeks to years after the procedure have been free of any related gynecologic complaints is reassuring that no chronic inflammatory process has occurred.

- In many instances, patients desiring pregnancy have been able to conceive.

- No precise data on fertility potential exist regarding patients treated by uterine packing.

- Uterine packing can be considered for control of hemorrhage secondary to uterine atony, placenta accreta, and placenta previa.

- In the single provided example of endomyometritis, packing of the uterine cavity was safely accomplished.

- There should be no inference made that this procedure must be used in all instances of postpartum hemorrhage.

- Because > 1000 cases where uterine packing was used for postpartum hemorrhage are available in the cited references, with a successful outcome in the great majority, the procedure seems reasonable for the control of postpartum hemorrhage.

- To use uterine packing early in the management of postpartum hemorrhage or as a "last resort" before abdominal surgery is a judgment best decided by the treating physician.

- The instrument used in this paper was a Torpin packer, which is a canister modification of the Holmes packer.

- DeLee et al. described using packing forceps with a hand in the uterus.

- Cavanagh used either uterine packing forceps or the Brodhead packer.

- Apparently no instrument is a "must have," but rather an effort should be made to pack the uterine cavity completely and uniformly.

- The interval until removal of the pack is not fixed and can vary depending on the clinical situation.

» The patient should be medically stable.

- In this report of nine patients the earliest removal was 5 h and the latest was 96 h.

- Accepting the experience of medical forefathers, 24 to 36 h seems reasonable.

- To be forced to perform major surgery, which may include a hysterectomy, under the worst of clinical conditions on a patient who desires more children is not an enviable position for any obstetrician.

- This is unfortunately the plight of the physician in some instances of postpartum hemorrhage.

- Having excluded genital lacerations and with placental removal, the integration of uterine packing into the management choices for the control of postpartum hemorrhage seems reasonable and presents little risk to the patient.]

---

27. At five weeks following a term normal spontaneous vaginal delivery, a patient has a curettage for delayed postpartum hemorrhage. The most likely interpretation of the tissue retrieved by that procedure is

    A. decidua.
    B. endometritis.
    C. involution of the placental bed.
    D. normal endometrium.
*E. retained placental tissue.

---

p. 18 (Khong T Y, Khong T K. Delayed postpartum hemorrhage: A morphologic study of causes and their relation to other pregnancy disorders. Obstet Gynecol 1993; 82:17)

27. [F & I: •Background: Postpartum bleeding occurring after the first 24 h, termed variously as secondary, late, or delayed bleeding, has received less attention than postpartum bleeding within the first 24 h, presumably because it usually causes maternal morbidity rather than mortality.

- Many causes may lead to delayed postpartum hemorrhage, but subinvolution of the placental bed may have "superceded all other etiologic factors as to frequency of incidence and gravity of consequences."

- The diagnosis is a pathologic one, requiring the histologic finding of subinvoluted placental bed vessels in the absence of retained fetal products.

- Although first recognized in 1945, relatively little has been written on the subject since 1961.

- Despite advances in the management of labor, no contemporary study has evaluated the incidence of this diagnosis or other causes of delayed postpartum hemorrhage.

- Although it is often assumed that delayed postpartum hemorrhage is due to retained products of conception, the frequency of detection of retained placental fragments ranges from 27-to-88%.

- Other common causes of delayed postpartum hemorrhage include placental polyps and infection.

- Objectives: To assess the various causes of delayed postpartum hemorrhage from a pathologic perspective.

- To test the hypothesis that subinvolution of the placental bed is associated with defective placentation.

- To examine the incidence of spontaneous abortion, fetal growth retardation (FGR), preeclampsia, and placenta accreta in previous pregnancies of women with subinvolution of the placental bed versus women with other causes of delayed postpartum hemorrhage.

- During normal placentation, the small-caliber spiral uterine arteries in the nonpregnant state are transformed by extravillous trophoblast into flaccid distended uteroplacental arteries to allow an adequate blood supply to the fetus and placenta.

- Defective placentation may underlie pregnancy disorders such as spontaneous abortion FGR preeclampsia, and placenta accreta, and aberrant maternal trophoblastic interaction in the placental bed may be a common pathogenetic feature.

- Postpartum hemorrhage is defined as delayed, secondary, or late when there is excessive blood loss from the genital tract after the first 24 h postpartum until 6 weeks after the birth.

  ° The upper limit is imposed because after 6 weeks, it is often difficult to determine whether bleeding is related to the previous delivery, to subsequent menstruation, or even to a spontaneous abortion of a new conception.

- Women were included whose hemorrhage occurred beyond the conventional upper limit of 6 weeks postpartum, for two reasons.

  ° First, bleeding may be a late phenomenon.

  ° Second, in those women who had involuted or subinvoluted placental bed, the morphology of the spiral arteries resembled that seen in the third trimester, with fibrinoid matrix in the walls of what were obviously previously distended uteroplacental arteries.

  ° Attribution of the bleeding to a subsequent pregnancy is unlikely.

  ° The morphology of the placental villi in the group with retained fragments was clearly that of the third trimester, with peripherally situated vasculosyncytial membranes, inconspicuous cytotrophoblast, and villous stroma, again rendering bleeding due to a subsequent pregnancy unlikely.

- It is difficult to discount the possibility that bleeding in the endometrium-only group could be due to subsequent menstruation when the bleeding occurred beyond 6 weeks.

- The definition of delayed postpartum hemorrhage is merely a subjective impression of an increased amount of bleeding after the first 24 hours, and up to 13% of patients may have persistent lochia at 60 days postpartum.

- Although some women in the decidua-only and endometrium-only groups may not have true postpartum hemorrhage for those reasons, why others should present with the symptom is not clearly understood because the hormonal influences on the puerperal uterus are not adequately known.

- It is inappropriate to compare pathologic causes of delayed postpartum hemorrhage with causes found in the literature, because changes in the management of labor and the western social trend toward smaller family size and older maternal age at the first pregnancy may affect the causes.

- **Results: Retained placental fragments were the most frequent histologic findings in tissue obtained at uterine evacuation for delayed postpartum bleeding.**

- Subinvoluted uteroplacental arteries were seen in 20 of 23 cases of retained placental fragments when maternal arteries were included in the curetted material.

- It is likely that the placental fragments prevent involution by a space occupying stenting effect, thereby allowing blood to percolate through these spiral arteries.

- Endometrial fragments were the next most frequent finding, followed by involuted placental bed and subinvoluted placental bed.

- Bleeding due to subinvolution of the placental bed can be explained as blood flowing through the patent or partially occluded vessels.

- Why women with an involuted placental bed present with hemorrhage is unclear, but this may be due to dislodgment of thrombi.

- Endometritis appears to be an **overstated** cause of postpartum hemorrhage.

- Less than 5% of cases were ascribable to endometritis, but there may have been more cases successfully treated by antibiotic therapy.

- Retained placental fragments were associated with an increased incidence of preeclampsia, FGR, spontaneous abortion, and placenta accreta in prior pregnancies.

- This is to be expected because retained placental fragments indicate a degree of placenta accreta, which has proven to be associated with abnormal maternal-fetal interaction in the placental bed.

- It could be argued that the choice of comparison subjects—those presenting with postpartum hemorrhage and endometrium only, decidua only, endometritis, or nondiagnostic tissue—may not be valid.

  ° These conditions are not known to be associated with aberrant maternal-trophoblastic interactions.

- A proportion of these women may not have true postpartum hemorrhage for the reasons stated earlier and would be expected to be comparable to women without postpartum hemorrhage insofar as controls are concerned.

- No relationship with previous adverse pregnancy complications could be found for women who had an involuted placental bed; this is in keeping with involution being a physiologic phenomenon.

- Subinvolution of the placental bed in the index pregnancy was also **not** associated with an increased incidence of preeclampsia, FGR, spontaneous abortion, or placenta accreta in previous pregnancies.

- This is somewhat surprising because this study confirmed previous morphologic studies that have hinted that subinvolution of the placental bed may be associated with an abnormal maternal-fetal relationship in the vessels in the placental bed.

- Intraluminally located endovascular trophoblast, pointing to an abnormal maternal-trophoblastic interaction at the placental bed vascular interface, has been reported in subinvolution of the placental bed but appeared more prominent in these cases; it also has been reported in the third trimester in preeclampsia and FGR.

- The discrepancy between the epidemiologic and morphologic findings is difficult to explain.

- Subinvolution of the placental bed may have less to do with abnormal maternal-fetal immunologic interactions and more to do with regression phenomena, such as necrosis and apoptosis, features that have not been studied systematically in relation to trophoblast disappearance postpartum.

- There are many other risks for postpartum hemorrhage.

•It is clear that subinvolution of the placental bed and retained placental fragments are major causes of delayed postpartum hemorrhage, and the latter may be associated with aberrant maternal trophoblastic interactions.]

---

28. Post-cesarean endometritis can be effectively prevented if

    A. there is a special skin prep with parachlorometaxylenol and saline lavage of the pelvic and subcutaneous tissue.
    B. there is a special skin prep with parachlorometaxylenol and no pelvic or subcutaneous irrigation.
    C. there is a standard skin preparation with povidone iodine and the normal saline lavage of the pelvic and subcutaneous tissue.
  *D. there is standard skin preparation and cefazolin irrigation of the pelvic and subcutaneous tissues.
    E. There is no evidence to show that either skin prep or pelvic lavage is effective in preventing endometritis.

---

p. 924 (Magann E F, Dodson M K, Ray M A, Harris R L, Martin, J N, Morrison J C. Preoperative skin preparation and intraoperative pelvic irrigation: Impact on post-cesarean endometritis and wound infection. Obstet Gynecol 1993; 81:922)

28. [F & I: •Background: The incidence of post-cesarean endometritis ranges from 20-to-85% in indigent patients.

•Subcutaneous wound infections occur in approximately 5% of patients following abdominal surgery and cesarean delivery.

•Intraabdominal and subcutaneous lavage with antibiotic solutions appears to reduce postoperative infectious morbidity in women at risk after cesarean birth.

•Operative antibiotic irrigation as an alternative method of prophylaxis against endometritis minimizes antibiotic exposure and is an inexpensive approach to a prevalent postoperative complication.

•Skin is impossible to sterilize.

•Proper preparation of an incision site involves removal of surface dirt and oil by a soap or detergent scrub plus application of a topical antimicrobial agent that will reduce the bacterial population to a minimal level.

•In nonpregnant surgical patients, the choice of surgical scrub and the duration of scrub time do not make any significant difference in the rate of wound infection in clean or clean-contaminated (such as cesarean skin incision) wounds.

•The time spent in skin cleansing varies considerably between hospitals and among obstetricians.

•Some obstetricians scrub the abdomen with a surgical scrub for 5 min or longer and then apply a bactericidal solution, whereas others scrub the incision area for 30-to-60 seconds followed by a bactericidal solution.

•Objective: To evaluate the effects of skin preparation alone and in combination with antibiotic irrigation in a socioeconomically disadvantaged population at high risk for the subsequent development of post-cesarean endometritis and wound infection.

•Methods: The study subjects were placed into one of four groups, involving the following: standard skin preparation (povidone-iodine surgical scrub [7.5%] followed by povidone-iodine [10%] solution) or special skin preparation (5-min scrub with parachlorometaxylenol followed by povidone scrub and solution), and either normal saline or antibiotic (cefazolin sodium, 1 g in 500 ml normal saline) irrigation of the pelvis and subcutaneous tissue at uterine closure and fascial closure, respectively.

•There were four treatment groups:

°standard preparation plus saline irrigation,

°standard preparation plus antibiotic irrigation,

°special preparation plus saline irrigation, and

°special preparation plus antibiotic irrigation.

•Prophylactic antibiotic irrigation of the pelvis and skin preparation have the potential to prevent postoperative infection.

•The bacterial contamination present at cesarean birth may be overwhelming and exceed host resistance, leading to postoperative infectious morbidity.

•This increases total costs and prolongs hospital stay through the use of multiple IV antibiotics and surgical wound debridement until the infection is resolved and the wound can be closed secondarily.

•A number of **obstetric factors** may contribute to a large bacterial inoculum:

°1) lengthy labor,

°2) rupture of the membranes and a long interval between rupture and operative delivery,

°3) a large number of vaginal examinations,

°4) the use of internal fetal scalp electrode and internal monitoring devices, and

°5) indigent status, regardless of race.

•**Operative factors** that affect post-cesarean infectious morbidity include

°the skill of the operating surgeon,

°procedure length,

°type of anesthesia,

°blood loss, and

°maternal obesity.

•**Antibiotic irrigation** of the pelvis and paracolic gutters appears to reduce the incidence of post-cesarean endometritis more than does saline irrigation.

•This study shows the superiority of antibiotic irrigation to saline irrigation for the reduction of post-cesarean endometritis.

•In nonpregnant surgical patients, a **prolonged abdominal scrub is not** superior to a 30-to-60-second scrub of povidone-iodine for preventing postoperative infection.

•This study did **not** find a difference in the incidence of subcutaneous infections even if the skin incision was irrigated with an antibiotic-containing solution before closure.

•Additional skin preparation with a surgical scrub was no better than a 30-to-60-second surgical povidone-iodine scrub followed by application of a povidone-iodine solution.

•Compared with standard preparation and saline irrigation, the combination of extra surgical scrub and antibiotic irrigation also did not reduce significantly the incidence of subcutaneous infection.

•Conclusion: Mechanical cleansing of the incision site with a surgical scrub in addition to an iodine surgical scrub and solution does **not** offer any distinct advantage in the reduction of post-cesarean endometritis or wound infection in this sample population.]

---

29. In mothers on methadone maintenance, neonatal plasma methadone levels are lower than maternal levels because

    A. extensive biotransformation takes place in the placenta.
    B. fetal enzymes are rapidly metabolized methadone.
    C. methadone levels are about the same in maternal and neonatal tissues.
    *D. placentally transferred methadone is rapidly stored in fetal tissues.
    E. plasma protein-bound methadone is increased in pregnancy.

---

p. 938 (Doberczak T M, Kandall S R, Friedmann P. Relationships between maternal methadone dosage, maternal-neonatal methadone levels and neonatal withdrawal. Obstet Gynecol 1993; 81:936)

29. [F & I: •Background: Not all infants born to opiate-using mothers have overt symptoms of withdrawal.

•In addition, when withdrawal does develop, its onset and course are unpredictable.

•A consistent relationship between neonatal opiate withdrawal and factors such as maternal drug dosage or maternal-neonatal plasma levels of a particular drug of dependence such as methadone has not been defined.

•Neonatal withdrawal has not correlated with maternal methadone dosage but does with neonatal plasma methadone levels.

•Both the onset and severity of neonatal opiate withdrawal might logically be related to the decrease in neonatal plasma methadone levels during the first 4 days of life, the time during which withdrawal usually becomes apparent.

•This hypothesis is based on the concept that plasma methadone levels reflect tissue stores of methadone, and that the unpredictability of opiate withdrawal could be related to varying rates of tissue clearance of methadone by the newborn infant.

•Neonatal plasma methadone levels obtained shortly after birth could be related to both maternal drug levels and maternal methadone dosages.

•If these relationships could be established, they would provide a scientific basis for management of the maternal methadone dosage late in pregnancy with the specific aim of ameliorating the severity of neonatal opiate withdrawal.

•Objective: To define the relationships between neonatal opiate withdrawal and drug related factors such as maternal methadone dosage, maternal and neonatal plasma levels, and the rate of decline of methdone in neonatal plasma.

•Results: A continuum of relationships exists between maternal methadone dosage, maternal methadone plasma level, initial neonatal methadone plasma level, rate of decline of that initial level, and ultimately the severity of withdrawal in the opiate-exposed neonate.

•Although a relationship between maternal methadone dosage just before delivery and maternal plasma methadone levels drawn on the day of delivery was found, there was considerable variability in the relationship of these two indices.

- This variability is most likely due to unmeasured maternal factors, such as irregular intake of methadone, poly-drug abuse, and pregnancy-associated physiologic alterations in hormone levels, plasma protein binding of methadone, and shifts in the body water-fat ratio, all of which may alter methadone pharmacokinetics and maternal plasma methadone levels.

- Maternal and neonatal plasma methadone levels drawn postpartum correlated significantly, but the neonatal levels were consistently lower than maternal levels.

- It is not obvious why neonatal methadone levels are so much lower, because plasma protein-bound methadone is decreased in pregnancy and increased amounts of free methadone are available for placental diffusion.

- In addition, fetal hepatic enzymatic activity is sluggish, and limited biotransformation of methadone takes place in the placenta.

- Lower neonatal plasma methadone levels are probably best explained by avid transfer of placentally transferred methadone into fetal tissue, as has been suggested by studies in animals showing rapid accumulation of methadone in fetal brain, liver, spleen, and lungs, associated with sharp declines in plasma methadone levels.

- Higher initial methadone levels were associated with more rapid declines of drug levels in methadone-exposed neonates.

- The presence of higher initial drug levels probably leads to more rapid depletion of tissue drug stores through the mechanism of enzyme induction and enhanced drug demethylation and cyclization in the liver.

- Animal studies have shown that higher methadone dosages lead to increased rates of hepatic metabolism of the drug, resulting in more rapid decreases in serum methadone levels.

- The rate of decrease in serum methadone levels correlated significantly with the acuity of the CNS withdrawal signs.

- This may be explained by animal studies, which have shown that methadone accumulates in the non-human primate brain during gestation, resulting in significantly higher brain levels compared with fetal plasma levels.

- Intrauterine exposure of the fetal brain to opiates promotes regional development of specific opiate receptors and suppresses neurotransmitter formation and function.

- A more rapid decline in methadone levels would produce a rapid shift of drug out of brain tissue, leading to increased availability of specific opiate receptors as well as rapid replenishment of neurotransmitters.

- In the presence of increased receptor sites, this replenishment of neurotransmitters would produce neuronal excitability, clinically manifested as CNS signs of withdrawal such as irritability, tremors, hyperreflexia, and possibly seizures.

- **Lowering methadone dosages late in pregnancy reduces the severity of neonatal withdrawal.**

- A relationship between the severity of neonatal withdrawal and the maternal methadone dose during pregnancy has been found.

- The amelioration of neonatal opiate withdrawal presents significant benefits to the mother and her infant.

- Neonates undergoing moderate to severe withdrawal often show excessive weight loss and slow return to birth weight, which may lead to prolonged hospitalization.

•When infants remain hospitalized, maternal-infant bonding is interrupted and the cost of hospitalization is increased.

•At present, no specific protocols to regulate methadone dosages in pregnant women have been established.

•Generally, medication regimens are individually determined based on those dosages that prevent the development of withdrawal symptoms in methadone-maintained women.

•Using maternal criteria, the literature generally recommends keeping methadone maintenance doses at 60 mg/day or higher to avoid maternal drug hunger and withdrawal during pregnancy.

•If reduction of the maternal methadone dosage during pregnancy is contemplated, it must always be done with extreme caution and with close medical-obstetric supervision to prevent fetal instability and withdrawal with possible fetal death.

•Dosage reduction carries the risk of maternal discomfort and self-medication with street drugs, thus increasing neonatal morbidity and eliminating any possible advantage of maternal dosage reduction.

•Although all 21 women were receiving methadone daily, 14 were poly-drug abusers, 13 of whom abused cocaine.

•Cocaine may affect the determination of methadone levels if the drug alters either the compartmentalization or metabolism of methadone.

•Because **cocaine** may affect neonatal neurobehavioral adaptation, the combination of opiates and stimulants may have complicated the clinical assessment of study infants.

•The findings related to opiate withdrawal were independent of poly-drug exposure.]

---

30. The major handicap associated with surviving neonates delivered at 24 weeks is

    *A. blindness.
    B. bronchopulmonary dysplasia.
    C. cerebral palsy.
    D. deafness.
    E. mental retardation.

---

p. 1731 (Silver R K, MacGregor S N, Farrell E E, Ragin A, Davis C, Socol M L. Perinatal factors influencing survival at twenty-four weeks' gestation. Am J Obstet Gynec 1993; 168:1724)

30. [F & I: •Background: The minimum fetal age beyond which survival is anticipated is not clearly defined.

•This is due in part to advances in neonatal care, which have resulted in the ability to save progressively smaller and younger infants.

•Marked differences in survival rates have been noted among low-birth-weight cohorts from different centers, even though they were managed contemporaneously.

•Such disparities have contributed to a lack of consensus with regard to the limit of fetal viability and, when published in retrospect, cannot account for the latest improvements in clinical care.

•Exogenous surfactant is an addition to the neonatal armamentarium that could further influence low-birth-weight survival because this cohort is at greatest risk of respiratory disease.

- Because clinicians also incorporate their own biases about the limits of viability in clinical decision making, survival advantages may be inadvertently extended to those neonates of greater gestational age (or estimated weight).

- This self-fulfilling prophecy could obscure the potential for improved outcome in the smallest infants and confound the interpretation of survival statistics because aggressive care may not be uniformly given at the lower limit of viability.

- Survivability during the twenty-fifth week of gestation was coincident with the availability of calf-lung surfactant extract, introduced as a single-dose, prophylactic therapy and available for infants delivered during this range of gestation.

- Objective: To identify those obstetric and neonatal factors associated with survival in infants delivered during this specific week of pregnancy.

- Gestational age is related to survival in low-birth weight infants.

- It was somewhat surprising to see this influence in this study because the entire cohort was confined to a single week of pregnancy.

- Even small delays in delivery (e.g., 1 to 2 days) can improve survival in this range of gestation.

- Aggressive attempts to delay delivery for a short time during the twenty-fifth week would seem an appropriate clinical recommendation on the basis of this observation.

- The issue of delivery method comprises two questions: (1) Can cesarean section favorably influence the outcome among infants who would have survived labor and vaginal delivery? (2) Will withholding cesarean section increase the likelihood of either intrapartum death or delivery of a compromised fetus?

- The former issue has been the focus of most retrospective reviews, and the consensus is that abdominal delivery by itself is not advantageous.

- A subset of the cesarean sections performed among survivors prevented intrapartum death, and that is the goal of emergency abdominal delivery when patients with more advanced gestations experience similar complications (e.g., cord prolapse).

- The willingness to consider cesarean delivery in response to standard obstetric indications may reflect a more general attentiveness to intrapartum events in these early pregnancies.

- This may explain why univariate analysis demonstrated a trend that favored cesarean section, although a majority of survivors were delivered vaginally.

- The influence of prompt neonatal resuscitation and intensive care is not usually considered when survival probabilities are assessed from an obstetric vantage point.

- Observations of infants delivered at 24 weeks would support that 26 weeks' gestation is a survival breakpoint and suggest that this is not just a categoric issue.

- Instead, the degree of which neonatal resuscitation is accomplished may also have an impact on survival.

- Once a point of viability is established at a particular center, the obstetric objective should include delivery of the infant in the most favorable condition possible within the guidelines of routine clinical care.

- It is then the responsibility of the neonatal team to proceed with a similar philosophy in keeping with the goal of an intact survival.

- Conclusion: Analysis of a cohort of infants delivered at 24 weeks' gestation has led to the conclusion that **gestational age** is the most predictive indication of survival.]

31. The correct order of restitutive maneuvers for the optimal management of shoulder dystocia is

   A. fundal pressure, McRoberts maneuver, release of posterior arm, Zavanelli maneuver.
   B. suprapubic pressure, McRoberts maneuver, release of posterior arm, Zavanelli maneuver.
   C. rotate the shoulders to the oblique, McRoberts maneuver, release of posterior arm, Zavanelli maneuver.
   D. suprapubic pressure, release of posterior arm, Zavanelli maneuver.
   *E. none of the above.

p. 1737 (Nocon J J, McKenzie D K, Thomas L J, Hansell R S. Shoulder dystocia: An analysis of risks and obstetric maneuvers. Am J Obstet Gynec 1993; 168:1732)

31. [F & I: •Background: Shoulder dystocia is an obstetric emergency that may result in substantial trauma to the neonate.

•Protocols for the management of shoulder dystocia abound.

•The literature contains conflicting information, especially regarding the predictability and management of shoulder dystocia.

•There is no absolute definition of shoulder dystocia.

•One definition includes any difficulty in extracting the shoulders after delivery of the head.

•A more precise definition indicates that "true" dystocia requires maneuvers to deliver the shoulders, in addition to downward traction and episiotomy.

•Reported cases of shoulder dystocia appear to be increasing.

•The prevalence is 0.15% to 1.7% of all vaginal deliveries, and it is quite variable, depending on the definition used.

•Objectives: To determine whether there is a risk profile for predicting or preventing shoulder impaction.

•To evaluate various management plans to disimpact a shoulder to determine which, if any, reduce the likelihood of a permanent injury.

•This should allow practitioners to select a reasonable management option consistent with their clinical judgment.

•The goals of this study were to place the predictable characteristics of patients with shoulder dystocia into a risk management format where the emphasis is on decision making.

•The incidence of reported shoulder dystocia increased from 1.2% to 1.8%.

•Although the increase was not statistically significant, there was an increase in attention to the problem.

•During July 1988 a departmental meeting was convened to address the appropriate documentation of shoulder dystocia, the risks, and management (especially the McRoberts maneuver).

•It was stressed that at all times during the management of the delivery the obstetrician should be careful to maintain the proper attitude of the infant's cervical spine to its shoulders.

•After this meeting there was an increase in the incidence of shoulder dystocia documented.

- The significant increase in the use of McRoberts maneuver after this meeting may also illustrate the effect of continuing medical education on clinical management.

- As expected, the study revealed that the larger the fetus the greater the likelihood that a shoulder will impact against the symphysis.

- What is striking is the number of shoulder dystocia cases that occurred in newborns weighing <4000 gm.

- In this respect, 92.4% of all vaginal deliveries accounted for 42.7% of all shoulder dystocias.

- **What is most important is that this single observation refutes the general notion that shoulder dystocia is always predictable and therefore preventable.**

- Conditions like diabetes and midforceps delivery after a prolonged second stage of labor become significant only in the presence of a large fetus, especially if there was a large newborn in a prior pregnancy.

- This study did **not** confirm that traditional risks, such as obesity, multiparity, and postdate pregnancy, were statistically significant or relevant for predictability.

- There was **no** association of shoulder dystocia with episiotomy, oxytocin use, or anesthesia.

- There are various techniques that can be used to relieve shoulder dystocia.

- **This study found no rationale for choosing one technique over another.**

- Nor is there a significant reason to suggest that the subjective degree of shoulder dystocia (mild, moderate, or severe) should be managed by any particular approach.

- There is no basis to suggest that the choice of anesthesia is related to shoulder dystocia or injury.

- There is no empiric evidence to suggest that the failure to perform an episiotomy is related to the outcome of shoulder dystocia.

- In spite of the fact that the **removal of the posterior arm** resulted in a higher incidence of brachial plexus injury, the clinical importance of this approach cannot be refuted.

  ° **It was the only procedure that resolved the impaction when other maneuvers failed.**

- For this reason all physicians who deliver babies should be competent in its use.

- The cohort of 19 patients with neonatal injury, but not coded for shoulder dystocia, was significantly different from those with dystocia.

- Statistically, they represent a different population, especially regarding the nature of the predominant injury (clavicular fractures) and the smaller size of the infants.

- There was also no evidence of prolonged labor, diabetes, or other risk factors in this group.

- It could be argued that documentation of injury at delivery influences the documentation of shoulder dystocia.

- In this study 29 of 33 brachial plexus injuries were documented in the delivery record by the obstetrician whereas only one of the clavicular fractures was noted.

  ° Most fractures (27/28) were discovered during the third infant examination (obstetric resident, then third-year pediatric medical student, then pediatric intern or resident).

°Although some portion of the "noncoded" group may represent underreporting of shoulder dystocia, this does not explain all of the injuries in this group.

°Thus it appears that a fractured clavicle or a brachial plexus injury can occur spontaneously.

•Many of the brachial plexus injuries were transient and resolved by discharge.

•More importantly, all but one had completely resolved by 6 months.

•The majority of such injuries in this study occurred on the left.

•All the brachial plexus injuries were Erb's palsies.

•Only one infant (3864 g) had residual mild arm weakness at 3 years old.

•If the newborns weighing >4000 g could have been accurately predicted, routine cesarean section would have prevented 106 shoulder dystocias but not one permanent injury.

•This study clearly indicates that shoulder dystocia is an **unpredictable** event, especially if the birth weight is <4000 g, and that infants at risk for permanent injury are virtually impossible to predict.

•Although the obvious relationship between shoulder dystocia and progressive fetal birth weight is valid, most of the traditional risk factors were found to have no predictive value.

•One exception exists: the history of a previous large infant is a highly significant statistical and clinical factor that cannot be ignored.

•Because the most significant factor consistent with shoulder dystocia is increasing fetal weight, one cannot fault the logic or clinical judgment in the selective use of cesarean section when there is objective evidence that the fetus weighs >4500 g.

•This study also reveals that any reasonable method to disimpact the anterior shoulder is an appropriate response to this obstetric emergency.

•Thus no protocol should serve as a substitute for clinical judgment.

•In this study permanent injury was uncommon.

•Regardless of the maneuver used to resolve the shoulder dystocia, at all times the obstetrician should be careful to maintain the proper attitude of the infant's cervical spine to its shoulders.

•From a risk management perspective it is imperative to document the reasonable basis for one's clinical judgment in the management of shoulder dystocia.]

---

32. Effects of elective amniotomy at term in an otherwise uncomplicated pregnancy include increased incidence of

    A. cesarean section.
    B. meconium passage.
    C. neonatal depression.
    D. prolonged decelerations.
    *E. none of the above.

---

p. 1830 (Garite T J, Porto M, Carlson N J, Rumney R J, Reimbold P A. The influence of elective amniotomy on fetal heart rate patterns and the course of labor in term patients: A randomized study. Am J Obstet Gynec 1993; 168:1827)

32. [F & I: •Background: Elective amniotomy is common in current obstetric practice.

- This practice seems to be the result of several factors, including the general belief that it facilitates the progress of labor, enables the placement of internal electrodes and pressure catheters for fetal heart rate (FHR) and contraction monitoring, and allows the clinician to know whether meconium is present.

- In recent years an increased appreciation of the relationship between oligohydramnios and fetal distress as a result of umbilical cord compression has been developed.

- The use of amnioinfusion to replace intrauterine fluid volume results in a decrease in the severity and frequency of FHR patterns consistent with umbilical cord compression (variable decelerations), as well as both decreased operative intervention for fetal distress and improved neonatal status at birth.

- The recognition of this relationship has led clinicians to wonder whether they are causing iatrogenic fetal compromise with elective amniotomy by creating oligohydramnios and its resultant complications.

- Very few data currently exist in modern obstetric practice to address this concern.

- Objective: To evaluate the effects of elective amniotomy on FHR patterns, operative intervention, and newborn condition, as well as the progress of labor in the setting of current practice.

- Practices become commonplace for various reasons, often without full knowledge of either the risk or the benefit.

- Such seems to be the case with amniotomy.

- In the mid-1970s and early 1980s, electronic monitoring came into wide acceptance in this country and now is used for the majority of patients in labor.

- Early technology did not provide high-quality external tracings, so it became commonplace to artificially rupture membranes to permit placement of an internal electrode, which usually provides an excellent tracing.

- Elective amniotomy is commonly performed be cause it can ascertain the presence or absence of meconium staining and because many believe that the practice accelerates otherwise normal labor.

- The effects of amniotomy on FHR patterns are an increased incidence of early, or type 1, decelerations with early amniotomy or early versus late spontaneous membrane rupture.

- Extensive information accumulated over the last 10 years has heightened appreciation of the relationship between oligohydramnios and fetal distress as a result of umbilical cord compression.

- A frequent and logical concern that is raised is that the common practice of amniotomy in normal labors might lead to iatrogenic oligohydramnios and subsequently result in many of the associated complications seen in patients with a more naturally occurring decrease in fluid volumes.

- This study does not directly address the question of whether artificial rupture of membranes leads to substantial or pathologic degrees of oligohydramnios in labor and, if so, with what frequency this occurs.

- This study does examine whether there are any clinically pertinent effects of this common practice.

- Two common practices were compared: totally elective amniotomy shortly after admission versus amniotomy only for a specific indication.

- Conclusions: First, the only apparent negative effect of elective amniotomy is a higher incidence of **mild and moderate variable decelerations** limited to the first stage of labor.

  ° It is very reassuring that there was no differences in the frequencies of more severe variable or prolonged decelerations or other abnormal FHR patterns, nor were there differences in any deleterious outcomes, including meconium passage, cesarean sections, operative vaginal deliveries, neonatal depression, or any definable neonatal complications.

°The fact that the observed abnormal patterns are limited to the first stage of labor should not be surprising.

•Other than oligohydramnios, only unusual events, such as true knots of the cord, short cords, or other cord abnormalities, are likely to lead to cord compression in the first stage of labor; thus any contribution from oligohydramnios will be more readily apparent.

•With respect to the study design, elective second-stage amniotomy was allowed in the intact group and thus no statements about its effect after complete dilatation can be made.

•Variable decelerations in the second stage of labor are quite common and are most frequently a result of cord (especially nuchal cord) entanglement.

°Any minor contribution from oligohydramnios might not be apparent.

°No differences have been shown in second-stage FHR patterns with oligohydramnios in studies that have measured amniotic fluid volume in labor.

•This study did not demonstrate an increased incidence either in meconium passage or in thick meconium in those patients subjected to elective amniotomy.

•The effect of elective amniotomy on the progress of labor is certainly significant, both clinically and statistically.

•Elective amniotomy appears to **shorten** the first stage of labor substantially; although no effect on the cesarean section rate was found (surprisingly low in both groups), there was much less need to augment labor with oxytocin in the elective amniotomy group.

•This effect was seen in both nulliparous and multiparous patients and does lend some support to at least one aspect of the active management of labor.

•Early amniotomy probably does contribute to the overall success of the active management of labor.

•The low cesarean section rate in both groups is remarkable and probably results from selection of a low-risk group.

•Patients with abnormal presentations, fetal distress on admission, premature rupture of membranes, induction of labor for any indication, and other common indications or predispositions for cesarean section present on admission were excluded from this study.

•Excluding patients with oligohydramnios on admission may also result in a decrease in the number of patients at risk of fetal distress.

•Eliminating fetal distress on admission defines >50% of patients who will require operative intervention for fetal distress at any time before delivery.]

33. Magnesium sulfate inhibits uterine contractions by

   A. decreasing extracellular calcium.
   B. down regulating oxytocin receptors.
   *C. elevating intracellular free magnesium.
   D. inactivating calmodulin.
   E. suppressing lysosomal metabolism.

---

p. 138 (Mizuki J, Tasaka K, Masumoto N, Kasahara K, Miyake A, Tanizawa O. Magnesium sulfate inhibits oxytocin-induced calcium mobilization in human puerperal myometrial cells: Possible involvement of intracellular free magnesium concentration. Am J Obstet Gynec 1993; 169:134)

33. [F & I: •Background: The contractile activity of smooth muscle is regulated by the intracellular level of free Ca^{2+}.

•The regulatory pathway leading to uterine contraction begins with an increase in the intracellular free Ca^{2+} concentration, which activates myosin light chain kinase and other calcium-dependent kinases.

•Magnesium sulfate has an inhibitory effect on uterine contraction in vivo and in vitro.

•Several clinical studies showed the effectiveness of the intravenous administration of magnesium sulfate in the treatment of preterm labor.

•The mechanisms of the tocolytic action of Mg^{2+} on the human myometrium are not thoroughly defined.

•Mg^{2+} may compete with Ca^{2+} for sites at the neuromuscular junctions, resulting in the inhibition of release of acetylcholine.

•Mg^{2+} itself may induce relaxation of the myometrium at the level of the muscle cell.

•Mg^{2+} is an important physiologic regulator of cell functions, possibly through its effect on Ca^{2+} movement.

•Oxytocin increases intracellular free Ca^{2+} concentration in human puerperal myometrial cells.

•The effects of a solution containing a high Mg^{2+} concentration on the intracellular free Ca^{2+} concentration have not been clarified.

•Objectives: To determine the effects of the extracellular free Mg^{2+} concentration on the changes in intracellular free Ca^{2+} concentration induced by oxytocin by means of a Ca^{2+}-sensitive fluorescent dye and a digital imaging microscopic system.

•Next, with a Mg^{2+} sensitive fluorescent dye to determine the intracellular free Mg^{2+} concentration in human puerperal myometrial cells under various conditions of extracellular Mg^{2+}.

•Then, to clarify which condition (i.e., normal intracellular free Mg^{2+} concentration with high extracellular Mg^{2+} or high intracellular free Mg^{2+} concentration with high extracellular Mg^{2+}) was essential for suppression of oxytocin-induced increases in intracellular free Ca^{2+} concentration.

•By measuring the changes in the intracellular free calcium and magnesium concentrations in cultured human puerperal myometrial cells with fluorescent dyes, the increase in intracellular free Ca^{2+} concentration induced by oxytocin was inhibited in a high extracellular Mg^{2+} solution and an increase in intracellular free Mg^{2+} concentration suppressed Ca^{2+} influx, probably through the calcium channels.

•Intravenous administration of magnesium sulfate is effective in preventing preterm labor.

- Results: A high extracellular Mg^{2+} solution inhibited the oxytocin-induced increase in intracellular free Ca^{2+} concentration at the level of human puerperal myometrial cells, whereas this Ca^{2+} mobilization was not affected by extracellular Mg^{2+} in the absence of extracellular Ca^{2+}.

- These data indicate that a high extracellular Mg^{2+} solution does not affect Ca^{2+} release from intracellular stores but mainly inhibits Ca^{2+} **influx** across the cell membranes of human puerperal myometrial cells.

- The increase in intracellular free Ca^{2+} concentration in myometrial cells induced by oxytocin was not inhibited 1 min after replacement of the normal solution with a 10 mmol/l extracellular Mg^{2+} solution, when extracellular Mg^{2+} was high and intracellular free Mg^{2+} concentration with high extracellular Mg^{2+} reduced the ocytocin-induced increase in intracellular free Ca^{2+} concentration to one fourth.

- Unlike nifedipine, it took 20 min for the effect of the high extracellular Mg^{2+} (10 mmol/l solution to be apparent.

- Clinically, intravenous administration of magnesium sulfate does not have an immediate effect.

  ° **It takes nearly 1 h to manifest a tocolytic action.**

- The question is how a high extracellular Mg^{2+} solution can have an inhibitory effect on intracellular free Ca^{2+} concentration.

- High extracellular Mg^{2+} itself with normal intracellular free Mg^{2+} concentration had **no** effect on Ca^{+2} mobilization.

- High intracellular free Mg^{2+} concentration with high extracellular Mg^{2+} was concomitant with suppression of Ca^{2+} influx induced by oxytocin in human puerperal myometrial cells.

- Oxytocin did not induce any change in intracellular free Mg^{2+} concentration in the human puerperal myometrial cells.

- Keeping intracellular free Mg^{2+} concentration constant may be preferable and may be important to maintain the functions and activities of cells.

- Elevated intracellular free Mg^{2+} concentration, caused by submaximal levels of high extracellular Mg^{2+}, may reduce cell functions, and it actually may have a calcium channel antagonistic effect.

- The increase in intracellular free Mg^{2+} concentration may block the calcium channels of the plasma membrane and inhibit Ca^{2+} influx.

- Administration of magnesium sulfate simultaneously with calcium blockers would not be preferable, because one enhances the other effect excessively, by similar mechanisms.

- At least one possible mechanism is suggested by which magnesium sulfate is effective in the inhibition of uterine contraction.

- A high level of serum Mg^{2+} may lead to a gradual increase in intracellular free Mg^{2+} concentration in myometrial cells.

- Elevated intracellular free Mg^{2+} concentration may proportionally block Ca^{2+} entry by calcium channels from the cytoplasmic aspect of the plasma membrane, and it may have a suppressive effect on the increase in intracellular free Ca^{2+} concentration, thereby resulting in relaxation of the myometrium.

- This finding may have defined one ot the roles of intracellular tree Mg^{2+} concentration as a modulator of cell functions.]

34. Routine weekly cervical examinations in twin gestations after 20 weeks is likely to result in

　　A. increased incidence of post-partum infections.
　　B. increased incidence of preterm labor.
　　C. increased incidence of ruptured membranes.
　　D. increased of neonatal sepsis.
　*E. none of the above.

---

p. 25 (Bivins, Jr. H A, Newman R B, Ellings J M, Hulsey T C, Keenen A. Risks of antepartum cervical examination in multifetal gestations. Am J Obstet Gynec 1993; 169:22)

34. [F & I: •Background: Routine antepartum cervical examination has been assessed as to its ability to predict premature labor in multifetal gestations.

　•There is little information regarding the possible detrimental effects of routine cervical examination on the initiation of preterm labor, premature rupture of membranes, bleeding, or other infectious complications in the multifetal gestation.

　•Objective: To report the frequency of these complications in a group of twin gestations receiving routine antepartum cervical examination and a second group receiving cervical examination tor obstetric indications only.

　•Routine antepartum cervical examination has been integrated into many preterm birth prevention programs and is a clinically useful predictor of patients at increased risk for preterm delivery.

　•Results: The data show a significant **reduction** in the frequency of premature rupture of membranes with routine cervical examination.

　•The reason for this reduction in premature rupture of membranes is unknown, but it may be a result of heightened cervical surveillance and the earlier detection and treatment of preterm labor.

　•The early detection and suppression of occult uterine activity may help avert the complication of preterm premature rupture of membranes.

　•When the obstetric outcome of those women attending the Twin Clinic was compared with a contemporary control group followed without routine antepartum cervical examination, there were significant reductions in the rates of very early (<30 weeks' gestation) and very-low-birth-weight (<1500 g) deliveries because of either preterm labor or premature rupture of membranes.

　•Cervical examination increases uterine activity.

　　°This may be caused by increased prostaglandin release.

　•A reasonable postulate would be that more frequent cervical examination would increase the rate of preterm delivery, especially in a group of women already at high risk.

　•The data do **not** support this postulate.

　•The preterm delivery rate was comparable between the patients in the Twin Clinic and those twin gestations followed up in the high-risk obstetric clinic who had cervical examinations for obstetric indications only.

　•There is also the theoretic risk of introducing bacteria into the cervical canal by digital examination, resulting in complications such as intraamniotic infection, neonatal sepsis, or a change in the cervical microflora that could lead to a higher incidence of postpartum infection.

•The risks of premature rupture of membranes, intraamniotic infection, or neonatal sepsis were not increased among the multifetal gestations receiving routine cervical examination.

•Because all cervical examinations were performed by a single examiner in the Twin Clinic it is conceivable that how the cervical examination was performed may be another important variable, potentially off-setting the presumed adverse effects of multiple examinations.

•The cervical examination technique does not vary significantly among examiners.

•Because almost all physicians would not hesitate to perform a cervical examination if the obstetric situation required, this study really addresses what incremental risks may be encountered if routine antepartum cervical examination is used.]

---

35. Spontaneous version of a twin pregnancy is influenced by

   A. amniotic fluid volume.
   B. birth weight discordancy.
   *C. gestational age.
   D. parity.
   E. placental location.

---

p. 1502 (Divon M Y, Marin M J, Pollack R N, Katz N T, Henderson C, Aboulafia Y, Merkatz I R. Twin gestation: Fetal presentation as a function of gestational age. Am J Obstet Gynec 1993; 168:1500)

35. [F & I: •Background: The decision regarding mode of delivery in a twin gestation is controversial and is dictated primarily by fetal position and presentation.

•Twin pregnancies are associated with an increased incidence of fetal malposition and malpresentation leading to an increased rate of cesarean section.

•Perinatal morbidity and mortality increase when the presentation in twins is other than cephalic-cephalic (presenting-nonpresenting twin).

•Despite the importance of fetal position and presentation for both management and outcome of twin gestation, the rate of spontaneous version as a function of gestational age is unknown.

•Objectives: To evaluate the rate of spontaneous version in twin gestation throughout the third trimester and to assess correlating factors.

•Results: The rate of spontaneous version in twin gestation significantly decreases as gestational age advances.

•The rate is as high as 60% early in the third trimester but, despite the significant decrease, remains relatively high (approximately 25% to 30%) even at term.

•This rate is much higher than the 5% cephalic version reported in singleton breech presentations at term.

•The mean gestational age in this twin population was 37 weeks, and the mean birth weight was 2640 g.

•Antepartum counseling concerning the mode of delivery in patients who have a cephalic-cephalic presentation at the initial evaluation is relatively simple because only a small proportion of these patients will experience spontaneous changes in fetal position and presentation.

•Antepartum counseling concerning other presentations should reflect the fact that they are relatively unstable.

•Spontaneous version in twin pregnancy is not influenced by parity, amniotic fluid volume, placental location, or birth weight discordancy.

•**Gestational age** and fetal presentation and position have a significant association with the rate of spontaneous version.

•Analysis of the data demonstrates that the presenting twin is less likely than the second twin to undergo spontaneous version.

•These data should be valuable to clinicians who use the presentation of the first twin as the primary determinant of the mode of delivery.

•In addition, the use of these data may result in a lower cesarean delivery rate if clinicians realize that malpresentations may resolve spontaneously before the onset of labor.

•The high rate of spontaneous version observed throughout the third trimester indicates that the final decision regarding mode of delivery should be decided at the onset of labor.

•This fact should be incorporated into the routine antepartum counseling of patients with twin gestation.]

---

36. Of the following the most common cause of preterm labor is

    A. cervical incompetence.
    *B. faulty placentation.
    C. fetal anomalies.
    D. immunologic factors.
    E. intrauterine infection.

---

p. 1482 (Lettieri L, Vintzileos A M, Rodis J F, Albini S M, Salafia C M. Does "idiopathic" preterm labor resulting in preterm birth exist? Am J Obstet Gynec 1993; 168:1480)

36. [F & I: •Background: Preterm birth is a major cause of perinatal morbidity and mortality and accounts for 6% to 10% of all births.

•This percentage has remained relatively unchanged over the past several decades despite aggressive tocolytic therapy and intensive investigation into the pathogenesis of preterm labor.

•In fact, as advances occur in the obstetric care of other maternal and fetal complications, the portion of perinatal morbidity and mortality due to preterm birth increases.

•Programs to prevent preterm birth have had little impact to date.

•Objective: To elucidate possible causes of preterm labor by studying all patients admitted with preterm labor and intact membranes who required tocolysis.

°The group of patients in whom tocolysis failed and who eventually had preterm delivery are the focus of this report.

•Approximately 1% of all deliveries are complicated by **abruptio placentae**, and 60% of these will result in a preterm birth.

•Antepartum hemorrhage from a **placenta previa** or abruptio placentae can be associated with preterm birth, and has been reported to be the highest risk factor.

•Results: 25 patients (50%) had clinical or histologic evidence of faulty placentation, with the majority (24) having abruptio placentae.

- All instances of suspected abruptio placentae were confirmed by histologic examination of the placenta.

- An association between abruptio placentae and **immunologic factors** was observed leading to the speculation that a chronic immunologic abnormality may first result in a decidual or implantation site abnormality and, as the pregnancy progresses, may lead to either chronic or acute abruptio placentae.

- This process can also be associated with **intrauterine infection**.

- Six patients had evidence of both abruptio placentae and intrauterine infection.

- Many studies have indicated that intrauterine infection occurs in patients in preterm labor but is often subclinical.

- Investigative efforts have centered on various laboratory and histologic means to predict infection (i.e., amniocentesis for Gram stain, culture, and glucose determination, serum C-reactive protein, etc.).

- Using a combination of amniotic fluid cultures and placental histologic type, evidence of intrauterine infection in 38% of patients in preterm labor was found.

- Positive amniotic fluid Gram stains and cultures were used as indication for delivery and may have slightly, but not significantly, interfered in the calculations of the incidences of the remaining groups of possible causes.

- Another area of preterm birth research that has recently evolved is that of immunopathology.

- The antiphospholipid antibody syndrome and the immunologic characteristics of recurrent pregnancy loss are gradually becoming more defined.

- The immunochemical characterization of preterm labor still needs further investigation.

- Three placental abnormalities are significantly more frequent in preterm labor patients: **chorionic vasculitis, decidual vasculopathy, and chronic villitis**.

- Two of these lesions—decidual vasculopathy and chronic villitis—are associated with abnormal **immunologic** events.

- Decidual vasculopathy has been associated with maternal autoimmune or alloimmune disorders, whereas chronic villitis is theorized to be due to a maternal-fetal immunopathologic condition or a congenital vital infection.

- In cases of decidual vasculopathy and chronic villitis, an antigenic stimulus from either maternal tissue (autoimmune) or fetoplacental unit (alloimmune) results in chronic inflammation and ultimately culminates in their respective lesions.

  ° These lesions can then result in defective placentation and ultimately result in preterm delivery.

- Immunopathologic condition of the placenta (decidual vasculopathy, chronic villitis) combined with positive maternal immunoserologic findings suggested a possible immunologic cause for 30% of patients in preterm labor.

- **Cervical incompetence** is associated with preterm birth.

- Eight of 50 patients (16%) had cervical incompetence.

- Interestingly, all patients with cervical incompetence also had evidence of an intrauterine infection.

- In those patients in whom cervical incompetence was diagnosed during this index pregnancy, it is difficult to ascertain whether a subclinical infection occurred first, leading initially to silent cervical dilatation and ultimately to preterm labor, or whether the cervical dilatation allowed microorganisms easier access, thereby predisposing the patient to an intrauterine infection.

•**Uterine anomalies**, significant physical trauma, major surgical procedures during pregnancy, and fetal anomalies are known to be associated with preterm labor.

•In general, these etiologic factors account for a small percentage of preterm births.

•In this study these groups of possible causes occurred in 6% to 14% of the patients.

•Maternal complications such as **systemic infection** are also associated with preterm labor.

•Although **preeclampsia** is generally associated with an indicated preterm delivery, it has also been associated with an increase in preterm labor.

°The mechanism is unclear, but perhaps the vasospasm with subsequent disruption of the vascular endothelium that occurs in preeclampsia leads to uterine ischemia, which then can result in defective placentation, abruptio placentae, fetal growth retardation, and in some cases preterm labor.

•Of increasing importance in today's society are certain maternal behaviors, notably the rising **drug use** during pregnancy.

•Two of the study patients had positive toxicology screens for **cocaine**.

•Toxicology screening should be considered for patients in preterm labor.

•With a thorough evaluation, most preterm labor can be potentially explained, since 96% of patients had at least one identifiable possible cause.

•Surprisingly, in 58% of patients in preterm labor, two or more causes were found; this finding supports the hypothesis that preterm labor has multiple causes and that efforts to focus only on one area (i.e., infection, immunology, etc.) may miss many of the causative agents.]

---

37. Which of the following are **fetal** effects of maternal ingestion of low-dose aspirin prophylactically?

    A. Decreased amniotic fluid.
    B. Myocardial dysfunction.
    C. Premature closure of the ductus.
    D. Thrombocytopenia.
    *E. None of the above.

---

p.1436 (Veille J, Hanson R, Sivakoff M, Swain M, Henderson L. Effects of maternal ingestion of low-dose aspirin on the fetal cardiovascular system. Am J Obstet Gynec 1993; 168:1430)

37. [F & I: •Background: Daily intake of low-dose aspirin may result in a decrease in the incidence of preeclampsia and fetal growth retardation and may improve the pregnancy outcome in women with positive lupus anticoagulant and anticardiolipin antibodies.

•Aspirin is a potent anti-inflammatory drug that inhibits the biosynthesis and release of prostaglandins in an effective manner throughout the body and that can readily cross the placenta.

•As little as 2 weeks of low-dose aspirin therapy can inhibit the platelet production of thromboxane.

•Prostaglandin synthetase inhibitors administered chronically during pregnancy may result in major systemic or regional alteration in fetal hemodynamics by their constricting effects on vascular smooth muscle.

- This could result in premature closure of the ductus arteriosus, myocardial dysfunction, or tricuspid regurgitation.

- Chronic maternal ingestion of nonsteroidal anti-inflammatory drugs could be potentially dangerous to the human fetus causing significant reduction in fetal weights, an increase perinatal mortality, and prolonged gestation.

- Objective: To analyze blood flow across the umbilical artery, the tricuspid and mitral valves, the descending aorta, and the fetal renal artery in a group chronically exposed to aspirin during pregnancy.

- A group of normal fetuses not exposed to aspirin were used as controls.

- Results: Blood flow across the fetal atrioventricular valves and the descending aorta is not significantly different in a group of fetuses exposed to aspirin early in gestation when compared with a group of fetuses not exposed to such a drug regimen.

- Even prolonged and early ingestion of low-dose aspirin to term does not adversely affect flow across the umbilical artery, the atrioventricular valves, and the descending aorta.

- None of the fetuses enrolled in this study had evidence of right-to-left shunting or impairment of diastolic or systolic ventricular function.

- Prolonged maternal ingestion of low-dose salicylates does not cause major hemodynamic changes in the human fetus.

- All fetuses had a Doppler echocardiography performed during the neonatal period.

- The first echocardiogram was done within the first 4 to 6 h after delivery, at 48 h, and at 6 weeks after delivery.

- None of the neonates had evidence of early ductal closure or abnormal right ventricular contractility.

- The Doppler shift obtained by pulsed Doppler has the advantage of comparing flow through a structure with some degree of precision.

- This Doppler shift, which is displayed as peak velocity and temporal velocity, can be influenced by many factors.

- One of these is the difference between atrial and ventricular diastolic pressures, which in turn influences flow.

- Valve mobility, heart rate preload, and diastolic relaxation of the ventricle can also influence flow across the atrioventricular or semilunar valves.

- The lack of differences among blood flow across the atrioventricular valves between the two groups suggests that the above-mentioned characteristics are not significantly affected by the daily maternal intake of low-dose aspirin.

- There was no evidence of tricuspid regurgitation; this may be difficult to assess because such a regurgitation jet may be small and fine.

- One of the most important values of pulsed Doppler ultrasonography is to quantify blood volume through a particular vascular structure.

- In this study the volume of blood through the cross-sectional area of the descending aorta was estimated.

•Peak flow velocity and velocity integral were not different between the two groups at any of the periods studied.

•The group exposed to aspirin did not show the increase observed in the control group with advancing gestational age.

•Flow across the descending aorta is mostly derived from the left ventricle and from ductal flow.

•Calculated flow across that structure also increased in both groups with advancing gestational age.

•When these flows were indexed to the estimated fetal weight, the group exposed to aspirin did not show the decrease observed in the control group.

•The babies receiving aspirin were significantly smaller in the third group.

•The absolute values of blood flowing through the fetuses exposed to aspirin is elevated throughout gestation when compared with the control group.

•This may be related to the direct or indirect effects of aspirin on ductal or aortic size.

•Finally, the analysis of fetal renal artery waveforms showed that this vascular bed did not respond differently after prolonged maternal intake of low-dose aspirin.

•None of the fetuses studied had absent diastolic flow of the fetal renal artery or decreased amniotic fluid.

•Although the peak systolic velocity-to-end-diastolic ratio were higher in the group exposed to chronic aspirin, this did not achieve significance, indicating that this particular regional circulation is not affected by such daily intake of aspirin and that such low doses may not significantly affect renal vascular resistance.

•Because this study was limited to low-dose aspirin, comments on the influence of higher doses or different prostaglandin inhibitors cannot be made or inferred.

•Chronic ingestion of low-dose acetylsalicylic acid from week 12 until delivery does not cause significant effects on central and regional fetal hemodynamics.]

---

38. The use of indomethacin in the treatment of preterm labor should be limited to those fetuses that are how many weeks old?

    A. 28
    B. 29
    C. 30
    D. 31
    *E. 32

---

p. 1353 (Moise Jr K M. Effect of advancing gestational age on the frequency of fetal ductal constriction in association with maternal indomethacin use. Am J Obstet Gynec 1993; 168:1350)

38. [F & I: •Background: **Indomethacin** is effective in the treatment of premature labor, forms of symptomatic hydramnios, and degenerating uterine leiomyomas.

•Enthusiasm for indomethacin has been tempered because of possible constriction of the fetal ductus arteriosus in as many as 50% of cases.

•It has been suggested that indomethacin use should be restricted to gestational ages of <34 weeks, after which constriction of the ductus is more likely to occur.

Obstetrics and Gynecology: Review 1994-Obstetrics References

- This recommendation was based on indirect data.

  ° Antedotal cases of **persistent fetal circulation** in newborns whose mothers ingested indomethacin involved fetal exposure late in gestation.

  ° Laboratory data revealed that this prostaglandin synthetase inhibitor does **not** cross to the fetus until late in pregnancy.

- Objectives: To determine whether indomethacin is associated with an increasing incidence of constriction of the fetal ductus arteriosus with advancing gestational age.

  ° To determine if the incidence of ductal constriction differed in singleton and multiple gestations.

- Both prostacyclin and prostaglandin E2 are important in maintaining the patency of the fetal ductus arteriosus.

- Prostaglandin synthetase inhibitors have been implicated in premature closure of the fetal ductus arteriosus.

- Constriction of the ductus in utero leads to a diversion of right ventricular output either in a retrograde fashion through the tricuspid valve (**tricuspid regurgitation**) or alternatively into the pulmonary arteries.

- An increase in pulmonary flow produces reactive **hypertrophy of the arterioles**.

- After birth relative **pulmonary hypertension** can cause right ventricular output to bypass the pulmonary circuit by way of the foramen ovale, leading to hypoxia and further pulmonary vasoconstriction.

- The condition produced by this scenario is known as **persistent fetal circulation** of the neonate.

- The earliest gestational age at constriction was 27 weeks.

- Indomethacin crosses the human placenta throughout gestation with a fetal-maternal gradient approaching unity.

- The human fetal ductus arteriosus is sensitive to the constrictive effects of indomethacin as early as the late second trimester.

- If the human ductus arteriosus becomes more sensitive to the constrictive effects of indomethacin as gestational age increases, one would expect to find a higher incidence of constriction in the latter portion of pregnancy.

- Results: A sharp increase in the incidence of ductal constriction at 32 weeks' gestation.

  ° At this point in the pregnancy approximately 50% of fetuses will be affected.

- Comparison of data between fetuses of singleton and multiple gestations revealed similar gestational age effects.

- In two of the five twin gestations in which ductal constriction was detected in at least one of the fetuses, only one member of the twin pair exhibited signs of ductal compromise.

- It would appear that the twin fetus is at a similar risk for ductal constriction as the singleton fetus, although this effect may vary between fetuses.

- Constriction of the fetal ductus arteriosus after maternal indomethacin use can occur at any time during gestation.

•Fact   °Detail   »issue   *answer

»Because of the high incidence of constriction that occurs after 32 weeks' gestation, the use of indomethacin should be restricted to gestational ages <32 weeks.

•Short-term use of indomethacin (<72 h) probably does not require monitoring of the patency of the ductus arteriosus by fetal echocardiography.

»Long-term use should involve initial assessment after 24 to 48 h, with weekly assessment thereafter.

•In multiple gestations all fetuses should undergo evaluation, because the finding of ductal patency in one fetus fails to guarantee the same in the remaining fetuses.]

---

39. Which of the following increase the risk of uterine rupture during attempted vaginal delivery after cesarean section?

    A. Epidural anesthesia.
    B. History of cesarean section previously for CPD.
    C. Macrosomia.
    *D. Two or more previous cesarean sections.
    E. Unknown uterine scar from previous cesarean section.

p. 1362 (Leung A S, Farmer R M, Leung E K, Medearis A L, Paul R H. Risk factors associated with uterine rupture during trial of labor after cesarean delivery: A case-control study. Am J Obstet Gynec 1993; 168:1358)

39. [F & I: •Background: Cesarean section is the most frequently performed surgical procedure in the United States.

•A high rate of 30% repeat operations has led to advocation of vaginal delivery after cesarean section.

•Labor after cesarean delivery is reasonably safe, but there is a finite risk of uterine rupture that is can be devastating for both the fetus and the mother.

•The reasons for routine repeat cesarean deliveries are multifactorial, but may reflect concern regarding the inability to predict uterine rupture.

•Objective: To investigate the risks of uterine rupture in patients undergoing trial of labor after cesarean section.

•In comparison with women who underwent trial of labor uneventfully, patients who had **excessive amounts of oxytocin, dysfunctional labor, and a history of two or more cesarean deliveries were at greater risk for uterine rupture.**

•Epidural anesthesia, macrosomia, a history of successful vaginal delivery after cesarean delivery, unknown uterine scar, and a history of prior cesarean delivery because of cephalopelvic disproportion were not associated with uterine rupture.

•Results: The overuse of oxytocin was associated with increased risk of uterine rupture.

•In the majority of subjects (74% or 40/54) oxytocin administration was started in the **latent phase** of labor solely because of the failure to abate uterine contractions despite hydration or sedation and the absence of cervical progression.

•Prolonged latent phase may be effectively terminated by therapeutic rest with a narcotic agent or by oxytocin stimulation.

- Although both modes of therapy are equally efficacious, oxytocin terminates prolonged latent phase promptly, whereas most patients who undergo therapeutic rest enter the active phase hours later.

- Ideally, patients should be observed for any progress in labor.

- **When a prolonged latent phase is recognized, then therapeutic rest with a narcotic agent should be offered.**

- The **judicious** use of oxytocin may simultaneously lower the incidence of uterine rupture and induce vaginal delivery in a well-selected population.

- **Arrest disorders** may predispose a patient to uterine rupture.

- The most common types of dysfunctional labor identified were active-phase arrest disorders (dilatation and descent).

- Different patterns of dysfunctional labor have different etiologic and prognostic implications.

    ° Arrest disorders have the worst prognosis for successful vaginal delivery.

- The majority of patients received oxytocin before they had dysfunctional labor (at 1 to 4 cm dilatation) and proceeded to have arrest disorders with adequate uterine activity.

- In general, most cases of arrest disorders occur with poor uterine activity, and it is reasonable to use oxytocin judiciously in these patients to establish adequate uterine activity.

    » **When arrest disorders fail to be resolved despite adequate oxytocin augmentation, termination of the trial of labor followed by cesarean section should be considered.**

- **Epidural anesthesia** was **not** associated with risk of uterine rupture.

- **Macrosomia** was **not** associated with increased risk of uterine rupture.

- **Uterine rupture was related to the number of prior cesarean deliveries.**

    ° Patients with two or more prior cesarean deliveries were at greater risk of uterine rupture than patients who had had one prior cesarean delivery.

    ° The incidence of uterine rupture in patients with two or three prior cesarean deliveries undergoing trial of labor was 2% (23/1165).

    ° 98% of the patients with two or three prior cesarean deliveries underwent trial of labor uneventfully.

- A history of **prior successful vaginal delivery after cesarean delivery** did **not** decrease the risk of uterine rupture.

- The same precautions should be used for all patients with a history of cesarean delivery whenever trial of labor is allowed.

- The majority of patients in the case and control groups had an **unknown type of uterine scar**, which did **not** seem to contribute any difference in the incidence of uterine rupture.

    » It remains prudent to document the type of uterine scar whenever possible.

- Patients who had a prior cesarean delivery because of cephalopelvic disproportion did **not** have increased risk of uterine rupture.]

Obstetrics and Gynecology: Review 1994-Obstetrics References

40. Which of the following in the most rapid and reliable test for the detection of group B streptococci which have colonized the reproductive tract of pregnant patients?

   *A. DNA probe.
   B. Enzyme immunoassay.
   C. Gram stain.
   D. Latex agglutination test.
   E. Todd-Hewitt broth culture.

p. 639 (Yancey M K, Clark P, Armer T, Duff P. Use of a DNA probe for the rapid detection of group B streptococci in obstetric patients. Obstet Gynecol 1993; 81:635)

40. [F & I: •Background: Group B streptococci are the most common cause of neonatal sepsis and result in significant morbidity and mortality, especially in preterm infants.

•The bacteria are transmitted perinatally to as many as 70% of neonates born to colonized mothers.

•Maternal colonization rates vary from 5-to-30%, and up to 60% of colonized women have intermittent carriage of the bacteria.

•Accordingly, antenatal cultures have not been effective in predicting intrapartum carriage.

•In general, approximately 60-to-70% of women with group B streptococcal genital colonization in the second trimester will remain colonized at the time of delivery, and up to 30% of women with negative second-trimester cultures will harbor group B streptococci in their genital tract at term.

•Vertical transmission of group B streptococci can be effectively reduced by timely intrapartum antibiotic prophylaxis.

•Intrapartum identification of women colonized with group B streptococci is critical.

•Standard culture methods commonly require 24-to-48 h for results.

•Rapid detection of group B streptococci antigens in clinical specimens by latex agglutination and enzyme immunoassays has been described.

•Although these rapid tests are generally sensitive in identifying heavily colonized patients, they remain relatively insensitive in specimens with a low bacterial inoculum.

°**Up to 90% of carriers have light colonization of the genital tract; thus a large percentage of carriers are missed by these rapid detection methods.**

•Nucleic acid probes for identifying microorganisms have a sensitivity equivalent to standard bacteriologic cultures.

•A commercial gene probe, the Accuprobe system, is available for identification of *streptococcus agalactiae*, or group B streptococci.

•The Accuprobe system has been used to confirm the identification of culture isolates from pediatric patients with suspected group B streptococcal infections and was found to be 100% accurate.

•Objective: To determine the accuracy of this DNA probe as a rapid diagnostic test to detect colonization of the female genital tract by group B streptococci.

•The likelihood that a neonate will develop early-onset group B streptococcal disease is directly related to gestational age, duration of labor, duration of ruptured membranes, and size of the maternal bacterial inoculum.

•Fact   °Detail   »issue   *answer

- Although infants born to heavily colonized women are generally at the greatest risk, there have been reports of significant morbidity and mortality from group B streptococcal disease in neonates born to lightly colonized parturients.

- Accordingly, an effective intrapartum screening method should have acceptable sensitivity for identifying specimens with a low inoculum.

- Current rapid detection methods, which generally have low sensitivity in lightly colonized women, have improved sensitivity in specimens with low inocula following growth amplification.

- The duration of growth amplification necessary to attain sensitivity of more than 50% varies greatly among previously reported rapid methods, with a range of 8-to-20 h.

- The Accuprobe had similarly good performance in specimens with low inocula after only 3.5 h of growth amplification.

- Growth amplification presumably improves sensitivity by increasing the number of group B streptococcal target rRNA strands available for hybridization.

- The DNA probe had acceptable performance with a cell density of at least 1×10^3 cells/ml in the specimen and was 100% accurate when group B streptococci were present in concentrations of 1×10^4 cells/ml or greater, which is considered light colonization by semiquantitative methods.

- Further testing using longer periods of growth amplification might increase sensitivity; any improvement would have to be interpreted in light of the potential impact of a delay in obtaining results.

- False-positive results were generally restricted to specimens that were **grossly contaminated with erythrocytes,** possibly because of nonspecific chemiluminescence from hemoglobin.

- This decrease in specificity in bloody specimens could obviously have a detrimental effect on the usefulness of the assay as an intrapartum screen.

- Intrapartum patients with vaginal bleeding could alternatively be screened using a rectal swab or a different rapid method.

- Although the current investigation was not designed to evaluate the clinical impact of the DNA method, the results from the test were 100% accurate in identifying women who subsequently delivered infants that developed group B streptococcal disease.

- This is in contrast to the results obtained from the central hospital laboratory, which reported negative maternal culture results from both of the women who delivered preterm neonates.

- These false-negative results characterize the insensitivity of standard culture methods using direct plating techniques rather than selective broth media.

- The potential impact of timely antibiotic chemoprophylaxis in these patients remains a matter of speculation.

- To be considered a useful screening test, the method should be sensitive, specific, easy to perform, inexpensive, and rapid enough to produce results in time to modify the natural course of the illness.

- The DNA probe methodology has several distinct advantages as a rapid screen when compared with other currently available methods, including a relatively rapid assay time, good overall sensitivity, and an objective end point that is easy to interpret.]

41. Approximately, what percentage of fetuses with trisomy 18 have congenital heart disease?

   A. 50
   B. 67
   C. 75
   D. 85
   *E. 99

p. 682 (Paladini D, Calabro R, Palmieri S, D'Andrea T. Prenatal diagnosis of congenital heart disease and fetal karyotyping. Obstet Gynecol 1993; 81:679)

41. [F & I: •Background: Structural cardiac abnormalities are among the most common congenital malformations, with an incidence of two to eight per 1000 live births.

   •Cardiac defects are responsible for 20% of perinatal deaths due to congenital malformations and greater than 50% of deaths in childhood from malformations.

   •The frequency of chromosomal abnormalities in infants with congenital heart diseases is estimated as 5-to-10% from postnatal clinic data.

   •With the introduction of fetal echocardiography in perinatal medicine, it is evident that the frequency of chromosomal anomalies in fetuses with cardiac structural defects is far higher than that reported for live births.

   °Several authors reported that 20-to-45% of fetuses with cardiac defects have an abnormal karyotype.

   °The high intrauterine mortality rate for fetuses with chromosomal abnormalities could account for such a discrepancy.

   •Objective: To determine the incidence of aneuploidy among fetuses with congenital heart disease diagnosed in utero.

   •The extensive use of fetal echocardiography has found that the incidence of chromosomal abnormalities among fetuses with congenital heart disease is higher than that reported for live-born infants.

   •Results: The incidence was 48% (15 of 31).

   •The incidence of associated chromosomal anomalies was also high for fetuses with isolated cardiac malformations (29.4%, five of 17).

   °In these five cases, the cardiac anomaly was the only phenotypic expression of the underlying genotypic alteration.

   •The frequency of chromosomal abnormalities in fetuses with congenital heart disease substantially exceeds the 0.3% risk for genetic abnormalities due to advanced maternal age alone.

   •The detection of a cardiac structural defect represents a stronger indication for fetal karyotyping than advanced maternal age.

   »Although it is not possible to perform fetal echocardiography on the general population, a screening view such as the **four-chamber view** should be considered as an integral part of the routine obstetric ultrasound examination.

   •In this series, an abnormal screening four-chamber view was found to be a major indication for fetal echocardiography, leading to the diagnosis of cardiac defects in 20% of cases.

Obstetrics and Gynecology: Review 1994-Obstetrics References

•Screening for chromosomal anomalies based only on advanced maternal age allows detection of only 20% of chromosomally abnormal fetuses.

°The remaining 80% occur in women younger than 35, and this is the age group in which fetal echocardiography does play a role.

•It is not possible to propose a screening procedure for chromosomal anomalies based on fetal echocardiography for two reasons:

°1) Congenital heart disease is present in up to **99% of cases of trisomy 13 and 18**, but in only 50% of Down syndrome cases; and

°2) fetal echocardiography is a level II examination that cannot be applied on a wide scale.

•When a cardiac structural defect is detected there is a **50% possibility for that fetus to be chromosomally abnormal**, and this fact may contribute substantially to the detection of chromosomal abnormalities in women less than 35 years of age.

°Fetal karyotyping should be offered whenever a fetal cardiac anomaly is diagnosed, regardless of maternal age.

°Fetal chromosomal evaluation is useful regardless of the gestational age at the time of diagnosis.

°Trisomy 18 detected in a fetus with an isolated ventricular septal defect affects dramatically the prognosis and, consequently, the management of labor and delivery.

°Conversely, a normal karyotype in a fetus with a surgically correctable lesion helps reassure the parents and definitely supports any resuscitative effort to transport the neonate to the cardiac surgery unit.

»Considering the high incidence of cardiac anomalies in fetuses with lethal trisomies (up to 99%), advanced gestational age should not represent a deterrent to offering fetal karyotyping.]

---

42. Which of the following carries the highest risk for premature labor?

   A. Chorioamnionitis
   B. Cigarette smoking
   *C. Multiple gestation
   D. Previous preterm labor
   E. Uterine anomalies

---

p. 755 (Heffner L K, Sherman C B, Speizer F E, Weiss S T. Clinical and environmental predictors of preterm labor. Obstet Gynecol 1993; 81:750)

42. [F & I: •Background: The incidence of preterm delivery has remained constant over the last 3 decades in spite of major advances in obstetric care.

•Preterm labor, preterm premature rupture of the membranes (PROM), and medical problems such as fetal distress, maternal bleeding, and preeclampsia remain the major causes of preterm delivery.

•Spontaneous deliveries occurring as a result of preterm labor and PROM account for at least two-thirds of premature infants.

•Reduction of the prematurity rate is a major goal of clinicians, investigators, and society because preterm and low birth weight infants contribute disproportionately to neonatal morbidity and mortality.

•From obstetric population surveys, several clinical and environmental factors appear to increase the risk of spontaneous preterm delivery.

•Fact   °Detail   »issue   *answer

- Objective: To assess the relative risks and interactions of specific clinical and environmental factors for preterm labor. To date, these data represent the largest epidemiologic analysis of risk for a single, rigorously defined cause of preterm delivery--preterm labor.

- Results: The clinical variables of **third-trimester bleeding, multiple gestation, and chorioamnionitis** carry a very **high** risk of preterm labor in pregnancy.

- The environmental exposures of cigarette smoking and drug use, in addition to the clinical variables of prior preterm delivery, bleeding in early pregnancy, uterine anomalies, maternal DES exposure, and urinary tract infection, pose a moderate risk for preterm labor.

- Although the medium-risk clinical variables and smoking and drug use each pose far less risk to a given gravida than do the high-risk variables, the lesser risk factors have a substantial impact on the population because of their higher prevalences.

- The changes in the odds ratios for the clinical variables when the cases were divided into those with and without **PROM** provide information on the relative importance of two potential causal pathways for preterm labor, infection and uterine overdistention.

- Though clinically apparent **chorioamnionitis** is a frequent occurrence among patients experiencing preterm PROM, it is often unclear whether it is the cause or the result of ruptured membranes.

  ° The fact that the odds ratio for chorioamnionitis as a preterm labor risk remains elevated in the absence of ruptured membranes confirms clinically what has been observed pathologically; intrauterine infection plays a substantial role in preterm delivery.

- **Bleeding** during early pregnancy is a risk for preterm labor only when preceded by ruptured membranes, consistent with the theory that disruption of fetal membrane adhesion to the uterine wall leads to ascending infection and ruptured membranes.

- The risk of preterm labor following a **urinary tract infection** is limited to women experiencing ruptured membranes before labor onset is consistent with the theory that abnormal colonization of both the urinary and genital tracts is responsible for the association.

- **Placental abruption** can be accompanied by histologic evidence of chorioamnionitis, and smoking and cocaine use—both of which can cause constriction of the uterine blood vessels—are risk factors for bleeding in pregnancy, including abruption

- The elevated risk for preterm labor documented among women with twins or with uterine anomalies confirms what clinicians have sensed previously; namely, that **overdistention of the uterus**, either by a multiple gestation or by the presence of a singleton in a woman with an abnormal uterus, puts the woman at risk for preterm labor and, to a lesser extent, for preterm PROM.

- Some causes of preterm labor can act through an infectious or inflammatory process (third-trimester bleeding and chorioamnionitis).

- 40-to-50% of preterm labor could be prevented by identifying exposures that increase the risk for these late complications and treating or preventing them before they occur.

- Emphasis should be placed on interventions early in the causal chain because once preterm labor has occurred, preterm delivery is likely despite aggressive attempts to stop it.

- Programs to reduce cigarette smoking and drug use could reduce the preterm labor rate by more than the 20% calculated for their independent effects because of their implicated roles in third-trimester bleeding.

- Because of the large risk for preterm labor attributable to twins (41%), programs for high-intensity management of multiple gestations may have a major public health impact.

•Other patients having a high risk for preterm labor are those who have had a prior preterm delivery.

°This is a relatively small, easily identifiable high-risk population who would likely participate in preventive strategies.

°Efforts to prevent recurrences in this group of women have been largely unsuccessful.

°Successful interventions in this group of women will reduce the prematurity rate by only 6%, half of what smoking-cessation programs during pregnancy might accomplish.

•Conclusions: Strategies to reduce the impact of the infrequent but high-risk conditions of third-trimester bleeding, twins, and infection should lower the prematurity rate substantially.

•Educational and interventional programs targeted to the much larger number of women who smoke and use drugs should also lower the preterm labor rate and, hence, the preterm delivery rate.]

---

43. At 36 weeks a patient presents with a blood pressure of 180/110, backache, blurred vision, and abdominal pain. Urinalysis is negative for protein, sugar and leukocyte esterase. Within 45 min her blood pressure in 110/70 with supportive treatment. The diagnosis is

   A. anxiety neurosis.
   B. chronic hypertension.
  *C. cocaine intoxication.
   D. pheochromocytoma.
   E. preeclampsia.

---

p. 549 (Towers C B, Pircon R A, Nageotte M P, Porto M, Garite T J. Cocaine intoxication presenting as preeclampsia and eclampsia. Obstet Gynecol 1993; 81:545)

43. [F & I: •Background: Statistics from the National Institute of Drug Abuse and the Drug Abuse Warning Network reveal that emergency room visits for medical problems and deaths related to cocaine use have increased drastically in the past 5-to-6 years.

•Prevalence surveys have not shown the same increase in the number of people who use cocaine.

•Before 1985, cocaine hydrochloride (the sulfate form) was the most common type of cocaine sold on the street.

°Many drug abuse programs have noted a marked change in the type of cocaine used.

°This change is in the direction of the more potent forms of cocaine such as "crack" and "free base" (the alkaloid forms).

•The increase in medical problems and deaths due to cocaine use may be related to inexperience with a very powerful drug.

•Medical complications from cocaine include cardiac arrhythmias, myocardial infarction, and seizures.

•In obstetrics, difficulties with premature labor, abruptio placentae, and small for gestational age infants have been reported.

•The cardiovascular effects of cocaine use include increases in heart rate and systemic blood pressure in the pregnant and nonpregnant state.

°The elevation of blood pressure may be a possible cause of abruptio placentae.

Obstetrics and Gynecology: Review 1994-Obstetrics References

•Objective: To report 11 cases of cocaine intoxication in the third trimester that presented as possible preeclampsia or eclampsia.

•Clinicians should be aware that cocaine intoxication can mimic preeclampsia.

•Because this drug can produce hypertension as well as symptoms of headache, blurred vision, and abdominal pain, it is easy to see how these patients were initially thought to have preeclampsia.

•The symptoms of abdominal pain and blurred vision may be caused by vasoconstriction of vessels that supply the gastrointestinal tract and retina, respectively.

•Headaches are thought to be due to hypertension.

•The clinical presentation of a cocaine-intoxicated patient can be impressive, the presence of seizures, may suggest a diagnosis of eclampsia.

•Two common traits of all the women in this report were the **rapid resolution of their hypertension** and symptoms and the **normal laboratory studies**.

»Preeclampsia should still be the initial diagnosis in any patient presenting in the third trimester with hypertension and symptoms of headache or abdominal pain.

°If the clinical picture appears to normalize rapidly, cocaine should be considered as a possible cause.

°Amphetamine abuse can also cause hypertension and the same clinical symptoms as seen with cocaine.

•Street drugs such as cocaine, amphetamines, and heroin are usually mixed with other drugs, such as lidocaine, procaine, and arsenic.]

---

44. The minimum dose of aspirin to effectively reduce the incidence of preeclampsia is

   *A. 80 mg.
   B. 100 mg.
   C. 160 mg.
   D. 250 mg.
   E. 500 mg.

(Two references.)
p. 1089   (Hauth J C, Goldenberg R L, Parker Jr R, Philips III J B, Cooper R L, DuBard M B, Cuuter G R. Low-dose aspirin therapy to prevent preeclampsia. Am J Obstet Gynec 1993; 168:1083)

44. [F & I: •Background: High-risk populations for preeclampsia or eclampsia encompass nulliparous women or those with chronic hypertension, diabetes mellitus, multifetal gestations, or chronic vascular disease.

•Preeclampsia is manifested by increased peripheral vascular resistance with arteriolar vasospasm and endothelial damage.

•The characteristic resistance to the pressor effects of the infusion of the potent vasopressor angiotensin II, which occurs in normal pregnancy, is not present in women with preeclampsia.

•As early as 24 to 28 weeks' gestation, 90% of women who subsequently become hypertensive are significantly more sensitive to an infusion of angiotensin II than are women who never become hypertensive.

- Except for a history or presence of the maternal medical and obstetric complications detailed above, a positive angiotensin II test (marked sensitivity) is the only reliable method to predict which nulliparous women are destined to develop preeclampsia later in pregnancy.

- Maternal sensitivity to angiotensin II infusion can be increased by cyclooxygenase inhibitors (such as 500 mg of acetylsalicylate [aspirin] or 25 mg of indomethacin given twice 2 h apart).

- Conversely, a low dose of aspirin (80 mg) causes refractoriness to the pressor effects of infused angiotensin II.

- A proposed mechanism of low-dose aspirin-induced maternal refractoriness to angiotensin II is an alteration in the maternal thromboxane A2 (TxA2)/prostacyclin (vasoconstrictor/vasodilator) ratio in favor of the vasodilator prostacyclin (as determined by measurement of their metabolites thromboxane B2 [TxB2] and 6-keto-prostaglandin F1α [PGF1α].

- Placental tissue of women with preeclampsia produced more TxB2 and less 6-keto-PGF1α than did placentas from women with normal pregnancies.

- Eicosanoids mediate vascular reactivity during pregnancy and altered production of these substances may lead to the development of preeclampsia.

- Objectives: To test the hypothesis that daily maternal prophylaxis with 60 mg of aspirin would significantly reduce the incidence of or ameliorate the severity of pregnancy-associated hypertensive disorders (encompassing pregnancy-induced hypertension, preeclampsia, and eclampsia).

- To assess fetal and newborn risks related to daily maternal aspirin therapy from 24 weeks' gestation until delivery.

- Methods: The patients were randomized to receive a daily 60-mg capsule of aspirin or an identical-appearing placebo containing a lactose filler.

- Before any project deliveries, hypertensive disorders were defined as follows:

  ° (1) **Pregnancy-induced hypertension**: *mild*, a diastolic blood pressure of ≥90 but <110 mm Hg on at least two occasions at least 1 h apart and before or during labor or within 12 h postpartum; *severe*, a diastolic blood pressure of >110 mm Hg on at least two occasions at least 1 hour apart and before or during labor or within 12 h postpartum. (If a study patient had a platelet count of <100,000/mm³ or an aspartate aminotransferase ≥100 U/l, she was considered to have *severe* pregnancy-induced hypertension even if the blood pressure criteria for severe pregnancy-induced hypertension were not met.)

  ° (2) **Preeclampsia**: mild, a diastolic blood pressure >90 but <110 mm Hg on at least two occasions at least 1 h apart and before or during labor or within 12 h post partum and proteinuria of ≥1 + on two or more occasions at least 1 h apart in the absence of a urinary tract infection or gross hematuria or ≥0.5 g per 24 h; *severe*, a diastolic blood pressure ≥110 mm Hg on at least two occasions at least 1 h apart before or during labor or within 12 h of delivery and proteinuria as defined for mild preeclampsia.

    °° One of the following was also present: headaches or visual disturbance, epigastric pain, oligura, thrombocytopenia, increased bilirubin, increased aspartate aminotransferase, fetal growth retardation, or proteinuria ≥ 3 to 4(+) or 4 g per 24 h.

    °° **Fetal growth retardation** was defined as a birth weight ≤ 10th percentile according to the growth standard of Brenner et al.

  ° In the research clinic blood pressure was determined with the patient seated and the cuff at heart level after the patient had rested for 5 min.

°A standard air or mercury sphygmomanometer was used with a standard (25 to 35 cm) or large adult cuff (33 to 47 cm) selected as determined by the patient's upper arm circumference.

°Korotkoff 1 and 5 were recorded unless Korotkoff 5 = 0; then Korotkoff 4 was used.

°If, at an antepartum clinic visit, the Korotkoff 5 was ≥90, the blood pressure was repeated after the patient had rested for 15 to 30 min. During initial evaluation at labor and delivery, similar equipment, patient position, and criteria were used; these aspects were not standardized throughout a subsequent labor, delivery, and postpartum period that encompassed up to 24 to 48 h.

•TxA2, whether of placental or platelet origin, is a powerful vasoconstrictor, whereas prostacyclin, of endothelial cell origin, is a potent vasodilator.

•In the placentas of women with preeclampsia, the production of TxA2 is increased and that of prostacyclin is decreased relative to their production in placentas from normal pregnancies.

•Whether this alteration in the placental production of these eicosanoids occurs after the onset of the clinical syndrome of hypertension, edema, and proteinuria or precedes and mediates the development of preeclampsia has not been determined.

•If a model for the development of preeclampsia presumes that there is an early and increasingly (with advancing gestational age) disparate ratio between maternal TxA2 and prostacyclin levels, then many clinical and physiologic observations regarding preeclampsia can be explained.

•Women with increased sensitivity to angiotensin II as early as 24 weeks' gestation have an increased incidence of preeclampsia.

•Both these phenomena would be expected if these women had an excessive level of an endogenous vasoconstrictor or a deficit of an endogenous vasodilator.

°Also, most pregnant women have a lowered total peripheral vascular resistance.

°This is probably because of an increase of various smooth muscle relaxants, including progesterone, prostacyclin, and endothelial-derived relaxing factor.

°Normal pregnant women tend to have an "underfilled" intravascular capacity as viewed by their renal and adrenal systems.

°Women with excessive vasoconstriction and increased peripheral resistance from early gestation would be expected to have a diminution of the normal increase of plasma and red blood cell volume.

°This lack of intravascular volume expansion commonly occurs in women with severe preeclampsia or eclampsia.

•A continued maternal imbalance of TxB2 and prostacyclin, favoring vasoconstriction, would explain the increased occurrence of uteroplacental insufficiency and the resultant fetal growth impairment that is common in women with severe preeclampsia or eclampsia.

•Finally, with worsening of the vasoconstrictor/vasodilator imbalance, the clinical syndrome of hypertension, edema, and proteinuria would become manifest.

•Sequelae of this syndrome, such as hepatic dysfunction, major motor seizures, endothelial disruption with microangiopathic hemolytic anemia, and thrombocytopenia can also be explained by excessive arteriolar spasm produced by an increased eicosanoid vasoconstrictor.

•If an imbalance in vasoconstrictor and vasodilator substances occurs before the overt clinical syndrome of preeclampsia and it either causes or mediates this illness, then pharmacologic prophylactic intervention before the clinical syndrome, aimed at reversing this imbalance, should ameliorate or prevent subsequent preeclampsia.

- The dosage of aspirin necessary to inhibit TxA2 synthesis without affecting prostacyclin synthesis is very low.

- Results: In patients taking the placebo median serum TxB2 levels increased by 28% from 24 weeks' gestation to delivery (mean 38.9 weeks) but decreased by 60% from 24 weeks' gestation to delivery (mean 39.1 weeks) in the women who received 60 mg of aspirin daily.

- Pharmacologic prophylaxis significantly reduced the incidence of preeclampsia in the aspirin group (five of 302 vs 17 of 302 in the placebo group).

- The severity of preeclampsia was also ameliorated, because severe preeclampsia developed in only one of 302 women who received aspirin compared with six of 302 who received placebo.

- Other than a reduction in preeclampsia in 12 of 302 women who received aspirin, no evidence of significant maternal, fetal, or neonatal benefit was found.

- Because the sample size was based on the end points of pregnancy-induced hypertension and preeclampsia, there was not sufficient power to find improvement, if present, in perinatal mortality or morbidity.

- The data were suggestive only of a positive effect of aspirin on fetal growth in that the mean birth weight of infants of aspirin-treated women was 3249 g compared with 3169 g in those who received the placebo (P = .08).

- Prescription of daily prophylactic low-dose aspirin therapy is dependent on several factors.

    ° First, although all the women in this study were medically at low risk, the fact that many were black and all were poor undoubtedly accounted for the relatively high background rate of preeclampsia.

    ° A middle-class white population would be expected to have a lower background risk of preeclampsia, and the effect of aspirin would probably be less dramatic.

    ° Second, universal aspirin prophylaxis in nulliparous women would be more attractive if an improvement in fetal or neonatal morbidity or mortality could be shown.

        °° Even if an improvement in the perinatal outcome cannot be demonstrated, universal aspirin prophylaxis might still be valuable.

    ° Treating 600 women with daily low-dose aspirin might well cost less than providing more intense medical care for the 12 additional women with preeclampsia.

    ° Finally, the question of universal aspirin prophylaxis in nulliparous women would not arise if there were better predictors of preeclampsia in nulliparous women with no other risk factors.

- In spite of the apparent efficacy of aspirin for preventing preeclampsia in this population, a good predictive test for preeclampsia would be extremely useful.

- In populations at high risk for preeclampsia because of poverty, race, and age, daily low-dose aspirin holds promise of achieving a substantial reduction in the incidence and severity of preeclampsia and perhaps an increase in birth weight.]

(Second reference)

p. 1164   (O'Brien W F, Krammer J, O'Leary T D, Mastrogiannis D S. The effect of acetaminophen on prostacyclin production in pregnant women. Am J Obstet Gynec 1993;168:1164)

[F & I: •Background: The recent interest in the use of aspirin for prevention of preeclampsia and other nonsteroidal anti-inflammatory agents for the inhibition of preterm labor has resulted in a need for greater understanding of the action and side effects of these drugs.

•The mechanism of action of nonsteroidal anti-inflammatory agents involves inhibition of the microsomal enzymes cyclooxygenase or prostaglandin synthetase.

•This inhibition accounts for the anti-inflammatory, antipyretic, and analgesic properties of these agents and for their gastric and hemorrhagic side effects.

•Acetaminophen (4-acetamidophenol), one commonly used agent, exhibits a unique profile.

•Acetaminophen is a potent antipyretic and analgesic but combats inflammation poorly, causes little gastric irritation, and has no obvious effect on the duration of bleeding.

•**This therapeutic profile is so favorable that it is the most widely used medication in pregnancy.**

•Prostacyclin (PGI2), may play an important role in normal and hypertensive pregnancies.

•Objective: To investigate the effect of acetaminophen on PGI2 production by endothelial cells in culture and by third-trimester pregnant women.

•PGI2 is produced primarily by endothelial cells and is antiaggregatory and vasodilatory.

•TxA2 is produced mainly by circulating platelets and is proaggregatory and vasoconstrictive.

•Normal pregnancy is associated with an increase in the production of PGI2.

°This increase is severely reduced in pregnancy-associated hypertension, which may be a result of the generalized endothelial cell dysfunction seen in these women.

•The resultant imbalance between PGI2 and TxA2 production is the target of low-dose aspirin prophylaxis.

•This therapy, which is based on the partial selectivity for TxA2 versus PGI2 production, appears to be beneficial in the prevention of proteinuric preeclampsia.

•Inhibition of prostaglandins and other arachidonic acid derivatives by acetaminophen appears to be related to the tissue studied.

•Nonsteroidal anti-inflammatory agents derive their anti-inflammatory, analgesic, and antipyretic properties by inhibition of prostaglandin synthetase is highly tissue specific.

°A potent inhibition of prostaglandin production in slices of cerebral cortex was felt to account for its antipyretic potency, whereas relatively low activity in spleen and platelets resulted in poor anti-inflammatory and antiaggregratory effect.

•Clinical studies of acetaminophen use during pregnancy have not shown any harmful effect on the mother or any increase in fetal malformations.

°These studies have been directed primarily at ingestion during the first half of pregnancy and have compared acetaminophen with aspirin ingestion.

•The recent development of reliable estimation of prostaglandin production by measurement of metabolites in the urine has allowed investigation of the effect of acetaminophen on vascular tissue.

•Results: Human endothelial cells in culture produced less prostacyclin when exposed to acetaminophen in concentrations of 10 or 100 µg/ml.

•These concentrations are pharmacologically appropriate, because the peak plasma level after a single dose of acetaminophen is approximately 10 µg/ml, and toxicity is not reached until plasma levels exceed 300 µg/ml.

•Inhibition caused by 100 µg/ml of acetaminophen was similar to 10 µg/ml of indomethacin, which is 10 to 20 times higher than typical plasma levels.

°Acetaminophen ingestion at recommended therapeutic doses (approximately 15 mg/kg) is associated with a significant **inhibition** of PGI2 production, as reflected in 2,3-dinor-6-keto-PGF1α excretion.

°The reduction in excretion appeared to occur in both normotensive and hypertensive women, although statistically significant only in the hypertensive group.

°There was no effect of acetaminophen ingestion in the smaller group of women in whom TxB2 metabolite was measured.

•**A disproportionate reduction in PGI2 and decrease in the PGI2/thromboxane ratio may adversely affect conditions in which abnormal platelet aggregation and vascular smooth muscle tone are suspected, especially preeclampsia.**

•A possible effect of acetaminophen ingestion, moreover, must be considered in studies of low-dose aspirin therapy in which PGI2 and thromboxane production is used as a measure of disease or therapy.]

---

45. The antibiotic to which *M. hominis* is sensitive and *U. urealyticum* is resistant is

    A. chloramphenicol
*B. clindamycin
    C. erythromycin
    D. quinolones
    E. tetracycline

---

p. 285 (Roberts S, Maccaro M, Faro S, Pinell P. The microbiology of post-cesarean wound morbidity. Obstet Gynecol 1993; 81:383)

45. [F & I: •Background: Wound infection after cesarean delivery occurs in 2-to-16% of patients depending on antibiotic prophylaxis, length of labor, duration of rupture of membranes, duration of internal monitoring, and number of vaginal examinations.

•Genital mycoplasmas have been isolated from wound infections in patients who have cesarean delivery.

•The Gram stain is highly specific but less sensitive in the prediction of post-cesarean endomyometritis and in the early detection of significant burn wound microbial growth.

•No study has attempted to evaluate Gram stain findings for the purpose of identifying possible genital mycoplasmal infection.

•Objectives: To better define the prevalence of genital mycoplasmas in post-cesarean wound infection and to use the Gram stain to predict subsequent culture results.

•Mycoplasms are small (0.2-to-0.3 um) pleomorphic organisms bounded only by a cell membrane with no evidence of a cell wall.

- Mycoplasmal colonization rates in the lower genital tract appear to be related to socioeconomic status; public hospital patients in one Boston-based study had *Ureaplasma* and *Mycoplasma* isolation rates of 76.3 and 53.6, respectively.

  ○ Their counterparts in private offices had significantly lower rates, at 52.9 and 21.3%, respectively.

- *Ureaplasma urealyticum* and *M. hominis* are causative in very few.

- *Mycoplasma hominis* will cause acute pyelonephritis and exacerbate existing chronic pyelonephritis, and may have a causative role in pelvic inflammatory disease.

  ○ It is frequently isolated from the blood of women with postpartum fever.

  ○ Cases of neonatal meningitis, brain abscess, and septic arthritis have been reported.

  ○ Several recent reports have described sternotomy wound infections caused by *M hominis*.

- **Ureaplasmas** are a rare cause of acute nonchlamydial epididymitis.

  ○ They are associated with chorioamnionitis, postpartum fever, and nongonococcal urethritis.

  ○ Despite a link with repeated spontaneous abortion and stillbirth in humans, a causal relationship has to be established.

- In vitro, *M. hominis* is sensitive to clindamycin, tetracyclines quinolones, and chloramphenicol and is **resistant to erythromycin, penicillins, and cephalosporins**.

- In vitro, *U. urealyticum* is susceptible to erythromycin, doxycycline, quinolones, or chloramphenicol is **resistant** to **clindamycin**.

- About 10% of ureaplasmas are **resistant** to tetracyclines in **nongonococcal urethritis**, but these patients usually respond to erythromycin.

- No bacteria were ever noted on Gram stain in the 16 exudates with genital mycoplasmas alone.

- In identifying infected wounds, a Gram stain that showed the presence of organisms only had a sensitivity of 0.55.

- Even though the positive predictive value was 1.0, the low sensitivity makes this a poor test for predicting wound microbiology before culture results.

- If the presence of greater than ten WBCs per 400x field is used to define wound infection with all types of organisms, then the sensitivity of the Gram stain result is 0.83 and the positive predictive value is 0.89.

  ○ This finding is consistent with inflammation.

- Specificity and negative predictive values drop from 1.0 to 0.72 and from 0.71 to 0.62, respectively, when considering genital *Mycoplasmas* and Gram stain findings in this way.

- Genital mycoplasmas are highly prevalent isolates in wound infections.

  ○ This probably relates to the prevalence of genital mycoplasmas in the lower genital tract of this population.

- Gram stain findings may become clinically more important as the pathogenicity of genital mycoplasmas in post-cesarean wound infections (if any) is better defined.

•The data support the opinion that most post-cesarean wound morbidity is due to contamination from the lower genital tract at the time of surgery.

•The low number of anaerobic isolates may reflect the efficacy of **cefotetan** as a prophylactic agent against anaerobes in this indigent population.

•In contrast, the high prevalence of *E. faecalis* obtained in wound exudates reflects the lack of activity of cephalosporins against this organism.

°Studies have reported an increase in enterococcal isolation in postoperative endometritis following cephalosporin prophylaxis.

•Conclusion: Genital mycoplasmas (*U. urealyticum* and *M. hominis*) were frequently isolated in wound exudates from post-cesarean patients.

»If adequate treatment of these wounds could be achieved without the increased morbidity (e.g., longer hospital stay) associated with opening incisions and healing by second intention, a simple diagnostic test such as the Gram stain would be clinically useful.]

---

46. Which of the following **single** oral GTT plasma glucose levels is associated with LGA infants?

    A. elevated fasting blood sugar
    B. elevated 1 h blood sugar
*C. elevated 2 h blood sugar
    D. elevated 3 h blood sugar
    E. All are associated with large for gestational age infants.

---

p. 347 (Berkus M, Langer O. Glucose tolerance test: Degree of glucose abnormality correlates with neonatal outcome. Obstet Gynecol 1993; 81:344)

46. [F & I: •Background: The oral 3-h glucose tolerance test (GTT) has become the standard means of diagnosing gestational diabetes mellitus.

•If the number of abnormal GTT values relates to the severity of disease, then one would expect increasingly higher glucose levels during pregnancy and greater morbidity associated with increasing numbers of abnormal GTT values.

•Gravidas with one abnormal value on the GTT have glucose profiles and adverse outcomes similar to those with gestational diabetes.

•In addition, it seems that there is an **increasing incidence of macrosomia with increasing 2-h values on the GTT even when patients are "normal."**

•Gravidas with abnormal 50-g screening values but normal GTTs have significantly higher insulin output and insulin-glucose ratios than women with normal glucose challenge tests.

•Their infants also have increased morbidity.

•These findings support the concept of a **continuum** of glucose abnormality; this continuum may well reflect the degree of abnormality of the GTT and extend to patients with three or four abnormal GTT values.

•A paucity of information exists relating the degree of abnormality (i.e., the number of abnormal test values) to pregnancy course and outcome, especially when there are more than two abnormal GTT values.

•Objective: To investigate whether the extent of glucose abnormality, as reflected by the number of abnormal GTT values, correlates with the level of carbohydrate intolerance during pregnancy, and whether increasing degrees of abnormality signify greater adverse outcome.

- The uniqueness of this study was the attempt to relate the number of abnormal GTT values to pregnancy outcome, including three or four abnormal GTT values.

- The incidence of LGA was **not** associated with the degree of GTT abnormality, but was similarly elevated **regardless of the number of abnormal GTT values**.

- This increased rate of LGA was related to the level of glucose control during the third trimester, when excess growth is initiated.

- The patients with poor control (fasting plasma glucose above 90, 2-h postprandial level above 120 mg/dl) constituted a group having an increased likelihood of delivering an LGA infant.

- The number of abnormal values on the GTT **does** reflect an increasingly aberrant glucose profile, expressed by mean glucose values, glucose excursion, and GTT periodicity.

- The level of control as expressed by mean fasting plasma glucose, 2-h postprandial, and overall mean glucose values was positively related to the number of abnormal GTT values.

- The mean glucose curves were significantly higher for increasing numbers of abnormal GTT values.

- These elevations mean that all the values were greater for subjects with more abnormal GTT values, including the values less than the National Diabetes Data Group maximum normal values, as well as being greater than the 0-abnormal group.

- Gestational diabetes can be identified in patients with positive glucose screening using the **GTT periodicity**.

- This descriptor of glucose tolerance can predict the disease, and its consequences.

- Prediction of glucose intolerance after pregnancy awaits long-term follow-up.

- The more carbohydrate intolerant the patient (increasing number of abnormal GTT values and increasing GTT periodicity), the **worse** the glucose control during the third trimester as reflected by weekly mean fasting and 2-h postprandial serum glucose values.

- Those subjects with poor glucose control all had significantly increased adverse outcomes.

- Because the subjects were not followed with weekly serum glucose measurements, it can only be speculated that the patients with one abnormal value and those with elevated weekly glucose values similarly contributed to the incidence of LGA infants, as the overall rate was not different from the rates in the other abnormal groups.

- In addition, there was no significant increase in the incidence of LGA neonates with good glucose control except for those with two abnormal GTT values, and there was a trend toward a decrease of LGA to normal levels with the greater use of insulin in patients with more GTT abnormality.

- Because it is no longer ethical to identify gravidas with gestational diabetes and not treat them, it is not possible to determine the outcome of these subjects based only on their diagnostic findings.

- Control of glucose during pregnancy becomes a confounding factor that influences the incidence of LGA.

- The mothers in this study who were poorly controlled, for whatever reason, represent a group as close to a non-intervention group as is possible to study today.

- Good control decreases the incidence of LGA to near normal.

•Only the patients with two abnormal GTT values and good control had a significantly greater incidence of LGA compared with controls.

•This finding may reflect the use of less insulin in this group, perhaps because their glucose values were lower initially than those of subjects with four abnormal GTT values.

•Even "relative hyperglycemia" in pregnant patients is associated with an increase in adverse outcome, primarily macrosomia.

•Greater insulin levels and higher insulin-to-glucose ratios, are a reflection of insulin resistance, in these "normal" patients.

•Even minor glucose abnormalities are associated with LGA infants, a classic complication related to the glycemic level, and there is a continuum of glucose abnormality associated with increased adverse outcome.

•The present study extends this continuum to patients with more than two abnormal GTT values and relates increasingly greater intolerance, hence the need for stricter glucose control to decrease the incidence of LGA infants, with the degree of abnormality on the GTT.]

---

47. Associated with hypothyroidism in pregnancy

   *A. gestational hypertension
   B. macrosomia
   C. maternal anemia
   D. post-date pregnancy
   E. postpartum hemorrhage

---

p. 352 (Leung A S, Millar L K, Koonings P P, Montoro M, Mestman J H. Perinatal outcome in hypothyroid pregnancies Obstet Gynecol 1993; 81:349)

47. [F & I: •Background: Pregnancy in hypothyroid patients is uncommon because of frequent anovulation.

•Although hypothyroid pregnancies can be associated with increased risks of miscarriage, stillbirth, preterm delivery, congenital anomalies, and developmental abnormalities, more recent investigations have described successful pregnancy outcomes in hypothyroid women.

•The differences in outcome may be partly attributed to various definitions for hypothyroidism or to small sample sizes that included hypothyroid patients with other medical illnesses.

•Objective: To report the pregnancy outcome in a large number of hypothyroid patients with no other concurrent illnesses and to investigate the relationship between severity of hypothyroidism and adverse outcomes.

•This study is the largest report on pregnancy outcome in gestations complicated by hypothyroidism.

•**Gestational hypertension** was significantly more common in hypothyroid patients than in the general population.

•Results: A higher incidence of gestational hypertension among overt hypothyroid patients (22%) than in subclinical hypothyroid subjects (15%) was found.

•The incidence of gestational hypertension was even higher in those who remained hypothyroid at delivery compared to those who became euthyroid before delivery in each group.

•The cause of this finding is unknown.

•Hypothyroidism is a recognized cause of reversible hypertension in nonpregnant women.

•Maternal anemia and postpartum hemorrhage were uncommon in this study.

•Gestational hypertension was the main cause of LBW in the hypothyroid women.

•The results provide a strong argument for expeditious diagnosis and treatment of hypothyroidism, as gestational hypertension with its attendant maternal and fetal sequelae occurred more commonly in the severely hypothyroid patients at presentation and in those who remained hypothyroid at delivery.

•Ideally, hypothyroid patients should be made euthyroid before delivery.

•For those with persistent hypothyroidism during pregnancy, the goal should be euthyroidism as indicated by normal serum TSH.]

---

48. Preeclampsia is associated with an increase in the effect of which substance on placental arteries?

    A. Angiotensin II.
    B. Endothelin.
    C. PGF2α.
    D. Prostacyclin.
 *E. None of the above.

---

p. 872 (Inayatulla A, Chemtob S, Nuwayhid B, Varma D R. Responses of placental arteries from normotensive and preeclamptic women to endogenous vasoactive agents. Am J Obstet Gynec 1993; 168:869)

48. [F & I: •Background: Preeclampsia complicates 6% to 8% of human pregnancies and is one of the major causes of maternal and fetal mortality and morbidity.

•Although the pathogenesis of preeclampsia is well defined, its cause remains obscure.

•There is evidence that the uteroplacental bed, especially the placenta, is involved in the genesis of preeclampsia.

•Placenta can contribute to preeclampsia by numerous mechanisms, including an overproduction of endothelin, an imbalance in the synthesis of vasoconstrictor and vasodilator eicosanoids, a disturbance in the renin-angiotensin-aldosterone system, an increase in serotonin, and so on.

•Objective: To test the hypothesis that preeclampsia may be associated with an increase in the responses of placental arteries to endogenous vasoconstrictors or a decrease in the responses to vasodilators.

•For this purpose vasoconstrictor activities of angiotensin II, norepinephrine, endothelin, serotonin, and PGF2α and vasodilator activities of a prostacyclin analog (Iloprost), ANF, and isoproterenol (a ß2-adrenergic receptor agonist) were determined.

•Results: Preeclampsia is not associated with an increase in the activity of vasoconstrictor agents or a decrease in the activities of vasodilator agents; **placental arteries** of preeclamptic women have more marked oscillations than those of normal pregnancies.

•**Umbilical** arteries are relatively refractory to the constrictor effects of angiotensin II.

•Because placental arteries do contain angiotensin II receptors, it would seem that the receptor-response coupling has not developed in fetal placental blood vessels.

•**Norepinephrine** exerted inconsistent effects on normal arteries and no effect on arteries from patients with preeclampsia.

•Because both angiotensin II and norepinephrine are potent vasoconstrictors of the maternal placental vascular bed, it would seem that there exist qualitative differences in the responsiveness of maternal and fetal placental arteries to certain vasoactive substances.

•Endothelin, PGF2α and serotonin caused concentration-dependent **contractions** of placenta arteries, and their maximal effects were equal to or greater than that caused by potassium.

•Among the **vasorelaxants, isoprenaline was ineffective**.

•Prostacyclin analog (**Iloprost**) and **ANF** caused concentration-dependent **relaxation**, although less than was often caused by sodium nitroprusside.

•Prostacyclin does not dilate maternal placental vessels, as reflected by blood flow measurement studies.

•As is the case with angiotensin II and norepinephrine, the responses of maternal and fetal placental vessels to prostacyclin also differ.

•Oscillations were more frequent in preeclamptic arterial strips when compared with normal strips.

•Oscillations of blood vessels are characteristics of the hypertensive state.

•Although oscillations were present in both normal and preeclamptic arteries, the greater magnitude of these oscillations in preeclampsia may be related to the hypertensive state.

•Quantitation of these oscillations by modern technologic advances may be diagnostic of preeclampsia.

°A complete and consistent suppression of these oscillations required concomitant treatment of tissues with both cyclooxygenase inhibitor, indomethacin, and the lipoxygenase inhibitor nordihydroguaiaretic acid; this suggests that leukotrienes also contribute to these oscillations, although their role in placental arteries seems minimal.

°The reason why oscillations were completely suppressed by indomethacin in tissues from preeclamptic women but not in arteries from normotensive women is not clear; it is possible that the cyclooxygenase pathway plays a much more important role in placental vessels during preeclampsia than during normotensive pregnancy.

•If the assumption that spontaneous oscillations are a contributory factor in pregnancy hypertension is correct, then their inhibition by indomethacin may provide another rationale for the beneficial effects of aspirin in pregnancy hypertension.]

---

49. Umbilical vessel oxytocin administration for retained placenta is to be undertaken. Which technique is likely to deliver the most oxytocin to the placental capillary bed?

    A. Allow the cord to bleed, clamp, inject 20 ml of saline with 20 units of oxytocin into the umbilical vein.
    B. Do not allow the cord to drain, clamp the cord, inject 20 ml with 20 units of oxytocin into the umbilical vein.
    *C. Do not allow the cord to drain, clamp the cord, inject 30 ml into the umbilical vein and milk the cord toward the placenta.
    D. Do not allow the cord to drain, clamp the cord, inject 30 ml with 20 units of oxytocin into the umbilical vein.
    E. Do not the allow the cord to drain, clamp the cord, inject 30 ml into the umbilical artery.

p. 795 (Pipingas A, Jofmeyr G J, Sesel K R. Umbilical vessel oxytocin administration for retained placenta: In vitro study of various infusion techniques. Am J Obstet Gynec 1993; 168:793)

49. [F & I: •Background: Retained placenta is a serious complication of childbirth.

•The injection of oxytocin into the umbilical vein has been suggested as a simple and safe method of treatment.

•Considerable disagreement exists in the literature concerning the effectiveness of umbilical vein administration of oxytocin for retained placenta.

•In a review of six rather small randomized control trials (numbers ranging from 30 to 60) the incidence of manual removal of the placenta was increased in two studies and reduced in four studies, the typical odds ratio for all the studies being 0.50 (95% confidence interval 0.30 to 0.83).

•A more recent study involving 220 women, 20 of whom were excluded from analysis, showed no reduction in the incidence of manual removal of the placenta.

•The volume, concentration, and route of oxytocin administered in these studies appears to have been chosen empirically.

•In the majority 10 IU of oxytocin in 20 ml of saline solution has been used, presumably because 20 ml syringes are readily available, with or without "milking" of the cord after injection.

•In one small study that showed the greatest benefit, 100 IU in 30 ml was used, and in one of the negative studies 10 IU in 10 ml was used.

•Objective: To determine the most efficient method of delivering infused fluid to the placental capillary vasculature.

•The most likely mechanism would be a direct action on the myometrium underlying the unseparated placenta.

•Injected oxytocic agents would need to reach at least the villous capillary level to be able to diffuse across to the maternal circulation to cause myometrial contraction.

•The technique most commonly reported, the injection of 20 ml of solution into the umbilical vein without previous bleeding, resulted in capillary demonstration in only one of five cases in this study (technique 3) and in two of five when the cord was "milked" after injection of 20 ml (technique 4).

•Injection into the umbilical artery (technique 5) is technically more difficult and on basic principles would seem not advisable because only half the placental surface would be reached.

•Injection into the umbilical vein after the cord was allowed to bleed (technique 2) produced consistent capillary filling but not a cotyledonary pattern with 30 ml, and it was technically somewhat difficult to introduce the needle into the collapsed vein.

•The introduction of an infant mucus-extraction catheter into the cut end of the umbilical vein (technique 1) was technically easy and effective in producing capillary filling, as well as a cotyledonary pattern, when 30 ml was used.

•This technique can also be easily used when the cord has broken or torn but is still accessible and the vein has collapsed.

•Conclusion: The following technique is recommended to ensure that infused oxytocin reaches at least the placental capillary bed:

  °1. Clean an area of umbilical cord if it has become soiled, cut the cord, and hold the edge of the cut surface with a pair of artery forceps or by hand.

°2. Introduce an infant feeding tube or mucus-extraction catheter into the cut end of the umbilical vein, advance it until resistance is felt, and then withdraw it about 5 cm.

°3. Compress the umbilical cord around the catheter to prevent back-flow and inject 30 ml of oxytocin solution.

°°Clamp the cord with the catheter in position.

°°If direct needle injection into the protruding cord is used, at least 30 ml should be injected and the fluid should be "milked" toward the placenta.

•Retained placenta is a condition associated with considerable maternal morbidity and risk.]

---

50. Following amniocentesis for genetic anomalies, a fetus is discovered to have a balanced translocation. What is the empiric risk for the fetus to have anomalies or develop mental delay?

    A. 0%
    B. .5%
    C. 1%
    D. 5
    *E. 10%

---

p. 15 (Clark B A, Kennedy K, Olson S. The need to reevaluate trisomy screening for advanced maternal age in prenatal diagnosis. Am J Obstet Gynec 1993; 168:812)

50. [F & I: •Background: Most referrals for prenatal diagnosis are for the increased risk of trisomies, particularly Down syndrome, associated with advanced maternal age.

•Prenatal diagnosis for genetic disease is time-consuming, involving either chorionic villus sampling (CVS) or amniocentesis, in vitro culture of cells, banding of chromosomes and, finally, microscopic analysis of cells arrested in metaphase.

•With the use of deoxyribonucleic acid (DNA) probes and fluorescence in situ hybridization, it is possible to screen interphase cells from amniotic fluid, chorionic villi and, potentially, fetal cells in the maternal circulation for numeric abnormalities with the promise of immediate results.

•The major genetic risk with advanced maternal age is a **trisomy**, a numeric chromosome abnormality.

•This maternal age effect is apparent in live births, at amniocentesis and chorionic villus sampling, and in spontaneous abortions.

•Trisomy screening may be the most important function of prenatal diagnosis and that the use of fluorescence in situ hybridization to screen interphase nuclei may eliminate the need for karyotype analysis.

•Although trisomies are the most important chromosome abnormalities to be screened, little discussion has been given to the background rate of structural chromosome abnormalities (duplications, deletions, inversions, insertions, and translocations) and the medical and reproductive consequences of missing these structural abnormalities by screening only for abnormalities in chromosome number.

•**As opposed to numeric abnormalities, structural abnormalities do not show a relation to maternal age.**

•Objective: To evaluate the impact of aneuploidy screening with DNA probes on a prenatal diagnosis and counseling program, by studying the karyotype of 7240 amniotic fluid samples referred for screening because of advanced maternal age alone.

- Numeric versus structural abnormalities were compared and the occurrence of the structural abnormalities determined.

- For women at risk, antenatal diagnosis of genetic disorders is now the standard of prenatal care.

- Advanced maternal age with its associated increased risk of a chromosome abnormality is the most common reason for prenatal diagnosis.

- The major risk is Down syndrome, followed by trisomies 13 and 18.

- The association of the sex-chromosome aneuploids such as XXY or XXX is not as striking.

- The frequency of **structural chromosomal abnormalities** (translocations, duplications, deletions, and inversions) has **not** shown a similar relation to advanced maternal age.

- Because their rates are stable across the maternal age range and their contribution to genetic morbidity is not as great as the trisomies, screening for structural abnormalities has not been considered important in prenatal diagnosis.

- The risk of trisomy associated with advanced maternal age is a source of patient anxiety and has fueled a demand for rapid prenatal diagnostic services.

- This anxiety has likely contributed to the popularity of CVS, which is done in the first trimester—this in spite of the questionable accuracy and safety of CVS with respect to amniocentesis.

- There is now a push to speed the screening for trisomies in prenatal diagnosis by using the technique of fluorescence in situ hybridization.

- Traditional cytogenetic methods are time-consuming, requiring the culturing of cells, the arrest of the cell cycle, and finally the staining and analysis of chromosomes in a karyotype.

- Fluorescence in situ hybridization exploits techniques of molecular biology and holds the promise of rapid results because interphase cells can be analyzed.

- Chromosome-specific DNA probes are labeled with fluorescent marker molecules.

- Fetal cells are treated and then fixed onto glass slides.

- The DNA in the fetal cells and the cloned probe are then denatured and the probe solution incubated with the fetal cells.

- In the process of hybridization some of the probe molecules find their complementary target in the fetal chromosomes.

- After being washed, the slides are visualized under a fluorescent microscope and the probe signals are analyzed.

- In general, for any chromosome-specific probe, normal cells show only two signals, and trisomic cells show three.

- By using either single or multiple chromosome-specific DNA probes that are chemically tagged to fluorescent markers, fluorescence in situ hybridization can detect numeric abnormalities of chromosomes 13, 18, 21, X, and Y in interphase cells.

- The potential of the fluorescence in situ hybridization technique with composite chromosome-specific probes has been shown.

- The risk of a structural chromosome abnormality is equal to that of a trisomy at age 37 years but is higher than the risk of trisomy in younger women.

•At age 35 years the risk of a structural chromosome abnormality is twice that of the risk of trisomy.

•This rate is higher than previously reported and suggests that, although not age-related, de novo and previously unrecognized but inherited structural chromosome abnormalities represent more of a risk than previously suspected.

•Structural chromosome abnormalities such as duplications, deletions, translocations, and inversions represent a significant genetic and reproductive risk.

•Duplications and deletions discovered at amniocentesis are **unbalanced**; these fetuses are at high risk for anomalies and developmental delay.

•Though balanced, **inversions** discovered at amniocentesis are at risk for unequal crossing-over during meiosis, producing unbalanced gametes.

°If familial, the presence-of inversions represents a risk for pregnancy loss or unbalanced conceptions in other family members.

°Apparently balanced translocations are not genetically neutral.

°The fetus discovered to have a new but apparently balanced translocation at amniocentesis is at risk.

°Because the translocation has never been inherited in a normal individual, it may be submicroscopically unbalanced.

°Apparently balanced translocations are associated with a **6% to 10% empiric risk of anomalies or developmental delay.**

°If familial, previously unidentified family members are at risk for unbalanced gametes and affected offspring.

•**The finding of a rate of structural chromosome rearrangements twice as high as trisomies at age 35 years in women not previously at risk, with 70% of these rearrangements familial but unrecognized before amniocentesis, suggests that numeric aneuploidy screening for trisomy alone is not adequate in a prenatal diagnosis program.**

•Fluorescence in situ hybridization aneuploidy screening would not routinely detect structural chromosome abnormalities that were twice as frequent as numeric aneuploidy at age 35 years.

•Until the reproductive risks and the impact of structural chromosome abnormalities identified at amniocentesis by high-resolution chromosome banding are known, routine use of fluorescence in situ hybridization for prenatal diagnosis should **not** be adopted without a prospective study of its accuracy and reliability compared with high-resolution karotype analysis.]

---

51. Which of the following antibiotics does NOT disrupt bacterial cell walls?

    A. ampicillin
    B. bacitracin
    C. cephalosporin
    *D. gentamicin
    E. vancomycin

---

p. 579 (Graham J M, Oshiro B T, Blanco J D, Magee K P. Uterine contractions after antibiotic therapy for pyelonephritis in pregnancy. Am J Obstet Gynec 1993; 168:577)

51. [F & I: •Background: In pregnancy acute pyelonephritis is a common disorder of the urinary tract, affecting approximately 2% of all pregnancies.

•Complications such as adult respiratory distress syndrome, hemolysis, and septic shock have been associated with this condition.

•Preterm labor occurs in patients with pyelonephritis, but the cause remains unknown.

•The initiation of uterine contractions in pyelonephritis may be related to the effects of bacteria or their by-products.

•The most common organisms isolated in pyelonephritis are gram-negative rods, of which *Escherichia coli* is the most frequent isolate.

•Gram-negative bacteria contain endotoxins that when released may stimulate the production of cytokines and prostaglandins.

•These inflammatory mediators are associated with uterine contractility and subsequent preterm labor.

•Objective: To investigate the role of pyelonephritis (extrauterine infection) in the pathogenesis of uterine contractility.

•To determine (1) the number of uterine contractions occurring in patients with pyelonephritis on admission and (2) whether the number of contractions is increased by antibiotic therapy.

•Results: Pregnant patients with pyelonephritis averaged eight contractions/hr on admission.

•The uterine contraction rate significantly increased in hours +1 to +4 after antibiotic administration.

•Patients with gram-negative bacteria accounted for this increase in contraction frequency.

•No increase in contraction frequency occurred in patients infected with gram-positive bacteria.

•A significant increase in contraction frequency occurred in hours +1 and +2 in the gram-negative group.

•There is an increase in hours +3 and +4 also, but these differences did not achieve statistical significance because of the smaller number of patients in the gram-positive group.

•An association has been suggested between uterine contractility and maternal bacterial infection, especially with gram-negative organisms.

•The lysis of gram-negative bacteria results in the release of **endotoxin** (lipopolysaccharide) into local tissues and, if in sufficient concentration, the bloodstream.

•In patients with premature rupture of membranes, lipopolysaccharide levels were higher for patients in labor compared with those not in labor.

•The liberated lipopolysaccharide stimulates the monocyte-macrophage system that results in tumor necrosis factor and interleukin-1 production.

•Eventually interleukin-6 is synthesized and, together with tumor necrosis factor and interleukin-1, stimulates decidual cells to produce prostaglandins.

•The released prostaglandins may stimulate uterine contractility.

•If sufficient prostaglandin production occurs, premature labor may ensue.

•This proposed mechanism of uterine contractility is obviously driven by the release of bacterial products, namely endotoxin.

•Any event that increases lipopolysaccharide release may result in increased uterine contractility.

•Antibiotics may increase lipopolysaccharide release and subsequently uterine contractility.

•The enhancement of the deleterious effects of lipopolysaccharide by administration of antibiotic therapy is well known in the general medical literature.

•The antibiotics that lyse the cell wall of gram-negative bacteria enhance the release of lipopolysaccharide and exacerbate the outcome of some patients with gram-negative sepsis.

•In theory the released lipopolysaccharide stimulates the monocyte-macrophages system to release cytokines and prostaglandins that may worsen end-organ damage and make shock refractory to medical management.

•Antibodies to ameliorate the lipopolysaccharide effect have been used.

•The use of antibiotics that do not lyse the cell wall, i.e., **aminoglycosides**, may not produce the lipopolysaccharide release or its subsequent side effects.

•Adult respiratory distress syndrome, hemolysis, and premature labor are associated with acute pyelonephritis.

•By enhancing lipopolysaccharide release, antibiotic therapy may increase the frequency of uterine contractions and may predispose to complications in pregnancies affected by maternal gram-negative bacterial infection.

•The release of lipopolysaccharide may be the initiating event that produces adult respiratory distress syndrome and hemolysis—the end result of an immune system out of control.

•Antibiotic therapy that lyses the bacterial cell wall may result in the release of a large bolus of lipopolysaccharide, which may initiate or increase the frequency of uterine contractions in pregnancies complicated by acute gram-negative infection.]

---

52. Clinically useful in discriminating true labor from false labor in the early third trimester

    A. bed rest
    *B. cervicovaginal levels of oncofetal fibronectin
    C. hydration
    D. morphine sedation
    E. observation of fetal breathing movements on ultrasound

---

p. 541 (Morrison J C, Allbert J R, McLaughlin B N, Whitworth N S, Roberts W E, Martin R W. Oncofetal fibronectin in patients with false labor as a predictor of preterm delivery. Am J Obstet Gynec 1993; 168:538)

52. [F & I: •Background: Distinguishing true from spurious labor is important, particularly when the gestation is remote from term.

•This distinction is critical because preterm delivery remains one of the major causes of neonatal mortality and morbidity.

•Clinically, as many as 50% of women who have false labor eventually deliver preterm.

- The differentiation of false from true labor is problematic because the only absolute differentiating factor is that in true labor the contractions lead to irreversible progressive cervical change and, ultimately, delivery.

- Sedatives such as morphine, parenteral administration of fluids, periods of rest, or fetal breathing movements on ultrasonographic examination are used to distinguish false from true labor with little to moderate success.

- Oncofetal fibronectin in cervicovaginal fluid has been suggested as a sensitive and specific correlate of early delivery.

  ° This type of fibronectin has been identified in amniotic fluid, placental tissue, and malignant cell lines.

  ° It can be detected by the monoclonal antibody FDC-6, which specifically binds oncofetal fibronectin.

- Clinically, this technique has been used to measure fetal fibronectin in the cervicovaginal secretions of women at risk for early delivery.

- Objective: To detail the effectiveness of oncofetal fibronectin obtained from cervicovaginal secretions in differentiating who would later have true preterm labor with subsequent early delivery in a population of women who had had an episode of false labor but were otherwise not at risk for preterm birth.

- The null hypothesis was that a positive fetal fibronectin would not discriminate the group of women who would deliver before term because of preterm labor from those who delivered at term.

- The accurate determination of whether a patient is in true preterm labor is important but difficult.

- The level of discomfort and the intensity and frequency of contractions does not allow distinction of uterine activity that results in false labor and does not single out those who are destined to deliver early.

- Although some investigators have revealed that a decreased interval between contractions is more often associated with true labor, the mean and SD of these measurements were too wide to make this a clinically valuable tool.

- Likewise, cervical dilatation at the time of observation for false labor has been noted to be less in those with false labor, but the large SD often results in data that are not clinically useful if dilatation is <1 cm.

- Analgesic administration, observation, hydration, and administration of subcutaneous tocolytics are frequently **not** predictive of women who have false labor but who are at risk of preterm delivery.

- Because clinicians do not have a good discriminator of false versus true labor, and because as many as 50% of women with "false labor" deliver early, the need for an accurate test is evident.

- Results: 64% of 14 patients delivered early with positive oncofetal fibronectin, whereas of patients with negative test results only one (7%) patient delivered early.

- The correlation of a positive fetal fibronectin test result with preterm delivery revealed a sensitivity of 90% and specificity of 82.5%.

- The most important feature of oncofetal fibronectin was the 93% negative predictive value in women with false labor.

- Conclusion: Positive fetal fibronectin test results in women between 24 and 34 weeks' gestation who have false labor indicates a significant risk for the subsequent development of true preterm labor and a high risk for early delivery.

•A negative fetal fibronectin test result is a good indication that subsequent preterm labor and early delivery are unlikely to occur.]

---

53. The drug of choice for postpartum endometritis caused by enterococcus is

   A. ampicillin
   B. cephalexin
   C. clindamycin
   D. gentamicin
   *E. none of the above

---

p.116 (Graham J M, Blanco J D, Oshiro B T, Magee K P, Monga M, Eriksen N. Single-dose ampicillin prophylaxis does not eradicate enterococcus from the lower genital tract. Obstet Gynecol 1993; 81:115)

53. [F & I: •Background: Enterococcus, a gram-positive bacterium, may cause endometritis after cesarean delivery.

•Higher rates of enterococcal isolation may occur after prophylaxis with cephalosporins because these drugs are ineffective against the enterococcus.

•Many antibiotics used to treat endometritis are not effective against enterococcus; ampicillin has been recommended for cesarean prophylaxis to eradicate enterococcus from the lower genital tract.

•Patients with endometritis and enterococcal isolation are less likely to respond to therapy with clindamycin and gentamicin and require the addition of ampicillin to achieve cure.

•Objectives: To identify the pre- and postoperative carriage rates of enterococcus in the lower genital tract of women undergoing a cesarean delivery and to determine whether a single intraoperative dose of ampicillin eradicates enterococcus.

•Postpartum endometritis is an ascending infection caused by organisms found in the lower genital tract.

•The role of the enterococcus in the pathogenesis of postpartum endometritis remains unclear.

•Women with postpartum endometritis who receive cephalosporin prophylaxis are likely to have positive enterococcus cultures when the clinical diagnosis of endometritis is made.

°These cases of endometritis may be less likely to respond to antibiotic therapy that is not effective against enterococcus.

°It has been suggested that ampicillin be used for cesarean prophylaxis to eradicate enterococcus from the genital tract.

•Results: 39.3% of women had enterococcus in the genital tract.

•Nine subjects had enterococcus recovered only in postoperative cultures.

°Contamination from the rectum may have occurred in the interval between the two cultures.

•Enterococcus was recovered from the genital tract in the majority of women (93.8%) who received cephalosporin prophylaxis.

•Postoperative culture rates remained high (70.5%) despite ampicillin prophylaxis.

•**The presumption that ampicillin will eliminate or drastically reduce the carriage rate of enterococcus is erroneous.**

»The prophylactic use of ampicillin should have a minimal impact on postoperative infections due to enterococcus.]

---

54. The approximate number of Down Syndrome cases that can be detected by prenatal testing using advanced maternal age (greater than 35 years) as a criterion is

   *A. 20
    B. 25
    C. 33
    D. 50
    E. 57

p. 72 (Chenge E Y, Luthy D A, Zebelman A M, Williams M A, Lieppman R E, Hickok D E. A prospective evaluation of a second-trimester screening test for fetal Down syndrome using maternal serum alpha-fetoprotein, hCG, and unconjugated estriol. Obstet Gynecol 1993; 81:72)

54. [F & I: •Background: Maternal age has been the primary means of identifying pregnancies at risk for trisomy, based on the association between advancing maternal age and increasing risk for a conception with aneuploidy.

•Using maternal age of 35 years or greater as the threshold for testing, only about 20% of Down syndrome pregnancies can be identified.

•When the risks for Down syndrome based on maternal age and MSAFP level are combined, the detection rate of Down syndrome pregnancies approaches 25-to-33%, at a false-positive rate of 5%.

•**Elevated** second-trimester maternal serum hCG levels is associated with fetal aneuploidy.

•Second-trimester unconjugated estriol (E3) levels are **lower** in the serum of women carrying Down syndrome fetuses.

•Combining all three analyses with maternal age, the potential detection rate is 67% for pregnancies affected with Down syndrome, at a false-positive rate of 7.2%.

•Objective: To determine whether the combination of all three biochemical markers and maternal age can be used as a screening protocol to detect Down syndrome pregnancies.

•Results: Seven more Down syndrome cases (22 versus 15) than expected were detected, even accounting for an expected 22% fetal loss.

•There were four cases of de novo D;G or G;G translocation Down syndrome, accounting for over half of the excess number of Down syndrome cases.

•De novo robertsonian translocations occur approximately once in 10,000 live births and are not associated with maternal age.

•The excessive number of Down syndrome cases cannot be fully explained although all cases were carefully reviewed to exclude ascertainment bias.

•None of the subjects received serum screening or level II ultrasound before entry into the study.

•The high detection rate observed may be attributed in part to the selection of a 1:195 risk for the cutoff.

•Eighteen of the 20 screen-positive Down syndrome cases had risks of 1:100 or greater.

- The mean risk for Down syndrome (+ 1 SD) was 1:67 (1:82); thus the selection of a 1:195 cutoff identified the majority of Down syndrome pregnancies.

- The average multiples of the median values for pregnancies unaffected by Down syndrome differed from the expected value of 1.00.

- The triple-marker screen identified several other chromosomal disorders besides Down syndrome.

   ° Three cases of trisomy 18 occurred in this study population.

   ° One case was detected through a positive screen designed to detect Down syndrome, an additional one would have been detected if suggested cutoffs for the triple-marker screen specific for trisomy 18 had been used, and one would have escaped detection under all conditions.

- The triple-marker screen performed well across all age groups, with acceptable rates of amniocentesis.

   ° One case of Down syndrome was detected for every 23 women offered amniocentesis, and one case was found for every 17 amniocenteses performed.

- The use of the triple-marker screen among women aged 35 and older provides a more accurate risk assessment for fetal Down syndrome than maternal age alone.

   ° Over half of the screen-negative women in this age group can avoid the risks of second-trimester amniocentesis.

- The use of the triple-marker screen could potentially result in major cost savings by decreasing the number of amniocenteses performed in this age group.

   » It should be offered with informed consent and counseling that stresses the limitations of serum screening (i.e., the potential for missed cases) and recognizes that only diagnostic testing (amniocentesis or chorionic villus sampling) can identify all chromosomal disorders.

- The triple-marker screen resulted in better test performance than either the double-marker screen (MSAFP and hCG) or the MSAFP test alone.

- Either the triple or the double-marker screen was clearly superior to MSAFP alone. Sensitivity and specificity will depend on the actual cutoff chosen.

   ° A cutoff may be selected based on a desired or acceptable false-positive rate (the number of women potentially requiring amniocentesis) or based on existing practice (such as the Down syndrome risk for a 35- or 37-year-old woman).

   ° The cutoff selected is, by definition, somewhat arbitrary and may be changed over time as test performance is evaluated.]

---

55. During pregnancy the terbutaline induced glucose intolerance is caused by

    A. decreased levels of C peptide.
    B. decreased levels of insulin.
    *C. increased insulin resistance.
    D. increased levels of pancreatic peptide.
    E. Terbutaline does not cause glucose intolerance in pregnancy.

---

p. 103   (Foley M R, Landon M B, Gabbe S G, O'Dorisio T M, Waxman M, Leard R, Iams J D. Effect of prolonged oral terbutaline therapy on glucose tolerance in pregnancy. Am J Obstet Gynec 1993; 168:100)

55. [F & I: •Background: ß2-Adrenergic agonists such as ritodrine and terbutaline are used in the treatment of premature labor.

•Terbutaline often is the preferred oral tocolytic agent because it is equally effective, is less expensive, and offers a more convenient dosing interval than ritodrine.

•Oral terbutaline may be a contributing factor in the development of gestational diabetes.

•The mechanism by which oral terbutaline causes an altered response to a glucose challenge is unknown.

•Objective: To describe the effects and reversibility of terbutaline induced changes in carbohydrate metabolism.

•Results: The anticipated difference between control and treatment areas under the curve for the 3-hour GTT after terbutaline therapy was significantly overestimated.

•Only 1 of 17 women (5.8%) had gestational diabetes after five days of terbutaline therapy.

•Oral terbutaline therapy increases the risk of gestational diabetes.

•The data showed a postchallenge increase in glucose, insulin, pancreatic polypeptide levels, and insulin/glucose ratios after 5 consecutive days of oral terbutaline therapy.

•With the exception of glucagon levels, which returned to baseline, these remained significantly elevated 7 days after cessation of therapy suggesting that **chronic oral terbutaline produces a prolonged metabolic effect.**

•The significantly increased postchallenge glucose level seen after terbutaline therapy appears to result from an **adrenergically mediated rise in glucagon levels and diminished insulin sensitivity**.

•The literature supports a rapid and sustained depression in glucagon levels after a glucose challenge with advancing gestation.

•The rise in glucagon levels is postulated to result from a direct effect of terbutaline.

•The elevated postchallenge glucose level observed may result from the **augmented gluconeogenesis and glycogenolysis produced by rising levels of glucagon.**

•The elevation in glucose and glucagon levels directly increases the secretion of insulin.

•The adrenergic stimulus produced by chronic terbutaline may directly stimulate the release of insulin (mediated by cAMP).

•This adrenergic stimulus may interrupt the normal extraction of insulin by the liver, resulting in elevated serum insulin levels without a concurrent increase in the byproduct of normal insulin production, C-peptide.

•Without a parallel increase in C-peptide, an alternative explanation for the observed elevated insulin level may be cross-reactivity of the insulin assay with the less potent proinsulin from which no C-peptide is produced.

•Pancreatic polypeptide functions primarily to regulate gastrointestinal functions such as exocrine pancreatic secretion and gallbladder emptying and is under vagal control.

• The increased insulin/glucose ratio appears to represent a terbutaline-induced, glucagon-mediated **insulin resistance**.

•That the serum terbutaline level drawn after therapy failed to correlate with any of the pertinent metabolic parameters strongly suggests that the effect produced is dose-independent.

•**Body mass index** did not correlate consistently with baseline measurements but did correlate significantly with **postchallenge insulin levels and insulin/glucose ratio**.

•Body mass index was not correlated with either fasting or postchallenge measures of glucagon.

•These results support the conclusion that patients with higher body mass indexes consistently produce larger amounts of postchallenge insulin and exhibit higher degrees of diminished insulin sensitivity as exemplified by consistently higher insulin/glucose ratios.

•The data support a dose-independent, terbutaline-induced glucose intolerance mediated by glucagon and caused by diminished insulin sensitivity.

•Patients taking oral terbutaline at between 24 and 32 weeks' gestation are at an increased risk for developing metabolic derangements consistent with glucose intolerance.

•Although there is no information to suggest that the metabolic disturbances induced by oral terbutaline contribute to an increase in perinatal morbidity or mortality, standard screening for glucose intolerance in patients receiving prolonged oral terbutaline is strongly supported, particularly if they exhibit other risks for gestational diabetes such as obesity (body mass index >29).]

---

56. Magnesium sulfate causes plasma endothelin-1 levels in preeclamptic pregnancies to decrease because of

   A. decreased production of angiotensin converting enzymes
   B. direct suppression of Et-1 production
   C. increased production of nitric oxide
   D. increased vasodilatation and release of prostacyclin
   *E. none of the above

p. 1558   (Mastrogiannis D S, Kalter C S, O'Brien W F, Carlan S J, Reece E A. Effect of magnesium sulfate on plasma endothelin-1 levels in normal and preeclamptic pregnancies. Am J Obstet Gynec 1992; 167:1554)

56. [F & I: •Background: Endothelium modulates cardiovascular homeostasis during normal pregnancy and endothelial cell damage is involved in the pathophysiologic characteristics of preeclampsia.

•The endothelium regulates the reactivity of vascular smooth muscle through production of both vasodilators and vasoconstrictors.

•Endothelin-1 (Et-1), the most potent naturally occurring vasoconstrictor yet identified, belongs to a group of peptides, the endothelins.

°There are at least three related peptides, endothelin 1, 2, and 3, which are products of separate genes and act via distinct receptors.

•Et-1 mainly acts as a **vasoconstrictor** that also has effects in other target organs such as brain, adrenal gland, lung, kidney, intestine, and uterus.

•Et-1 may be involved inthe etiology of hypertensive diseases.

•Several lines of evidence implicate endothelial cell injury as a basic pathogenetic mechanism in preeclampsia, resulting in impaired synthesis of vasodilators and a possible increase in the production of vasoconstrictors.

- Before labor, women with preeclampsia have higher plasma Et-1 concentrations when compared with normal antepartum women.

- Magnesium sulfate infusion in antepartum patients with preeclampsia decreased the concentration of Et-1 in plasma.

- Objectives: To determine whether the effect of magnesium sulfate on Et-1 concentration is limited to preeclampsia and whether this effect is mediated via inhibition of Et-1 release by the endothelial cell.

- Preeclampsia is a hypertensive disorder unique to pregnancy that is characterized by generalized vasoconstriction.

- Et-1 concentrations in pregnancy are influenced by gestational age, presence or absence o labor, and the administration of magnesium sulfate.

- The possible mechanisms for the increased Et-1 levels in preeclampsia include:

  ° (1) Because there is disruption and destruction of the anatomic boundaries between the endothelium and smooth muscle layer, Et-1 can leak into the circulation from its local environment with subsequently high peripheral blood levels.

  ° (2) An abnormal production of Et-1 by the affected endothelium could be a primary mechanism for the increased levels locally or in the bloodstream.

    °° Excessive production of Et-1 could be the product of placental or fetal tissue in preeclampsia with possible increased diffusion into the maternal circulation.

  ° (3) Last, a defect of endothelin clearance could be a mechanism for increased levels in preeclampsia.

- The increased Et-1 concentrations that observed in preeclampsia are not necessarily related to the degree of vasoconstriction (emphasizing the not-well-studied paracrine effects of Et-1).

- The simultaneous production of endothelium-derived relaxing factors or vasodilatory prostaglandins by the endothelium may have a possible cooperative effect, supported by the following laboratory observations:

  ° (1) When pharmacologic concentrations of Et-1 are added to cultures of human umbilical cord endothelial cells, there is an increase in prostacyclin release

  ° (2) Et-1 causes the release of nitric oxide (endothelial cell relaxing factor).

    °° These properties may counterbalance its vasoconstrictive effects in vivo and serve as a complex feedback mechanism.

    °° The exact process of the release of the vasoactive substances is not known at this time.

    °° Prostacyclin levels are relatively reduced in preeclampsia, therefore an abnormality of endothelin-prostacyclin interaction could exist.

- Magnesium sulfate is considered the standard antiseizure prophylaxis in preeclampsia by the majority of obstetricians and gynecologists in the United States.

  - Some of its pharmacologic properties suggest vasoactive effects through interaction with vasoactive peptides and/or direct vasodilatation.

  - When given intravenously as a bolus, it has a transient hypotensive effect that is not observed with continuous infusion.

•Magnesium sulfate added to isolated umbilical arteries and veins obtained from normal term deliveries decreased the basal tension of these vessels in a dose-dependent manner.

•An increase in renal prostacyclin production was found in patients in preterm labor after magnesium sulfate infusion.

•An in vitro study has suggested that magnesium might increase the prostacyclin production from endothelial cells.

•Intravenous administration of magnesium sulfate significantly vasodilated maternal intracranial vessels distal to the middle cerebral artery as evidenced by a decreased Pourcelot index without significantly affecting the other maternal or fetal vessels that were studied.

•Results: A lowering of plasma Et-1 concentration in patients during magnesium sulfate infusion was observed, which was limited to women with preeclampsia.

°Lower Et-1 levels might be associated with a higher degree of vasodilatation in response to magnesium sulfate infusion in preeclampsia, at least in some vessels.

°The effect of magnesium sulfate on Et-1 levels does not appear to be a characteristic of normal endothelial cells.

°When endothelial cells in culture were exposed to magnesium sulfate, the release of Et-1 did not differ from that of controls.]

---

57. In late pregnancy the increased uterine activity seen between midnight and 2:00 a.m. is secondary to

    A. decreased maternal progesterone
    B. increased maternal catecholamines
    C. increased maternal estrogen
    *D. increased maternal oxytocin
    E. increased maternal prostaglandins

---

p. 1562 (Fuchs A, Behrens O, Liu H. Correlation of nocturnal increase in plasma oxytocin with a decrease in plasma estradiol/progesterone ratio in late pregnancy. Am J Obstet Gynec 1992; 167:1559)

57. [F & I: •Background: Uterine activity in pregnant women exhibits a marked diurnal rhythm.

•Increased activity occurs at night time with a peak around midnight.

•This biorhythm may be the reason why the hour of labor onset also shows a 24-h rhythm with a peak between midnight and 2 AM.

•In animals no correlation was found between the nocturnal uterine activity and maternal catecholamines or prostaglandins or with amniotic fluid prostaglandins.

•Maternal and fetal plasma steroid hormones exhibited marked diurnal variations; progesterone in phase and estrone phase shifted in relation to uterine activity.'

•Uterine responsiveness to oxytocin also exhibited a 24-h rhythm, which coincided with the rhythm in uterine activity.

•Administration of specific oxytocin antagonists abolished the midnight peak in uterine activity in pregnant animals, which strongly suggested that oxytocin was responsible for the 24-h rhythm in uterine activity in pregnant subhuman primates.

•Objectives: To examine whether plasma concentrations of oxytocin exhibit diurnal variations in women in late pregnancy.

- To examine the possible influence of ovarian and adrenal steroids on plasma oxytocin levels the concentrations of plasma estradiol, progesterone, and cortisol were measured in the same samples as for oxytocin.

- Results: Plasma concentrations of oxytocin exhibit a nocturnal peak and early morning nadir in women in late pregnancy.

- The peak concentrations of oxytocin in women were of similar magnitude as those measured after a 4 to 16 mU bolus of oxytocin was injected into women in late pregnancy.

- These injections elicited uterine contractions, indicating that comparable oxytocin concentrations are capable of stimulating uterine contractions in women at or very near term.

- Oxytocin may be responsible for the nocturnal increase in uterine activity in pregnant women.

- In the human, prostaglandin secretion is maximal in the daytime and significantly lower at nighttime, as indicated by urinary excretion rates, suggesting that prostaglandins may not provide the primary stimulus for the midnight peak in uterine activity in women, although the participation of prostaglandins in the nocturnal augmentation of myometrial contractions cannot be ruled out.

- What factors in turn regulate oxytocin secretion in pregnant women is not known.

- The strong correlation between the ratio of estradiol to progesterone suggests that ovarian hormones participate in the regulation of oxytocin secretion in women.

- Those steroids that are produced by maternal adrenals or depend on maternal or fetal adrenal precursors (cortisol and estradiol) are likely to exhibit circadian variations whereas those synthesized de novo in the placenta (progesterone) are less likely to exhibit such variations.

- The significant nocturnal increase in plasma progesterone could perhaps be due to variations in the production of precursor cholesterol by maternal liver or to a direct interaction between circulating cortisol and progesterone.

- In the early morning hours, when cortisol levels are maximal, the cortisol-binding protein in plasma is fully saturated with cortisol; hence progesterone may be more rapidly metabolized than at midnight when, at low cortisol levels, a substantial proportion of progesterone is bound to the cortisol-binding protein.

- Conclusion: Concentrations of oxytocin in the plasma of women in late pregnancy exhibit significant daily rhythms with a nocturnal peak.

- The oxytocin peak is temporally associated with a peak in uterine activity which may in turn be associated with the onset of spontaneous term and preterm labor, both of which show a significant peak around midnight and early morning hours.]

---

58. What percentage of functioning nephron mass is lost when serum creatinine is 0.8 mg/dl during gestation?

    A. 15
    B. 20
    C. 25
    D. 33
    *E. >50

p. 122   (Stettler R W, Cunningham F G. Natural history of chronic proteinuria complicating pregnancy. Am J Obstet Gynec 1992; 167:1219)

58. [F & I: •Background: Although proteinuria complicating pregnancy-induced hypertension is common, characteristically it recedes postpartum, and usually there are no adverse sequelae.

•Chronic proteinuria that is discovered during pregnancy in most cases antedates conception and signifies any of a number of glomerulopathic syndromes that may be quite serious.

•Coincidental hypertension or renal dysfunction, as opposed to proteinuria, are the prime determinants of pregnancy outcome in women with renal disease.

•Pregnancies complicated by the nephrotic syndrome or nephrotic-range proteinuria are associated with excessive adverse maternal and fetal outcomes.

•Objective: To evaluate varying degrees of chronic proteinuria as a predictor of pregnancy outcome and the long-term prognosis for these women.

•Protein excretion of up to 300 mg per day may accompany normal pregnancy, but levels in excess of this are considered pathologic.

•A minimum value of 500 mg per day excluded questionably significant cases.

°Diabetic pregnancies or those with evidence of preeclampsia at presentation were excluded from this study.

•The nephrotic syndrome in its purest form is characterized by proteinuria, edema, hypoalbuminemia, and hyperlipidemia.

°The syndrome has multiple causes, all of which characteristically damage the glomerular endothelium and cause abnormal filtration.

°The clinical spectrum that results is from excessive glomerular leakage of proteins, with the hallmark of nephrotic syndrome being protein excretion of more than 3.5 gm/1.73 m^2/day.

•Results: Only one third of women had proteinuria sufficient enough to satisfy the classic definition of the nephrotic syndrome, and only a few of these had other stigma of the syndrome.

•Perhaps a term such as "proteinuric nephrosis" describes these women better but, whatever term is chosen, these women whose pregnancies were complicated by persistent but asymptomatic proteinuria had significantly **increased adverse perinatal and long-term outcomes.**

•Except for a threefold increased incidence of preeclampsia, isolated proteinuria is usually associated with a good pregnancy outcome.

•When there was coexisting renal insufficiency or chronic hypertension—factors that commonly coexist with renal disease-adverse pregnancy outcomes were increased significantly.

°The incidences of preeclampsia, preterm delivery, and fetal growth retardation were increased markedly.

•Renal insufficiency is associated with adverse pregnancy outcomes; although the incidence of associated complications is lower than that for pregnancies complicated by chronic renal insufficiency, most women now described had only mild renal dysfunction.

°For example, the median serum-creatinine level among these women was 1.1 mg/dl.

°Although this value is less than the 1.4 mg/dl commonly cited to define clinically significant renal dysfunction, serum creatinine >0.8 mg/dl during gestation suggests a loss of ≥50% of the functioning nephron mass and indicates renal insufficiency.

- Antecedent hypertension complicated about 40% of these pregnancies with chronic proteinuria, and this alone is associated with an increased incidence of preeclampsia and fetal growth retardation.

- Superimposed preeclampsia is difficult to diagnose when there is preceding proteinuria, and this is made even more difficult when there is also underlying hypertension.

- Preeclampsia was defined as worsening hypertension or proteinuria or onset of characteristic symptoms with and without laboratory abnormalities such as thrombocytopenia and elevated serum hepatic transaminase concentration.

- Using this definition, superimposed preeclampsia was diagnosed in 60% of pregnancies that reached viability.

- In women with renal dysfunction, the incidence of superimposed preeclampsia ranges from 10% to 60%; when there is chronic hypertension, the incidence is as high as 80%.

- Moreover, it seems likely that these two factors of renal insufficiency and hypertension are additive in their effects on gestation.

- Although the early pregnancy loss rate, including therapeutic abortions, was only 12%, the stillbirth rate was 7% and there were two neonatal deaths among 53 infants born alive.

- The perinatal mortality rate of 108 per 1000 for the study group, although not prohibitive, represents significant morbidity for these women.

- In nonpregnant patients, persistent proteinuria is a marker for renal disease, and the long-term prognosis is worse than that for patients with intermittent proteinuria.

- Specifically, of the 21 women with extended follow-up, more than half required chronic dialysis or renal transplantation within a mean of 5 years.

- Although there is bias in that women with severe disease were more likely to return for follow-up, the 11 women with renal failure still represent 20% of all of those who had persistent proteinuria during pregnancy.

- Daily urinary protein excretion correlates with the rate of deterioration of renal function.

- All 21 women who underwent renal biopsy had intrinsic renal disease.

    ° Microscopic examination showed a heterogeneous spectrum of renal diseases.

    ° Investigations of nonpregnant patients with isolated proteinuria have found evidence of renal structural aberrations in 40% to 100%; with persistent proteinuria this incidence increases.

- In these patients the most common histopathologic patterns were membranous glomerulonephritis and focal sclerosing glomerulonephritis, two common primary glomerular lesions associated with asymptomatic proteinuria.

    ° Most patients with focal sclerosing glomerulonephritis and persistent proteinuria progress to end-stage renal disease or death within 10 years; only 20% to 30% of those with membranous glomerulonephritis do so.

- The significance of proteinuria of <500 mg per day was not addressed.

- This lesser degree of proteinuria is not characteristically associated with renal dysfunction; coexisting renal disease is common when proteinuria exceeds this level.

- Postural orthostatic proteinuria may occur in women of reproductive age and can increase during pregnancy.

°Among the 53 women, only one demonstrated orthostatic proteinuria.

°Differentiating this entity from constant proteinuria is most important because the long-term prognosis for orthostatic proteinuria is significantly better.

•Proteinuria exceeding 500 mg per day should alert the clinician to the possibility of adverse pregnancy outcome.

•Specifically, the risks for preeclampsia, preterm delivery, and fetal growth retardation are increased markedly.

•Although pregnancy outcomes are acceptable, the perinatal mortality rate is increased at least fivefold compared with uncomplicated pregnancies.

•Perhaps the most important finding is that long-term maternal morbidity is significant and there is at minimum a 20% incidence of progression to end-stage renal disease.

•Postpartum renal evaluation is of paramount importance in such women.

•In only two women was there documented spontaneous remission of persistent chronic proteinuria after delivery; thus it appears that the hasty acceptance of proteinuria as "gestational" is ill-advised.]

---

59. The greatest sensitivity in predicting subsequent clinical infection in patients with premature rupture of the membranes is

   *A. amniotic fluid glucose level
   B. Gram stain
   C. leukocyte esterase estimation
   D. limulus amebocyte lysate assay
   E. white blood count

p. 1248   (Coultrip L L, Grossman J H. Evaluation of rapid diagnostic tests in the detection of microbial invasion of the amniotic cavity. Am J Obstet Gynec 1992; 167:1231)

59. [F & I: •Background: Microbial invasion of the amniotic cavity is frequently found in patients with preterm labor with intact membranes and preterm premature rupture of the membranes.

•The microbial invasion of the amniotic cavity is a risk for maternal and neonatal infections and noninfectious complications.

•The culturing of amniotic fluid is a means of identifying patients at risk for infectious morbidity.

•Rapid, inexpensive techniques such as the Gram stain, leukocyte esterase assay, *Limulus* amebocyte lysate assay, and intraamniotic glucose level determination are recommended for their value in supplying the information needed to make timely management decisions.

•The **Gram stain** is the most frequently used rapid diagnostic test for detecting intraamniotic infection.

°Sensitivity and positive predictive value of this test range from 0% to 84.6% and 0% to 100%, respectively.

°The Gram stain is the standard against which other tests are compared.

•The presence of **leukocyte esterase activity** reflects the presence of activated neutrophils and has been used as a rapid bedside test for intraamniotic infection.

°Sensitivity ranges from 19% to 94%

•The *Limulus* amebocyte lysate assay, a test for bacterial endotoxin, has a sensitivity of 69% in the detection of microbial invasion of the amniotic cavity; the combined use of the *Limulus* amebocyte lysate and the Gram stain increases the sensitivity to 95.6%.

•Low intraamniotic fluid glucose level may be a sensitive indicator of amniotic fluid infection.

•Objective: To evaluate the diagnostic performance of several rapid diagnostic tests, including the Gram stain, leukocyte esterase, *Limulus* amebocyte lysate assay, and intraamniotic glucose level measurement in the detection of intraamniotic infection as defined by a positive amniotic fluid culture or by clinical infection within 24 h of amniocentesis.

•The rapid diagnosis of intraamniotic infection is problematic.

•To allow the opportunity for intervention, a test should detect infection before it is clinically apparent.

•Indeed, if a condition can be diagnosed clinically, further testing is redundant.

•The test should be rapid, inexpensive, and capable of being performed in a hospital at any time of the day.

•The ultimate value of a test will be whether or not it is efficient enough to warrant the risks of intervention.

•Ideally, the test would be 100% sensitive with a negligible false-positive rate.

•Because such a test is not currently available, it must be acknowledged that any optimal testing scheme will be influenced by gestational age and the course of action (i.e., antibiotics or delivery).

•A low amniotic fluid glucose level has been found to have comparable or greater efficiency than the Gram stain for the detection of intraamniotic infection.

•Results: Amniotic fluid glucose concentration is significantly **decreased** in preterm labor patients with intraamniotic infection (whether defined by a positive amniotic fluid culture or clinical infection) and in patients with preterm premature rupture of the membranes who developed clinical infection.

•The precise mechanism of this decrease in amniotic and other body fluids is unclear but probably involves glucose metabolism by both microorganisms and polymorphonuclear leukocytes analogous to the presumed pathogenesis of the decreased cerebrospinal fluid glucose level in central nervous system infection.

•Patients with many or moderate polymorphonuclear leukocytes noted on Gram stain were more likely to have an amniotic fluid glucose level <10 mg/dl than were those with few polymorphonuclear leukocytes.

•Assuming that clinical infection represents a continuum of a progressive inflammatory response triggered by proliferating bacteria, it is logical that more advanced disease (i.e., clinical infection as opposed to asymptomatic patients with positive amniotic fluid cultures) would be characterized by more drastic reductions in glucose concentration.

•This may well explain the more marked decrease and greater prevalence of low glucose concentration found in patients destined to have clinical infection than in those with positive cultures.

•In patients with preterm premature rupture of the membranes who had positive cultures, glucose levels did not significantly decrease.

°There are several plausible explanations.

°The sample size (n = 29) may have been too small to detect a difference.

°Positive cultures may have been detected before there was a significant polymorphonuclear response, that is, very early in the inflammatory continuum and before significant glucose metabolism.

°Finally, glucose metabolism may be somewhat microorganism dependent.

°Viral meningitis, for example, is not associated with decreased cerebrospinal fluid glucose levels.

•Microorganisms traditionally presumed to be virulent, such as *S. agalactiae,* were associated with very low glucose levels (median 1.5 mg/dl), in contrast to *U. urealyticum* (median 16 mg/dl).

•In patients with preterm premature rupture of the membranes 7 (50%) of 14 amniotic fluid cultures were positive for *U. urealyticum,* an uncommon neonatal pathogen but common cervical isolate that is **not detectable by Gram stain.**

•Amniotic fluid white blood cell counts with differential in conjunction with amniotic fluid glucose concentration and quantitative microbiologic examination may help clarify the relationship between these entities.

•The false-positive low glucose levels warrant emphasis.

°Eleven of 15 patients with false-positive glucose (threshold <10 mg/dl) had other evidence of infection, suggesting false-negative cultures possibly caused by particularly fastidious microorganisms, very small inoculum size, or faulty laboratory technique.

°Two patients had a positive *Limulus* amebocyte lysate assay and delivered at term with no other symptoms of infection.

°Although meticulous sterile technique was used, because both glucose analysis and *Limulus* amebocyte lysate assay for endotoxin were carried out on thawed specimens, it is conceivable that bacterial contamination of the fluid occurred after retrieval.

•Although leukocyte esterase has been regarded as a sensitive test for intraamniotic infection, it was not found useful.

•Leukocyte esterase, a product of polymorphonuclear leukocytes, may be a marker of advanced infection and as such is not useful.

•Likewise, the data do not support the routine use of the *Limulus* amebocyte lysate assay, as many intraamniotic infections cannot be attributed to Gram-negative or endotoxin-producing organisms and thus may go undetected.

•An optimal testing scheme must consider the consequences of a false-positive result.

•Should the treatment of a positive test result be delivery rather than antibiotics, gestational age becomes a critical issue.

•Appropriate testing at very early gestational ages might include **two** positive test results (i.e., positive Gram's stain and a low glucose level) or a lower glucose level (i.e., 2 mg/dl rather than 15 mg/dl).

•In more advanced gestations, when the risk of prematurity lessens, not missing an infection (maximizing sensitivity) may be more important than being right all the time (tolerating a higher false-positive rate).

•Receiver-operator characteristic curves may serve as a guide for the clinician to select the appropriate testing scheme.

•Conclusion: The initial screen for infection with either a glucose concentration or Gram stain.

•The precise glucose level and the need for a confirming alternative test will be determined by the clinicians' tolerance of a given false-positive rate.]

---

60. Predictive of learning deficits in the older child (9 to 11 years)

    A. fetal asphyxia
 *B. intrauterine growth retardation
    C. newborn encephalopathy
    D. newborn infections
    E. newborn respiratory complications

---

p. 1504   (Low J A, Handley-Derry M H, Burke S O, Peters R D, Pater E A, Killen H L, Derrick E J. Association of intrauterine fetal growth retardation and learning deficits at age 9 to 11 years. Am J Obstet Gynec 1992; 167:1499)

60. [F & I: •Background: The effect of fetal growth retardation on neurodevelopmental outcome is unknown.

•Growth retardation is a heterogeneous entity that has a range of severity.

•Two studies have assessed preterm SGA children at age 8 years, and one study has assessed term SGA children in their adolescent years.

•SGA children continue to have smaller body measurements than their peers.

•There is no increased incidence of major handicaps.

   °The evidence in regard to minor neurodevelopmental disability, emotional development, and school performance is contradictory.

•Objectives: To assess the school performance of SGA children at 9 to 11 years of age.

•To examine the association of the biologic variables (fetal and newborn complications identified in the perinatal period) and the environmental variables (socioeconomic factors and early home environment) with learning deficits assessed between 9 and 11 years of age.

•The children were a selected population who had experienced one or more fetal or newborn complications during the perinatal period.

•The children assessed at age 9 to 11 years had advantages in relation to those lost to follow-up.

•The incidence of fetal or newborn complications at birth was similar.

•The socioeconomic status and home environment were more favorable and they had fewer motor and cognitive deficits at age 4 years.

•Learning deficits were determined by assessment of reading, spelling, and mathematic skills.

•Most children, when assessed, were in grade 4 or 5.

•By the end of grade 3 children should have well-established **decoding skills** and be showing increased speed and efficiency of reading.

•From grade 4 onward the child is required to **read independently** to obtain new information.

- In spelling, most children in grade 2 will be able to spell by using phonetic structures.

- This gives them the basis to rapidly increase their spelling vocabulary.

- In mathematics, the child should be able to add and subtract by the end of grade 3 with a good understanding of place value and regrouping.

- Results: 77 children studied were shown to have learning deficits.

  ° The deficits were equally distributed between reading, spelling, and arithmetic.

  ° There was a major learning deficit in 34 children, which corresponds to more than two grade levels below that expected for age.

- The children with learning deficits had less favorable measures of cognitive development with lower full-scale IQ scores on the Wechsler Intelligence Scale for Children.

- The children with learning disabilities also had an **increased frequency and range of behavioral and emotional** development problems identified by their teachers.

  ° The most significantly different behavioral characteristics of the children with learning deficiencies as determined by the Achenbach form and Connor's Teacher Rating Scale were **increased inattention and anxiety**.

- Examination of the biologic variables demonstrates that certain fetal and newborn complications (fetal asphyxia, newborn respiratory complications, newborn infection, and newborn encephalopathy) that are associated with motor and cognitive deficits at age 1 and 4 years are **not** predictive of learning deficits at age 9 to 11 years.

  ° Fetal growth retardation, which previously had not been a predictor of motor or cognitive deficits at age 1 and 4 years, is associated with learning deficits that can be assessed at age 9 to 11 years.

- Features of growth-retarded children that may influence outcomes, including the severity of the growth retardation, maturity at birth, and the sex of the child, were **not** shown to be related to learning deficits.

- Comparison of the growth-retarded children with and without learning deficits indicated **no difference in the severity of the growth retardation as expressed by weight and length of either the newborn at birth or the child at age 9 to 11 years**.

- Head circumference in appropriate-for-gestational-age children during the first year has been proposed as a predictor of cognitive abilities in school.

- Head circumference in the growth-retarded children with learning deficits was **smaller** than in those with normal academic achievement, but the differences were **not statistically significant**.

  ° This is in keeping with an earlier report that subnormal head size in growth-retarded children may not have an associated adverse effect on outcome.

- The incidence of learning deficits in the growth-retarded children was the same in children born preterm and at term, as well as in both boys and girls.

- The association between growth retardation and learning deficits may be mediated through low IQ scores or behavioral problems.

- There was no association between growth retardation and low full-scale IQ scores in the total population.

°Although low IQ scores are associated with learning deficits, it is unlikely they represent the explanation for the association between growth retardation and learning deficits.

•The children with learning deficiencies are described as inattentive and anxious.

•The group differences, although significant, are modest in degree.

•There was a relationship between socioeconomic indicators and learning deficits.

°The parents' education and the father's Blishen Score were related to learning deficits in these children at age 9 to 11 years.

°The association with socioeconomic factors suggests interactions with environmental factors.]

---

61. A patient is admitted at term with a vertex presentation. Active management of labor is to be undertaken. Success in achieving vaginal delivery includes all of the following EXCEPT

   A. development of chorioamnionitis.
   *B. maternal height.
   C. need for oxytocin augmentation.
   D. the station of the vertex on admission.
   E. use of epidural anesthesia.

---

p. 943 (Peaceman A M, Lopez-Zeno J A, Minogue J P, Socol M L. Factors that influence route of delivery-Active versus traditional. labor management Am J Obstet Gynec 1993; 169:940)

61. [F & I: Background: Physician practice style has been implicated as the single most important factor that influences whether a patient is delivered vaginally or by cesarean section.

•Other factors found to influence the route of delivery in traditional labor management include maternal age, height, payor status, cervical dilatation rate after admission, maximum infusion rate of oxytocin, epidural anesthesia, development of chorioamnionitis, pelvic size, and birth weight.

•Active management of labor may lower the cesarean section rate in nulliparous patients.

•Studies using both historical and randomized concurrent controls have found the efficacy of this labor management scheme in decreasing the incidence of dystocia.

•Objectives: To identify whether the risks for cesarean delivery differ between actively managed patients and patients with traditional labor management and that patient characteristics or medical interventions that predict an increased risk for cesarean section could be identified in both schemes.

•Data was analyzed for actively managed patients and from patients in a concurrent traditionally managed control group to determine obstetric factors that influence the route of delivery.

•Actively managed patients (n = 346) underwent amniotomy within 1 hour of admission if membranes were intact, and oxytocin augmentation was initiated when cervical dilatation was <1cm/hr.

•When used, oxytocin was initiated at a rate of 6 mU/min and was increased by increments of 6 mU/min every 15 min until either seven contractions occurred every 15 min or a maximum infusion rate of 36 mU/min was reached.

•For traditionally managed patients (n = 354) the timing of amniotomy, frequency of cervical examinations, and criteria for the diagnosis of protracted labor were left to the managing obstetrician.

•If arrest of dilatation or labor protraction was identified, oxytocin infusion was begun at 1 mU/min, and the dose was increased by 1 or 2 mU/min at 15-min intervals until eight uterine contractions occurred every 20 min.

- The decision to deliver by cesarean section for secondary arrest disorders or for fetal acidemia was made by the attending obstetrician.

- Chorioamnionitis was diagnosed on the basis of maternal fever (≥38° C) and either uterine tenderness, fetal tachycardia, or maternal tachycardia without another identifiable source.

- It was hypothesized that, as with traditional labor management schemes, patient characteristics on presentation in labor might foretell an increased risk for cesarean delivery when an active management of labor protocol is used.

- In univariate and multivariate analyses of patients with active management the only patient characteristic on **admission** associated with an increased risk of cesarean section was the observation of the **fetal presenting part above the station -1**.

- Other factors relating to labor that were also associated with higher rates of cesarean birth were **epidural anesthesia** and clinical **chorioamnionitis**.

- The need for oxytocin, especially when the maximum infusion rate was >18 mU/min, was a marker for increased risk of abdominal delivery with univariate analysis, but logistic regression did **not** identify the need for oxytocin to be independently associated with route of delivery in this group.

- With use of active management of labor maternal age, gestational age, pregravid weight, and total weight gain did **not** influence the likelihood of delivery by cesarean section.

- Nor were race or payor status different between the two groups.

- Patients delivered vaginally were taller, but this small difference was no longer significant after controlling for confounding variables with logistic regression.

- The presence of ruptured membranes on admission, cervical dilatation on admission, and the rate of cervical dilatation in the first 2 h of labor also were **not** found to influence route of delivery.

- Some similarities were identified between actively managed patients and traditionally managed patients in the risks for cesarean section.

- In contrast to the actively managed group, **birth weight, maternal height, and payor status** were identified with multiple logistic regression as being associated with higher rates of cesarean birth in the **traditionally** managed group.

- Maternal age, gestational age, and cervical dilatation on admission were also related to route of delivery with univariate analysis, but with logistic regression these factors were **not** found to be independently associated with cesarean delivery.

- **These data suggest that the increased risk of cesarean section associated with certain patient characteristics can be diminished with active management of labor.**

- Physician practice styles are also known to influence the route of delivery.

- With active management physician-controlled factors should have less of an influence.

- With traditional labor management **increasing birth weight** has been associated with an **increased risk of cesarean section**.

- With both univariate and multivariate analysis no significant contribution of fetal weight to the route of delivery when active management of labor was used was found.

•Although the number of patients studied is insufficient to exclude a contribution of birth weight to route of delivery when active management is used, the contention was that with this labor management scheme the development of dystocia is related more to uterine contractility than to fetal size.

•The effect of **epidural anesthesia** on the incidence of dystocia in labor remains controversial.

•A higher proportion of patients receiving epidural anesthetics for pain management during labor were delivered by cesarean section with both active management and traditional management; multivariable analysis confirmed this association.

•Given the similarities between the actively managed patients delivered vaginally and those delivered by cesarean section in the timing of epidural induction, the data support the contention that epidural anesthesia increases the risk of cesarean birth.

•**Chorioamnionitis** has previously been linked to an increased incidence of cesarean section.

•The data confirm the association between amnionitis and dystocia; whether intra-amniotic infection is a cause or a result of prolonged labor could not be determined.]

---

62. True statements about the standing position in pregnancy at term include all of the following EXCEPT

    A. a decrease in maternal cardiac output.
    B. a decreased incidence of fetal heart rate accelerations.
    C. an increase in fetal vessel resistance.
    *D. an increased incidence of inferior vena cava compression with the vertex engaged.
    E. diminished venous return.

---

p. 187 (Schneider K T M, Bung P, Weber S, Huch A, Huch R. An orthostatic uterovascular syndrome-A Prospective, longitudinal study. Am J Obstet Gynec 1993; 169:183)

62. [F & I: •Background: In a recent pilot study 33 of 55 women examined in the last trimester while standing motionless and unsupported were found to have cyclic maternal heart rate accelerations with a mean cycle length of 105 seconds and a mean amplitude of 27 beats/min.

•Measurements in the femoral vein showed that when there was a sharp decrease in blood flow velocity, maternal heart rate increased.

•Spontaneous uterine contractions then occurred, followed by an increase in femoral blood flow velocity and normalization of the maternal heart rate.

•In eight of the 33 cases with this orthostatic "uterovascular syndrome" the fetal heart rate (FHR) showed a decrease in oscillation amplitude.

•The uterus compresses the pelvic vessels when a woman is standing.

•The maternal tachycardia is a compensation for the reduced preload.

•Objective: To investigate the interaction between maternal hemodynamics and uterine activity for pregnant women in the upright position.

•The hemodynamic changes in the upright position increased with gestational age and increasing size of the uterus.

•Spontaneous contractions, probably by changing the shape or position of the uterus, released the blocked venous return flow, leading to normalization of maternal hemodynamics.

- In contrast to the nonpregnant state, orthostatic regulation in pregnant women is complex, and no steady state was reached in the measurements in 71% of the women examined at 38 weeks' gestation.

- The maternal heart rate acceleration amplitude increased with advancing gestational age and with duration of standing.

- **Uterine compression of pelvic vessels and hemodynamic regulation.**

- Invasive investigations of venous pressure revealed that, when a pregnant women is standing, the uterus might compress pelvic vessels.

- The leg venous pressure in both the upright and the supine position is three times greater in pregnancy.

- The greatest risk of compression of the inferior vena cava is when the fetal head is at the level of the promontory.

- Once the fetal head is engaged, there is no longer significant compression.

- In the upright position near term the anatomic situation is comparable.

- When a pregnant woman near term is standing, engagement of the fetal head releases compression, allowing return flow.

- Similarly, when a pregnant woman leans forward, the uterus is lifted away from the spine, also resulting in return venous flow.

- Uterus volume or weight is related to the observed circulatory changes.

- In patients with larger uteri, the impedance of venous return flow begins earlier in pregnancy and is more pronounced.

- Postpartum venous return flow is again normal.

- The trigger mechanism of the increased uterine contractility in the upright position is yet unknown.

- In the supine position only strong (labor) contractions can lift the uterus from the spine.

- Supine hypotensive syndrome can only occur when the uterus is relaxed and takes 3 to 7 min to reach its peak.

- During labor there is no time for it to develop.

- The situation is similar in the upright position in pregnancy, when there is a significantly increased contraction frequency (the intervals between contractions are usually under 4 min).

- Most (80%) of the contractions in the upright position were not felt by the women.

- Yet hemodynamic effects were observed.

- Uterine contractions cause return flow to the vena cava and such an effect is even assumed for the Alvarez waves.

- It is not necessary for the whole uterus to be lifted, but even in the standing position collapse can occur if contractions are insufficient.

- **Implications for the fetus.**

•When women are tilted by an angle of 70 degrees, there is a decrease (23%) in the distribution of technetium 99 concentration, compared with the left lateral recumbent position.

•This is attributed to a diminished venous return flow with increased pooling in the legs.

•Doppler ultrasonographic investigations also show an increase in the resistance in the fetal vessels when the mother changes to the upright position.

•Pregnant women with jobs requiring standing have a higher risk of low birth weight and stillbirth.

•In the upright position, and in spite of compensatory maternal tachycardia, there is a decrease in maternal cardiac output and a decrease in FHR accelerations.

•Thus placental perfusion may be reduced when a pregnant woman is standing.

•**Clinical significance.**

•Several cases of orthostatic collapse have been related to orthostatic uterovascular syndrome.

•Such patients should wear compression stockings and rest in the left lateral recumbent position.

•The increase in uterine contractility in the upright position also justifies bed rest if there are signs of premature labor.

•Because maternal standing can also cause fetal stress, it might also be used as a test for fetal hypoxia.]

---

63. Increased physiologic effects in preeclampsia all of the following EXCEPT

   *A. calcitonin gene-related peptide.
   B. endothelin.
   C. plasma fibronectin.
   D. thromboxane.
   E. total plasma activator inhibitors.

p. 164 (Kraayenbrink A A, Dekker G A, van Kamp G J, van Geijn H P. Endothelial vasoactive mediators in preeclampsia. Am J Obstet Gynec 1993; 169:160)

63. [F & I: •Background: Injury of vascular endothelial linings appear to be important in the pathogenesis of preeclampsia.

•Increased levels of factor VIII-related antigen to factor VIII coagulation activity, increased levels of fibronectin, and a disturbance of the thromboxane A2 (TXA2)/prostacyclin (PGI2) balance all support the hypothesis that endothelial cell damage, which may be caused by an immune maladaptation, is intimately involved in the pathogenesis of preeclampsia.

•This hypothetic immune maladaptation may result in endothelial dysfunction by oxygen-free radicals or neutrophil elastase production.

•**Endothelin**, a potent vasoconstrictor peptide produced by the vascular endothelium, may cause vasospasm with respect to intimal injury, subsequent platelet aggregation, and thrombin formation and therefore in the pathophysiology of preeclampsia.

•**Calcitonin gene-related peptide**, an extremely potent vasoactive peptide that causes profound vasodilation in man, is increased during normal pregnancy, and it may regulate blood flow in the placental vasculature and in fetal development.

- In theory a decreased level of calcitonin gene-related peptide could contribute to preeclamptic vasospasm.

- Objective: To evaluate the extent to which these three vasoactive mediators (endothelin, calcitonin gene-related peptide, and TXA2/PGI2) are involved in the pathophysiology of preeclampsia.

- In the past decade increasing evidence has been adduced to support the hypothesis that endothelial cell injury and disturbed endothelial cell function is of major importance in the pathogenesis of preeclampsia.

- The increased levels of plasma fibronectin, a disturbance of tissue-plasminogen activator and plasminogen activator inhibitor balance, and a disturbance of the TXA2/PGI2 balance point in the direction of endothelial damage.

- Direct evidence is provided by the characteristic morphologic lesions of preeclampsia: glomerular endotheliosis and ultrastructural changes in placental bed and uterine boundary vessels.

- Serum from preeclamptic patients is cytotoxic to endothelial cells in vitro.

- Consistent with the reversal of the clinical condition after delivery, cytotoxic activity in serum of preeclamptic women is reduced after 24 to 48 h post partum.

- In contrast, in normal pregnant women cytotoxic activity of serum increases after delivery.

- Advances in the understanding of endothelial physiologic and pathophysiologic conditions have led to the concept that endothelium has profound effects on the regulation of vascular tone, vascular remodeling, and the activation of platelets and the coagulation cascade.

- Endothelial injury can lead to the secretion of potent mitogens and vasoactive factors through increased production of peptide growth factors by endothelium itself or by stimulating the release of stored products by activated platelets.

- **Platelet-derived growth factor**, one of the mitogens, is also a potent vasoconstrictor.

- Sera from preeclamptic women obtained before delivery have increased mitogenic activity compared with that from normal pregnant women.

- In addition, this increased mitogenic activity disappears within 24 to 48 h after delivery.

- Whether this increased serum mitogenic activity results from the release of mitogens directly from injured endothelial cells or indirectly from the activated platelets has not yet been established.

- One of the possible mitogens might be endothelin, which may underlie systemic disorders associated with endothelial damage.

- Animal studies have shown that, apart from its local vasoconstrictor activity on the underlying smooth muscle, endothelin can cause induction of the release of potent vasodilator substances such as PGI2 and endothelium-derived relaxing factor, which limit the pressor activity of any endothelin reaching the circulating blood.

- In humans endothelin shares in common with other vasoactive hormones, such as angiotensin II, norepinephrine and vasopressin, the ability to activate phospholipase C, an initial event that leads to vascular smooth muscle contraction.

- Up until now, an increasing amount of data concern the role of endothelin in normotensive human pregnancy and preeclampsia.

- Results: Suggest that endothelin is involved in preeclamptic vasoconstriction.

- The extreme hypertension and multiple organ failure that occurred in six patients with severe preeclampsia (the syndrome of **hemolysis, elevated liver enzymes, and low platelets**) might be related to the very high levels of endothelin in these patients.

- The finding that endothelin levels are only markedly increased in severe preeclampsia suggests that an increase in venous plasma endothelin levels does **not** precede the clinical development of the disease.

- It might be that the increased levels of endothelin in severe preeclampsia are either the cause or just a consequence of extensive endothelial damage.

- Evidence of this endothelial damage could also be found by means of significantly elevated plasma fibronectin levels.

- To support or refute this hypothesis, longitudinal follow-up of venous plasma endothelin levels in an adequate number of patients is obligatory.

- The **lung** inactivates 30% to 50% of the circulating endothelin in one pass.

- Because of this one would expect lower plasma endothelin levels in the arterial than in the venous circulation.

- Significant higher levels in the arterial circulation were found.

- This suggests continuous arterial production and receptor binding of endothelin in the peripheral arterial circulation (small arteries and arterioles).

- The importance of endothelin in the early pathogenesis of preeclampsia still remains uncertain.

- Plasma levels of calcitonin gene-related peptide showed a wide range in normotensive and preeclamptic women.

- Mean levels were lower in preeclamptic women compared with normotensive women, but this decrease was not significant and there was no relation with the clinical condition in the individual patient.

- Calcitonin gene-related peptide may be a vasodilator in normotensive pregnancy, but it appears not to be directly involved in the pathophysiology of preeclampsia.

- The ratio of $TXB_2/6$-keto-$PGF_{1\alpha}$ was significantly elevated in preeclampsia compared with normotensive pregnancy.

- These results indicate a disturbed balance between TXA_2 and PGI_2 produced by platelets and the endothelium.

- Evidence for significantly elevated TXA_2 production was not found.

- Endothelial cell dysfunction in preeclampsia is not only manifested in an imbalance between vasodilator and vasoconstrictor eicosanoids but also in an increase in endothelial endothelin release.

- Although mean urinary excretion levels of PGI_2 metabolites were significantly lower in preeclampsia, the actual urinary excretion of stable PGI_2 metabolites was not decreased to such an extent that it supports the concept of PGI_2 deficiency as primary change in the pathophysiology of preeclampsia.

- These findings support the concept of a generalized endothelial cell dysfunction in preeclampsia.

- Animal studies support the hypothesis that endothelium-derived relaxing factor is the major vasodilator in man.

- If this holds true in human pregnancy, vascular PGI_2 synthesis might be just a pivotal rescue mechanism of the uteroplacental circulation in those pregnancies where uteroplacental perfusion is endangered because of inadequate conversion of spiral arteries to uteroplacental arteries and a decrease in uteroplacental endothelium-derived relaxing factor release with subsequent vasoconstriction, platelet activation, and TXA2 release.

•Severe preeclampsia with fetal growth retardation or fetal death will then only occur when uteroplacental PGI2 synthesis, as the critical rescue mechanism, is deficient.]

---

64. Predictors of severe meconium aspiration syndrome (i.e. prolonged ventilation) include all of the following EXCEPT

  A. delivery by cesarean section.
  B. fetal heart rate abnormality.
  C. intubation in the delivery suite for resuscitation.
  D. low Apgar score.
 *E. presence of meconium below the cords.

---

p. 66 (Hernandez C, Little BB, Dax J S, Gilstrap III L C, Rosenfeld C R. Prediction of the severity of meconium aspiration syndrome. Am J Obstet Gynec 1993; 169:61)

64. [F & I: •Background: Despite aggressive obstetric and pediatric approaches to intervention, meconium aspiration syndrome remains a significant cause of neonatal morbidity and mortality.

• Meconium-stained amniotic fluid occurs with increasing frequency as gestation advances and is noted in 10% to 15% of all deliveries.

•Meconium-stained amniotic fluid reflects the occurrence of fetal hypoxia or asphyxia.

•Meconium aspiration syndrome may occur in 10% to 30% of all infants with meconium-stained amniotic fluid and in 1% to 3% of all live infants.

•Irrespective of the time of aspiration, meconium aspiration syndrome results in varying degrees of respiratory distress or respiratory failure as a result of airway obstruction, alveolar inflammation, and impaired gas exchange.

•Although the mortality rate for meconium aspiration syndrome has declined from ≈50% to 4% to 18% in recent years, the severity of meconium aspiration syndrome and the risk of death cannot always be predicted.

•To determine which infants are at risk of meconium aspiration syndrome, various investigators have attempted to correlate intrapartum and neonatal events with the occurrence of meconium aspiration syndrome.

•Factors that may distinguish the fetus and neonate at risk of meconium aspiration syndrome include the presence of thick meconium, fetal heart rate (FHR) abnormalities, umbilical arterial pH level ≤7,15, 1- and 5-min Apgar scores ≤5, and the presence of meconium in the trachea (97% specificity, 50% sensitivity).

•No one has attempted to relate predictive factors to either the severity of meconium aspiration syndrome or the subsequent need for ventilatory support.

•Such information would permit identification and intensive observation not only of those pregnant women most at risk but also of those neonates who will require intensive management and support.

•Objectives: To determine whether the severity of meconium aspiration syndrome could be predicted.

•To determine whether the need for neonatal ventilation and for prolonged ventilation (>3 days) could be predicted.

- A secondary objective was to examine both the need for extracorporeal membrane oxygenation therapy and the outcome in infants with meconium aspiration syndrome who were eligible for extracorporeal membrane oxygenation therapy but who were managed with conventional therapy in a large tertiary teaching hospital.

- Through examination of perinatal events, several investigators have attempted to predict which infants are at risk of meconium aspiration syndrome; none have sought to predict the severity of the disease or the need for ventilatory support.

- The ability to predict severity of meconium aspiration syndrome would be invaluable in the first few minutes after delivery because it would permit recognition of those infants who will require intensive neonatal resuscitation, direct transfer to a neonatal intensive care nursery, or active intervention to prevent the sequelae of this disease.

- Identifiable prognostic signs for significant or severe meconium aspiration syndrome would, perhaps, be most important in the triage of infants not born in tertiary referral hospitals.

- Results: 18% of deliveries of live infants were associated with meconium-stained amniotic fluid, a value that was unchanged from year to year.

- Of these neonates, 1% had meconium aspiration syndrome (82/8003) that required admission to the special care nursery, 48% (39/82) had severe meconium aspiration syndrome that required mechanical ventilation, and the mortality rate was 5% (4/82).

- A number of infants with subclinical disease or with only minor respiratory symptoms were excluded from the study because they required little or no oxygen supplementation and they were not admitted to the special care nursery.

- Thus the reported incidence of meconium aspiration syndrome may actually be underestimated, whereas the incidence of severe disease is overestimated.

- Significant differences, determined by univariate analyses, between the nonventilated and ventilated groups suggest that infants with FHR abnormalities during labor, delivery by cesarean section, low Apgar scores, and intubation in the delivery suite for immediate resuscitation might have more severe degrees of perinatal hypoxia or asphyxia and an increased risk of severe meconium aspiration syndrome.

- Notably, this was not associated with a difference in the consistency of meconium-stained amniotic fluid or the presence of meconium below the vocal cords, factors previously considered to be important predictors.

- Although univariate analysis will determine significant associations, only stepwise logistic regression analysis, which examines the interaction between variables and their relationship to an outcome, can be used to determine those variables that might predict the occurrence of severe meconium aspiration syndrome.

- In this instance the presence of fetal tachycardia, an Apgar score of ≤ 6 at 5 min, respiratory distress that requires intubation in the delivery suite, a shortened interval between meconium detection and delivery, and delivery by cesarean section identified the fetus at risk of meconium aspiration syndrome severe enough to require mechanical ventilation.

- This model correctly predicted 72% of the infants who would require ventilation and 64% of the infants who would not require ventilation.

- The relatively high sensitivity of this model would certainly aid in making timely referrals of newborn infants most at risk of severe meconium aspiration syndrome.

- Although these predictions may be incorrect in approximately one third of the cases, this should not hinder its use because overdiagnosis would not be detrimental if it resulted in increased recognition.

•The odds ratio for fetal tachycardia suggests that if tachycardia were present, the risk of neonatal ventilation would increase 26-fold.

•The presence of **fetal tachycardia** cannot be totally explained by a concomitant diagnosis of chorioamnionitis because there were relatively few patients with this diagnosis.

•Fetal tachycardia has previously been identified as a risk for the occurrence of meconium aspiration syndrome, and the finding that this feature also predicts the severity of disease underscores the likelihood that it reflects a fetal response to hypoxia and is thus a possible marker for ensuing acidosis.

°For example, in fetal sheep acute episodes of hypoxia or asphyxia are associated with increases in FHR during the recovery phase.

•The univariate analyses of the groups ventilated <3 days versus ≥3 days were **not** informative.

•By means of a weighted logistic regression analysis, several predictors of prolonged neonatal ventilation were identified.

•This model predicted which infants would not require prolonged ventilation (specificity 91%) more accurately than it predicted those infants who would (sensitivity 67%).

•Overall, this model correctly predicted need of prolonged ventilation in 83% of the cases and thus would be especially useful to the pediatrician in identifying and managing infants with severe meconium aspiration syndrome.

•Interestingly, once again the presence of meconium below the vocal cords did not correlate with severity of disease.

•An umbilical artery pH value of <7.20 increased the risk of prolonged ventilation fourfold.

•The occurrence of an ominous FHR tracing had an even greater impact and increased the risk of prolonged ventilation 24-fold.

•The 16-fold increase in risk associated with an LGA infant likely reflects the fact that term and postterm infants are most often affected by meconium aspiration syndrome.

•No association between fetal growth retardation and severity of meconium aspiration syndrome was found.

•The observation that an **Apgar score** >4 at 1 min was a risk for predicting the need for prolonged ventilation may seem puzzling at first.

•A substantial number of infants who subsequently have meconium aspiration syndrome have acceptable 1-min Apgar scores.

•The survival of patients eligible for extracorporeal membrane oxygenation therapy managed by hyperventilation therapy was 50% (2/4).

•This is significantly increased from the predicted 10% to 20% survival rate, based on historical data, if extracorporeal membrane oxygenation is not used.]

65. Factors predisposing to preeclampsia all of the following EXCEPT

    A. advanced maternal age.
*B. cigarette smoking.
    C. family history of hypertension.
    D. high body mass.
    E. multiparity.

p. 1464 (Lehrer S, Stone J, Lapinski R, Lockwood C J, Schachter B S, Berkowitz R, Berkowitz G S. Association between pregnancy-induced hypertension and asthma during pregnancy. Am J Obstet Gynec 1993; 168:1463)

65. [F & I: •Background: Pregnancy-induced hypertension is a major cause of maternal mortality, intrauterine growth retardation, and perinatal mortality.

•Pregnancy-induced hypertension is also an important component of preeclampsia, a disorder of pregnancy characterized by hypertension, proteinuria, edema, and at times thrombocytopenia and disturbances of liver function.

•Objective: To report that asthma during pregnancy may be a risk factor for pregnancy-induced hypertension.

•Pregnancy-induced hypertension and preeclampsia are closely related, and various factors predispose to preeclampsia: nulliparity, history of preeclampsia in a multiparous woman, black race, high body mass, family history of hypertension, and advanced maternal age.

•**Only cigarette smoking is protective.**

•Some of these factors also predispose to pregnancy-induced hypertension.

•There are at least three possible explanations for the association of pregnancy-induced hypertension and asthma during pregnancy.

•One is that the medicines used to treat the asthma, specifically **glucocorticoids**, might cause the pregnancy-induced hypertension.

°Only **aerosol** glucocorticoids were used in the pregnant asthmatics studied here.

°Administered in this form, the glucocorticoid side effects are minimal.

°Also, glucocorticoids increase the risk of **gestational diabetes**.

°Because there was no correlation between gestational diabetes and asthma during pregnancy in this study, glucocorticoid use is unlikely to be a confounding variable.

°In addition, a study of 85 corticosteroid-dependent patients with respiratory disease showed that the prevalence of hypertension was not greater in these patients than in the general population.

•**Aspirin** might then be a confounding variable because of aspirin-induced asthma.

°However, use of aspirin during pregnancy in these patients was extremely rare.

°It was used as an anticoagulant in women with lupus, but these women were excluded from this study.

•A second possible explanation for the association of pregnancy-induced hypertension and asthma during pregnancy is that the **stress of the hypertension** brings on asthma attacks, or vice versa.

Obstetrics and Gynecology: Review 1994-Obstetrics References

•A third possibility is that both are caused by **a circulating factor** affecting smooth muscle reactivity.

•The causes of the altered vascular smooth muscle reactivity associated with pregnancy-induced hypertension are unknown.

•One mechanism proposed is **vascular endothelial cell dysfunctional circulating substances** that stimulate the production of growth factors, such as **platelet-derived growth factor**, have been implicated in this dysfunction.

•In addition, circulating lipid peroxides, endothelin, and serotonin are under study, although the findings have not been consistent.

•Another hypothesized mechanism holds that the vasoconstriction in pregnancy-induced hypertension is the result of a **relative or absolute deficiency of vasodilating prostaglandins**.

•As is pregnancy-induced hypertension, asthma is characterized by abnormal smooth muscle reactivity and constriction, although airways are involved rather than arteries.

•In addition, asthma is the most prevalent obstructive pulmonary disease during pregnancy.

•**Twenty-nine percent of pregnant asthmatics report reduction in frequency or severity of asthma attacks during pregnancy, 22% report an increased number of attacks, and the remaining 49% report no change.**

•Constriction of airway smooth muscle during asthma attacks may be caused by the **local release of bioactive mediators.**

°Among the substances implicated are platelet-activating factor, histamine, acetylcholine, kinins, adenosine, tachykinins, and leukotrienes.

°Of interest is the fact that leukotrienes are also implicated in the genesis of pregnancy-induced hypertension.]

---

66. All of the following drugs may be safely prescribed in pharmacologic doses upon indication for a breast-feeding mother EXCEPT

    A. diclofenac.
    B. flurbiprofen.
    C. ibuprofen.
    D. mefenamic acid.
    *E. naproxen.

---

p. 1398 (Ito S, Blajchman A, Stephenson M, Eliopoulos, Joren G. Prospective follow-up of adverse reactions in breast-fed infants exposed to maternal medication. Am J Obstet Gynec 1993; 168:1393)

66. [F & I: •Background: Human milk is the most appropriate of all milks for the human neonate because of its nutritional and immunologic advantages.

•The psychologic benefits of breast-feeding for mothers and infants are widely recognized, and successful breast-feeding is a satisfying experience for both.

•As women increasingly choose to breast-feed, more opportunities arise for infants to be exposed to maternal medications.

•Objective: To report the results of a prospective cohort study evaluating the clinical outcomes of infants breast-fed by women who were taking various medications.

Obstetrics and Gynecology: Review 1994-Obstetrics References

- Results: There have been no previous studies of cloxacillin, cefaclor, alprazolam, salbutamol, and many antihistamines.

- Exposures of breast-fed infants to a drug via breast milk depend on timing of breast-feeding relative to the dosing, the maternal dose, the dosing interval, and the duration of therapy.

- These factors were not analyzed because mothers and infants were not supervised directly during the therapy and breast-feeding and because the follow-up interviews were not intended to be immediate and frequent enough.

- The risks for development of adverse reactions in each drug group are currently unknown.

- These factors, as well as data on drug concentrations in milk and infant's blood, need to be carefully assessed with regard to any drugs with suspected effects on breast-fed infants.

- Results: The data are reassuring in that no adverse reaction was severe enough to require consultation or a visit to a physician.

- Although long-term neonatal effects caused by low-level drug exposure (e.g., antiepileptics and antipsychotics) need to be assessed, the findings suggest that, for most drugs, short-term clinical effects are **not** substantial.

- In contrast, mild and transient minor adverse outcomes were reported by the breast-feeding women to have occurred in as many as 11% of the infants.

- The drug groups had different profiles of adverse reactions compatible with their pharmacologic effects.

- These signs appear too mild to pose risks significant enough to outweigh the benefits of breast-feeding.

- In the **antibiotics** group **diarrhea** was the most commonly reported adverse reaction in the infants.

  ° The milk plasma ratio of the penicillins and cephalosporins is generally <0.2.

  ° Assuming a daily milk intake of 1000 ml, the infant dose via breast milk is estimated to be as low as 0.1% to 0.3%, at most, of the maternal dose on a weight basis.

  ° Although erythromycin has a milk/plasma ratio of 0.48, the estimated infant dose is still <1% of the weight-based maternal dose.

  ° It seems unlikely that such a small dose would result directly in gastrointestinal irritability; these amounts may be capable of changing intestinal flora.

  ° This trend has been shown in infants receiving antibiotics intravenously but has not been investigated in breast-fed infants exposed to maternal antibiotics.

  ° It is also possible that some maternal illnesses for which antibiotics were prescribed may have been viral in nature and may have caused gastrointestinal symptoms in the infants.

  ° Even if a causal relationship between maternal antibiotics and gastrointestinal effects in babies could be established, in most cases the mild nature of the symptoms would not justify discontinuation of breast-feeding during antibiotic therapy.

- In the **analgesics** group acetaminophen formulations containing codeine were associated with drowsiness in 5 of 26 cases (all the infants were younger than 1 month).

  ° **Codeine** has a milk plasma ratio of about 2.12

°**Morphine**, an active metabolite of codeine, is also detected in breast milk with a milk plasma ratio of 1:4.

°On a weight basis, 6.8% of the maternal dose of codeine is estimated to be ingested by the infants.

°This dose, when given for a short duration, is still too low to be likely to have any effect on the infant.

°A potential risk should be considered, especially in the early neonatal period, when the elimination half-life is prolonged.

•Because they are weak acids, **nonsteroidal anti-inflammatory drugs** do not usually achieve high concentrations in milk; amounts of ibuprofen, naproxen, and salicylate in breast milk ingested by infants are reportedly <0.6%, 1.1%, and 2.2% of the maternal dose on a weight basis, respectively.

•Intermittent use of these drugs seems compatible with breast-feeding.

•The results support this argument in showing **no substantial adverse effects** in the infants breast-fed by women who used these medications.

•Continuous high-dose therapy may be of concern.

•Because of their relatively short elimination half-lives, low concentrations in milk, and absence of active metabolites, four drugs were listed as suitable (ibuprofen, flurbiprofen, diclofenac, and mefenamic acid); **naproxen** and several other drugs were **not** recommended for nursing women because of their long elimination half-lives; salicylates, fenoprofen, and ketoprofen were also listed as unsuitable because their glucuronide conjugates may be cleaved, thereby releasing active drugs or metabolites.

•There are no published data regarding concentrations of **antihistamines** in milk and their effects on breast-fed infants.

•This study found minor adverse effects, mostly irritability, with an average incidence of 7%.

•Drowsiness was reported in only one case of diphenhydramine use.

•The mildness of these reactions suggests that breast-feeding should not be discontinued during treatment with these drugs.

°Drowsiness was reported in one of the five cases in which alprazolam was being taken.

°The symptom was mild and resolved spontaneously despite continued therapy.

°Lorazepam, another member of the benzodiazepine group, reportedly results in an infant dose of 2% to 6% of the maternal dose on a weight basis with no sedative effect.

°Breast-feeding is probably safe if nursing mothers take benzodiazepines for a short period.

»On the basis of these results, there is no need to discontinue breast-feeding during therapy with these maternal medications.

•Indications for treatment with drugs should be assessed as carefully as they are for other patient populations.

•These results should not be generalized to **premature** infants because pharmacokinetics and pharmacodynamics in this age group are often different from those of term infants.]

67. All of the following affect the maternal homeostatic response to hypermagnesemia EXCEPT

    A. 1α,25-dihydroxycalciferol.
*B. calcitonin.
    C. dietary intake of fortified cow's milk.
    D. exposure to sunlight.
    E. parathyroid hormone.

p. 1175 (Cruikshank D P, Chan G M, Doerrfeld D. Alterations in vitamin D and calcium metabolism with magnesium sulfate treatment of preeclampsia. Am J Obstet Gynec 1993; 168:1170)

67. [F & I: •Background: Magnesium is an important component of calcium homeostasis, along with vitamin D, parathyroid hormone, calcitonin, and phosphorus.

•Understanding the maternal homeostatic response has remained incomplete because vitamin D levels have not been measured.

•Inactive vitamin D precursors are synthesized in the skin by the action of ultraviolet radiation on 7-dehydrocholesterol producing cholecalciferol (vitamin D3,) or are obtained in the diet as ergocalciferol (vitamin D2).

•Cholecalciferol and ergocalciferol have essentially identical activity and potency in humans and will be considered together as calciferol.

•In the liver calciferol is hydroxylated at carbon 25 to 25-hydroxycalciferol, a relatively weak compound, blood levels of which are dependent mainly on sunlight exposure and dietary intake.

•25-Hydroxycalciferol is further hydroxylated in the proximal renal tubule to the active compound 1α, 25-dihydroxycalciferol, blood levels of which are stringently regulated by various positive and negative feedback loops involving calcium, parathyroid hormone, and other ions and hormones and to a minimal extent, if at all, by diet and sunlight exposure.

•1α, 25-dihydroxycalciferol is thought to be a hormone rather than a vitamin; it acts on skin, parathyroid glands, and the kidneys, but its principal actions are on the gut and bone.

•In the gut 1α, 25-dihydroxycalciferol increases calcium absorption, whereas in bone, in association with parathyroid hormone, it activates osteoclasts and causes release of calcium into the circulation.

•In normal adult humans ionized calcium levels are closely regulated minute to minute.

•Any fall in calcium levels elicits almost immediately increases in 1α, 25-dihydroxycalciferol and parathyroid hormone levels, and their effects on gut, kidney, and osteoclasts begin within 20 min.

•Objective: To characterize the response of maternal and fetal calcium homeostasis, especially the vitamin D response, to magnesium sulfate treatment of preeclampsia, to further the understanding of the effects and potential side effects of such therapy.

•Results: Baseline values of 1α, 25-dihydroxycalciferol in both preeclamptic and control subjects are above the normal nonpregnant range and that significant increases in both maternal and fetal levels occur in response to magnesium sulfate treatment.

•Elevated maternal levels during normal pregnancy are caused in part by the increased maternal parathyroid hormone level in pregnancy, which promotes the conversion of 25-hydroxycalciferol to 1α, 25-dihydroxycalciferol, and in part by placental production of 1α, 25-dihydroxycalciferol.

•On the basis of whole organ weight, the term placenta synthesizes more 1α 25-hydroxycalciferol (1.2 µg/day) than the kidneys (0.8 to 1.0 µg/day).

- The time of onset and the regulation of placental synthesis of 1α, 25-dihydroxycalciferol are unknown but 1α, 25-dihydroxycalciferol of placental origin can enter both the maternal and fetal circulations.

- Fetal levels are lower than or similar to maternal levels, the latter being more consistent with findings in control subjects.

- Fetal 1α, 25-dihydroxycalciferol is derived from three sources.

  ° Fetal renal production accounts for two thirds of blood levels; the balance comes from placental synthesis and transport.

- Both the maternal and fetal kidneys respond to the magnesium-induced fall in serum calcium and rise in parathyroid hormone concentration with increased 1α, 25-dihydroxycalciferol synthesis, although it is possible that some of the increase in both compartments is caused by altered placental synthesis.

- The finding that preeclamptic subjects had significantly **lower** levels of 25-hydroxycalciferol before magnesium sulfate treatment than did control subjects could possibly be explained on the basis of subclinical hepatic dysfunction in preeclamptics because 25-hydroxylation of vitamin D precursors occurs in the liver.

- None of the subjects had evidence of hepatocellular damage, and the rise in maternal 25-hydroxycalciferol concentrations after magnesium infusion speaks against this hypothesis.

  ° There is no evidence that their sunlight exposure was different from controls.

  ° It may be possible that by chance their dietary intake was remarkably different than control subjects, in light of recent studies showing huge (500-fold) differences in the amounts of vitamin D in various samples of fortified cow's milk.

- In normal pregnant women 25-hydroxycalciferol levels are the same as in nonpregnant subjects.

- Fetal levels in normal pregnancy are the same as or slightly lower than maternal and significantly correlated with them, suggesting ready passage of 25-hydroxycalciferol across the placenta.

- At first glance it seems inconsistent that preeclamptic subjects should have lower baseline levels of the substrate, 25-hydroxycalciferol, but develop higher levels of the product, 1α, 25-dihydroxycalciferol, after magnesium sulfate treatment.

  ° In both treated and control subjects there is an order of magnitude difference between the levels of 25-hydroxycalciferol and 1α, 25-dihydroxycalciferol (nanograms per milliliter vs picograms per milliliter), and the findings underscore the profound and rapid effect of falling serum ionized calcium levels on 1α, 25-dihydroxycalciferol concentration.

- The finding of significantly lower baseline parathyroid hormone concentrations in preeclamptic subjects than in controls confirms the previous finding of depression of maternal parathyroid hormone levels in term pregnant women with essential hypertension.

- These associations between hypertension in pregnancy (a well recognized high aldosterone state) and reduced maternal parathyroid hormone concentrations seem even more intriguing in light of the finding that hypertensive nonpregnant adults with hyperaldosteronism have depressed parathyroid hormone levels, whereas adults with low-aldosterone essential hypertension have normal or elevated parathyroid hormone levels.

- These links lend credence to the suggestion that calcium supplementation during pregnancy reduces maternal mean arterial pressure and the incidence of preeclampsia, although the molecular basis remains to be elucidated.

•Magnesium sulfate treatment leads to marked maternal hypercalciuria, which in turn causes a fall in serum ionized and total calcium levels, to which the mother responds by increasing levels of parathyroid hormone.

•Increased maternal levels of parathyroid hormone and 1α, 25-dihydroxycalciferol rapidly exert their effects on maternal bone, gut, and kidney to prevent more clinically significant maternal hypocalcemia.

•The complexity of the hormonal control of calcium homeostasis is underscored by the **lack of correlation** between either 1α, 25-dihydroxycalciferol or parathyroid hormone and the various ions and hormones.

•This same lack of correlation has been found in nonpregnant, normally pregnant, and lactating adults and in normal neonates.

•The higher fetal than maternal levels of parathyroid hormone in treated subjects suggests that the fetal parathyroids respond to lowered serum ionized and total calcium levels by increasing serum parathyroid hormone levels, which together with the rise in fetal 1α, 25-dihydroxycalciferol prevents even more marked fetal hypocalcemia.

•Unlike 1α, 25-dihydroxycalciferol, **parathyroid hormone does not cross the placenta** so that umbilical venous levels are entirely of fetal or placental origin.

•The elevated fetal 1α, 25-dihydroxycalciferol and parathyroid hormone levels in treated subjects explains the observation that the offspring of magnesium sulfate-treated preeclamptic women rarely develop clinically significant hypocalcemia and in fact may have higher serum calcium concentrations than control infants.

•These fetal biochemical responses may also help explain the osteolytic lesions recently described in the bones of infants exposed in utero to long-term magnesium sulfate tocolysis, although chronic magnesium sulfate therapy may elicit different maternal and fetal responses than the short-term effects.

•Maternal levels of the ions and hormones reach a relatively steady state by 12 h of magnesium sulfate infusion.

•Calcitonin is not involved in the homeostatic response to acute hypermagnesemia.

•Conclusion: Maternal hypermagnesemia causes relative maternal hypocalcemia, which elicits an increase in maternal 1α, 25-dihydroxycalciferol and parathyroid hormone levels.

•The fetuses of such women have reduced calcium levels, to which they respond with elevations of 1α, 25-dihydroxycalciferol and parathyroid hormone as well, thus preventing more marked fetal and neonatal hypocalcemia.]

---

68. The rapid eye test used in the screening of substance abuse includes all of the following EXCEPT

    A. evaluation of pupil size
    B. testing for corneal reflexes
    *C. testing for frequency of blinking
    D. testing for nystagmus
    E. testing reaction of pupil to light

---

p. 355 (Burke M S, Roth D. Anonymous cocaine screening in a private obstetric population. Obstet Gynecol 1993; 81:354)

68. [F & I: •Background: The population using cocaine is frequently 20 to 30 years old, which includes women in the childbearing years.

•The prevalence of illicit drug use in the obstetric population is 7.5 to 20.5%.

- Positive urine toxicology rates are as high as one-quarter of clinic patients and as low as one per 100 in a military obstetric population.

- The use of cocaine in pregnancy is associated with placental abruption, preterm delivery, fetal distress, stillbirth, and congenital malformations.

- In addition, long-term neurobehavioral effects in infants exposed to cocaine have been suspected.

- The economic expense of cocaine use is estimated to increase the cost of neonatal care four to eight times, especially if social evaluation and foster-care placement are required.

  ° National estimates are about $500 million.

- Routine history alone identifies only a small proportion of those who have used cocaine.

- Based on the severity of the effects of cocaine and the inability to identify patients by medical history, some have recommended universal substance screening at the first prenatal visit.

- Another suggested approach is to screen all patients who received no prenatal care, who have preterm labor or preterm birth, or who deliver an infant with a 1-min Apgar score of 6 or less.

- Objective: To evaluate the prevalence of cocaine use in a wide distribution of private patients.

- Results: The results of this anonymous screening of urine samples obtained at prenatal visits and admissions to delivery units in a large metropolitan area suggest that universal screening in this population would **not** be cost-effective.

- A similar trial would be advisable to establish the need for this expensive testing in any community considering universal screening.

- The use of an appropriate history and physical examination for initial drug screening in pregnant patients is encouraged.

- A **history** of drug use or a combination of lack of prenatal care and cigarette use can predict a positive cocaine urine test with a 70% positive predictive value and a 94.9% negative predictive value.

- Additional clues identified in the study were a history of preterm rupture of the membranes (PROM), low birth weight infants, and positive syphilis serology.

  ° These historical identifiers are most useful in a population with a **high** prevalence rate.

- In populations with a low prevalence of cocaine use, these indicators helped predict the absence of a positive drug screen.

- Some physical examination findings are associated with cocaine use.

- The **rapid eye test**, used routinely by law enforcement personnel, is performed in a quiet setting and contains five parts: general observation of the patient, evaluation of pupil size, testing the reaction of the pupil to light, testing for nystagmus, and testing for corneal reflex.

- In patients who have used cocaine or amphetamines, the rapid eye test will show a dilated pupil with slow or decreased reaction to light and a decreased corneal reflex.

- Very high doses of cocaine may constrict rather than dilate the pupil.

- A false-positive result has been reported to be infrequent.

• The goal of detecting substance abuse during pregnancy is to improve the perinatal outcome by encouraging **discontinuation** of use.

• Detection of users is only the first step in improving outcome.

• Few treatment centers will work with pregnant patients and even fewer will treat those who are covered by Medicaid or have no insurance.

• The availability of treatment centers will not increase until a need for them has been identified.

» Evaluation of every patient during prenatal care and at admission for delivery by appropriate questions during history-taking is recommended.

• In addition, some physical findings can be used to identify the patient at risk.

• Women who are evaluated for specific high-risk problems in pregnancy, including preterm labor and delivery, PROM, fetal growth retardation, or placental abruption, should be considered at increased risk for substance abuse.

• Urine toxicology screening should be considered in these patients.]

---

69. The Doppler indices of placental function are affected by all of the following EXCEPT

   *A. diabetes mellitus
   B. erythroblastosis fetalis
   C. intrauterine growth retardation
   D. preeclampsia

---

p. 650 (Salvesen D R, Higueras M T, Mansur C A, Freeman J, Brudenell J M, Nicolaides K H. Placental and fetal Doppler velocimetry in pregnancies complicated by maternal diabetes mellitus. Am J Obstet Gynec 1993; 168:645)

69. [F & I: •Background: Doppler studies of the placental and fetal circulations have improved the understanding of the cardiovascular adjustments in different fetal-maternal conditions.

• In intrauterine growth retardation (IUGR) caused by uteroplacental insufficiency, impedance to flow in the uteroplacental and fetoplacental circulations is increased.

• There is an association between fetal hypoxemia and acidemia and redistribution in the fetal circulation in favor of the brain and at the expense of the viscera.

• In red blood cell isoimmunization, the fetus is subjected to varying degrees of anemic hypoxia (decreased oxygen content caused by anemia but usually normal partial pressure of gases).

• Impedance to flow in the placental and fetal circulations is normal; these fetuses have a hyperdynamic circulation, as demonstrated by increased blood velocity in the fetal descending thoracic aorta and middle cerebral artery in proportion to the degree of fetal anemia.

• Objective: To investigate a third model of fetal-maternal disease, that of maternal diabetes mellitus, where some fetuses are polycythemic and acidemic, in the presence of a normal PO_2.

• Results: In pregnancies complicated by maternal diabetes mellitus the uteroplacental and fetoplacental circulations are essentially **normal**, except in those cases complicated by preeclampsia or IUGR.

• The fetal acidemia in uncomplicated diabetic pregnancies is probably metabolic in origin, and the tendency for fetal acidemia and hypoxemia in those pregnancies complicated by diabetic nephropathy may also either be a consequence of poor glycemic control or of altered placental transfer.

•Although in this study there were significant associations between Doppler parameters and umbilical venous blood pH and PO_2, because the Doppler measurements were essentially normal in those without preeclampsia or IUGR, they did not provide a clinically useful prediction of the degree of metabolic derangement in the fetus.

•In IUGR caused by uteroplacental insufficiency fetal acidemia is associated with Doppler evidence of fetal blood flow redistribution.

•The absence of redistribution in many of the acidemic fetuses suggests that this hemodynamic alteration occurs only with the severe or chronic fetal acidemia observed in placental insufficiency.

•The degree of fetal acidemia was relatively mild.

•Because fetal blood pH is significantly associated with maternal blood glucose concentration, it is possible that the degree of fetal acidemia is liable to acute fluctuations related to short-term maternal glycemic control.

•It is also possible that the fetal blood flow redistribution observed in IUGR is a consequence of metabolic derangements that do not accompany the fetal acidemia of pregnancies complicated by maternal diabetes mellitus.

•In anemic fetuses of pregnancies complicated by red blood cell isoimmunization, the increased blood flow velocity is caused by decreased blood viscosity with consequent increased venous return and cardiac output.

•Although in fetuses of diabetic mothers blood viscosity is increased as a consequence of polycythemia, the fetal descending thoracic aorta and middle cerebral artery mean velocity were normal.

•There was no significant association between the degree of fetal polycythemia and these Doppler indices.

•This finding suggests that the increase in hematocrit observed in this study may not have been sufficient to adversely affect blood viscosity.

•Conclusions: In pregnancies of women with diabetes mellitus, in spite of fetal acidemia and polycythemia the results of Doppler studies of the placental and fetal circulations are essentially normal except in those complicated by IUGR or preeclampsia.

•The extent to which poor diabetic control is associated with alteration in the fetal circulation remains to be determined.]

---

70. Associated with a decreased length of pregnancy predicted by Naegele's rule all of the following EXCEPT

    A. age less than 19
    *B. alcohol
    C. coffee consumption greater than 5 cups per day
    D. low educational achievement
    E. multiparity

p.483 (Mittendorf R, Williams M A, Berkey C S, Lieberman E, Monson R R. Predictors of human gestational length. Am J Obstet Gynec 1993; 168:480)

70. [F & I: •Background: Naegele's rule—a nineteenth-century algorithm that predicts the date of confinement and the length of pregnancy—is a point estimate that does not consider biologic variability.

- Identifying risks which determine gestational duration and variability may have practical applications in obstetrics and public health.

- To control for confounding factors, any study of the length of pregnancy must contain many observations (pregnant women) and information on risks.

- Objective: To identify the important variables that modulate the length of pregnancy.

- In previous studies, although a number of variables were associated with birth weight, very few risks were found to be associated with length of pregnancy.

- Results: History of miscarriage and in utero exposure to DES are associated with gestational duration.

- 17 other variables were also found to be statistically significant in the application of multiple linear regression for predicting the length of pregnancy.

- Multiparity is significantly associated with decreased length of pregnancy.

  ° Multiparity reduces the length of pregnancy by a mean of 3.1 days.

  ° A history of even one delivery shortens subsequent gestations.

- Age is statistically significantly associated with gestational length.

  ° Nearly 22% of women <19 years of age had preterm deliveries.

- Black race was associated with a decrease in length of pregnancy of 2.5 days.

  ° 14.4% of black women but only 8.6% of nonblack women were delivered of preterm infants.

- Educational level was found to be statistically significant.

  ° Use of prenatal care in the first trimester and welfare status (a risk factor known to be associated with birth weight) were not significant.

- Cigarette smoking—modeled as a continuous variable (with control for other variables with which smoking may be correlated) was found **not** to be associated with gestational duration.

- Mothers who gave any history of alcohol consumption during pregnancy had longer pregnancies than did nondrinking mothers.

  ° Those who drank also had fewer preterm deliveries.

  ° The harmful consequences of alcohol consumption on fetal neurologic development outweigh any modest prolongation in gestational duration.

- When modeling coffee consumption as a continuous variable, each cup drunk daily shortened gestation by 0.39 days (95% confidence interval -0.16 to -0.62 days).

  ° The mother who drinks five cups of coffee every day during her pregnancy loses, on average, about 2 days (0.39 x 5 = 1.95 days) in total gestational length.

- In this linear regression gestational length is predicted by the sum of the risk terms.

- By means of a linear equation gestational lengths for mothers with different risks can be computed.

  ° For example, a 30-year-old white primiparous woman who had some college education and a ponderal index of 20 (1.65 m in height, prepregnancy body weight of 54.5 kg) would have a predicted length of gestation of 282.6 days—from the first day of the last menstrual period to the estimated date of confinement.

°An otherwise identical white mother with a history of cervical incompetence who is having her third delivery would have a different predicted length of pregnancy— 260.7 days.

°This model more precisely estimates the length of pregnancy in women with different risks than does Naegele's rule.]

---

71. Infants who develop major neurological deficits are likely to have all of the following EXCEPT

    A. hypercarbia
    B. infection
    C. late decelerations
    *D. metabolic acidemia
    E. oligohydramnios

---

p. 1512   (Goodwin T M, Belai I, Hernandez P, Durand M, Paul R H. Asphyxial complications in the term newborn with severe umbilical acidemia. Am J Obstet Gynec 1992; 167:1506)

71. [F & I: •Background: Population-derived statistical lower limits of normal umbilical artery pH range from 7.10 to 7.20.

•An umbilical artery pH below these levels is not correlated with Apgar scores or with evidence of short and long-term end-organ asphyxial sequelae.

•The risk of neonatal asphyxial complications may not correlate with pH until the arterial level falls below 7.00 with a significant metabolic component.

•The severely acidemic infant destined to develop hypoxic ischemic encephalopathy may have a marked depression of the 5-minute Apgar score (≤3).

•A pH < 7.00 has been associated with a significantly increased frequency of early neonatal seizures and neonatal death, although the Apgar score appeared to be less specific than previously suggested.

•The risk of neonatal asphyxial sequelae associated with a cord pH of <7.00 and the predictive value of the Apgar score for these complications is unknown.

•Objective: To describe the neonatal asphyxial complications with severe umbilical acidemia (pH <7.00) in term infants, with particular attention to cerebral dysfunction.

•The relationship of the type and degree of acidemia to asphyxial complications was examined along with the predictive value of the Apgar score.

•A profile of those infants with confirmed major neurologic deficit was constructed.

•Results: The degree of umbilical artery acidemia correlates with asphyxial end-organ injury in the term newborn with severe acidemia (pH < 7.00).

°Because it is unlikely that a pH in this range would be found in the absence of fetal distress or some degree of newborn depression (the indications for umbilical blood sampling in this study), it is probable that the numbers here approximate the absolute risk for asphyxial injury associated with this degree of acidemia.

•A predominant respiratory acidemia was not uncommon especially among infants with a pH ≤6.90 (22/58 38%).

°There was a trend toward a **lower** incidence of seizures and hypotonia among these infants.

- Below a pH of 6.90, this effect was not apparent.

- The profound hypercarbia seen with a respiratory or mixed acidemia in this pH range has few parallels in pediatric or adult medicine.

- Its particular contribution to the pathologic sequence in perinatal asphyxia is unknown, but it may act in synergy with hypoxemia to exacerbate tissue ischemia.

- A number of independent deleterious effects of **hypercarbia** are found in both animal models and man, including altered cerebral blood flow, seizures, myocardial depression, dysrhythmias, pulmonary vasoconstriction, and decreased oxygen availability caused by a right shift in the oxyhemoglobin dissociation curve.

- The **highest incidence of seizures** was found among infants with a **mixed** acidemia, including a significant respiratory component, a pattern suggestive of chronic or subacute partial asphyxia followed by a predelivery episode of acute total asphyxia.

- It is noteworthy that **no** infants with a **pure metabolic acidemia** developed seizures or were abnormal at discharge.

- Other factors can predispose newborn seizures or result in neonatal hypoxia confounding the intrapartum contribution to neurologic morbidity.

  ° For example, the incidence of infants delivering after term was more than twice the expected rate.

  ° Three of the five infants with seizures and neonatal death had specific confounding factors.

  ° Among survivors who developed hypoxic ischemic encephalopathy the incidence of infection (1/34), trauma (1/34), and distinct neonatal asphyxia (2/34) was low.

  ° The confluence of cardiopulmonary, renal, and cerebral injury manifesting shortly after birth identifies asphyxia as the probable major pathophysiologic factor.

- Although a significant insult occurred during the intrapartum period, the adverse outcomes were not necessarily preventable.

  ° 14 of 15 infants with confirmed abnormal outcome (five neonatal deaths and 10 major neurologic deficit) had evidence of possible fetal compromise (e.g., abnormal FHR, oligohydramnios) or preexisting pathologic process, usually of unknown duration, present on arrival in the labor and delivery area.

- The Apgar score has limitations in diagnosing perinatal asphyxia.

- Among infants with a cord pH <7.00 Apgar scores of ≤3 should be observed to attribute neonatal cerebral dysfunction and subsequent permanent neurologic injury to intrapartum events.

- The findings suggest that even in the pH range below 7.00, a 5-min Apgar score ≤3 has only moderate predictive value for hypoxic ischemic encephalopathy.

- This is not surprising, because some infants with hypoxic ischemic encephalopathy, in particular those with a history of intermittent hypoxia, may have injury limited to the cortex.

  ° This will affect tone but not brainstem functions controlling color, heart rate, and some reflexes.

- Although follow-up was not complete, it is possible to describe a profile of the infants who died in the neonatal period or survived with major neurologic deficit.

•The most common pattern is that of a fetus with evidence of distress or compromise at initial evaluation (e.g., oligohydramnios, significant decelerations, infection who then experiences a near-total interruption of gas exchange, as suggested by the degree of hypercarbia.

•A profound acidemia (usually <6.80) associated with marked hypercarbia is seen at birth.

•This is followed by multiorgan system dysfunction, including hypoxic ischemic encephalopathy.]

---

72. Using decreased amniotic fluid glucose as marker for intraamniotic infection, all of the following can be responsible for false positive tests EXCEPT

    A. advanced gestational age
    B. fetal growth retardation
    C. placental insufficiency
    D. preeclampsia
    *E. ureaplasma colonization of amniotic cavity

---

p. 1019   (Meyer W J, Gauthier D W. Effect of time and storage temperature on amniotic fluid glucose concentration. Obstet Gynecol 1992; 80:1017)

72. [F & I: •Background: Intrauterine infection is an important cause of preterm labor and preterm rupture of membranes (PROM).

•Its accurate detection is important in selecting appropriate clinical management and may improve perinatal outcome in these conditions.

•Because clinical signs and symptoms do not correlate well with amniotic fluid (AF) cultures, several rapid methods of predicting intrauterine infection have been proposed.

•**Gram stain** and **leukocyte esterase** activity lack sensitivity compared with AF cultures, which limits their clinical usefulness.

•AF glucose concentration may be a more accurate method of detecting intra-amniotic infection than is the Gram stain.

•Serum glucose concentration decreases over time at room temperature because of glycolysis.

•Objective: To determine the effects of time and storage temperature on AF glucose concentration.

•Measurement of AF glucose is a rapid and inexpensive method of detecting intraamniotic infection.

  °False-positive results can occur.

•Several factors may alter the AF glucose concentration and predispose to false-positive results.

  °Pregnancies complicated by **placental insufficiency, fetal growth retardation, and preeclampsia** are associated with **decreased** AF glucose levels.

  °AF glucose levels **decrease** with advancing gestational age.

  °In addition to these factors, investigators have described a "gray zone" of AF glucose concentrations of 13 to 21 mg/dl in patients at or before 34 weeks gestation; in this range, glucose concentrations in noninfected samples overlap those of infected samples.

•These factors limit the universal use of a single, immediate determination of glucose concentration in making clinical decisions regarding delivery of a preterm infant.

- **Results:** AF glucose concentration is stable in uninfected samples regardless of the storage temperature.

  ° Infected samples had a significantly **lower** baseline glucose concentration, which then continued to decrease over time at both room temperature and at 37 C.

  ° All samples with positive cultures except one demonstrated a significant decrease in glucose concentration within 2 h, whereas none of the culture-negative samples exhibited a significant decrease.

  ° Although the exact etiology of decreased AF glucose concentration in patients with intra-amniotic infection is unknown, it may be that bacteria and/or activated neutrophils use the glucose as a metabolic substrate.

  ° The rate of decline in glucose concentration may also be related to differences in the type and concentration of bacteria present.

- A single sample positive for *Ureaplasma* alone did not have any decrease in glucose concentration, a finding that reflects this organism's failure to use glucose as a metabolic substrate.

- Glucose concentration of stored, unfrozen AF does not change over 12 h in the absence of intra-amniotic infection.

- It is possible that sequential measurement of AF glucose concentration from the same sample may rapidly and correctly identify those patients with active intraamniotic infection, eliminate false-positive results, and allow early clinical intervention.

- This would be especially important in women with medical or pregnancy complications that may alter the AF glucose concentration and lead to false-positive results.

- Rapid identification of patients with active intraamniotic infection before the development of overt clinical signs of chorioamnionitis may allow aggressive intrauterine medical therapy, possibly preventing sepsis, premature birth, and neonatal sequelae.]

PERINATAL MEDICINE

Directions: Each of the questions or incomplete statements below is followed by several suggested answers or completions. Select the BEST answer in each case.

1. The best predictive measurement in fetal urine for postnatal renal function is

   A. ammonium.
   B. chloride.
   C. sodium.
   D. ß2 microglobulin.
   E. urea.

2. An elevated uterine artery resistance index is most closely related to

   A. elevated middle cerebral artery resistance index.
   B. maternal blood pressure.
   C. maternal parity.
   D. maternal weight.
   E. placenta ischemic changes.

3. The vascular refractoriness to exogenous angiotensin II during pregnancy is due to

   A. diminished affinity of angiotensin II receptors.
   B. down regulation of angiotensin II receptors is a function of angiotensin II level.
   C. increased catabolism of angiotensin II.
   D. occupation of angiotensin II receptors by endogenous peptide applies when concentration is elevated during pregnancy.
   E. reduction of vasoconstrictor effective angiotensin II by vasodilator substances.

4. Electrocardiographic changes associated with a normal pregnancy include

   A. 15 degree left axis deviation.
   B. Q wave in lead AVF.
   C. Q wave inverted in lead III.
   D. S-T segment elevation in lead II.
   E. T wave inverted in lead III.

5. Which of the following has the best predictive value for identifying patients at risk for preeclampsia?

   A. Analysis of parental HLA loci.
   B. Angiotensin sensitivity test.
   C. Doppler screening of the uterine artery
   D. "roll over" test.
   E. Serum uric acid.

6. A para 1001 delivers an infant with congenital heart block. Antibodies to SS-A/Ro and SS-B/La are detected in her serum. The outcome of subsequent pregnancies can be improved by maternal administration of

   A. dexamethasone
   B. gamma globulin and prednisone
   C. methotrexate
   D. plasmapheresis and prednisone
   E. none of the above

7. Which of the following pregnancy-related conditions is associated with low serum fibrinogen, lower serum glucose and diabetes insipidus?

   A. Acute fatty liver of pregnancy.
   B. HELLP syndrome.
   C. Hemolytic uremic syndrome.
   D. Intrahepatic cholestasis of pregnancy.
   E. Thrombocytopenic purpura.

8. True statements about pregnancy in a patient who has a successful heart transplant include

   A. birth control pills are the preferred method of contraception.
   B. cyclosporine is teratogenic.
   C. epidural anesthesia is contraindicated.
   D. the risk to the fetus in the patient who had a cardiomyopathy is between 25% and 50% that the fetus will also have a cardiomyopathy.
   E. the transplacental heart responds to vagal but not catecholamine stimuli.

9. The most sensitive method for detecting antepartum maternal use of cocaine is

   A. amniotic fluid analysis.
   B. fetal urine analysis.
   C. maternal urine analysis.
   D. meconium (from amniocentesis) analysis.
   E. fetal hair analysis.

10. The major estrogen formed by human fetal membranes is

    A. conjugated estriol.
    B. estradiol.
    C. estrone.
    D. unconjugated estriol.
    E. All estrogens are produced in about the same amount.

11. Which of the following is particularly effective in protecting the fetus from viral infections?

    A. B-lymphocytes.
    B. Interferon gamma.
    C. Neutrophils.
    D. T-lymphocytes.
    E. Transplacental transfer of maternally-derived immunoglobulins.

12. The discrepancy in size in pregnancies complicated by twin-twin transfusion syndrome is caused by

    A. disproportionate distribution of maternal uterine blood vessel.
    B. increase blood viscosity in the recipient twin.
    C. increase hematocrit in the recipient twin.
    D. placental vascular communication.
    E. progressive vascular obliteration of tertiary resistance vessels.

13. In the human fetus, nephrogenesis is complete by

    A. 14 weeks
    B. 20 weeks
    C. 28 weeks
    D. 32 weeks
    E. 36 weeks

14. At 18 weeks, amniotic bands are identified in an otherwise normal pregnancy. The pregnancy is at risk for

    A. chorioamnionitis.
    B. low birth weight infant.
    C. oligohydramnios.
    D. posterior placenta.
    E. premature rupture of the membranes.

15. Which placental abnormality is associated with twin-twin transfusion syndrome?

    A. Battledore placenta.
    B. Bipartite placenta.
    C. Circumvallate placenta
    D. Placenta succenturiata
    E. Velamentous insertion of the cord.

16. Short-term ritodrine infusion used for tocolysis raises

    A. serum cholesterol
    B. serum glucagon
    C. serum insulin
    D. serum placental lactogen
    E. serum triglycerides

17. The earliest time that the fetus can respond to tissue hypoxia by increasing erythropoietin production is

    A. 20 weeks
    B. 22 weeks
    C. 24 weeks
    D. 26 weeks
    E. 28 weeks

18. In which condition is there increased monocyte secretion of thromboxane?

    A. pregnancy-induced hypertension
    B. chronic hypertension in pregnancy
    C. normal nonpregnant state
    D. normal pregnancy
    E. all about the same

19. True statements about the prenatal diagnosis of gastroschisis include

    A. Associated with a 20% incidence of trisomy.
    B. Bowel dilation is a marker of bowel damage.
    C. Elective cesarean section improves outcome.
    D. Etiology of intestinal damage is ischemia.
    E. Intestinal damage most likely occurs during delivery.

20. Clinically useful in evaluating renal function in fetuses with obstructive uropathy, fetal urinary

    A. calcium
    B. creatinine
    C. osmolality
    D. potassium
    E. urea

21. Increased thromboxane in the pathogenesis of preeclampsia in the diabetic patient is generated by

    A. kidney
    B. liver
    C. lung
    D. placenta
    E. platelets

22. A fetus at risk for developing distress is being evaluated sonographically three times a week. At 28 weeks, end diastolic velocity is noted to be absent. The most powerful predictor of the time interval between the absence of end diastolic velocity and the need for delivery is

    A. change in amniotic fluid volume
    B. decrease in middle cerebral artery pulsatility index
    C. gestational age
    D. severity of intrauterine growth retardation
    E. umbilical artery pulsatility index

23. Which of the following maternal-fetal HLA relationships is associated with pregnancy-induced hypertension?

    A. Fetus does not have the HLA-DR antigens allogeneic to its mother.
    B. Mother does not have the HLA-DR antigens allogeneic to her fetus.
    C. Neither the fetus nor the mother have allogeneic antigens to each other.
    D. The fetus and the mother both have allogeneic antigens to each other.
    E. none of the above

24. A 30-year old patient has a maternal serum alpha-fetoprotein at 16 weeks reported as 6 multiples of the median. Amniotic fluid alpha-fetoprotein is reported is reported as 15 multiples of the median and acetylcholine determination is within normal limits. Ultrasound evaluation of the fetus reveals no abnormalities. The next best step in the management of this patient is

    A. culture the amniotic fluid for acid-fast bacilli
    B. obtain alpha-fetoprotein for karyotype
    C. offer mother termination of pregnancy
    D. repeat amniotic fluid alpha-fetoprotein in two weeks
    E. repeat ultrasound in two weeks

25. The main site of erythropoietin in the fetus is

    A. bone marrow
    B. kidney
    C. liver
    D. lung
    E. spleen

26. At 30 weeks a fetus is noted to have nonimmune hydrops. Umbilical venous pressure is normal. The LEAST likely cause of the condition is

   A. fetal tachyarrhythmia
   B. hypoalbuminemia.
   C. parovirus infection.
   D. tetralogy of Fallot.
   E. viral myocarditis.

27. All of the following are increased in the large for gestational age fetus EXCEPT

   A. C peptide.
   B. IGF I.
   C. IGF II.
   D. IGFBP-1.
   E. none of the above.

Directions: Each group of numbered words or phrases is preceded by a list of lettered statements. MATCH the lettered item most closely associated with the numbered word or phrase. Each item may be used once, more than once, or not at all.

Items 28-30.

   A. chorioamnionitis
   B. placental vasculopathy
   C. chronic villitis
   D. abruptio placentae
   E. none of the above

28. polymorphonuclear leukocytes

29. occlusive thrombi

30. mononuclear cell infiltrates

Directions: Each set of lettered headings below is followed by a list of numbered words or phrases. For each numbered word or phrase select:

   A. if the item is associated with *(A) only*
   B. if the item is associated with *(B) only*
   C. if item is associated with *both (A) and (B)*
   D. if item is associated with *neither (A) nor (B)*

Items 31-33.

In a twin gestation:

   A. chorionic villus sampling.
   B. amniocentesis (16-18 weeks)
   C. both
   D. neither

31. fetal loss rate about 10%

32. increased incidence of twin-twin contamination

33. preferred method in the event of discordant results require termination of affected twin

Items 34-36.

In the treatment of pregnancy-induced hypertension:

   A. nicardipine
   B. nifedipine
   C. both
   D. neither

34. more selective dihydropyridine derivative

35. can be infused IV

36. reduced rate of fetal growth retardation

Items 37-39.

In the affected fetus:

   A. septated cystic hygroma
   B. nonseptated cystic hygroma
   C. both
   D. neither

37. usually 1 to 5 centimeters

38. regresses before the 16th week of gestation

39. non-immune hydrops

Items 40-42.

A. dihydralazine
B. labetalol
C. both
D. neither

40. effective antihypertensive in pregnancy

41. antiarrhythmic

42. decreases diastolic filling time

Items 43-44.

A. acute fatty liver of pregnancy
B. HELLP syndrome
C. both
D. neither

43. periportal necrosis

44. numerous fat droplets

Directions: For each of the questions or incomplete statements below, ONE or MORE of the answers or completions given is correct. In each case select:

A. if only 1, 2, and 3 are correct
B. if only 1 and 3 are correct
C. if only 2 and 4 are correct
D. if only 4 is correct
E. if all are correct

45. Elective cesarean section in cases of antenatally diagnosed gastroschisis decreases neonatal morbidity by

1. avoiding intestinal ischemia during labor.
2. decreasing bacterial contamination of the exposed intestines.
3. decreasing physical damage to the intestine during delivery.
4. decreasing the incidence of fetal distress if vaginal delivery is anticipated.

46. Sources of amniotic fluid platelet activating factor include

1. fetal lung.
2. fetal liver.
3. fetal kidney.
4. maternal macrophages.

47. Likely to be associated with aneuploidy in the early second trimester fetus with cystic hygroma

1. septation.
2. multiple structural anomalies.
3. size greater than 15 mm.
4. "space suit" sign.

48. Early surveillance (before 32 weeks) of pregnant diabetic patients should be undertaken if there is concomitant

1. proteinuria.
2. hypertension.
3. systemic lupus erythematosus
4. diabetics of at least class R or F.

49. Rapid intravenous crystalloid infusion into a pregnant patient causes increased blood flow to

1. skin.
2. kidney.
3. skeletal muscle.
4. placenta.

50. True statements about diabetes and vascular function during pregnancy include

1. Blood vessels from nonpregnant diabetic women produce less prostacyclin than blood vessels from healthy subjects.
2. Platelets from nonpregnant women and women with gestational diabetes produce greater amounts of thromboxane than platelets from nondiabetic women and nondiabetic pregnant women.
3. Hydrogen peroxide produces a prostaglandin mediated contraction that is larger in placental vessels from women with gestational diabetes compared to normal women.
4. Responses to hypoxia in the diabetic patient originates and changes in the production of vasoactive mediators produced by the endothelium.

51. Effects of acoustic stimulation on fetal behavior include

1. tachycardia.
2. increased swallowing.
3. decreased breathing.
4. fetal heart rate acceleration.

52. Effects of acoustic stimulation on fetal behavior include

    1. tachycardia.
    2. increased swallowing.
    3. decreased breathing.
    4. fetal heart rate acceleration.

53. Associated with the development of peripartum cardiomyopathy

    1. increased maternal age
    2. twin gestation
    3. preeclampsia
    4. terbutaline

54. Viruses which may be responsible for triggering the development of diabetic mellitus in genetically susceptible patients include

    1. Coxackie B
    2. mumps
    3. rubella
    4. CMV

55. Associated with fetal chylothorax

    1. Down syndrome
    2. Turner syndrome
    3. Noonan syndrome
    4. generalized lymphangiectasis

56. In pregnancies complicating diabetic nephropathy

    1. the fetus has hematologic changes and alterations in fetal heart rate patterns similar to the intrauterine growth retarded fetus secondary to decreased placental perfusion
    2. there is not hypoxia induced redistribution in the fetal circulation
    3. the diagnosis of fetal hypoxemia may be obscured
    4. there is impedance to flow in the uterine artery

57. Conditions associated with nonimmune hydrops include

    1. congenital heart block
    2. fetomaternal hemorrhage
    3. twin-twin transfusion syndrome
    4. fetal hypoproteinemia

58. Platelet activating factor

    1. increases PGE2 function in the amnion.
    2. stimulates myometrial contraction.
    3. is a proinflammatory agent.
    4. is responsible for the vascular refractoriness to pressor agents during pregnancy.

59. Protein S is known to be decreased in

    1. warfarin therapy
    2. chronic liver disease
    3. seminated intravascular coagulation
    4. pregnancy

60. Effects of ritodrine include

    1. fetal tachycardia
    2. neonatal hypoglycemia
    3. maternal tachyarrhythmias
    4. increase in maternal glycogenolysis

61. True statements about glycated hemoglobin and glycated albumin during pregnancy include

    1. glycated albumin is increased in the first to the third trimester
    2. fructosamine begins to fall in the second trimester
    3. glycated hemoglobin of light erythrocytes is lower in the second and third trimester
    4. glycated hemoglobin of dense erythrocytes is low in the first and second trimester and elevated in the third trimester

62. Substances with a strong affinity for collagen include

    1. hyaluronic acid
    2. dermatan sulfate
    3. chondroitin sulfate
    4. fibronectin

63. Clinically useful in the management of pulmonary edema secondary to left ventricular contractile dysfunction

    1. diltiazem
    2. captopril
    3. propranolol
    4. furosemide

64. Anticonvulsant drugs which induce microsomal enzymes to degrade vitamin K1 include

    1. phenobarbital.
    2. phenytoin.
    3. carbamazepine.
    4. valproic acid.

65. Causes of hypertension developing in patients following orthotopic liver transplants include

    1. use of corticosteroids
    2. use of cyclosporin A
    3. nulliparity
    4. graft rejection

66. Effective in relaxing human myometrium

    1. cyclooxygenase inhibitors.
    2. ß agonists.
    3. calcium channel blockers.
    4. potassium channel openers.

67. Amino acid N-methyl-D-aspartate receptors are involved in

    1. epilepsy.
    2. ischemic brain damage.
    3. Huntington's disease.
    4. Alzheimer's disease.

68. The tachyphylaxis that occurs with ritodrine infusion during the treatment of preterm labor is secondary to

    1. decline in ß2-receptor density
    2. production of PGF2α
    3. uncoupling of the receptor with adenylyl cyclase
    4. production of PGE

69. Changes which accompany preeclampsia include

    1. altered platelet membrane function
    2. reduced antioxidant systems in red blood cells
    3. endothelial cell dysfunction
    4. platelet aggregation

PERINATAL MEDICINE REFERENCES

Directions: Each of the questions or incomplete statements below is followed by several suggested answers or completions. Select the BEST answer in each case.

---

1. The best predictive measurement in fetal urine for postnatal renal function is

   A. ammonium.
   B. chloride.
   C. sodium.
   *D. ß2 microglobulin.
   E. urea.

---

p. 819 (Muller F, Dommergues M, Mandelbrot L, Aubry M, Nihoul-Fekete C, Dumez Y. Fetal urinary biochemistry predicts postnatal renal function in children with bilateral obstructive uropathies. Obstet Gynecol 1993; 82:813)

1. [F & I: •Background: Dilation of the fetal urinary tract is an anomaly commonly detected by routine obstetric sonography.

•Unilateral dilatation of a ureter or renal pelvis carries a good postnatal functional prognosis, provided the contralateral kidney is normal.

•The outcome for bilateral urinary tract dilations is variable.

•Fetal and neonatal death can result from renal dysplasia and pulmonary hypoplasia, and although up to half of fetuses with low or bilateral obstructions survive, as many as 50% develop renal failure.

•Perinatal death can be anticipated when prenatal ultrasound shows severe oligohydramnios associated with hyperechogenic renal parenchyma or subcortical cysts.

•Biochemical characteristics of fetal urine have been determined by ultrasound-guided sampling in the fetal renal pelvis or bladder.

•Renal dysplasia, renal failure at birth, and pulmonary insufficiency are related to **high** sodium chloride levels in the fetal urine.

•Neither prenatal sonography nor urine electrolytes have been evaluated for their capacity to predict postnatal renal failure among survivors.

•Sensitive prognostic markers would be of great use for prenatal management.

•Intrauterine uro-amniotic shunting procedures have been performed over the past decade for decompression of the fetal urinary tract.

•It is difficult to select patients who would optimally benefit from prenatal intervention.

•Objective: To evaluate prenatal predictors of postnatal renal function.

•100 fetuses with bilateral uropathies were investigated prenatally by both ultrasound and fetal urine sampling.

•No intrauterine shunting was performed.

•The data base for the correlation between pre and postnatal data compromised 42 infants with isolated bilateral uropathies who survived the first year of postnatal life and had adequate follow-up of their renal function.

•Fact   °Detail   »issue   *answer

- The management of prenatally diagnosed uropathies is controversial, in large part because their natural history is not thoroughly understood.

- Obstruction of the urinary tract can be associated with a spectrum of alterations of the renal parenchyma.

- In the severest cases, bilateral renal dysplasia leads to terminal renal failure in utero.

- The absence of urine output is responsible for severe oligohydramnios, which in turn leads to pulmonary hypoplasia (Potter sequence) and fetal or perinatal death.

- In milder cases progressive renal failure may still occur in childhood despite appropriate neonatal surgical correction of the urinary tract obstruction.

- This has been particularly well documented in cases of posterior urethral valves.

- Finally, some infants survive with no evidence of renal dysfunction in childhood.

- Fetal or perinatal death can be anticipated when hyperechogenic renal cortex, cortical cysts, and/or severe oligohydramnios are detected in utero by ultrasound.

- Fetal urine sampling under ultrasound guidance is used to obtain additional information on fetal kidney function.

- Fetal urinary sodium or chloride values in excess of 100 mmol/l are highly predictive of fetal or perinatal death from terminal renal or pulmonary failure.

- Although the majority of fetuses with urinary sodium values below 100 mmol/l survive into the neonatal period, little has been reported concerning their postnatal renal function.

- Available data do suggest the possibility of significant morbidity in many of these children.

- Markedly elevated fetal urinary sodium and chloride are predictive of severe renal dysplasia, as are very high fetal urinary levels of calcium, phosphorus, glucose, total protein, and ß2 microglobulin, or extremely low levels of creatinine and urea.

- At the start of the study, it was thought that the isolated finding of a fetal urinary sodium value above 100 mEq/L should be a potential indication for termination of pregnancy, but all fetuses with higher values were found to have severe oligohydramnios in the second trimester.

- Information from fetal urinalysis did not alter obstetric management in any case.

- The surviving children were divided into two groups according to whether their last serum creatinine value during the second year of life was greater or less than 50 μmol/l.

- Despite its potential disadvantages (interindividual variability and gross evaluation of renal function), serum creatinine was used as the single end point because of its availability.

- In young children, serum creatinine measurements may be more accurate than clearance measurements, which are impaired by incorrect sampling.

- The cutoff level of 50 μmol/l corresponds to 2 SDs above the mean value in healthy children.

- Group I consisted of infants with strictly normal renal function, whereas group II comprised children potentially at risk of renal failure.

- These groups did not differ significantly in terms of anatomical sampling site, gestational age at the time of sampling, prenatal management, or postnatal therapy.

- Forty-one of the 42 surviving children in this series were males, which is only partly accounted for by the frequency of posterior urethral valves in this population.

- Posterior urethral valves, the most common lesion in this series, led to the highest proportion of survivors with high serum creatinine after 1 year of age.

- Prenatal ultrasound **failed** to distinguish this etiology accurately from other causes of bilateral urinary dilatation with a better prognosis.

  ° It was not possible to distinguish megacystis due to reflux from enlarged bladder due to urethral valves.

- Sonographic predictors of postnatal renal dysfunction (moderate oligohydramnios and abnormal structure of the renal parenchyma) were found to be specific but lacked sensitivity.

- Except for glucose, all fetal urinary compounds measured were better predictors of renal function in the second year of life than was prenatal sonographic evaluation of AF volume or of renal parenchyma, because of higher sensitivity.

- The most sensitive fetal urinary compounds were sodium, chloride, ß2 microglobulin, and urea.

- Fetal urinary **ß2 microglobulin** had the best combination of sensitivity and specificity when correlated with serum creatinine values during the second year of life.

- Although sodium and chloride values greater than 50 mEq/L and urea less than 8.6 mmol/l were sensitive, they were not as specific as ß2 microglobulin.

- Concentrations of the latter did not vary significantly as a function of gestational age, thereby enhancing the clinical value of this assay.

- Conclusion: ß2 microglobulin is probably the best single fetal urinary compound to measure for prediction of renal function in fetuses with obstructive uropathies.

- Urinary ß2 microglobulin levels may reflect renal tubular reabsorption, but the pathophysiology of the increased urinary output of ß2 microglobulin in fetuses with compromised kidneys has not yet been found.

- Experimental ligation of the ureter in the fetal lamb during the first 70 days of gestation has shown that high pressures in the urinary tract during fetal development may create histologic alterations of the renal parenchyma similar to those observed in human obstructive uropathies.

- This finding supports the hypothesis that intrauterine decompression of the urinary tract may prevent ongoing renal damage.

- Intrauterine percutaneous drainage of the bladder or kidney has been advocated to restore urinary flow, relieve intrapelvic pressure, maintain AF volume, and prevent pulmonary hypoplasia.

- **Renal dysplasia** may also result from a primary defect in nephrogenesis, unrelated to elevated hydrostatic pressure in the renal pelves, or irreversible damage secondary to an obstructive lesion may already have occurred before therapy.

- In such circumstances, no benefit can be expected from intrauterine therapy.

- Intrauterine shunting is not likely to restore normal renal function in the presence of second-trimester severe oligohydramnios, as a consequence of irreversible renal dysplasia.

- Invasive prenatal therapy is not justified for fetuses who, even if untreated, will have normal postnatal renal function.

• These patients would be needlessly exposed to the risk of several complications resulting from shunt placement, including premature birth, chorioamnionitis, and fetal death.

• The best indication for uroamniotic shunting procedures is clearly to prevent postnatal renal failure in at-risk fetuses whose kidneys have not yet been irreversibly damaged.]

2. An elevated uterine artery resistance index is most closely related to

- A. elevated middle cerebral artery resistance index.
- B. maternal blood pressure.
- C. maternal parity.
- D. maternal weight.
- *E. placenta ischemic changes.

p. 497 (Iwata M, Matsuzaki N, Shimizu I, Mitsuda N, Nakayama M, Suehara N. Prenatal diagnosis of ischemic changes in the placenta of the growth-retarded fetus by doppler flow velocimetry of the maternal uterine artery. Obstet Gynecol 1993; 82:494)

2. [F & I: •Background: A growth-retarded fetus has an increased risk of perinatal morbidity and mortality.

• Recent advances in ultrasound imaging techniques for monitoring fetal growth have made it possible to assess and manage growth-retarded fetuses.

• Doppler flow velocimetry studies show abnormal waveforms in the umbilical or uteroplacental artery to be useful in the assessment of high-risk growth retarded fetuses, pregnancy-induced hypertension, and fetal asphyxia.

• Abnormalities of the uteroplacental circulation may be related to acute or chronic placental insufficiency, leading to preterm delivery, fetal distress, or fetal death.

° Not all placentas of growth retarded fetuses show such pathologic changes.

• Few studies have examined the relationships among the pregnancy outcomes with high-risk fetal growth retardation (FGR), pathologic changes in the placenta, and Doppler flow velocimetry of the fetomaternal circulation.

• Objective: To examine the relationship between the placental pathologic changes and risks, including the uterine artery resistance index.

• Placentas of growth-retarded fetuses have characteristic histologic features, including placental ischemia, high syncytial knot count, placental infarction, intervillous fibrin deposition, basement membrane thickening, stromal fibrosis and edema, apparent placental hypovascularity, and villous maturation.

° These changes may lead to acute or chronic fetal hypoxia, resulting in FGR, fetal distress, or fetal death.

• Ischemic changes in the placenta are closely related to preterm delivery of growth-retarded fetuses.

• No other placental pathologic changes, including thrombosis, chronic villitis, or immature villi, had such a direct association with the clinical course of growth-retarded fetuses.

• Placentas with ischemic changes were associated with a higher incidence of cesarean delivery for fetal distress and worse results in the cord blood gas measurements than the placentas without ischemic changes.

• Although growth-retarded fetuses have been classified into types I (symmetrical) and II (asymmetrical), the findings suggest the possibility of classifying them as high risk (ischemic placenta) and low risk (nonischemic placenta) based on Doppler flow velocimetry.

- The uterine artery resistance index is the best diagnostic index in terms of sensitivity, specificity, and positive predictive value for the antenatal detection of ischemic placentas in growth-retarded fetuses.

- Linear discriminative analysis supported this conclusion, as an ischemic placenta correlated most closely with a high uterine artery resistance index.

- Doppler flow velocimetry of the fetoplacental circulation is useful for prenatal evaluation of high-risk growth-retarded fetuses.

- The flow velocity of the fetal middle cerebral artery is useful for detecting hypoxia of growth-retarded fetuses, because of the fetal brain-sparing effect.

  ° These resistance indexes of the umbilical and middle cerebral arteries were less useful than that of the uterine artery for prenatal detection of placental ischemic changes in growth-retarded fetuses.

- The flow velocity waveform of the uterine artery has been proposed as a useful measure for the detection of high-risk growth-retarded fetuses.

- An abnormal uterine artery resistance index at 16 to 18 weeks' gestation may predict outcome in cases of hypertensive complications of pregnancy, FGR, or fetal asphyxia.

- Ideally, fetuses at increased risk of antepartum or intrapartum hypoxia should have periodic monitoring, first by ultrasonographic biometry to confirm FGR and then by measurement of the uterine artery resistance index.

- Placental pathologic changes leading to abnormalities of the fetomaternal circulation are associated with growth retardation.

  ° Such placentas showed arterial abnormalities such as decreased number, abnormal wall thickening, or obliteration, vascular and connective tissue alterations, or impaired trophoblastic invasion of the placental bed, resulting in elevated circulatory resistance in the uteroplacental unit with consequent placental ischemic changes.

- These circulatory abnormalities can be detected by Doppler velocimetry as elevated resistance in the fetal umbilical artery, maternal uterine artery, or fetal middle cerebral artery.

- Among these, **the uterine artery resistance index is the most sensitive to placental ischemic changes associated with a high risk of premature delivery and fetal distress.**

- An abnormal umbilical systolic-diastolic ratio in growth-retarded fetuses precedes a pathologic nonstress test, associated with a high risk of preterm vaginal and preterm cesarean delivery.

- The time interval between these events appears to be variable.

- In placentas with ischemic changes, an abnormal uterine resistance index and fetal distress occurred within 1 week of each other.

- In contrast, placentas without ischemic changes showed a normal uterine artery resistance index with a normal nonstress test, and preterm delivery was rare.

- **A normal uterine artery resistance index in a growth retarded fetus should serve as an indicator of term delivery.**]

3. The vascular refractoriness to exogenous angiotensin II during pregnancy is due to

    A. diminished affinity of angiotensin II receptors.
    B. down regulation of angiotensin II receptors is a function of angiotensin II level.
    C. increased catabolism of angiotensin II.
    D. occupation of angiotensin II receptors by endogenous peptide applies when concentration is elevated during pregnancy.
*E. reduction of vasoconstrictor effective angiotensin II by vasodilator substances.

---

p. 385 (Langer B, Barthelmebs M, Grima M, Coquard C, Imbs J. In vitro vascular reactivity of the rat utero-fetal-placental unit. Obstet Gynecol 1993; 82:380)

3. [F & I: •Background: The presence in tissue of several components of the renin-angiotensin system has given rise to the concept of the tissular renin-angiotensin system, which could operate at the utero-feto-placental level.

    •During human pregnancy, the renin-angiotensin system is activated on a major scale.

    •Plasma renin activity increases more than 50% in human pregnancy.

    •In pregnant women, this activation is accompanied by the development of relative refractoriness to the systemic pressor effect of hormones, in particular angiotensin II.

    •Reduced vascular reactivity to angiotensin II, a normal feature of pregnancy, disappears in preeclamptic subjects.

    •Objectives: To compare vascular reactivity to two vasoconstrictors, norepinephrine and angiotensin II, in pregnant and nonpregnant rats and to explore the local role of the angiotensin I-converting enzyme by also testing angiotensin I.

    •Results: Significant differences in uterine flow and vascular resistance during pregnancy was found, which are classic physiologic features; the rat preparation responded to various vasoconstrictor drugs and retained the capacity to convert angiotensin I to angiotensin II.

    •Vasopressor responses with angiotensin I show that vasoconstriction induced by this peptide is linked exclusively to its transformation into angiotensin II by the angiotensin I-converting enzyme and results from interaction with the angiotensin II receptors.

    •Ramiprilat, a converting enzyme inhibitor, reduced angiotensin I pressor response markedly, and saralasin, a competitive antagonist of the angiotensin II receptors, suppressed it completely.

    •Results with ramiprilat show that in the perfused uterus, angiotensin I metabolism operates exclusively through the angiotensin I-converting enzyme.

    •In pregnant uteri, the maximum vasopressor response to angiotensin II was lower than in nonpregnant uteri.

    •Hypotheses have been advanced to explain the vascular refractoriness to exogenous angiotensin II during pregnancy include:

        °1) occupation of the angiotensin II receptors by endogenous peptide, whose plasma concentration is elevated during pregnancy;

        °2) down-regulation of the angiotensin II receptors as a function of the angiotensin II level;

        °3) diminished affinity of the angiotensin II receptors;

        °4) increased catabolism of angiotensin II; and

°5) reduction in the vasoconstrictor effect of angiotensin II by vasodilator substances.

•These results cannot be explained by the first three hypotheses.

•The endogenous angiotensin II level might be very low after in vitro perfusion with a medium deprived of renin substrate or angiotensin I, whereas captopril administration did not to restore angiotensin II responsiveness in gravid rats.

•Despite a higher plasma angiotensin II concentration during pregnancy, no evidence of down-regulation of angiotensin II receptors was found in either uterine or systemic arteries, and the maximum vasoconstriction in response to angiotensin I remained unchanged.

•The affinity of the angiotensin II receptor was also unchanged during pregnancy, as was the apparent affinity, measured by the 50% effective concentration.

•Vascular hyporesponsiveness was not specific for angiotensin II and was also found with norepinephrine and vasopressin.

•The fourth hypothesis is also invalid, refractoriness to angiotensin II is not related to changes in the metabolic clearance of the peptide.

•The apparent lack of refractoriness to angiotensin I should be related to a lower catabolism of endogenous angiotensin II.

•The concentration-response curve for angiotensin II did not shift to the right, as would be expected in this case.

•Thus, only the final hypothesis can explain these results.

•Although clear evidence for regulation of the uteroplacental blood flow by prostaglandins is lacking, the refractoriness of sheep uterine arteries to angiotensin II reflects vessel production of **prostacyclin**.

•These results with angiotensin II are consistent with this finding.

•The results with angiotensin I were unexpected.

•The lack of refractoriness to this peptide points to a difference in responsiveness to endogenous and exogenous angiotensin II.

•The measurements of tissular angiotensin I-converting enzyme activity revealed a low level of activity in the different samples, compared to values measured in the rat aorta.

•This should be balanced by the fact that the proportion of vascular tissue, and thus of endothelial cells, is lower in the myometrium.

•Contrary to what was expected, enzyme activity was also low in the placenta, where there is a higher proportion of vascular tissue.

•The enzyme activity measured in the presence of ramiprilat is evidence of the inhibition of the converting enzyme in the perfused uterus.

•Unexpectedly, this inhibition appears to be less marked in the placenta and embryo.

•Free diffusion of the angiotensin-converting enzyme inhibitors to the embryo has been reported.

•The results also show that converting-enzyme activity in the myometrium—most probably in the endothelial cells—was not modified by pregnancy.

Obstetrics and Gynecology:Review 1994-Perinatal Medicine References

•The results in rats confirm the vascular refractoriness to angiotensin II observed clinically.

•They show that this refractoriness exists in the uterine vascular bed and persists in a denervated in vitro model.

•Tissular, probably endothelial, angiotensin I-converting enzyme permits in situ synthesis of angiotensin II.

•This local system could thus participate in regulation of the fetal flow in the placenta.]

---

4. Electrocardiographic changes associated with a normal pregnancy include

    A. 15 degree left axis deviation.
    B. Q wave in lead AVF.
    C. Q wave inverted in lead III.
 *D. S-T segment elevation in lead II.
    E. T wave inverted in lead III.

---

p. 281 (Sheikh A U, Harper M A. Myocardial infarction during pregnancy: Management and outcome of two pregnancies. Am J Obstet Gynec 1993; 169:279)

4. [F & I: •Background: The incidence of all cardiac lesions in women of reproductive age is 0.4% to 4.5%.

•The estimated incidence of myocardial infarction in this age group is <0.1%, with an incidence during pregnancy estimated at 0.01%.

•Fewer than 100 cases of myocardial infarction during pregnancy have been reported.

•Because of the relative scarcity of data about this complication during pregnancy, management has been empirically determined.

•The normal physiologic adaptations to pregnancy increase cardiac work load and may increase the risk of significant intrapartum morbidity and mortality in patients with myocardial infarction.

•This has prompted many to use invasive central monitoring, including pulmonary artery catheterization to guide control of preload and afterload during labor and delivery.

°This type of monitoring is associated with its own risks.

•Objective: To present two cases of myocardial infarction during pregnancy with good outcomes in which the patients were managed without pulmonary artery catheterization.

•Both patients had enzyme, electrocardiographic, and echocardiographic evidence of acute myocardial infarction.

•They did well during labor and delivery and postpartum.

•The mode of delivery was determined by obstetric indications.

•Intrapartum and postpartum management was based on the patients' physical examinations, signs, and symptoms.

•The perinatal mortality rate with maternal myocardial infarction may be as high as 34%, whereas maternal mortality ranges from 28% to 50%.

•**The mortality rate increases the closer to delivery that the myocardial infarction occurs, with the highest rates in those who infarct during labor.**

•The greatest risk for perinatal mortality was maternal outcome.

Obstetrics and Gynecology: Review 1994-Perinatal Medicine References

- A number of physiologic changes that add to the cardiac work load occur during normal pregnancy.

- Blood volume increases from 6 weeks of gestation and rises rapidly until midgestation, where it is 33% higher than in the nonpregnant patient.

- After midgestation blood volume rises gradually, and by term it has increased by 49%.

- The increase in volume correlates with both the weight of the products of conception and the maternal weight gain.

- Multigravid women and multifetal gestations experience larger increases in volume, with a rise of up to 60% to 70% occurring in the latter group.

- Cardiac output also increases beginning at 10 weeks of gestation.

- By 20 to 24 weeks cardiac output has risen 30% to 50%.

- **Cardiac output** is affected by posture, with a significant drop in output occurring on a move from the lateral to the supine position.

- **Heart rate** also increases during pregnancy, rising by 10 to 20 beats/min at term.

  ° In multifetal gestation the rise in heart rate occurs earlier than in a singleton gestation and may increase by 40% over nonpregnant values.

- The **systemic vascular resistance** decreases as a result of the low resistance circulation of the uterus and the decreased vasomotor tone associated with increased levels of progesterone, estrogen, prolactin, and prostacyclin.

- Additional cardiac changes include an increase in the preejection period (the time between onset of the electric signal and ejection of blood) and a decrease in the left ventricular ejection time (the actual time spent in ejection of blood from the left ventricle).

- Some have interpreted this as evidence of enhanced cardiac activity.

- **Oxygen consumption** increases during the course of pregnancy with a higher arteriovenous oxygen difference in late gestation.

  ° This reflects the increased metabolic demands of mother and fetus.

- Labor is associated with a significant increase in the **central venous pressure** and thus cardiac **preload**, as a result of transfusion of 300 to 500 ml of blood from the uterus during contractions.

- Heart rate, cardiac output, systemic vascular resistance, and blood pressure also increase during labor in the unanesthetized woman.

- Cardiac output increases approximately 35% immediately after cesarean section and also increases, although to a lesser degree, after vaginal delivery.

- In spite of the pregnancy-related increase in cardiac workload neither patient subsequently experienced cardiac failure.

- Efforts to decrease cardiac strain, including restricting activity, correcting anemia, and monitoring for signs of infection, may have helped reduce the chances of cardiac failure.

  ° These patients were able to tolerate the increased cardiac stress because they still had good cardiac function, as demonstrated by diagnostic imaging, after infarction.

•Fact   °Detail   »issue   *answer

Obstetrics and Gynecology: Review 1994-Perinatal Medicine References

- The amount of cardiac function remaining after infarction appears to be an important predictor of prognosis.

- Myocardial infarction is caused primarily by coronary artery obstruction or vasospasm.

- There are up to 40 disorders that may act by one or both of these mechanisms to cause infarction including hypercholesterolemia, hypertension, diabetes mellitus, hypothyroidism, systemic lupus erythematosus, syphilis, and cocaine abuse.

- Cigarette smoking and a history of preeclampsia independent of chronic hypertension are also risks.

- There is some speculation that the high estrogen levels present during pregnancy result in increased cholesterol and hypercoagulability and thus predispose pregnant patients to coronary artery disease.

- The rarity of coronary artery disease during pregnancy suggests that these factors alone are not sufficient.

- Myocardial infarction may occur in some pregnancies as a result of vasospasm triggered by renin release from the chorion.

- The diagnosis of myocardial infarction is based on clinical and laboratory findings.

- Typical symptoms include substernal chest pain with radiation to the arm or neck and respiratory symptoms, diaphoresis, nausea, and vomiting.

- The **differential diagnosis** in pregnancy includes other more common disorders, including reflux esophagitis, premature labor, hiatal hernia, cholelithiasis, costochondritis, and pneumonia.

  ° The diagnosis of myocardial infarction may initially be missed.

- Confirmatory laboratory tests include cardiac enzyme analysis, electrocardiogram, and diagnostic imaging.

- The serum **aspartate aminotransferase** level is specific for infarction, rising within 8 to 12 h.

  ° Aspartate aminotransferase is also abnormal in patients with liver, skeletal muscle, and biliary tract diseases.

- Serum **lactate dehydrogenase** levels also increase after myocardial infarction and typically peak 24 to 48 h after the event and return to normal within 7 to 14 days.

  ° There are five subfractions, of which lactate dehydrogenase-1 is found elevated in 95% of cases of myocardial infarction.

  ° Lactate dehydrogenase may be mildly elevated in 18% of normal pregnancies, but lactate dehydrogenase-1 is unaffected.

- Serum **creatine kinase** rises 6 to 8 h after infarction and peaks within 24 h.

  ° There are several creatine kinase isoenzymes, with the MB fraction being specific for myocardial injury.

- Occurrence of infarction is frequently confirmed by electrocardiogram.

- Normal changes that occur in association with pregnancy should be kept in mind.

- These changes include a 15-degree left axis deviation, Q and inverted T waves in lead III, and Q waves in lead AVF.

- **Elevation or depression of the ST segment or inversion of Q or T waves in other leads are suggestive of ischemia or infarction.**

- **Combining an electrocardiogram with exercise, as in a treadmill test, allows assessment of cardiac reserve.**

- **Three frequently used modes of diagnostic imaging are echocardiography, angiography, and radionuclide scans.**

- **Abnormal cardiac motion and blood flow patterns seen after infarction can be detected by echocardiography.**

- **In addition, ventricular ejection fraction (an estimate of ventricular function) can be measured by echocardiography.**

- **Normal ventricular ejection fraction is >65%.**

- **Coronary angiography is useful for detecting coronary artery disease or thrombosis.**

   ° The disadvantage is the exposure of the fetus to radiation.

   ° Shielding the maternal abdomen minimizes fetal exposure to radiation; it should be kept in mind that fetal exposure to total doses of radiation >0.05 Gy increases the risk of childhood cancers.

- **Cardiac catheterization should be avoided during the first 14 weeks of gestation, if possible.**

- **Radionuclide scans are very useful in assessing cardiac function.**

   ° **They are contraindicated during pregnancy because of the unacceptably high dose of radiation to the fetus.**

- **Management of myocardial infarction in pregnancy can be divided into short-term, long-term, intrapartum, and postpartum care.**

- **The primary goals are decreasing cardiac strain, preventing extension of infarction, increasing oxygenation, and preventing myocardial infarction-associated complications such as thrombosis.**

- **Care of these patients is best provided through a team approach with cardiologists, anesthesiologists, and perinatologists.**

- **An acute myocardial infarction warrants aggressive intervention.**

- **Some have recommended disregarding the fetus in planning maternal resuscitation and management in early gestation.**

- **Beginning in the late second trimester the gravid uterus can impede blood return through the inferior vena cava and should be laterally displaced during resuscitation.**

- **Initial management of the patient with an acute myocardial infarction depends on the severity of symptoms.**

- **In the absence of cardiac arrest, arrhythmias, congestive heart failure, or severe symptoms, treatment with oxygen, nitroglycerin, heparin, and morphine should be initiated, in addition to continuous electrocardiographic monitoring.**

- **Pulmonary artery catheterization is helpful in the pharmacologic management of cardiogenic shock.**

- **Intravenous medications, including dopamine; antiarrhythmic agents such as lidocaine, procainamide, or quinidine; diuretics; ß-blockers; and calcium channel blockers have been used in pregnancy.**

Obstetrics and Gynecology: Review 1994-Perinatal Medicine References

- Direct-current cardioversion may also be used in pregnancy at the same voltage used for resuscitation of nonpregnant patients.

- **Thrombolytic therapy is relatively contraindicated** because of the increased incidence of fetal and maternal hemorrhage.

- After the acute infarction, consideration needs to be given to long-term maintenance of the stabilized patient.

- Evaluation of cardiac reserve by exercise testing is helpful.

- Some have suggested that submaximal exercise levels be used in the pregnant patient.

- Follow-up echocardiography can assess recovery of cardiac function.

- Low-dose aspirin, dipyridamole, and heparin have been used to prevent thrombosis.

- If antihypertensive therapy is necessary, methyldopa or labetalol and other ß-blocking agents can be used.

- **Hydralazine** causes reflex tachycardia and is **relatively contraindicated** in patients with a recent myocardial infarction.

- The safety of calcium channel blockers during pregnancy is still being investigated.

- Issues to consider in intrapartum management include mode of delivery, maternal monitoring during labor and delivery, and methods of minimizing cardiac stress.

- Delivery by cesarean section should be determined solely on obstetric indications.

- Elective cesarean section is preferable when prolonged labor is anticipated and myocardial infarction has occurred within 4 days of delivery.

- Shortening the second stage of labor with forceps to minimize maternal strain has been recommended.

- Monitoring during labor and delivery should include continuous blood pressure, pulse, and fetal heart rate recordings and possibly continuous electrocardiogram and pulse oximetry.

- Up to 50% of patients may have reversible arrhythmias, and 1.5% may have other significant complications as a result of pulmonary artery catheterization.

- Because of these risks, central monitoring should be reserved for critically ill patients or those who have suffered a recent myocardial infarction.

- Measures should be taken to decrease maternal oxygen consumption and cardiac strain by providing adequate analgesia and sedation, decreasing maternal shivering by providing a higher ambient temperature or warming intravenous fluids, and providing supplemental oxygen.

- The issues of anxiety and pain relief are especially important in the laboring patient who has had a myocardial infarction.

- Both are associated with significant catecholamine release, resulting in increased cardiac work.

- Anxiety can be adequately diminished by reassuring the patient and by judicious use of sedatives like opioids and promethazine.

- Epidural anesthesia effectively decreases pain during labor while causing less hypotension and sympathetic blockade than seen with subarachnoid anesthesia.

Obstetrics and Gynecology:Review 1994-Perinatal Medicine References

°Spinal anesthesia has been safely used for both cesarean section and labor in patients after myocardial infarction.

•General anesthesia has also been used but is associated with a significant increase in blood pressure during intubation.

°Adequate control of blood pressure preoperatively and during induction of anesthesia is extremely important.

•The normal postpartum course is associated with significant **fluid shifts** from the interstitial to intravascular space and autotransfusion from the uterus.

•Reinfarction and maternal mortality rate may be higher in the early puerperium as a result of this increased cardiac stress.

»In the absence of signs or symptoms of heart failure or recurrent myocardial infarction, close monitoring of maternal symptoms, blood pressure, pulse, and urine output allows adequate assessment of the maternal state.

•These two cases support the belief that control of preload and afterload by pharmacologic manipulation does not require guidance by pulmonary artery catheter measurements when patients are more than 1 month beyond their myocardial infarction, have demonstrated good myocardial function, and have good cardiac reserves.

•For these patients, invasive hemodynamic monitoring appears to constitute an unnecessary risk.

•The mode of delivery should be determined by obstetric indications.]

---

5. Which of the following has the best predictive value for identifying patients at risk for preeclampsia?

    A. Analysis of parental HLA loci.
    B. Angiotensin sensitivity test.
*C. Doppler screening of the uterine artery
    D. "Roll over" test.
    E. Serum uric acid.

---

p. 82 (Bower S, Bewley S, Campbell S. Improved prediction of preeclampsia by two-stage screening of uterine arteries using the early diastolic notch and color doppler imaging. Obstet Gynecol 1993; 82:78)

5. [F & I: •Background: Preeclampsia is a leading cause of maternal and fetal morbidity and mortality.

•It is associated with a high incidence of emergency cesarean delivery, fetal growth retardation, placental abruption, and preterm delivery.

•Not all pregnancy-induced hypertension is harmful, and mild hypertension without proteinuria is associated with a good fetal outcome.

•Preeclamptic pregnancies have high impedance in the uteroplacental circulation and a reduction in the volume of flow, which result from failed trophoblastic invasion of the spiral arteries in the early second trimester.

•Uteroplacental vascular resistance can be assessed by Doppler ultrasound, and impedance indices measured by Doppler have been evaluated as an early screening test for preeclampsia.

•Using continuous-wave Doppler ultrasound, inclusion of an early diastolic notch in the definition of an abnormal flow velocity waveform improves the sensitivity for predicting preeclampsia.

Obstetrics and Gynecology: Review 1994-Perinatal Medicine References

°It does not reduce the high false-positive rate, presumably because the early diastolic notch can persist in some normal pregnancies up to 24 to 26 weeks.

•Objective: To determine whether a second-line investigation, using color Doppler of the uterine artery and identifying a notch in the flow velocity waveform, would improve specificity while maintaining sensitivity for the prediction of preeclampsia.

•The assessment technique for preeclampsia was modified by performing a second-line investigation at 24 weeks using color Doppler imaging.

°This allows accurate identification of the main uterine arteries, with the apparent crossover point of the uterine and external iliac arteries providing a convenient, standard landmark.

•Methods: Each subject was examined in the semirecumbent position after 10 min of bed rest.

•Color Doppler imaging was used to identify the left and right uterine arteries and to perform pulsed Doppler studies.

•By placing the transducer in the lower lateral quadrant of the uterus and angling it medially, the crossover of the external iliac artery and main uterine artery was identified, and the range gate was placed over the entire diameter of the uterine artery 1 cm distal to this site.

•The quality of the flow velocity waveform obtained was maximized by using the smallest possible angle of insonation (range 15-50°) and accepting only those waveforms with a sharp, clear outline.

•The angle of insonation was then determined on the frozen image.

•When five consecutive waveforms of satisfactory quality had been obtained, the resistance index was measured using an on-screen cursor for each flow velocity waveform. {Resistance index = $(S - D)/S$.}

•The mean value of the five waveforms was used for subsequent analyses.

•This study recruited 2430 women, representative of the local population, for the largest unselected screening study published to date.

°Outcome details were not available for 240 (9.9%), reflecting the mobile nature of the inner-city population.

°The timing of the first-stage screen at 18 to 22 weeks was governed by availability.

°At this stage, the diastolic notch had a higher sensitivity, but lower specificity, than a high resistance index in predicting all proteinuric hypertension.

°The low specificity and high false-positive rate may be due to the persistence of the notch until 24 to 26 weeks in some normal pregnancies.

°This was the rationale for performing two-stage screening.

•Subjects with proteinuric pregnancy-induced hypertension were divided into those with and without significant proteinuria to define genuine preeclampsia more accurately.

•The justification for analyzing preeclampsia separately from the rest of pregnancy induced hypertension is the significant difference in clinical outcome.

•In this study population, 40% of the preeclamptic women delivered infants who were below the fifth percentile for gestation, 40% required early delivery, and 18% required neonatal intensive care; in the nonpreeclamptic hypertension group, the risks of these complications were low.

•The predictive properties of the diastolic notch were markedly better for preeclampsia at both stages of screening, but especially at stage two.

•Fact   °Detail   »issue   *answer

•A notch at the second test had a high sensitivity (78%) and specificity (96%) for development of preeclampsia.

•The risk to the patient was increased 68-fold.

•The use of the diastolic notch increased the sensitivity and specificity while reducing false-positive rates.

•The improved predictive values in this study may result from the use of color Doppler imaging, which allows accurate visualization of vessels and also provides a reference point for sampling the uterine artery.

°Good reproducibility between continuous-wave Doppler ultrasound and color Doppler imaging has previously been noted, at least with experienced operators.

•The improvement in results may also be due to the difference in definition of an abnormal flow velocity waveform.

•The diastolic notch is caused by a reflected wave of high amplitude returning from a uteroplacental bed with high vascular resistance.

•In this study, the notch was recorded only as being present or absent.

•No objective measurement of the diastolic notch has been proposed.

•A high concordance rate has been reported between two experienced operators independently assessing the same series of taped waveforms for the presence or absence of a diastolic notch.

•All women who delivered before 34 weeks for maternal complications of preeclampsia were identified by a notch in the uterine waveform at both stages of screening, but not by a high resistance index.

•This finding emphasizes the discriminatory nature of the former test in predicting those women with clinically significant disease.

•Two-stage screening with color Doppler and the early diastolic notch successfully predicts clinically significant preeclampsia.

•This may allow more appropriate targeting of antenatal care and therapeutic intervention, such as aspirin treatment to modify the disease; this should be tested in randomized controlled trials.

•If these results are confirmed, Doppler screening of the uterine artery could become part of routine care.

•**No other method of predicting preeclampsia has combined such good predictive values with simple, noninvasive methodology.**]

---

6. A para 1001 delivers an infant with congenital heart block. Antibodies to SS-A/Ro and SS-B/La are detected in her serum. The outcome of subsequent pregnancies can be improved by maternal administration of

   A. dexamethasone
   B. gamma globulin and prednisone
   C. methotrexate
   D. plasmapheresis and prednisone
   *E. none of the above

p. 15 (Julkunen H, Kaaja R, Wallgren E, Teramo K. Isolated congenital heart block: Fetal and infant outcome and familial incidence of heart block. Obstet Gynecol 1993; 82:11)

6. [F & I: •Background: Congenital heart block without anatomical cardiac malformations is an uncommon but potentially fatal disease of infants born to mothers with an autoimmune disease, in which maternal antibodies to SS-A/Ro and/or SS-B/La autoantigens cross the placenta and damage fetal cardiac tissue.

•Evidence of this immunomediated pathogenesis for congenital heart block is based on the almost invariable finding of SS-A/Ro or SS-B/La antibodies in mothers of children with congenital heart block and the demonstration of the corresponding antigens in fetal heart conduction cells.

•Inflammation, immunoglobulins (Igs), and complement are found in affected fetal hearts.

•A woman with antibodies to SS-A/Ro or SS-B/La can have either an affected or a healthy child.

•The risk of recurrence of congenital heart block is not known with certainty, but is low, but may be as high as 33%.

•In addition to the risk of having another affected child, these mothers may have an increased risk of spontaneous abortions and stillbirths.

•Although the outcome of infants affected with congenital heart block is generally favorable, deaths during the first year of life are reported.

•Objective: To determine the 1-year outcome of infants with isolated congenital heart block, the risk of fetal loss in mothers of affected children, and the familial incidence and risk of recurrence of congenital heart block.

•Results: The prevalence of congenital heart block in all siblings of the affected children was 4% in this study, and the risk of recurrence of congenital heart block was 8%.

•The presence of maternal anti-SS-A/Ro or anti-SSB/La may be a prerequisite for the development of congenital heart block.

•Only a minority of women with these antibodies (about 0.5% of women with anti-SS-A/Ro) will deliver an infant with congenital heart block.

•A mother can have both healthy and affected children, and there have been reports of twins who were (as in this study) discordant for congenital heart block.

•More than just the presence of antibodies is required for development of congenital heart block.

•Additional risks may include maternal systemic lupus erythematosus or primary **Sjogren syndrome** (risk up to 5%), genetic features of the infant and/or mother, and environmental exposures during the index pregnancy, such as intrauterine **viral infection**.

•One risk may be **high levels** of anti-SS-A/Ro, although the importance of anti-SS-B/La has also been emphasized.

•The suggestion that a history of a previous affected child confers the greatest risk for congenital heart block is **not** supported by this or an earlier study.

•Mothers of children with congenital heart block appeared to have a slightly increased risk of fetal loss compared with controls, and this risk was not associated with anticardiolipin antibodies.

•Antibodies to SS-A/Ro are implicated in spontaneous abortions or fetal deaths in some women.

•One stillbirth and one spontaneous abortion occurred after the 15th week of gestation.

°In these two cases, antibodies to SS-A/Ro and/or SS-B/La may have contributed directly to the fetal deaths.

- The treatment of the fetus diagnosed in utero with isolated congenital heart block is usually expectant.

- Fetal hydrops, often preceded by pericardial effusion or ascites, is a sign of poor outcome and requires more active treatment.

- Adrenergic or anticholinergic drugs have been used because they may increase the fetal cardiac output.

- In contrast to a traditional belief that hydrops in congenital heart block is caused by low-output cardiac failure, an immune mechanism for the serious effusions has been proposed.

- Fetuses have been treated in utero with steroids that are not metabolized by the placenta, such as dexamethasone or betamethasone.

    ° Prednisone or prednisolone may work by decreasing maternal antibody levels.

- Attempts to reduce the amount of harmful maternal antibodies by plasmapheresis, in addition to steroid administration has been attempted.

- Fetal paracentesis and fetal ventricular pacing have also been used.

- In a viable fetus, the **best** treatment may be **elective premature delivery** and immediate postnatal pacing if fetal hydrops develops.

- Prophylactic treatment for congenital heart block in women with previous affected children has also been used.

- The goal of prophylaxis is to diminish the quantity of pathogenic maternal antibodies transmitted to the fetus.

- Two women were treated with corticosteroids and plasmapheresis, and one was given intravenous gamma globulin and prednisone.

- All three pregnancies were successful.

- In view of the low risk of recurrence of congenital heart block found in this study, prophylactic therapies, at least those with potentially serious side effects, should **not** be recommended.

- Because of the widespread use of ultrasound examination during pregnancy, the diagnosis of fetal heart block is now usually made in utero.

- This is likely to improve outcome by diminishing the frequency of unnecessary premature cesarean delivery.

- Seven emergency cesareans were performed because of suspected fetal distress, the majority before the 1980s and none after 1985.

- Although infants with congenital heart block can be delivered vaginally, there are inherent difficulties in fetal monitoring.

- Conventional fetal heart rate recordings **cannot** be used to diagnose fetal distress, and fetal scalp blood sampling for pH and acid-base measurements gives information at the time of the sampling only.

- Doppler assessment of the umbilical artery waveform velocity must be corrected for the slow heart rate.

- Signs of fetal hydrops indicate elective cesarean delivery.

•An infant with congenital heart block may die within a few hours after birth, and some fetuses may die in utero from cardiac failure.

•Congenital heart block may remain undiagnosed in cases of stillbirth and early neonatal death.

•The 15% mortality rate during the first year of life found in this study is most likely an underestimate.

•The prognosis seems to be good for children who survive infancy.]

---

7. Which of the following pregnancy-related conditions is associated with low serum fibrinogen, lower serum glucose and diabetes insipidus?

   *A. Acute fatty liver of pregnancy.
   B. HELLP syndrome.
   C. Hemolytic uremic syndrome.
   D. Intrahepatic cholestasis of pregnancy.
   E. Thrombocytopenic purpura.

---

p. 1687 (Sibai B M, Ramadan M K. Acute renal failure in pregnancies complicated by hemolysis, elevated liver enzymes, and low platelets. Am J Obstet Gynec 1993; 168:1682)

7. [F & I: •Background: Hemolysis, elevated liver enzymes, and low platelets is a complication of severe preeclampsia-eclampsia.

•The incidence among patients with preeclampsia ranges from 4% to 14%.

•Pregnancies complicated by this syndrome have a poor maternal and perinatal outcome.

•Maternal mortality ranges from 0% to 24%.

•The mothers are at increased risk for pulmonary edema, adult respiratory distress syndrome (ARDS), abruptio placentae, disseminated intravascular coagulopathy, ruptured liver hematomas, and acute renal failure.

•**Acute renal failure** is an extremely rare complication of preeclampsia-eclampsia.

•The incidence in pregnancies complicated by the syndrome of hemolysis, elevated liver enzymes, and low platelets is unknown because of the paucity of large series dealing with this subject.

•The development of acute renal failure in such pregnancies was only presented as case reports.

•The obstetrician must be prepared to counsel these women regarding the outcome in this pregnancy, future pregnancies, and any potential long-term effects from acute renal failure or its complications.

•Objective: To describe the maternal-perinatal outcome, subsequent pregnancy outcome, and remote prognosis in 32 women who had this complication.

•Methods: Laboratory evaluation included serial determination of renal function tests, coagulation profile, and liver function tests.

•**Disseminated intravascular coagulation** was defined as the presence of thrombocytopenia (<100 x 10^3/mm^3), low fibrinogen (< 300 mg/dl), positive fibrin split products (≥40 µg/dl), and prolonged prothrombin and partial thromboplastin times.

•Severe **ascites** was defined as the presence of ascitic fluid estimated as >1000 ml at cesarean section, laparotomy, ultrasonography, or computerized tomographic scanning of the abdomen.

•A computed tomographic scan of the abdomen was performed in 11 of these women.

- Management consisted of administration intravenous magnesium sulfate to prevent and control convulsions and bolus doses of hydralazine and nifedipine or continuous infusion of sodium nitroprusside to control severe hypertension.

- Magnesium sulfate was discontinued after diagnosis of acute renal failure.

- Blood and blood products were used as needed to correct coagulation abnormalities.

- Laparotomies were performed in case of intraabdominal bleeding.

- In addition, all patients received careful monitoring of electrolyte and acid-base status, fluid restriction, and special renal diet.

- Ion-exchange resin for hyperkalemia and dialysis were used when appropriate.

- The association of pregnancy with hemolysis, elevated liver enzymes, low platelets, and renal failure is an unusual complication occurring particularly in the postpartum period.

- The incidence of acute renal failure in patients with the syndrome of hemolysis, elevated liver enzymes, and low platelets in this study is 7.3%.

- The majority of patients had derangement of multiple organ systems such as the cardiovascular, pulmonary, and central nervous systems.

- In addition, these pregnancies were associated with multiple obstetric complications such as abruptio placentae, fetal death, disseminated intravascular coagulation, postpartum hemorrhage, and sepsis.

  ° 84% had disseminated intravascular coagulation,

  ° 44% had abruptio placentae,

  ° 44% had pulmonary edema,

  ° 13% had either cardiorespiratory arrest or cerebral injury, and

  ° 6% had ruptured liver hematomas.

- These findings underscore the importance of close observation of patients with this syndrome throughout labor, delivery, and postpartum.

- It also emphasizes the need for referral of such patients to tertiary care centers with appropriate intensive care facilities.

- All patients received various amounts of colloid and crystalloid infusions to correct significant hypovolemia or disseminated intravascular coagulation.

- Five patients required additional surgical procedures to control intraabdominal bleeding.

- 31 of the 32 patients received significant amounts of blood and blood products as therapeutic measures to control the above complications.

- These findings emphasize the importance of these complications and their management as a factor in the development of acute renal failure, pulmonary edema, and ARDS in some of the patients.

- These pregnancies are associated with poor maternal and perinatal outcome.

  ° Four patients (13%) died and 10 (31%) had severe renal failure requiring dialysis.

  ° Only one of the 32 patients studied had **bilateral cortical necrosis**.

Obstetrics and Gynecology: Review 1994-Perinatal Medicine References

°The perinatal mortality was 34% and eight of the 11 perinatal deaths were caused by abruptio placentae.

°72% of the deliveries were preterm, and 31% of the infants were growth retarded.

•The cause of the syndrome of hemolysis, elevated liver enzymes, and low platelets remains uncertain, the prognosis variable, and the therapy speculative.

•As a result, patients with delayed postpartum resolution of the syndrome with renal insufficiency represent a management dilemma.

•There are several ways to treat or reverse the syndrome and its complications including heparin, low-dose aspirin, thromboxane synthetase inhibitors, and prostacyclin infusions.

•Exchange **plasmapheresis** with fresh-frozen plasma has been advocated.

°A progressive elevation of bilirubin or creatinine associated with hemolysis and thrombocytopenia may be an indication for plasmapheresis.

•All patients studied had evidence of progressive microangiopathic anemia, persistent thrombocytopenia, and elevations in creatinine with azotemia.

°Many of them had evidence of multiorgan dysfunction.

•Exchange plasmapheresis was not used in the management of any of these patients.

•All surviving patients with pure preeclampsia had complete resolution of the syndrome by discharge, and all of them had normal renal function within 6 weeks after the acute episode.

°Early initiation of plasmapheresis may result in unnecessary treatment.

•There are minimal data describing subsequent pregnancy outcome and long-term prognosis after the syndrome of hemolysis, elevated liver enzymes, and low platelets and acute renal failure.

•Results: Patients with the syndrome are at increased risk for developing **preeclampsia** in subsequent pregnancies.

•The risks were particularly increased in those women who had preexisting chronic hypertension.

•In these women the risk of having preeclampsia in subsequent pregnancies was 50%, and the risk of perinatal death was 60%.

•One of four women in this group had one subsequent pregnancy complicated by hemolysis, elevated liver enzymes, and low platelets and another complicated by acute renal failure.

•The number of subsequent pregnancies is too small to draw any conclusions.

•Subsequent pregnancy outcome was generally favorable in women **without** preexisting chronic hypertension.

°In such women the risk of having subsequent preeclampsia was 10%, and none of the 10 subsequent pregnancies of more than 20 weeks' duration were complicated by hemolysis, elevated liver enzymes, and low platelets or by renal failure.

°These women should **not** be counseled against future pregnancies for fear of recurrence.

•There are few case reports that describe the long-term effects of the syndrome and acute renal failure on maternal blood pressure or renal function.

•Fact   °Detail   Page 452   »issue   *answer

•All surviving patients without preexisting chronic hypertension had reversible acute tubular necrosis with full recovery.

•The patients were followed up for an average of 4.6 years; none had any evidence of residual renal damage.

•None of these patients had chronic hypertension on follow-up.

•Two of five surviving patients with preexisting chronic hypertension required chronic dialysis on follow-up.

•One other patient had an elevated serum creatinine (1.7 mg/dl) after 1 year of follow-up.

•Conclusions: Pregnancies complicated by the syndrome of hemolysis, elevated liver enzymes, and low platelets and acute renal failure require a well formulated management plan.

•The development of this syndrome is an indication for delivery.

•In view of the high maternal and perinatal complications, such patients should be referred to a tertiary care center where maternal and neonatal intensive care facilities are available.

•Subsequent pregnancy outcome and long-term prognosis are usually favorable in those patients who develop this syndrome in the absence of preexisting chronic hypertension.]

---

8. True statements about pregnancy in a patient who has a successful heart transplant include

   A. birth control pills are the preferred method of contraception.
   B. cyclosporine is teratogenic.
   C. epidural anesthesia is contraindicated.
   *D. the risk to the fetus in the patient who had a cardiomyopathy is between 25% and 50% that the fetus will also have a cardiomyopathy.
   E. the transplacental heart responds to vagal but not catecholamine stimuli.

p.34 (Baxi L V, Rho R B. Pregnancy after cardiac transplantation. Am J Obstet Gynec 1993; 169:33)

8. [F & I: •Background: An increasing number of patients have undergone successful cardiac transplantation with a 1-year survival rate of 85% and a 5-year survival rate of 65%.

•As more cardiac transplant patients attempt to lead normal lives and those women of child-bearing age seek to become pregnant, questions arise regarding the feasibility of pregnancy after cardiac transplantation.

•Patients who have undergone cardiac transplant for cardiomyopathic conditions should be made aware of the risk of recurrence to the fetus of 50% for familial types and 25% for sporadic types.

•Eight successful pregnancies after cardiac transplantation and two after cardiopulmonary transplantation have been reported in the English and French literature.

•One patient, who discontinued her immunosuppressive medication, died of rejection 5 months after delivery.

•The immunosuppressive agents act by inhibiting cellular immunity by lowering the maternal T lymphocyte count and the T4/T8 ratio.

•Cord blood T cell counts and T4/T8 ratios are normal.

•Cyclosporine crosses the placenta and is decreased in cord blood compared with maternal blood.

•In therapeutic doses none of these immunosuppressive agents are teratogenic in humans.

•The transplanted heart is denervated and responds to circulating catecholamines but **not** to vagal stimulus.

•Epidural anesthesia is preferred.

•The patient should be watched for arrhythmia, which may be caused by catecholamines or may be a sign of rejection.

•In addition, these patients are predisposed to atherosclerosis.

•The presence of renal compromise may increase the risk of preeclampsia.

•In the presence of decreased creatinine clearance, the dosage of renally excreted antibiotics should be reduced.

•Cesarean section should be reserved for obstetric indications.

•Contraception should be limited to barrier methods or sterilization.]

---

9. The most sensitive method for detecting antepartum maternal use of cocaine is

*A. amniotic fluid analysis.
B. fetal urine analysis.
C. maternal urine analysis.
D. meconium (from amniocentesis) analysis.
E. fetal hair analysis.

---

p. 787 (Jain L, Meyer W, Moore C, Tebbett I, Gauthier D, Vidyasagar D. Detection of fetal cocaine exposure by analysis of amniotic fluid. Obstet Gynecol 1993; 81:787)

9. [F & I: •Background: Cocaine abuse during pregnancy is associated with an increased incidence of spontaneous abortion, abruptio placentae, stillbirth, prematurity, low birth weight, and abnormal neonatal neurologic development.

•Teratogenic effects of cocaine exposure occur but a consistent pattern of effects when cocaine is used during pregnancy has not been found.

•The failure to identify gestational cocaine abuse may be a serious limiting factor in studies that rely on maternal self-reporting or urine toxicology screens.

•Testing of newborn hair and meconium have been proposed as alternative screening methods.

°These methods are technically difficult and cannot be used when cocaine-related complications are suspected before birth.

•Objective: To assay AF for cocaine and its metabolites and to compare this assay with conventional methods of drug screening.

•The recreational use of cocaine has reached epidemic proportions in the United States.

•Concomitantly, there has been a rise in the number of pregnant women who abuse cocaine.

•Delineation of the risks associated with prenatal cocaine abuse is complicated by inadequate methods of identifying the gestational cocaine abuser and an inability to quantitate the amount of fetal exposure.

•Self-reports are unreliable in identifying and quantifying substance abuse.

- The interval between exposure and sampling and the biologic variability in cocaine degradation affect the sensitivity of screening methods.

- The short half-life of cocaine and its metabolites in urine is a major limiting factor of urine screening for cocaine use.

- There is evidence that cocaine and its metabolites may be concentrated in various body compartments over time.

  ° Radioimmunoassay of newborn hair and gas chromatography-mass spectrometry of meconium were more sensitive than immunoassay of newborn urine in identifying the cocaine-exposed infant.

  ° These methods will only identify infants exposed within the last 12 weeks of pregnancy and are **not** useful in the presence of antepartum complications suspected to be cocaine-related.

- Analysis of AF may be useful when such antepartum complications occur and delivery of the infant is not anticipated.

- The ability of AF analysis to reveal temporal relationships of cocaine use based on history is not known.

- The interval between exposure and delivery varied from less than 1 day to 8 weeks, but could not be objectively confirmed.

- A method of analysis involving solid-phase extraction and high-performance liquid chromatography that is sensitive for the detection of cocaine and benzoylecgonine in AF has been developed.

- When compared to AF analysis, conventional maternal and neonatal urine toxicology screens would have missed 39 and 65%, respectively, of the exposed infants in this study.

- The principle metabolites of cocaine are benzoylecgonine, ecgonine, and ecgonine methyl ester, of which benzoylecgonine is the major urinary metabolite.

- Benzoylecgonine was the only metabolite detected in the body fluids examined.

- Ecgonine and ecgonine methyl esther were not detected because they do not absorb ultraviolet light and could not be detected using high-performance liquid chromatography.

- After acute administration, cocaine is rapidly absorbed and metabolized by plasma and tissue cholinesterases principally to benzoylecgonine.

- Cocaine appears in maternal urine within 2 h of administration, whereas benzoylecgonine appears later (4 to 8 hours) and is eliminated more slowly.

  ° This finding could explain why there was one patient in this study who had positive maternal urine for cocaine but negative AF studies.

  ° This patient, who had acute abdominal pain and vaginal bleeding, claimed use of cocaine immediately before admission to the hospital.

  ° It is also possible that this represents a false-negative AF test.

- The concentration of benzoylecgonine in AF was several times higher than in neonatal urine.

- High levels of benzoylecgonine in AF may be secondary to transplacental transport of maternally formed benzoylecgonine and/or delayed elimination and fetal recirculation.

- After transplacental transfer and metabolism of cocaine by placental and fetal cholinesterases, fetal urinary excretion of benzoylecgonine into the AF may occur.

•The AF may act as a reservoir for benzoylecgonine, and fetal swallowing of AF could lead to recirculation of benzoylecgonine.

•Benzoylecgonine is a more powerful contractile agent than cocaine or norepinephrine.

•It is possible that recirculation of benzoylecgonine could lead to prolonged fetal exposure and may contribute to the observed teratogenic and perinatal complications attributed to prenatal cocaine use.

•Research into the recovery of cocaine and benzoylecgonine from the AF of patients at less than 32 weeks' gestation is needed to clarify fetal metabolism of cocaine.

•The use of solid-phase extraction procedures offers a highly efficient, rapid, reproducible alternative to traditional liquid-liquid extractions for drug testing.

•The results suggest the potential application of AF analysis for determination of gestational cocaine exposure.]

---

10. The major estrogen formed by human fetal membranes is

    A. conjugated estriol.
    B. estradiol.
 *C. estrone.
    D. unconjugated estriol.
    E. All estrogens are produced in about the same amount.

p. 1377 Mitchell B F, Wong S. (Changes in 17ß,20α-hydroxysteroid dehydrogenase activity supporting an increase in the estrogen/progesterone ratio of human fetal membranes at parturition. Am J Obstet Gynec 1993; 168:1377)

10. [F & I: •Background: In most mammalian species estrogen stimulates changes that increase myometrial contractility, whereas progesterone causes myometrial quiescence and the onset of labor is preceded by an increase in the estrogen/progesterone ratio in the maternal circulation.

•These changes occur in species that are dependent on the placenta and in those dependent on the ovary for sex steroid synthesis during pregnancy, suggesting that this may be a common mechanism regulating labor onset in all species.

•The increase in estrogen/progesterone ratio leads to changes that stimulate uterine contractility which include

    °an increase in prostaglandin synthesis,

    °an increased synthesis of myometrial oxytocin receptors, and

    °an increase in myometrial gap junction formation.

• In humans the situation is unknown because measurements of circulating estrogen and progesterone during late pregnancy do not show a significant change in the absolute concentrations or in the ratio of estrogen to progesterone.

•Both estrogen and progesterone are synthesized within human amnion, chorion, and decidua.

•These "fetal membranes" are also the major sites of synthesis of the stimulatory prostaglandins at parturition.

•Local changes in estrogen and progesterone formation, not reflected in the maternal circulation, may significantly influence human parturition.

- The major estrogen formed by human fetal membranes is **estrone**.

- Estrone can be converted within these tissues to the much more active estrogen, estradiol, by the enzyme 17β-hydroxysteroid dehydrogenase.

- Locally synthesized progesterone can be converted within these tissues to the completely inactive metabolite 20α-dihydroprogesterone by the enzyme 20α-hydroxysteroid dehydrogenase.

- A single site on the enzyme 17β,20α-hydroxysteroid dehydrogenase catalyzes both reactions.

  ° An increase in the reductive activity of this enzyme would both "activate" estrone to estradiol and "inactivate" progesterone to 20α-dihydroprogesterone, thus causing a marked increase in the "biologically active" estrogen/progesterone ratio.

- 17β,20α-hydroxysteroid dehydrogenase is an important regulator of stimulation of estrogen receptor activity, which has a major effect on the biologic potency of sex steroids in target tissues.

- Objective: To investigate these enzyme activities with particular attention to changes that occur around the time of parturition.

- Results: Show changes supporting the hypothesis of a local paracrine system within human fetal membranes producing an increase in the estrogen/progesterone ratio of these tissues around the time of labor onset.

- Both chorion and amnion tissues contain 17β,20α-hydroxysteroid dehydrogenase activity to interconvert C18 or C21, steroids. {See diagram of steroid metabolism on p.171.}

- Although the enzyme is reversible, both the kinetic and explant experiments demonstrate that the oxidative activity predominates, favoring formation of the weaker estrogen and the more potent progestogen.

- This suggests that the primary role of the enzyme may be to promote uterine quiescence.

- The data from the explant experiments for both tissues show significant changes in the direction of 17β,20α-hydroxysteroid dehydrogenase activity around the time of labor onset.

- Using the explant culture system to determine the net metabolism of estrogens and progestogens by this enzyme, the reductive activity was increased, leading to an approximate doubling both of the relative formation of the more active estrogen estradiol and the inactive progestogen 20α-dihydroprogesterone.

- This shift in activity would result in a significant increase in the estrogen/progesterone ratio of both chorion and amnion.

- For both substrates in both tissues, these changes in the "activation ratios" were caused by approximately equal contributions from increases in reductive and decreases in oxidative activities.

- The factor(s) leading to these changes around the time of parturition may be an important component of the mechanism regulating myometrial contractility.

- These experiments cannot distinguish whether the changes occurred before or after the onset of labor and thus whether they may be a cause or result of the increase in uterine activity.

- Although formation of the weaker estrogen and stronger progestogen still predominates after spontaneous labor onset, the data suggest a shift occurs, favoring a relative increase in the more active estrogen and a decrease in the more potent progestogen.

- This may be reflected in amniotic fluid, where a significant increase in estradiol and a decrease in progesterone around the time of labor onset occurs.

•A paracrine system within fetal membranes that increases the local estrogen/progesterone ratio at parturition.

•Although the kinetic studies do not reveal major changes in the kinetic parameters of 17,ß20α-hydroxysteroid dehydrogenase activity around the time of labor onset, **in chorion, the most active of the tissues**, the apparent maximal velocity with estradiol as substrate in both microsomes and cytosol was significantly lower after labor than before.

°This suggests that a shift in equilibrium toward production of the more active estrogen (estradiol) occurs around the time of labor onset.

•The data demonstrated the enzyme in both the cytosolic and microsomal subcellular fractions of both chorion and amnion.

•When estrone is used as substrate, the data suggest most of the activity is in the cytosol, although the highest specific activity is in the microsomes.

°In the placenta controversy remains about the subcellular distribution of the enzyme.

•These findings could be compatible with two separate enzymes or with a conformational change in the microenvironment, leading to an increase in the maximal velocity of a single enzyme.

°If the latter explanation is correct, then the regulation of translocation of the enzyme between the cytosol and the microsomal membranes may be an important factor in regulating the enzyme activity.

•Many studies have addressed the regulation of this enzyme in human placental tissue.

•Several C18, C19, and C21 steroids will inhibit the activity of the placental enzyme, usually demonstrating competitive kinetics.

•Whereas prostaglandins of the E and F series cause inhibition of the oxidation of 20α-dihydroprogesterone, the reverse reaction is stimulated by prostaglandin F2α.

°This increase can be blocked by cycloheximide, suggesting it involves synthesis of new enzyme.

°Additionally, cofactor availability may be a determinant of the net activity.

•It is likely that several locally produced factors regulate the velocity and direction of 17ß,20α–hydroxysteroid dehydrogenase.

•The factors that regulate the redox environment of this enzyme in human amnion and chorion and may influence the estrogen/progesterone ratio in these tissues around the time of parturition are not known.

•Abnormalities of the timing of parturition remain a major problem in clinical obstetrics.]

11. Which of the following is particularly effective in protecting the fetus from viral infections?

   A. B-lymphocytes.
 *B. Interferon gamma.
   C. Neutrophils.
   D. T-lymphocytes
   E. Transplacental transfer of maternally derived immunoglobulins.

p. 1445 (Abbas A, Thilaganathan Buggins A G S, Layton D M, Nicolaides K H. Fetal plasma interferon gamma concentration in normal pregnancy. Am J Obstet Gynec 1993; 168:1414)

11. [F & I: •Background: Analysis of lymphocyte subpopulations in fetal blood by means of flow cytometry has shown that natural killer cells are the major circulating leukocyte in the first trimester of pregnancy.

•The function of the natural killer cells is to confer innate immunity on the fetus at a stage of development when cell-mediated and humoral immune responses are immature.

•Interferon gamma (IFN-γ), a lymphokine with proved antiviral activity, has in both in vitro and in vivo studies the ability to substantially increase the cytolytic and secretory activity of natural killer cells.

•Objective: To determine whether plasma IFN-γ is present in the fetal circulation and, if so, whether its concentration is elevated in early pregnancy.

•Results: IFN-γ is present in the fetal circulation from as early as 12 weeks and plasma concentration decreases exponentially with advancing gestation.

•IFN-γ does not cross the placenta and no patient had history or clinical evidence of recent infection; observed alterations with gestation in fetal plasma IFN-γ concentration likely reflect physiologic changes with fetal development.

•Possible sources of IFN-γ in the fetal circulation are T lymphocytes, natural killer cells, monocytes, and tissue macrophages.

•Fetal macrophages are functionally immature, and production of IFN-γ is impaired.

•In early pregnancy, when the fetal plasma IFN-γ is high, the fetal T Lymphocyte and monocyte counts are low.

•The most likely source of fetal plasma IFN-γ is natural killer cells, which are also high in early pregnancy and decrease with advancing gestation.

•An alternative source may be the **placenta**, because tissue culture studies have documented the presence of IFN-γ messenger ribonucleic acid in trophoblasts.

•**A possible role for IFN-γ is protection of the fetus from viral infection.**

•Innate host defense against viral infection, which is the major function of IFN-γ in adults, would be especially important in the fetus in early pregnancy, when there is a sparsity of circulating neutrophils, low levels of both T and B lymphocytes, and poor transplacental transfer of maternally derived immunoglobulins.

•IFN-γ has direct antiviral properties that are are mediated by its effects on cellular metabolism and viral ribonucleic acid expression.

•Additionally, IFN-γ may confer antiviral properties on the fetus by increasing natural killer cell production and cytotoxicity.

•IFN-γ also protects uninfected host cells from natural killer cell cytotoxicity while increasing the sensitivity to lysis of host cells expressing viral antigens.

•Results: Circulating IFN-γ is present in relatively high concentrations in early fetal life.

•This is compatible with the hypothesis that in early fetal development immunity is provided by innate rather than adaptive mechanisms.]

12. The discrepancy in size in pregnancies complicated by twin-twin transfusion syndrome is caused by

    A. disproportionate distribution of maternal uterine blood vessel.
    B. increase blood viscosity in the recipient twin.
    C. increase hematocrit in the recipient twin.
  *D. placental vascular communication.
    E. progressive vascular obliteration of tertiary resistance vessels.

p. 558 (Giles W, Trudinger B, Cook C, Connelly A. Placental microvascular changes in twin pregnancies with abnormal umbilical artery waveforms. Obstet Gynecol 1993; 81:556)

12. [F & I: •Background: Placental microvascular disease is associated with abnormal umbilical artery waveforms in singleton pregnancies and in cases of autosomal trisomy.

•Affected placentas have a reduced number of small arterial vessels in the tertiary stem villi.

•In the ovine model, fetal placental vascular obliteration with microsphere embolization of the umbilical circulation caused the same umbilical Doppler waveform change.

•In the late second to early third trimester, obliteration of 60 to 90% of the small arterial vessels is required before a significant rise in fetal placental blood flow resistance is observed; once this point is reached, the resistance rises sharply.

•The origin of fetal umbilical vascular changes could be primary or in response to a change in the uteroplacental circulation.

•The vessel count may be low because of an obliterative process or because the vessels were never present in the first place.

•In twin pregnancy, the members of a pair may show discordant growth and this may be associated with differences in umbilical Doppler studies.

•The fetuses share the intrauterine environment and the two placentas rely on the same maternal uterine circulation, although they are discrete and implanted in different, though often contiguous, loci.

•If the umbilical placental lesion is due to uteroplacental ischemia, it is unlikely that what has been described as a generalized vascular lesion would be restricted to one placenta.

•There is also disagreement about whether discordant fetal size and the twin-twin transfusion syndrome are associated with discordant umbilical Doppler studies.

•Objective: To determine whether there is a relationship between umbilical artery Doppler waveforms and placental histology in twin pregnancies.

•Results: In twin pregnancy, abnormally increased umbilical Doppler markers of resistance are associated with a significant decrease in the mean number of small arterial vessels present in the tertiary stem villi of the placenta, confirming previously reported results in singleton pregnancy.

•The twin placentas were not similarly affected with the histopathologic vascular lesion.

•Because there were ten sets of unlike-sex twins, it is likely that 20 of the 41 twin pairs were dizygotic (if it is assumed that the dizygotic group contained equal numbers of like and unlike-sex pairs).

•These approximations are consistent with the known chorionicity detected by microscopic assessment of the dividing membranes.

•If the explanation for reduced resistance vessels were failure to develop rather than obliteration, this finding should be similar in both members of a monozygotic pair.

•It can be argued that there were approximately equal monozygotic (21 of 41 pairs) and dizygotic (20 of 41 pairs) twins.

•If the origin of the placental vascular lesion were absence of small arteries during formation of the placenta (i.e., the resistance vessels were never present), then one would expect a disproportionately higher number of twin pairs exhibiting both SGA size and abnormal placental vasculature.

•This was not the case.

•The findings support the hypothesis that progressive vascular obliteration accounts for the depletion of tertiary villi resistance vessels.

•With respect to the question of uteroplacental versus fetal etiology, it appears that the origin of this vascular problem is fetal (i.e., in the fetal placental component).

•If the lesion followed uteroplacental constraint, then such discordancy would be unlikely and both placentas would be expected to be similarly affected.

•The findings are relevant to the problem of twin-twin transfusion syndrome.

•There is usually little difference between the umbilical S/Ds for each twin in cases of twin-twin transfusion.

•There were no major differences in the vessel counts for the two known twin-twin transfusion syndrome cases despite discordancy in birth weights.

•Abnormalities of umbilical Doppler waveforms are primarily associated with a placental vascular lesion, and it is not likely that factors such as high blood viscosity or hematocrit could account for this.

•In twin-twin transfusion syndrome, the size discrepancy results from the hematologic mismatch of the placental vascular communication between the siblings, rather than from any placental microvascular obliteration.]

---

13. In the human fetus, nephrogenesis is complete by

    A. 14 weeks
    B. 20 weeks
    C. 28 weeks
    D. 32 weeks
    *E. 36 weeks

---

p. 562 (Mari G, Kirshon B, Abuhamad A. Fetal renal artery flow velocity waveforms in normal pregnancies and pregnancies complicated by polyhydramnios and oligohydramnios. Obstet Gynecol 1993; 81:560)

13. [F & I: •Background: Following the 20th week of gestation, the amniotic fluid (AF) volume is controlled mainly by the fetus through the processes of urination and swallowing.

•With ultrasound imaging, the fetal renal circulation and fetal urine production can be easily assessed.

•Objective: To test the hypothesis that the fetal kidney plays an important role in the genesis of many cases of polyhydramnios and oligohydramnios, by studying flow velocity waveforms of the fetal renal artery in normal pregnancies and pregnancies complicated by either polyhydramnios or oligohydramnios.

•In the human fetus, nephrogenesis is complete at 35 weeks' gestation.

- Mechanisms regulating the fetal renal blood flow are not known, although prostaglandins produced by the fetal kidney may be involved.

- In fact, in the human fetus, prostaglandin inhibitors decrease urine output without altering renal vascular resistance.

- Results: The fetal renal artery PI decreases with advancing gestation.

[PI = (peak systolic velocity - lowest diastolic velocity)/ average velocity over entire cycle.]

- The changes with advancing gestation, due mainly to a decrease of renal vascular resistance and an increase in renal perfusion if the pressure remains unchanged, are associated with an increased fetal urine output.

- This is probably due to increased renal perfusion.

- As human pregnancy progresses beyond the 20th week, the fetus seems to become the primary source of both AF production and elimination through the processes of urination and swallowing, thereby controlling the volume.

- Although polyhydramnios and oligohydramnios occur for various reasons, the results suggest that in twin gestation, renal perfusion may be involved.

- The twin gestations with polyhydramnios in one sac and oligohydramnios in the other sac represent an optimal model to assess the relationship between fetal renal artery velocimetry and the amount of AF.

- In the twins studied, oligohydramnios could have been a consequence of decreased renal perfusion and decreased urine output; polyhydramnios may have been due to increased renal perfusion and increased urine output.

- The findings are corroborated by those reported in the anemic fetus, which showed a decrease of the renal artery PI soon after intravascular transfusion.

- This observation suggests an increased renal perfusion soon after intravascular transfusion.

- The eight sets of twins investigated may have had twin-twin transfusion syndrome.

- This diagnosis is generally confirmed at birth with demonstration of vascular anastomoses between the circulations and anemia in the growth-retarded twin.

- The pathophysiology of this syndrome is not well understood.

- Dichorionic pregnancies with fetal anemia in one of the twins and no evidence of vascular anastomosis have been observed.

- Eleven therapeutic amniocenteses were performed during this gestation.

- Even though the twins were monochorionic, no evidence of vascular anastomosis was noted between them at birth, and the initial hematocrit was 47% in both twins.

- In another case of twin gestation, the presence of interplacental vascular anastomoses was confirmed at birth; the hematocrit was 46% in both twins.

- In the oligohydramnios-polyhydramnios group, there were three fetal and five neonatal deaths.

- The renal artery PI was abnormal in two twins who died.

- The renal artery PI in the twins studied did not seem to be a good predictor of adverse perinatal outcome.

•Renal tubular sensitivity to vasopressin increases with advancing gestation.

•A higher renal perfusion early in gestation will be associated with a higher urine output, whereas later in gestation, increased renal perfusion can be more easily associated with a lower urine output due to the vasopressin action.

•The etiology of AF reduction differs between growth-retarded fetuses and post-term pregnancies.

•In the former group, the reduction of AF volume appears to be related to Doppler-detectable changes in renal vascular resistance, whereas in the latter group, there appear to be other changes such as an increased capability of tubular reabsorption.

•The group with oligohydramnios included three deaths, and the renal artery PI was abnormal in all three.

»In singleton fetuses, renal blood flow decreases when hypoxemia is prolonged.

•Oligohydramnios in these fetuses is probably a consequence of decreased renal perfusion.

°The worst fetal outcome would be anticipated in those SGA fetuses with abnormal renal artery PI and oligohydramnios.

°Fetal renal perfusion is not the only factor that can influence the AF volume.

°Other factors such as tubular reabsorption may act in the pathogenesis of oligohydramnios and polyhydramnios.]

---

14. At 18 weeks, amniotic bands are identified in an otherwise normal pregnancy. The pregnancy is at risk for

    A. chorioamnionitis.
 *B. low birth weight infant.
    C. oligohydramnios.
    D. posterior placenta.
    E. premature rupture of the membranes.

---

p. 566 (Wehbeh H, Fleisher J, Karimi A, Mathony A, Minkoff H. The relationship between the ultrasonographic diagnosis of innocent amniotic band development and pregnancy outcomes. Obstet Gynecol 1993; 81:565)

14. [F & I: •Background: Ultrasonographic diagnosis of a band within the uterine cavity is uncommon.

•Amniotic sheets or bands have been described as aberrant sheets of tissue, often amnion and chorion, having a free edge within the amniotic fluid.

°They may be associated with "amniotic band syndrome," which presents as a variety of fetal malformations in nonembryonic distribution.

°Bands causing no fetal anomalies or restriction of fetal movements are known as "**innocent amniotic bands**" or "intrauterine shelves."

•Objective: To evaluate the association between the ultrasonographic diagnosis of an innocent amniotic band and pregnancy outcome, obstetric factors or complications, and factors that might predispose to the development of bands.

°An innocent amniotic band is defined as ultrasonographic diagnosis of a band or sheet that did not restrict fetal movement or show any evidence of fetal malformation.

•Amniotic band syndrome, a rare occurrence, results in a variety of fetal malformations.

Obstetrics and Gynecology:Review 1994-Perinatal Medicine References

•Amniotic band syndrome may represent an inherent developmental defect in embryogenesis.

•Some studies have shown that in the presence of normal fetal motion, lack of fetal attachment to the band, and normal fetal anatomy on ultrasonic examination, amniotic band syndrome probably presents little risk of fetal abnormalities.

°Amniotic bands occurring under these circumstances have been labeled "innocent amniotic bands."

•Results: There is an association between the development of innocent amniotic bands and negative pregnancy outcome, specifically preterm delivery and LBW offspring.

•In 11 of the 17 women who underwent repeat ultrasound examination, the amniotic band had disappeared at follow-up.

°The mechanism of this disappearance remains unknown but might be due to rupture or compression of the band by the enlarging fetus.

°The significance of the disappearance of innocent amniotic bands might necessitate early and repeated ultrasonographic examinations.

•The chief limitation of the study is sample size.

•Given this limitation, the study power was calculated in terms of the smallest detectable odds ratio that could be expected among the outcome measures not associated with amniotic band development.

°Using $\alpha = 0.05$ and $1-\beta = 0.80$, the estimated smallest detectable odds ratio ranged from 4.24 for spontaneous abortion to 6.74 for PROM.

•The study was restricted to inner-city Afro-American women.

°Although this group of women is known to be at risk for preterm delivery and LBW, the use of controls matched for race and for institution in which medical service was rendered makes it unlikely that selection bias affected these results.

°In addition, the controls were matched to each case by gestational age at the first sonogram, thus precluding any bias caused by unequal lengths of follow-up.

•Conclusion: The diagnosis of an amniotic band on routine ultrasound examination may be associated with adverse perinatal outcome, specifically preterm delivery and LBW.]

---

15. Which placental abnormality is associated with twin-twin transfusion syndrome?

    A. Battledore placenta.
    B. Bipartite placenta.
    C. Circumvallate placenta.
    D. Placenta succenturiata.
  *E. Velamentous insertion of the cord.

---

p. 574 (Fries M H, Goldstein R B, Kilpatrick S J, Golbus M S, Callen P W, Filly R A. The role of velamentous cord insertion in the etiology of twin-twin transfusion syndrome. Obstet Gynecol 1993; 81:569)

15. [F & I: •Background: Twin-twin transfusion syndrome is a severe complication of monozygotic twinning.

- It arises in diamniotic, monochorionic gestations presumably as the result of arteriovenous anastomoses between the circulation of one twin (the donor) and that of its co-twin (the recipient), leading to a circulatory disequilibrium.

- Although cross-circulation occurs almost universally in monochorionic gestations, these abnormal pregnancies may develop an uncompensated arteriovenous anastomosis.

- As a result of the transfusion, the donor twin becomes growth-retarded and oliguric and develops oligohydramnios, whereas the recipient twin becomes plethoric and polyuric and may demonstrate hydramnios, cardiomegaly, and frank hydrops.

- Historically, the diagnosis of twin-twin transfusion syndrome has been made postnatally, based on intertwin differences in cord blood hemoglobin of 5 g/dL or greater, weight differences of 15% or greater (using the heavier twin as 100%), and pathologic demonstration of transplacental shunting.

  ° Similar differences in cord blood hemoglobin and birth weight were found in both monochorionic and dichorionic twin gestations.

- The sonographic antepartum diagnosis of twin-twin transfusion syndrome has been based on the observation of amniotic fluid (AF) and fetal weight discrepancies in a monochorionic gestation.

- Occasionally, this disparity in sac size may be so great that the oligohydramnic twin is fixed to the uterine wall—a "stuck" twin.

- Withdrawal of a significant volume of AF from the hydramniotic sac may reverse this phenomenon, although the mechanism is not understood.

- Because of the increased incidence of velamentous cord insertions in twin gestations, the abnormal cord insertion may underlie the development of this severe complication of twinning.

- Objective: To evaluate the prevalence of velamentous insertion of the cord in diamniotic-monochorionic and monoamnioticmonochorionic placentas.

- Velamentous or membranous cord insertions are more common in twin than in singleton pregnancies, presumably as a result of the competition for uterine space by the enlarged placentation site.

- The data support this concept but also indicate a significantly **greater** frequency of velamentous insertions in diamniotic-monochorionic pregnancies that show twin-twin transfusion syndrome.

- Twin-twin transfusion syndrome may develop as a consequence of uteroplacental insufficiency affecting the donor twin.

- In this explanation, **increased resistance** in the placental circulation of the donor would lead to greater shunting of blood to the recipient through the common vascular channels.

- In a twin pregnancy complicated by a velamentous cord insertion, compression of the cord by folding or direct pressure on the membranes supporting the cord insertion could obstruct both arterial and venous blood flow, establishing a circuit that potentiates the development of the transfusion syndrome.

- Such a phenomenon is best visualized in cords that insert through the intervening amnion dividing the twins.

- An early disparity could be established in the AF volume of both sacs by vascular shunting from one twin to another.

- If this leads to hypervolemia, polyuria, and mild hydramnios in the recipient twin, the expanding sac could exert hemodynamically significant pressure on the velamentously inserted cord.

- Compression of the cord may impair blood flow to the nonhydramnic fetus.

•This fetus, because of its reduction in blood supply, would be oliguric and growth-retarded.

•More placental blood flow would be shifted through the common vascular channels to the hydramnic twin, which would become progressively more polyuric.

•The continually expanding hydramnios would exert more compressive force on the velamentously inserted cord, further impinging on blood flow to the oligohydramnic fetus and amplifying the hemodynamic disparity.

•The significance of the intervening membrane in the development of severe hydramnios/oligohydramnios is supported by observation of the cases of monoamniotic-monochorionic gestations, which have the same theoretical potential for twin-twin transfusion syndrome as diamniotic-monochorionic gestations.

•In this series, despite a large inter-twin weight difference, significant hydramnios did not occur in the monoamniotic gestations.

•The merit of amniocentesis in twin-twin transfusion syndrome may be prolongation of pregnancy by reduction in the volume of hydramnios, which often leads to preterm labor and delivery.

»The mechanism whereby large-volume amniocentesis causes placental decompression of the oligohydramnic twin is mediated by improvement in blood flow in the velamentously inserted cord after reduction in the size of the compressing hydramnic sac.

°This could only be accomplished effectively by very large and repetitive amniocenteses.

•The data indicate that velamentous cord insertions are significantly more common in monochorionic-diamniotic twin gestations complicated by twin-twin transfusion syndrome than in similar gestations without this syndrome.

•Those patients with the transfusion syndrome and velamentous cord insertions had a poorer outcome, with significantly earlier deliveries.

•The sonographic observation of a velamentous cord insertion in a monochorionic-diamniotic pregnancy with marked inter-sac disparity in AF volume may be a cause for increased perinatal concern and may also predict the response to amniocentesis therapy if this is initiated early enough and in large enough volumes.

•Continued careful pathologic review of the placentas from twin-twin transfusion syndrome pregnancies is critical to establish the true frequency of velamentous insertion in this high-risk condition and the utility of the sonographic observation of this phenomenon.]

16. Short-term ritodrine infusion used for tocolysis raises

    A. serum cholesterol
    B. serum glucagon
*C. serum insulin
    D. serum placental lactogen
    E. serum triglycerides

p. 1280 (Rouse D J, Widness J A, Weiner C P. Effect of intravenous ß-sympathomimetic tocolysis on human fetal serum erythropoietin levels. Am J Obstet Gynec 1993; 168:1278)

16. [F & I: •Background: Erythropoietin is a glycoprotein hormone produced and released in response to hypoxemia.

•Because it does not cross the placenta, umbilical cord blood erythropoietin is of fetal origin.

- Maternal conditions and complications known to be associated with elevated umbilical cord blood erythropoietin include labor, preeclampsia, rhesus isoimmunization, diabetes mellitus, and alcohol abuse.

- The presumed underlying mechanism of the erythropoietin elevation in these human conditions is fetal hypoxemia.

- Induction of hypoxemia in ovine fetuses results in predictable, progressive increases in fetal erythropoietin.

  ° Because the infusion of the ß-sympathomimetic agent ritodrine into ovine fetuses results in fetal hypoxemia, it was hypothesized that ß-sympathomimetic tocolysis would result in increased umbilical cord blood serum erythropoietin concentrations.

- Objective: To determine whether ß-sympathomimetic tocolysis is associated with alteration of fetal serum erythropoietin.

- Results: ß-sympathomimetic tocolysis was associated with increased levels of erythropoietin in fetal serum at delivery.

- Terbutaline and ritodrine are commonly used tocolytic agents structurally similar to epinephrine.

- Because both are relatively selective ß-agonists that are equally efficacious when administered intravenously, the results of patients receiving either were included.

- It was anticipated that ß-sympathomimetic drugs most likely act to increase fetal serum erythropoietin production by one of several mechanisms:

  ° (1) acceleration of maternal or fetal metabolism resulting in decreased tissue oxygenation,

  ° (2) reduction in fetal oxygen delivery as a result of decreased uterine or placental blood flow, or

  ° (3) stimulation of fetal erythropoietin synthesis directly by ß-agonist.

- With respect to the first two possibilities, hypoxemia is a potent stimulus for erythropoietin production.

- Of the three possible mechanisms by which ß-sympathomimetics could act to increase fetal serum erythropoietin levels, the most likely is that ß-sympathomimetics cause various metabolic effects that themselves can result in tissue hypoxia.

- ß-Sympathomimetics have a variety of maternal metabolic effects in human pregnancy.

- The short-term effects of ritodrine infusion on maternal metabolism include raised blood glucose and insulin but not elevated glucagon, triglycerides, cholesterol, placental lactogen, or chorionic gonadotropin.

- Maternal lactate levels are elevated in patients undergoing ritodrine tocolysis.

  ° This suggests that inadequate tissue oxygenation associated with ß-sympathomimetic use.

- Because ritodrine and terbutaline freely cross the human placenta, fetal ß-sympathomimetic levels are comparable to those in the maternal circulation.

- Relative to maternal studies, there are fewer human data on the metabolic effects of ß-sympathomimetics in the fetus.

- The lack of difference of umbilical artery PO_2 observed at delivery is not unexpected because umbilical artery PO_2 is a relatively insensitive indicator of the inadequacy of tissue oxygenation in the presence of the acute effects of labor or superimposed anesthesia.

- The marginally lower umbilical vein PO$_2$ in the group 1 fetuses may have been caused by a type 1 statistical error.

- In addition to the possibility that ß-sympathomimetics act directly to cause metabolic perturbations that result in an increase in serum erythropoietin is the possibility that ß-sympathomimetics induce an increase in serum glucose or insulin that in turn results in hypoxemia:

- In human insulin-dependent pregnancy antepartum glucose control is directly related fetal erythropoietin.

- The larger umbilical venous base deficit and lower umbilical venous PO$_2$ in group 1 compared with group 2 may have been a reflection of decreased uterine blood flow caused by the administration of ß-sympathomimetic drugs closer to the time of delivery.

  ° Alternatively, these laboratory findings could reflect maternal lactic acidemia.

- The third possible mechanism by which ß-sympathomimetics could increase fetal serum erythropoietin levels is direct stimulation of erythropoietin synthesis.

  ° This may be a result of enhanced erythropoietin production by the kidney in nonpregnant animal treated with ß-agonists.

  ° Alternatively, enhanced renal erythropoietin release may result from increased sensitivity of erythropoietin-producing cells to small decrements in oxygen tension as a consequence of ß-agonist administration.

- The data are consistent with the speculation that a ß-sympathomimetic stimulus to erythropoietin production exists that, when withdrawn, results in a fall in serum erythropoietin to basal levels.

- Because the half-life in pregnancy of ß-sympathomimetic ranges from 2.6 to 3.7 h, it is likely that the pharmacologic and metabolic effects of these agents will cease within a few hours after treatment has been stopped.

- Although the half-life of fetal human erythropoietin is unknown, in the neonatal period erythropoietin half-life is 2.6 to 3.7 h.

- The serum erythropoietin levels in group 2 ß-sympathomimetic tocolysis discontinued ≥24 from delivery were comparable to those measured in group 1 and group 2 levels fell after withdrawal of the ß-sympathomimetic stimulus.

- Because magnesium sulfate was administered to such a large proportion of both groups of study patients, its possible role as an explanation for the differences must be considered.

  » The statistically significant difference between the groups in duration of magnesium therapy and the near-significant difference in cessation of magnesium therapy-to-delivery interval are not of physiologic significance.

- Magnesium sulfate may actually increase uterine blood flow.

- Conclusions: There is a temporal relationship between maternal intravenous ß-sympathomimetic administration and fetal serum erythropoietin levels.

- The mechanism(s) of the erythropoietin elevation in the proximately tocolyzed group remains to be elucidated.

- The most attractive hypothesis is that maternal ß-sympathomimetic administration causes fetal hypoxemia, which in turn causes erythropoietin production to rise.

•Because elevations in serum erythropoietin likely reflect fetal hypoxemia, it would seem prudent to use the administration of ß-sympathomimetic tocolytics with caution and to carefully assess fetal well-being while using these agents.]

17. The earliest time that the fetus can respond to tissue hypoxia by increasing erythropoietin production is

- A. 20 weeks
- B. 22 weeks
- C. 24 weeks
- *D. 26 weeks
- E. 28 weeks

p. 618 (Snijders R J M, Abbas A, Melby O, Ireland R M, Nicolaides K H. Fetal plasma erythropoietin concentration in severe growth retardation. Am J Obstet Gynec 1993; 168:615)

17. [F & I: •Background: Antenatal studies involving fetal blood samples obtained by cordocentesis and Doppler investigations have found that in some small-for-gestational-age (SGA) fetuses at least two factors contribute to tissue hypoxia.

•First, there is hypoxemic hypoxia (low blood oxygen content) caused by reduced uteroplacental perfusion and oxygen transport to the fetus.

•Second, ischemic hypoxia occurs in the splanchnic, renal, pulmonary, and musculoskeletal tissues as a result of redistribution in fetal blood flow with preferential shunting to the brain, heart, and adrenals.

•In adult life tissue hypoxia increases renal production of erythropoietin.

•The resulting increase in erythropoietin concentration induces a rise in red blood cell mass by stimulating proliferation, differentiation, and maturation of erythroid precursors.

•During fetal life plasma erythropoietin concentrations increase in response to hypoxia.

•Studies examining umbilical cord blood from human pregnancies at delivery have established that plasma erythropoietin levels are increased in patients where intrauterine hypoxia is suspected.

•In most mammals fetal erythropoietin production occurs in the **liver** with a gradual switch to the **kidney** around the time of birth.

•Hematopoietic maturation and the switch from liver to kidney as the predominant site of erythropoietin production varies in different species.

•Findings from animal studies may not reflect human physiologic conditions.

•Similarly, because response to tissue hypoxia or effects on erythropoiesis may be altered around the time of birth or by the process of delivery itself, findings from postnatal human studies may not reflect antenatal physiologic responses.

•Objective: To determine whether hypoxemia induces an increase in plasma erythropoietin concentration in human fetal life and, if so, whether this response stimulates fetal erythropoiesis.

•Results: In pregnancies complicated by severe intrauterine growth retardation fetal plasma erythropoietin concentration is increased and the degree of increase is significantly associated with the degree of fetal **acidemia**.

•These findings are in keeping with data from postnatal, adult, and animal studies and establish that in human fetal life erythropoietin production in response to tissue hypoxia occurs from at least 26 weeks' gestation.

Obstetrics and Gynecology:Review 1994-Perinatal Medicine References

- There was no significant association between Δ-erythropoietin and Δ-PO_2.

- This implies that the deficit in umbilical venous blood oxygen tension does not provide an accurate prediction of the degree of tissue hypoxia, which is produced by a combination of decreased tissue perfusion and blood oxygen content.

- Umbilical venous acidemia causes a right shift in the hemoglobin-oxygen saturation curve, which for a given PO_2 results in reduced blood oxygen content.

- In the SGA fetuses increased erythropoietin production was associated with erythroblastosis but not with an increase in the number of erythrocytes.

- In normal human fetal life the number of circulating erythroblasts decreases exponentially with gestation, reaching a plateau at 24 to 26 weeks' gestation.

- This decrease coincides with the switch from hepatic to medullary erythropoiesis.

- With liver erythropoiesis erythroblasts enter the peripheral circulation freely, whereas with marrow erythropoiesis the nucleated erythroid precursors are confined to the parenchyma in which hematopoiesis takes place.

- Erythroblastosis in SGA fetuses may be caused by a delay in the switch from hepatic to marrow erythropoiesis.

- Such a developmental delay would not explain the correlation between increased plasma erythropoietin and increased numbers of circulating erythroblasts.

- More plausible explanations for the erythroblastosis of SGA fetuses include erythropoietin-mediated premature release of red blood cells from the bone marrow or recruitment of hepatic erythropoiesis; the data of the current study do not allow distinction between these hypotheses.

- Blood pH is widely accepted as an index of fetal oxygenation.

- The finding that the degree of increase in plasma erythropoietin was more strongly associated with the degree of erythroblastosis than with acidemia suggests that the erythroblast count may provide a better measure of tissue oxygenation.

  ° Supportive evidence is provided by the finding that neonatal asphyxia is more accurately predicted by the presence of erythroblastosis than by low pH in cord blood at delivery.]

---

18. In which condition is there increased monocyte secretion of thromboxane?

    A. pregnancy-induced hypertension
    *B. chronic hypertension in pregnancy
    C. normal nonpregnant state
    D. normal pregnancy
    E. all about the same

---

p. 666 (Hawkins T, Jones M P, Gallery E D M. Secretion of prostanoids by platelets and monocytes in normal and hypertensive pregnancies. Am J Obstet Gynec 1993; 168:661)

18. [F & I: •Background: Pregnancy-induced hypertension (preeclampsia), the most common medical complication of pregnancy, is a multisystem disorder.

- Although much circumstantial evidence is presented for an immunologic cause, direct evidence for such a theory is still lacking.

- Results of in vitro studies of classic measures of cell-mediated immunity are conflicting.

•Fact   °Detail   Page 470   »issue   *answer

- Increased **monocyte procoagulant activity**, which has been found in women with pregnancy-induced hypertension, could be the trigger activating the maternal clotting system.

- Abnormal arachidonic acid metabolism may be significant because of reports of prevention or amelioration by prophylactic therapy with low-dose aspirin.

- An abnormality of this nature could also have its origin in alteration of certain aspects of cell-mediated immunity.

- Circulating immune cells could be implicated in the production of factors that damage or activate endothelial cells (recently described in serum from women with pregnancy-induced hypertension) either directly or by prior stimulation of platelet activation.

- Objective: To examine the function of peripheral blood monocytes and platelets in normal pregnant women and in those with pregnancy-induced hypertension, particularly in relation to their procoagulant propensity.

- Because women with chronic essential hypertension are well-recognized to be at particular risk of having "superimposed preeclampsia," a group of women with chronic hypertension was also included for study.

- Alterations in maternal cell-mediated immunity occur in normal pregnancy.

- These alterations include reduced natural killer cell activity and the elaboration of inhibitors that block interleukin-2 production by specific T cells.

- T-lymphocytes in early pregnancy decidua do **not** express interleukin-2 receptor; whether this is the result of the effect of a local inhibitor or represents an inherent inability to produce interleukin-2 receptor in response to appropriate stimuli (e.g., interleukin-2, interleukin-1, or interferon-γ) is not certain.

- In pregnancy-induced hypertension there are fewer data about the function of immune cells.

- No consistent alteration has been described in mononuclear cell numbers, a relative increase in numbers of peripheral blood monocytes (OKM1-positive cells) in women with preeclampsia has been found.

- Increased procoagulant activity has been found in peripheral blood monocytes from women with preeclampsia; such an abnormality could be the trigger activating the clotting system.

- The results presented here support and extend earlier reports.

- Peripheral blood monocytes from normal women secrete low but measurable amounts of PGI2, and PGE2, and thromboxane, and they respond in vitro to both arachidonic acid and the calcium ionophore A23187 by increases in secretion of some of these substances.

- Basal levels of secretion of these substances were the same in peripheral blood monocytes collected from normal women in the third trimester of pregnancy as in nonpregnant women, and responses to the stimuli arachidonic acid and A23187 were similar.

- Basal PGE2 levels were similar to those of normal pregnancy in pregnant women with either pregnancy-induced hypertension or chronic essential hypertension, as were the responses to arachidonic acid, A23187, or a combination of these two stimuli.

- Prostacyclin, as estimated by assay of its stable endproduct 6-keto-PGF1α, was produced in low but measurable amounts by peripheral blood monocytes from all groups of subjects.

- There were no real differences among the groups in basal levels or in their responses to the stimuli used.

•Basal monocyte thromboxane production was similar in control and normal pregnant subjects; it was significantly increased in women with hypertension whether their hypertension was pregnancy induced or essential in origin, with no further augmentation in response to arachidonic acid or A23187, suggesting prior activation of the monocytes of these subjects.

•This would lead to the expectation that a biologic effect in the direction of vasoconstriction and coagulation, as is seen clinically in pregnancy-induced hypertension; women with chronic essential hypertension are known to be at high risk of having the same clinical abnormalities.

•Whether this heightened reactivity is an inherent feature of monocytes from women who have pregnancy-induced hypertension, or whether it is a response to the pathophysiologic events that result in the clinical disorder cannot be determined from these results.

•Results for platelets show some similarities and some important differences from monocytes in the pattern of thromboxane secretion.

•Basal secretion was markedly increased in those with chronic essential hypertension, with a wide scatter of values and no significant response to the addition of arachidonic acid or A23187.

•Basal levels in platelet supernatants from normal subjects, both pregnant and nonpregnant, were almost undetectable, and intermediate levels were found in the group with pregnancy-induced hypertension.

•In contrast to results for peripheral blood monocytes, there was augmentation seen in response to both arachidonic acid and A23187, alone and in combination in those with pregnancy-induced hypertension.

•Although at first sight the lack of gross elevation in basal thromboxane secretion seems contradictory for a condition characterized by activation of the coagulation system, this finding is in keeping with reports of reduced platelet malondialdehyde production in women with pregnancy-induced hypertension.

•It is possible that earlier in vivo events included increased thromboxane release, causing platelet aggregation, degranulation, and disaggregation.

•Responsiveness to the stimuli used seemed to be enhanced compared with normal pregnant subjects, perhaps indicating continuing increased reactivity in this disorder.

•Prospective study of women destined to have this disorder will clarify this situation.]

---

19. True statements about the prenatal diagnosis of gastroschisis include

    A. About a 20% incidence of trisomy.
  *B. Bowel dilation is a marker of bowel damage.
    C. Elective cesarean section improves outcome.
    D. Etiology of intestinal damage is ischemia.
    E. Intestinal damage most likely occurs during delivery.

---

p. 55 (Langer J C, Khanna J, Caco C, Dykes E H, Nicolaides K H. Prenatal diagnosis of gastroschisis: Development of objective sonographic criteria for predicting outcome. Obstet Gynecol 1993; 81:53)

19. [F & I: •Background: Prognosis for the infant born with gastroschisis depends mainly on the condition of the bowel at birth.

•Many infants have only a mild degree of bowel damage and do well after primary surgical repair.

•A substantial proportion with gastroschisis have more severe intestinal damage, requiring staged repair or resection of necrotic or atretic segments.

- These infants often have severe intestinal hypoperistalsis and poor absorptive capacity and may require prolonged or permanent parenteral nutrition, with its attendant risks of infection, growth retardation, metabolic disturbances, and severe liver disease.

- Routine prenatal screening, using maternal serum alpha-fetoprotein and obstetric sonography, has led to the detection of gastroschisis before birth in many cases.

- Gastroschisis has been identified as early as 12 weeks' gestation and can be readily differentiated from omphalocele.

- Accurate prenatal diagnosis provides an opportunity to alter the mode and timing of delivery to prevent intestinal damage.

- Thus far, **no studies have clearly demonstrated an advantage to routine cesarean delivery for gastroschisis.**

- Three groups have suggested that **preterm delivery** may prevent ongoing damage and improve outcome, although the data have not been convincing.

- The etiology of intestinal damage in gastroschisis is unknown.

- Recent experimental studies in the fetal lamb have suggested the following:

    ° 1) Most of the damage is caused by **constriction** of the bowel at the abdominal wall defect;

    ° 2) maximal damage occurs late in gestation; and

    ° 3) preterm repair partially reverses the damage.

- The mechanism of constriction-induced damage appears to be **mechanical obstruction** rather than ischemia.

- Mechanical obstruction can be identified prenatally by **sonographic evidence of bowel dilatation and bowel wall thickening.**

- Objective: To assess the accuracy of objective sonographic features in predicting outcome for the fetus with gastroschisis.

- Intestinal damage in fetuses with gastroschisis occurs **before** delivery, most likely during the last few weeks of gestation.

- Although there was a significant increase in time to oral feeding in infants who had a bowel diameter of more than 17 mm, the variability of this index made it difficult to use in individual cases.

- This variability also explains the disappointing results in previous small series.

- The combined effect of gestational age and bowel diameter was interesting, generating a threshold line above which 100% of infants had prolonged hypoperistalsis.

- The need for bowel resection in gastroschisis may result from intestinal atresia, necrosis, or both.

- Many cases with early dilatation result from atresia, a condition that is not necessarily associated with a poor outcome.

- This may explain in part the direction of the threshold line, which permits a larger bowel diameter at early gestational ages and implies that **late onset of dilatation may be more concerning than early onset.**

- Preterm delivery may be advantageous for preventing ongoing bowel damage, but it does add the multiple risks of prematurity.

°The two infants born before 34 weeks both had complications that may have been related to premature delivery.

°The risks of prematurity must be weighed against the potential advantages of preterm delivery for infants with gastroschisis.]

20. Clinically useful in evaluating renal function in fetuses with obstructive uropathy, fetal urinary

*A. calcium
B. creatinine
C. osmolality
D. potassium
E. urea

p.177　　(Lipitz S, Ryan G, Samuell C, Haeusler M C H, Robson S C, Dhillon H K, Nicolini U, Rodeck C H. Fetal urine analysis for the assessment of renal function in obstructive uropathy. Am J Obstet Gynec 1993; 168:174)

20. [F & I: •Background: Posterior urethral valves are membranous structures in the posterior urethra that may result in a lower urinary tract obstructive uropathy.

•Male fetuses are affected almost exclusively.

•Some of these fetuses are candidates for in utero vesicoamniotic shunting.

•The success rate of prenatal treatment depends primarily on good case selection.

•Once other anomalies have been excluded, the degree of renal damage that has already occurred is the major determinant of outcome.

•The prenatal assessment of renal reserve becomes a critical factor in providing realistic counseling for these parents and particularly in the selection of fetuses for in utero treatment.

•At present the two most acceptable methods of assessing fetal renal function are

°(1) the ultrasonographic evaluation of fetal renal parenchyma and volume of amniotic fluid and

°(2) electrolyte determination in fetal urine.

•Both methods have false-positive and false-negative results and are far from satisfactory.

•Newer methods include the measurement of low-molecular-weight plasma proteins (e.g., ß2-microglobulin and microalbumin) and kidney-derived enzymes (e.g., N-acetyl-ß-D-glucosaminidase).

•Urinary ß2-microglobulin in particular may be important in the assessment of fetal renal function.

•ß2-Microglobulin is a low-molecular-weight protein that is filtered freely by the glomeruli; under normal circumstances >99.9% is resorbed and metabolized in the proximal tubules.

•In renal disease in which there is damage to this segment of the nephron, increased quantities of ß2-microglobulin are excreted in the urine.

•The fetus with renal damage acts as a "salt loser", and the urinary electrolyte concentrations, osmolality, and ß2-microglobulin are elevated.

•Objective: To determine the value of several of these indexes, including ß2-microglobulin, N-acetyl-ß-D-glucosaminidase, and microalbumin, in the assessment of prenatal renal function in cases of posterior urethral valve and their potential role in the selection of such cases for in utero shunting.

- Methods: The 25 fetuses were divided into four groups according to the pregnancy outcome.

- Group A consisted of nine fetuses who underwent termination of pregnancy or had intrauterine fetal death; in all nine the diagnosis of posterior urethral valve was confirmed at the postmortem examination and dysplastic kidneys were found on histologic examination.

- Group B comprised seven fetuses who died postnatally; in all seven the postmortem examination confirmed the diagnosis of posterior urethral valve and the histologic diagnosis of renal dysplasia.

  ° In five of the seven, pulmonary hypoplasia was the primary cause of death and was a contributing cause in the other two.

- Group C consisted of seven live neonates in whom the diagnosis of posterior urethral valve was confirmed clinically (by micturating cystourethrogram) and who had some degree of renal damage as defined by their glomerular filtration rate (greater than expected for their age and weight), serum creatinine level (>70 mmol/l after the first week of life), dimercaptosuccinic acid scan result (< 40% differential function and decreased uptake), and need for peritoneal dialysis.

- Group D comprised two neonates in whom the diagnosis of posterior urethral valve was confirmed clinically and who had normal renal function.

- Early or prolonged lower urinary tract obstruction leads to renal damage, mainly in the region of the tubules.

- This impairs the ability of the kidney to resorb certain electrolytes and results in the production of hypertonic urine.

- Fetal urine can be easily aspirated under ultrasonographic guidance to measure various indexes of renal function.

- Substances that have been suggested, include Na^+, Ca^{++}, osmolality, urea, creatinine, and ß2-microglobulin.

- Na^+ and Ca^{++} are the best predictors taking gestational age into account when interpreting the Na^+ results.

- Results: The Na^+ and Ca^{++} levels were significantly higher in all fetuses who died as neonates than in the survivors where they were generally within the normal range.

- This discrimination is good mainly for survival, because seven of the nine survivors had some degree of renal impairment.

- **ß2-microglobulin may be a particularly helpful indicator in that it is a more sensitive marker of renal function than most urinary electrolytes; it is independent of gestational age.**

- Only fetuses in group D had ß2-microglobulin values close to a normal range, while all fetuses in group C had levels that were considerably higher.

- There was a significant difference in the values between groups B and C and, excepting one fetus, all fetuses with levels >13 mg/l died as neonates.

- The fetuses in group C had values well above the normal range.

  ° All of these infants are alive with some degree of renal compromise.

  ° This suggests that the normal range needs to be further clarified, particularly with respect to gestation, and also that values of ≤13 mg/l are compatible with survival.

- Correction of ß2-microglobulin values for urinary creatinine did not improve its predictive ability.

•In children and fetuses other markers such as N-acetyl-ß-D-glucosaminidase and microalbumin may be sensitive indicators of renal function.

•Apart from the finding that both fetuses in group D had N-acetyl-ß-D-glucosaminidase levels well below the rest, no other correlation between these levels and the eventual outcome of the pregnancies was found.

°At present there are no normal ranges established for N-acetyl-ß-D-glucosaminidase or microalbumin in fetuses.

•Although the numbers were small in each group, there was no obvious benefit to those fetuses who were shunted.

•ß2-Microglobulin is not a readily available assay in most units because it is both expensive and time consuming.

°It is a useful adjunct to the estimation of Na^+ and Ca^{++}.

°It may help to distinguish those fetuses who would survive with some degree of renal dysfunction from those who would die as neonates.

°This information would be of great help in counseling parents and in the selection of cases for in utero treatment.

°6 of 9 fetuses in group A had ß2-microglobulin >1.5 but <13 mg/l; these may have been the fetuses who would have survived, although with some degree of renal dysplasia.]

---

21. Increased thromboxane in the pathogenesis of preeclampsia in the diabetic patient is generated by

   A. kidney
   B. liver
   C. lung
   D. placenta
   *E. platelets

---

p. 86 (Van Assche F A, Spitz B, Hanssens M, Van Geet C, Arnout J, Vermylen J. Increased thromboxane formation in diabetic pregnancy as a possible contributor to preeclampsia. Am J Obstet Gynec 1993; 168:84)

21. [F & I: •Background: Pregnant diabetics have an increased incidence of preeclampsia.

•Preeclampsia was found in 9.9% of diabetic pregnancies compared with 4.3% in controls.

•The decision of how to diagnose preeclampsia in these women is a difficult one.

•Objectives: To measure the urinary metabolites of TXA2, in pregnant women with type I diabetes without clinical vascular complications at assay and to test the hypothesis that a higher TXA2 production contributes to the increased incidence of preeclampsia in pregnant women with diabetics.

•Results: Pregnant women with type I diabetes without clinical vascular complications have **higher** levels of TXA2 metabolites in the urine as compared with levels in control primigravid women.

•Seven women >6 months after delivery had the same level of 11 dehydro-TXB2 in the urine as nine control women.

°Platelets of diabetic patients have an increased capacity to produce TXA2.

•TXA2 biosynthesis is higher in normal pregnant women than in nonpregnant subjects, largely as a result of platelet activation.

•In normal primigravid women, urinary excretion of 2,3-dinor-TXB2 is also about twice as high as what was previously found in normal adult men.

•The increased capacity of platelets of diabetics to produce TXA2 together with the "physiologic" platelet activation of pregnancy could explain the high levels of urinary TXA. metabolites in pregnant diabetic women.

•Endothelial factors can precede vascular complications in the nonpregnant and in the pregnant diabetic state.

•Nonpregnant type I diabetic patients have an increased vasopressor responsiveness to angiotensin II.

•Primigravid women with absence of angiotensin II refractoriness, a known risk factor for preeclampsia, also have a significantly higher urinary excretion of 2,3-dinor-TXB2.

•Increased systemic production of TXA2 during pregnancy seems to be a predictor of preeclampsia.

•These findings help explain why preeclampsia is more frequent in diabetic pregnancy.

•This study confirms the role of an increased TXA2 formation in the pathogenesis of preeclampsia.

•Because treatment with low-dose aspirin provides protection against preeclampsia, it could be of interest to investigate further if prophylactic suppression of TXA2 synthesis could be useful in diabetic pregnancies.]

---

22. A fetus at risk for developing distress is being evaluated sonographically three times a week. At 28 weeks, end diastolic velocity is noted to be absent. The most powerful predictor of the time interval between the absence of end diastolic velocity and the need for delivery is

    A. change in amniotic fluid volume
    B. decrease in middle cerebral artery pulsatility index
 *C. gestational age
    D. severity of intrauterine growth retardation
    E. umbilical artery pulsatility index

---

p. 48 (Arduini D, Rizzo G, Romanini. The development of abnormal heart rate patterns after absent end-diastolic velocity in umbilical artery: Analysis of risk factors. Am J Obstet Gynec 1993; 168:43)

22. [F & I: •Background: Doppler ultrasonography is used to study umbilical artery velocity waveforms as a reflection of placental vascular resistance.

•Qualitative changes in indices of flow and perinatal complications may be associated.

•The **absence of end-diastolic velocity** is the finding with the greatest clinical interest, and it is frequently associated with fetal hypoxemia, acidemia, and poor perinatal outcome.

•There is no assessment on the time interval elapsing between the occurrence of absent end-diastolic velocity and evidence of abnormal heart rate patterns requiring early delivery.

•The interval between these two events may range from 0 day to 7 weeks.

•The variable length of this interval may have resulted from fetuses already with absent end-diastolic velocity at the first recording, thus not allowing a proper timing of the onset.

•Objectives: To report experience on 37 fetuses in which a shift from presence to absence of end-diastolic velocity in the umbilical artery was evidenced by serial Doppler recordings.

- To determine the factors related to the length of the interval between the onset of absent end-diastolic velocity in the umbilical artery and delivery, which may prove useful in predicting the occurrence of abnormal heart rate tracings.

- Although absent end-diastolic velocity in umbilical artery may be secondary to structural or chromosomal anomalies and uteroplacental insufficiency, both the criteria of selection and pregnancy outcome strongly point to the latter explanation.

- These fetuses were came from a population of high-risk fetuses with abnormal Doppler findings suggestive of the presence of the brain-sparing effect (i.e., increased umbilical artery vascular resistance associated with decreased middle cerebral artery vascular resistance) and subsequently developing absent end-diastolic velocity.

- Absent end-diastolic velocity may occur at a stage of uteroplacental insufficiency after the Doppler-detectable brain-sparing effect.

- Absent end-diastolic velocity usually precedes the onset of abnormal heart rate patterns in such fetuses.

- The duration of this time interval differs considerably among fetuses, and occasionally late decelerations appear close in time to the development of absent end-diastolic velocity.

- The longitudinal design allowed accurately dating the onset of absent end-diastolic velocity (with a maximum inaccuracy of 3 days), thus allowing evaluation of factors that may identify subsets of fetuses with a different likelihood of developing fetal distress.

- Stratifying patients according to gestational age at diagnosis of absent end-diastolic velocity, presence or absence of hypertensive diseases, and presence or absence of pulsations allowed identification of pregnancies whose risk of developing fetal distress was higher and closer to the first occurrence of absent end-diastolic velocity.

- **Gestational age** proved to be the most powerful predictor of the duration of the time interval between absent end-diastolic velocity and delivery, with longer time intervals in early gestation than in later pregnancy.

- The reasons for this difference are unknown.

- A possible explanation might be that smaller fetuses have lower nutritional and oxygen requirements, allowing them to develop a longer metabolic adaptation at absent end-diastolic velocity in umbilical artery before the development of hypoxemia and acidemia, causing abnormal heart patterns.

  ° Different explanations as a sensibility of fetal chemoreceptors varying with gestational age cannot be excluded.

  ° The presence of maternal hypertensive complications affected the duration of the time interval irrespective of the gestational age.

  ° This might be caused by a quicker deterioration of placental function in the presence of hypertension or by the effect of maternal hypertensive treatments on fetal circulation.

  ° The latter hypothesis is unlikely, because the drugs used (nifedipine and hydralazine) seem to minimally affect fetal hemodynamics.

- The presence of **pulsations in umbilical vein** was significantly related to the occurrence of abnormal heart rate patterns independent of gestational age and hypertension.

- The significance of umbilical vein pulsations in the human fetus is still unknown, but it may be that they are an expression of cardiac decompensation leading to abnormal heart filling and resulting in increased reverse flow during atrial contraction in the inferior vena cava.

•The abnormal reversal of the venous blood velocities would then extend beyond the ductus venosus into the umbilical vein causing these pulsations.

•The data support this hypothesis by showing significant relationship between the peak velocity in aorta and pulmonary artery, the percent reverse flow in inferior vena cava and umbilical vein pulsations.

•All these changes may be expressions of the same phenomenon because their simultaneous assessment in the multivariate analysis did not improve the significance in determining the duration of the time interval.

•Namely, all these findings may represent a deterioration of cardiac function, leading to a decrease of peak velocities at the outflow levels and an increase of reverse flow in inferior vena cava and umbilical vein pulsations.

•As a consequence of these central abnormal flow patterns, the return of blood from the placenta to the heart might be impaired, further reducing the supply of oxygen and nutrients in these fetuses and thus explaining the onset of abnormal heart rate patterns.

•The lower umbilical artery pH at birth and the higher perinatal mortality found in fetuses with pulsations further validate this concept.

•Finally, the absence of significant correlations between the other Doppler and ultrasonographic indices investigated and the occurrence of fetal distress suggests a limitation of these measurements in the longitudinal monitoring of fetuses with absent end-diastolic velocity in umbilical artery.]

---

23. Which of the following maternal-fetal HLA relationships is associated with pregnancy-induced hypertension?

   *A. Fetus does not have the HLA-DR antigens allogeneic to its mother.
   B. Mother does not have the HLA-DR antigens allogeneic to her fetus.
   C. Neither the fetus nor the mother have allogeneic antigens to each other.
   D. The fetus and the mother both have allogeneic antigens to each other.
   E. none of the above

---

p. 1011   (Hoff C, Peevy K, Giattina K, Spinnato J A, Peterson R D A. Maternal-Fetal HLA-DR relationships and pregnancy-induced hypertension. Obstet Gynecol 1992; 80:1007)

23. [F & I: •Background: Women with pregnancy-induced hypertension (preeclampsia or eclampsia) often have immunologic and vascular changes that may result from a dysfunctional maternal immune response to fetal or trophoblastic factors.

•Lower plasma levels of antipaternal antibody have been found in women with pregnancy-induced hypertension compared with normotensive controls.

•Women with pregnancy-induced hypertension have reduced in vitro lymphocyte activity, lower plasma levels of T lymphocytes, higher plasma levels of immune complexes and complement, and elevated deposits of immune complexes and immunoglobulins (Igs) in renal glomerular and placental vessels.

•The immune complex deposits, lymphocyte infiltrations, and placental vascular changes associated with pregnancy-induced hypertension are similar to those found in rejected renal allografts.

•Increased parental and maternal-fetal HLA sharing is associated with a higher prevalence of pregnancy-induced hypertension.

•This finding is consistent with the hypothesis that fetal homozygosity for recessive genes linked to HLA loci influences the development of pregnancy-induced hypertension.

- Women receiving blood transfusions before pregnancy have a lower prevalence of pregnancy-induced hypertension.

- Together, these findings suggest that a **lack of HLA allosensitization** may increase the risk for pregnancy-induced hypertension.

- The prevalence of pregnancy-induced hypertension was found to be **higher** among nonconsanguineous marriages in an inbred Turkish population, women changing spouses, and women impregnated by men from a different racial group.

- An increased prevalence of pregnancy-induced hypertension has also been found among women with the HLA-DR4 and the A30 and DR5 antigens, suggesting the existence of susceptibility genes in linkage disequilibrium with these HLA alleles.

- Objectives: To examine the direction of maternal-fetal HLA relationships to clarify their risk for pregnancy-induced hypertension.

- In particular, to determine whether the potential for maternal HLA allosensitization (the fetus has HLA antigens allogeneic to its mother) decreases the risk for pregnancy-induced hypertension, whereas lack of HLA allosensitization (mother and fetus share HLA antigens) increases this risk.

- Results: The lower prevalence of pregnancy-induced hypertension in women with the HLA-DR4 antigen was not significant in contingency-X^2 analysis and only marginally significant in multiple logistic regression analysis.

- HLA homozygosity at the four loci was not significantly associated with pregnancy-induced hypertension in either contingency-X^2 or multiple logistic regression analysis.

- These findings tend to contradict the existence of recessive genes closely linked to the HLA complex which increase the risk for pregnancy-induced hypertension.

- The existence of non-HLA-linked recessive genes influencing pregnancy-induced hypertension is still a distinct possibility.

- When associations were examined between maternal-fetal HLA relationships and pregnancy-induced hypertension, risk was significantly increased when the fetus did not have HLA-DR antigens allogeneic to its mother, but the mother had an HLA-DR antigen allogeneic to her fetus (maternal allogenicity).

- Otherwise, no differences in risk were observed for the other three types of maternal-fetal HLA-DR relationships.

- The manner in which maternal-fetal relationships were categorized is based on evidence in humans that when allogenicity exists, either mother or fetus, or both, can be exposed to each other's alloantigens.

- Especially relevant to the findings is evidence that maternal alloantigens (e.g., HLA, Gm, and Km) can gain access to the fetal circulation, resulting in fetal tolerization or allosensitization.

- This raises the question of how such an occurrence could lead to the development of pregnancy-induced hypertension and associated placental pathology.

- Although this model is not proven, it is based on published findings.

- The model assumes the existence of maternal allogenicity and the following events:

    ° 1) Maternal HLA-DR allosensitization does **not** occur; maternal B and T-cell immunosuppressive networks at the maternal-fetal interface that are potentially activated by HLA allosensitization are not initiated.

°°This is reflected in lowered peripheral blood levels of antipaternal antibody and decreased signs of cell-mediated activation compared with the majority of pregnancies, in which maternal allosensitization by fetal HLA-DR alloantigens is a more common occurrence.

°°In the women who are not allosensitized, the potential for a local maternal cytotoxic immune response against fetal and trophoblast non-HLA antigens is not suppressed and remains wholly intact.

°2) Maternal HLA-DR alloantigens cross the placenta after the fetus has developed self/nonself and immune competence; the fetus becomes allosensitized to these antigens.

°3) Fetal anti-maternal HLA IgG antibody is produced and crosses the placenta in the reverse direction.

°°The fetal IgG carries Gm, Km, or other allotypic markers of paternal origin that are allogeneic to the mother.

°4) The mother mounts a humoral response against the fetal alloantibody at the maternal-fetal interface.

°°The maternal humoral response results in increased production of immune complexes and complement, and some of these pass into the general maternal circulation.

°°At the maternal-fetal interface, this reaction causes increased amounts of immune-complex depositions and damage to the placental vasculature.

°°These and other pathologic events triggered by the maternal response to allotypic fetal antibody contribute to the development of pregnancy-induced hypertension.

•To summarize, the findings and hypothetical model are consistent with the hypothesis that a lack of maternal HLA sensitization to fetal HLA-DR alloantigens increases the risk for pregnancy-induced hypertension.

°Specifically, the findings imply that when maternal allosensitization cannot occur, risk is increased when the fetus is potentially sensitized to maternal HLA-DR alloantigens at the same time.

°The reason these findings have not been observed in previous studies may involve either a focus on parental HLA sharing or a failure to examine the direction of maternal-fetal HLA relationships.]

---

24. A 30-year old patient has a maternal serum alpha-fetoprotein at 16 weeks reported as 6 multiples of the median. Amniotic fluid alpha-fetoprotein is reported is reported as 15 multiples of the median and acetylcholine determination is within normal limits. Ultrasound evaluation of the fetus reveals no abnormalities. The next best step in the management of this patient is

   A. culture the amniotic fluid for acid-fast bacilli
   B. obtain alpha-fetoprotein for karyotype
   *C. offer mother termination of pregnancy
   D. repeat amniotic fluid alpha-fetoprotein in two weeks
   E. repeat ultrasound in two weeks

---

p. 1332   (Hogge W A, Hogge J S, Schnatterly P T, Sun C J. Blitzer M G. Congenital nephrosis: Detection of index cases through maternal serum α-fetoprotein screening. Am J Obstet Gynec 1992; 167:1330)

24. [F & I: •Background: Congenital nephrosis is an uncommon disorder in non-Finnish populations with an incidence of approximately 1 in 40,000.

•In spite of this relative rarity, antenatally four cases of congenital nephrosis have been detected during the last 4 years of the maternal serum α-fetoprotein (AFP) screening programs.

•Congenital nephrosis of the Finnish type is a rare, autosomal recessive disorder, and most reports of prenatal detection have followed the birth of an index case.

•Because of widespread screening of pregnancies with maternal serum AFP, most fetuses with congenital nephrosis should be detected.

•In these four cases the range was from 6 to 16 multiples of the median.

•The majority of cases would be found if an amniotic fluid AFP level of ≥10.0 multiples of the median (with a normal acetylcholinesterase value) was chosen as the diagnostic criterion.

•Because the correlation between maternal serum AFP levels and AFP levels in the amniotic fluid is poor, it would appear that all patients with an unexplained maternal serum AFP level of ≥5.0 multiples of the median should have amniotic fluid studies if a high rate of detection is to be achieved.

•Although congenital nephrosis is associated with a severe, diffuse proteinuria in the neonate, measurement of other protein constituents of amniotic fluid was not helpful for confirmation of the diagnosis.

•Children with congenital nephrosis have a very poor prognosis, in spite of the availability of renal transplantation.

•AFP studies offer the possibility of prenatal diagnosis in the index case, offering the family the option of pregnancy termination, if desired.

•In cases of elevated maternal serum AFP with unexplained and marked elevations of amniotic fluid AFP levels and normal acetylcholinesterase levels, the diagnosis of congenital nephrosis must be considered, regardless of ethnic origin.]

---

25. The main site of erythropoietin in the fetus is

    A. bone marrow
    B. kidney
    *C. liver
    D. lung
    E. spleen

---

p. 1295 (Thilaganathan B, Salvesen D R, Abbas A, Ireland R M, Nicolaides K H. Fetal plasma erythropoietin concentration in red blood cell-isoimmunized pregnancies. Am J Obstet Gynec 1992; 167:1292)

25. [F & I: •Background: In red blood-isoimmunized pregnancies fetal anemia results from antibody-coated red blood cell destruction in the fetal reticuloendothelial system.

•In severe anemia there is fetal macrocytosis and erythroblastosis, which are a consequence of extramedullary hematopoiesis.

•In mild to moderate anemia the increased fetal cardiac output and hyperdynamic circulation prevent tissue hypoxia, release of erythropoietin, and therefore increased hematopoiesis.

•Erythropoietin may also be produced with small hemoglobin deficits, but recruitment of extramedullary erythropoiesis occurs only when a particular threshold is reached.

•Objective: To investigate the relationship between fetal anemia, erythropoietin concentration, and erythroblastosis in red blood cell-isoimmunized pregnancies.

•The human fetus is capable of responding to anemic hypoxia by increasing erythropoietin production from at least 20 weeks' gestation, but this response does not occur until the hemoglobin deficit is >7 gm/dl.

•In fetal life the erythropoietin response to anemic hypoxia may be suppressed because of reduced fetal oxygen requirement, decreased hepatic responsiveness to hypoxia, the presence of other unspecified erythrogenic factors. or an erythropoietin inhibitory substance.

•The finding that the mean erythropoietin concentration only exceeds the normal range when the anemia is severe suggests that in mild to moderate anemia oxygenation of the liver, which is the main site of erythropoietin production in the fetus, is maintained.

•This may be a consequence of the increased cardiac output and peripheral perfusion.

•When the hemoglobin deficit is >7 gm/dl compensatory cardiovascular adjustments are not sufficient to prevent tissue hypoxia.

•Similar to findings in anemic fetuses, some growth-retarded fetuses have an increased fetal plasma erythropoietin concentration with reduced venous blood pH and increased erythroblast count.

•In these cases tissue hypoxia presumably results from a combination of hypoxemic hypoxia, caused by reduced uteroplacental perfusion and oxygen transfer, and ischemic hypoxia, caused by redistribution of fetal blood to the brain at the expense of the viscera.

•Blood pH is widely accepted as an index of fetal oxygenation.

•Although in both the anemic and hypoxic-ischemic hypoxia models of human fetal hypoxia an increase in erythropoietin was associated with acidemia and erythroblastosis, better prediction of erythropoietin concentration was obtained from the degree of erythroblastosis.

•Impaired fetal oxygenation may be more accurately predicted by the presence of erythroblastosis than by a low blood pH.]

---

26. At 30 weeks a fetus is noted to have nonimmune hydrops. Umbilical venous pressure is normal. The LEAST likely cause of the condition is

   *A. fetal tachyarrhythmia
    B. hypoalbuminemia.
    C. parovirus infection.
    D. tetralogy of Fallot.
    E. viral myocarditis.

---

p. 822 (Weiner C P. Umbilical pressure measurement in the evaluation of nonimmune hydrops fetalis. Am J Obstet Gynec 1993; 168:817)

26. [F & I: •Background: Nonimmune hydrops fetalis is a diagnostic and therapeutic challenge with a perinatal risk of morbidity and mortality in excess of 50%.

•The list of abnormalities associated with this disorder is lengthy.

•Unfortunately, the direct mechanism by which many of these abnormalities might cause hydrops is obscure.

•Some abnormalities associated with nonimmune hydrops fetalis are not the actual cause but rather are linked to another unrecognized problem that causes the hydrops.

•Cardiac malformations are among the most common causes because they are often found in hydropic fetuses.

°Cardiac malformations are one of the most common birth defects and only seldom are associated with nonimmune hydrops fetalis.

°The presence of a heart defect does not prove that the hydrops results from heart failure.

•There are at least three pathophysiologic mechanisms that might produce hydrops.

°The first possible mechanism is **inadequate cardiac output** as a secondary effect of either obstructed or diverted outflow, inadequate blood return, inadequate ventricular filling, or inadequate ionotropic force.

°°Indirect, noninvasive findings consistent with heart failure in some fetuses with nonimmune hydrops fetalis include regurgitant blood flow across one or both atrioventricular valves or venous flow reversal in the inferior vena cava.

°°Direct evidence has been lacking.

°°Inadequate cardiac output causing heart failure would increase the fetal central venous pressure as it does postnatally.

°°In the absence of cord or hepatic distortion, the umbilical venous pressure corrected for the amniotic fluid pressure may be thought of as a surrogate for the central venous pressure.

°°A fetus with nonimmune hydrops fetalis in association with heart failure will have an **elevated umbilical venous pressure**.

°The second possible direct mechanism for hydrops is a **lymphatic malformation** such as that found in association with cystic hygroma, Noonan's syndrome, pulmonary or peritoneal lymphangiectasia, or a lymphatic-venous anastomosis.

°°The **umbilical venous pressure will be normal** in these instances unless the collection of lymph interferes with cardiac return.

°The third possible direct mechanism for hydrops is **liver or peritoneal disease** causing an exudative ascites or hypoproteinemia, such as might result from overwhelming viral hepatitis or peritonitis.

•Objective: To examine the hypothesis that by measuring umbilical venous pressure nonimmune hydrops fetalis of cardiac origin could be distinguished from that of noncardiac origin.

•Increased umbilical venous pressure probably results from either an intracardiac or extracardiac process that has interfered with either cardiac return or output.

•If the hypothesis is true, effective therapy for nonimmune hydrops fetalis of cardiac origin should be associated with a reduction in the umbilical venous pressure.

•This is the first report where the measurement of the umbilical venous pressure was applied to the diagnosis and treatment of nonimmune hydrops fetalis.

•When elevated umbilical venous pressure normalized with therapy producing a reversal of hydrops substantiates the conclusion that inadequate cardiac output was the direct mechanism for hydrops in two thirds of the fetuses studied.

•There were several common causes of inadequate cardiac output.

•The least controversial was the cardiac arrhythmia where the production of hydrops and its resolution with correction of the arrhythmia are well documented.

Obstetrics and Gynecology: Review 1994-Perinatal Medicine References

- Evaluation of several nonhydropic fetuses with either a tachyarrhythmia or a bradyarrhythmia found that none had an elevated umbilical venous pressure.

- In the pregnancy presented where the hydrops was associated with a large pericardial effusion, probably the result of a viral infection, arterial puncture allowed documentation of a very low umbilical arterial pressure consistent with cardiac tamponade.

- Severe anemia in association with either human parvovirus, massive fetal-to-maternal transfusion, or immune hemolysis was also associated with an elevated umbilical venous pressure.

    ° Correction of the anemia led to normalization of the umbilical venous pressure and prompt resolution of the hydrops.

    ° This finding is consistent with high-output failure, where myocardial dysfunction is a secondary effect of hypoxemia.

- In the instance of fetal hemolytic anemia the umbilical venous pressure corrects far too rapidly for the immune hydrops to be explained solely by hepatomegaly and portal vein obstruction.

- In the three fetuses with nonimmune hydrops fetalis secondarily to twin-to-twin transfusion syndrome, heart failure developed because of polycythemia and hyperviscosity.

    ° A decrease in hematocrit while total protein concentration was maintained led to the resolution of the hydrops.

    ° Partial exchange transfusion is standard postnatal therapy.

- The four fetuses without hydrops but with a major cardiac defect and the one fetus with noncardiac hydrops and a ventricular septal defect demonstrate that the simple **presence of a heart malformation does not mean it is the cause of the hydrops**.

- Thoracic abnormalities were also commonly associated with nonimmune hydrops fetalis.

- Mediastinal deviation presumably decreased cardiac return, causing low-output failure.

- When the deviation was a secondary effect of a fluid-filled mass, aspiration allowed the mediastinum to shift to a more normal position, and the umbilical venous pressure promptly declined and the hydrops resolved if the drainage was maintained.

    ° If the fluid reaccumulated or the thoracoamniotic shunt was either dislodged or obstructed, the hydrops returned.

- A low umbilical arterial pressure was also observed in one fetus with nonimmune hydrops fetalis associated with a hydrothorax.

    ° This too was presumably corrected because the umbilical venous pressure was normal after drainage.

- These observations are clinically relevant.

- **Hydrothoraces most commonly occur during the late second to early third trimester** when the human lung has already adequately differentiated to support life.

- Thus the risk of a hypoplastic lung caused by compression at this stage of gestation is low.

    ° Hydrothoraces may be drained by the placement of a thoracoamniotic shunt.

- The measurement of umbilical venous pressure will enhance selection.

- If the hydrothorax has developed after 24 to 25 weeks and the umbilical venous pressure is normal or fails to normalize after aspiration of the hydrothorax, there is no physiologic reason to expect either cardiac or pulmonary benefit from long-term drainage.

- **Heart failure is not the only cause of an elevated umbilical venous pressure.**

- Care must be taken to identify the vessel accurately and to be sure that the needle aperture is not up against the vessel wall.

- Experience with a nonhydropic fetus who had tetralogy of Fallot demonstrates that a cardiac malformation that permits the transmission of arterial pressure to the venous system will also **elevate** the umbilical venous pressure in spite of adequate cardiac output.

- The pathophysiologic condition underlying hydrops in the absence of heart failure was not always clear.

- Although the **hypoproteinemia** has been suspected as a cause of hydrops, it was not a reproducible finding in the current study nor was it confined to fetuses with hydrops unrelated to inadequate cardiac output.

  ° In the instances where the low protein concentrations were associated with an elevated umbilical venous pressure, this condition may have resulted from either hemodilution, loss of protein into ascitic or thoracic fluid, or hepatic congestion and decreased synthesis.

  ° The infusion of albumin into the fetus to treat nonimmune hydrops fetalis should be undertaken cautiously.

- Potential fetal therapy was not formulated for fetuses with hydrops that was noncardiac in origin.

  ° In most instances the degree of hydrops was stable and other tests of fetal well-being were normal.

- Treatment of fetal infection would minimize fetal damage by limiting the progress of the infection.

- The hydrops associated with fetal viral infection can have multiple causes.

  ° In the current limited experience viral infection caused inadequate cardiac output by severe anemia (human parvovirus) and possibly by cardiac tamponade.

  ° This unit has previously documented hydrops in association with viral myocarditis.

  ° In three other infected fetuses the nonimmune hydrops fetalis was unassociated with an elevated umbilical venous pressure.

  ° In all three the fetal aminotransferase levels were markedly elevated.

  ° In two fetuses hepatic calcifications developed; one died postnatally of liver failure.

  ° It is unclear whether hydrops in the latter three cases resulted from an inflammatory process of the peritoneum or from liver disease.

  ° Ultrasonographic evidence of infection may be transient.

  ° Isolated pericardial effusion and nonimmune hydrops fetalis has spontaneously resolved associated with cytomegalic virus.]

27. All of the following are increased in the large for gestational age fetus EXCEPT

    A. C peptide.
    B. IGF I.
    C. IGF II.
    *D. IGFBP-1.
    E. None of the above.

p. 96 (Verhaeghe J, Van Bree R, Van Herck E, Laureys J, Bouillon R, Van Assche F A. C-peptide, insulin-like growth factors I and II, and insulin-like growth factor binding protein-1 in umbilical cord serum: Correlations with birth weight. Am J Obstet Gynec 1993; 169:89)

27. [F & I: •Background: There is extensive, although largely indirect, evidence that insulin and the **insulin-like growth factors** I (IGF-I) and 11 (IGF-II) have a role in the regulation of fetal growth and weight gain.

•Insulin is secreted by fetal pancreatic B-cells primarily during the second half of gestation and is believed to primarily stimulate somatic growth and adiposity through classic endocrine modes of action.

•The insulin-like growth factors, structurally proinsulin-like polypeptides, are produced by virtually all fetal organs from early development onward and are potent stimulators of cell division and differentiation; they probably act in an autocrine and paracrine manner.

•IGF-II is produced in far larger quantities than IGF-I in most fetal organs, yet serum IGF-II levels are not altered in newborns with intrauterine growth retardation (IUGR).

•The insulin-like growth factors circulate bound to specific binding proteins, particularly IGFBP-1 and IGFBP-2 in the fetus.

•IGFBP-1 and IGFBP-2 concentrations are increased in newborns with IUGR.

•This is interesting, because these binding proteins can modulate the action of the growth factors: IGFBP-1 was reported to inhibit the action of IGF-I in vitro.

•IGFBP-1 levels are inversely regulated by insulin in adults, but it is unknown whether this also occurs during fetal life.

•Many of the above data were derived from either pathologic conditions (severe IUGR, pancreatic agenesis, diabetes) or experimental procedures in nonprimate species (severe fasting, uterine artery ligation, pancreatectomy).

•Objective: To measure C-peptide, IGF-I, and IGF-II concomitantly in about 538 cord sera, and IGFBP-1 in part of these sera, including all gestational ages in the third trimester and over a large range of birth weights.

•Results: Cord serum IGF-I, IGF-II, and C-peptide concentrations are all positively correlated with birth weight and that IGF-I shows the best correlation.

•IGF-I levels are **decreased in SGA** newborns and **increased in LGA** compared with AGA newborns.

•Cord serum IGF-II levels are sixfold to tenfold higher than IGF-I levels, but the quantitative differences between SGA and LGA newborns, although present, are smaller.

•**C-peptide concentrations** are not different between SGA and AGA newborns but are clearly increased in LGA newborns.

- Cord serum IGFBP-1 is negatively correlated with birth weight, but IGFBP-1 levels do not seem to be regulated by insulin in the fetus.

- After birth, serum IGF-I concentrations largely reflect the hepatic IGF-I production, which is regulated by at least three variables: growth hormone, nutrition, and insulin.

- In the human fetus, IGF-I is produced by the liver and other organs; cord serum IGF-I levels—consistently lower than adult levels—reflect the "overflow" of the IGF-I produced by the tissues; IGF-I in the fetus is believed to act primarily in an autocrine and paracrine mode.

- If the uteroplacental blood flow is a reflection of the fetal nutrition, then there is good reason to assume that this uteroplacental supply line (the bulk as well as the composition) regulates fetal IGF-I production.

- Cord serum IGF-I levels increase with gestational age until 38 to 39 weeks as the uteroplacental blood flow does but decrease thereafter at a time when the uteroplacental blood flow is generally assumed to be dropping.

- Second, IGF-I levels are markedly lower in SGA newborns and in those neonates in whom IUGR ensued as a result of uteroplacental "vascular" pathologic conditions.

- IGF-I production in the fetus may be regulated by insulin, because transient diabetes in human neonates and pancreatectomy in ovine fetuses result in decreased serum IGF-I levels.

- Serum IGF-I levels were increased in newborns with high C-peptide levels, and cord serum C-peptide and IGF-I concentrations were correlated.

- The correlation could be indirect, simply because of the difference in mass, because the individual effects of gestational age and birth weight on serum C-peptide and IGF-I levels were dissimilar.

- Cord serum IGF-II concentrations are manyfold higher than IGF-I concentrations, reflecting the increased IGF-II production by fetal organs.

- In the multiple regression analysis a positive correlation was found between birth weight and serum IGF-II, which probably explains the correlation between gestational age and IGF-II when birth weight is not taken into account.

- A significant increase in cord serum IGF-II levels in LGA infants was found compared with both SGA and AGA infants.

- The differences in cord serum IGF-II concentrations between term SGA or AGA and LGA newborns and between preterm and term AGA newborns are much smaller than those of IGF-I.

- The data would suggest that, in the fetus, a submaximal IGF-II production is achieved before the third trimester and that this tissue synthesis is less dependent on external factors such as the uteroplacental supply line.

- This is consistent with reports showing that liver IGF-II messenger ribonucleic acid concentrations are unchanged in growth-retarded rat fetuses.

- Serum IGF-II levels of human adults are also independent of their nutritional status.

- Cord serum C-peptide levels did not increase during the third trimester.

- Fetal B-cell activity is well established at 28 weeks; in second-trimester newborns C-peptide levels were lower.

- C-peptide concentrations were higher in LGA than in AGA newborns and were higher in newborns with a birth weight of ≥3500 gm than in 2000 to 3499 gm newborns.

- This is compatible with the long-recognized association between fetal hyperinsulinemia and somatic overgrowth (macrosomia), sometimes referred to as the Pedersen-Freinkel hypothesis.

- Because samples from diabetic patients were excluded from this analysis, it is possible that smaller or more transient degrees of maternal (and fetal) hyperglycemia may result in a stimulation of fetal insulin secretion.

- A difference in cord C-peptide levels between SGA and AGA newborns was not found, indicating that a slower fetal growth rate is not primarily caused by a subnormal fetal insulin secretion.

- This does not refute previous observations that IUGR resulting from a severe impairment of uteroplacental blood flow can result in decreased insulin secretion, as reported in human and rat fetuses.

- ICFBP-1 is synthesized in many fetal organs but particularly in the liver.

- IGFBP-1 levels in cord serum are increased in preterm and in SGA newborns compared with term AGA newborns.

- This supports previous data obtained in human newborns and in experimental animals in which uterine artery ligation or maternal fasting result in increased fetal serum ICFBP-1 and liver IGFBP-1 messenger ribonucleic acid concentrations.

- Insulinlike-growth factor peptides and insulin-like growth factor binding proteins are distributed within the same cells of the human fetus and because IGFBP-1 inhibits the action of IGF-I in vitro.

- IGFBP-1 may be the "somatomedin inhibitory substance" found in the plasma of premature and SGA newborns.

- In human adults IGFBP-1 is inversely regulated by insulin, nutrition, and growth hormone, the same factors that are responsible for a decreased hepatic IGF-I synthesis.

- Although the data in fetuses are compatible with a role for the uteroplacental supply line (i.e., nutrition) in IGFBP-1 production, the current study indicates that there is little reason to believe that ICFBP-1 is regulated by insulin levels in the fetus; indeed, there was no correlation between cord serum C-peptide and IGFBP-1 in 131 cord samples with a wide range of C-peptide levels, not even when samples with the lowest and highest C-peptide concentrations were selected.

- Thus the inverse relationship that exists between birth weight and cord serum ICFBP-I is not mediated through insulin.]

Obstetrics and Gynecology: Review 1994-Perinatal Medicine References

Directions: Each group of numbered words or phrases is preceded by a list of lettered statements. MATCH the lettered item most closely associated with the numbered word or phrase. Each item may be used once, more than once, or not at all.

Items 28-30.

    A. chorioamnionitis
    B. placental vasculopathy
    C. chronic villitis
    D. abruptio placentae
    E. none of the above

28. polymorphonuclear leukocytes   Ans: A

29. occlusive thrombi   Ans: B

30. mononuclear cell infiltrates   Ans: C

---

p.586 (Arias F, Rodriquez L, Rayne S C, Kraus F T. Maternal placental vasculopathy and infection: Two distinct subgroups among patients with preterm labor and preterm ruptured membranes. Am J Obstet Gynec 1993; 168:585)

28-30. [F & I: •Background: There is a strong association between infection of the amniotic cavity and preterm labor and premature rupture of membranes.

•In preterm labor with **intact** membranes 22% of the patients who were delivered preterm had positive amniotic fluid cultures, and 12.5% of those with positive amniotic cultures had clinical chorioamnionitis.

•With premature rupture of membranes, 55% of patients have infection.

•The strength of this association is such that many believe that a cause-effect relationship is present.

•Not all patients with preterm labor or premature rupture of membranes have infection; conditions other than infection could produce these problems.

•Objectives: To find explanations for the occurrence of preterm labor and premature rupture of membranes, by studying the clinical characteristics and the placental histologic features of women who were delivered preterm because of preterm labor or premature rupture of membranes and comparing these findings with those of women who had an uncomplicated prenatal course and were delivered at term.

•**Definitions.** Patients were considered to have **infection** if one or more of the following could be demonstrated:

•(1) positive amniotic fluid Gram stain or cultures;

•(2) positive subchorionic placental cultures;

•(3) positive central cultures (blood, spinal fluid, tracheal aspirate) of the neonate, obtained shortly after birth;

•(4) severe (grade III) histologic chorioamnionitis.

•Patients were considered to have maternal **placental vasculopathy** if they had characteristic vascular lesions in the decidual spiral arteries and uneven accelerated villi maturation, multiple syncytial knots, and placental infarcts or the placental weight was <10th percentile for gestational age.

•A newborn was classified as **growth retarded** if the birth weight was <10th percentile for gestational age and the nursery stay was consistent with the clinical impression of intrauterine malnutrition.

Obstetrics and Gynecology: Review 1994-Perinatal Medicine References

- A patient was considered to have **chronic villitis** if the placenta exhibited the characteristic histologic findings with mononuclear cell infiltration and there was no clinical, histologic or laboratory evidence of acute infection.

- Histologic **chorioamnionitis** was characterized by the presence of polymorphonuclear leukocytes, with or without necrosis, in the fetal membranes and the subchorionic fibrin plate.

  ° The degree of severity was graded as slight (grade I), moderate (grade II), or severe (grade III) on the basis of the number and extent of infiltrating neutrophils.

- Maternal **placental vasculopathy** was diagnosed when segments of spiral arteries attached to the maternal surface of the placenta failed to show the presence of adaptive changes and remained as small, muscular vessels with well-defined walls, containing recent or old organized thrombi, mural or occlusive.

  ° Additional histologic criteria were the presence of uneven accelerated maturation of the chorionic villi, large numbers of multinucleated syncytial knots, and multiple placental infarcts.

- A mixed lesion was diagnosed when features of infection and maternal placental vasculopathy were present in the same specimen.

- **Chronic villitis** was diagnosed when areas of chronic inflammation with mononuclear cell infiltrates and areas of fibrinoid necrosis affected clusters of villi.

- Results: The presence of two well-defined subgroups among patients with preterm labor and premature rupture of membranes was identified.

  ° One of them is characterized by the presence of bacterial infection of the products of conception and the other by the presence of placental vascular abnormalities consisting of lack of adaptive changes in the decidual portion of the spiral arterioles and presence of uneven accelerated maturation of villi, multiple syncytial knots, and placental infarcts.

- The finding of an association between chorioamniotic infection and preterm labor and premature rupture of membranes is not surprising.

- This association is found so frequently that the possibility of a cause-effect relationship between infection and preterm labor and premature rupture of membranes is widely accepted among experts in this field.

- The changes in the maternal vascular compartment of the placenta in patients with preterm labor and premature rupture of membranes are similar to those found in patients with preeclampsia, in those with fetal growth retardation, and in some patients with repetitive second-trimester fetal death.

  ° Naeye originally described the association between these placental changes and spontaneous preterm delivery in patients without hypertension during pregnancy.

- Fetal growth retardation is a common finding in patients who are delivered preterm.

- Alterations in maternal and fetal artery flow velocity waveforms in patients in preterm labor and there is evidence indicating that those changes reflect vascular alterations of the placenta.

- Decidual vasculopathy occurs more frequently than chorioamnionitis in patients delivered preterm in all gestational age groups.

- All the evidence accumulated in the literature points to the possibility that a deficiency in the ability of the trophoblastic cells to produce adaptive changes in the spiral arterioles leads to inadequate and uneven uteroplacental blood flow with production of accelerated maturation, increased syncytial knots, thinning of the syncytiotrophoblast, fibrotic villi, and infarcts in those areas of the placenta affected by low flow.

- What is unknown at the present time is the nature of the link between the failure to establish adequate hemochorial placentation and its clinical expression.

• This enigma is of singular importance because it may explain why preeclampsia develops in some of these patients and some others have fetal growth retardation without hypertension, preterm labor, or preterm rupture of membranes.

• Another possibility, unsupported by evidence, is that the changes observed in the placenta are unrelated to the clinical picture shown in these patients.

• In addition to the obvious differences in laboratory findings patients with chorioamniotic infection and patients with maternal placental vasculopathy and either preterm labor or premature rupture of membranes seem to have a different clinical course and a different prognosis.

• Patients with preterm labor or premature rupture of membranes who have **infection** are delivered earlier, have smaller babies, have more severe morbidity, and have greater mortality than patients with preterm labor or premature rupture of membranes who do not have infection and have maternal placental vascular abnormalities.

• Correlation between placental histologic type, placental cultures, amniotic fluid Gram stain, amniotic fluid cultures, and clinical findings is not perfect.

• A similar imperfect correlation exists between decidual vasculopathy and clinical findings.

» It is tempting to speculate that in 60% to 70% of patients preterm labor and premature rupture of membranes are the result of infection and maternal placental vasculopathy.

• If this is true, strenuous efforts to inhibit preterm uterine activity and prolong pregnancy may be inappropriate, not only because of their lack of effectiveness but also because prolongation of pregnancy will keep the fetus in a hostile environment and potentially may cause more harm than good.]

Directions: Each set of lettered headings below is followed by a list of numbered words or phrases. For each numbered word or phrase select:

    A. if the item is associated with *(A) only*
    B. if the item is associated with *(B) only*
    C. if item is associated with *both (A) and (B)*
    D. if item is associated with *neither (A) nor (B)*

Items 31-33.

In a twin gestation:

    A. chorionic villus sampling.
    B. amniocentesis (16-18 weeks)
    C. both
    D. neither

31. fetal loss rate about 10%   Ans: B

32. increased incidence of twin-twin contamination   Ans: A

33. preferred method in the event of discordant results require termination of affected twin   Ans: A

---

p.55 (Wapner R J, Johnson A, Davis G, Urban A, Morgan P, Jackson L. Prenatal diagnosis in twin gestations: A comparison between second-trimester amniocentesis and first-trimester chorionic villus sampling. Obstet Gynecol 1993; 82:49)

31-33. [F & I: • Background: Prenatal diagnosis of a twin pregnancy has unique problems: The a priori genetic risk must be recalculated; tissue retrieval from each fetus must be assured; the potential for discordant results must be addressed.

- Second-trimester amniocentesis is a reliable and safe sampling procedure for twin gestations despite limited experience on which to base procedure-related risk estimates.

- Only recently has the feasibility of chorionic villus sampling (CVS) for evaluating twin gestations been explored.

- Objective: To evaluate the relative risks of these two sampling techniques, by comparing second trimester amniocentesis to first-trimester CVS in the genetic evaluation of twin gestations.

- Results: CVS is at least as safe as amniocentesis.

- The amniocentesis pregnancy loss rate of 2.9% and total fetal loss rate of 9.3% are consistent with those described in the majority of contemporary studies, and demonstrate the inherent risks associated with multiple gestations.

- Even though CVS was performed at a gestational age 4 to 6 weeks earlier than amniocentesis, the overall pregnancy loss rate of 3.2% was similar to that of amniocentesis.

- If only chromosomally normal fetuses and placentas are included, the CVS total fetal loss rate of 3.9% was significantly less than the 9.3% loss rate following amniocentesis.

- The major difference in total fetal loss between the sampling techniques was related to an increased incidence of intrauterine death of a single fetus in the amniocentesis group.

- Of the 13 fetal losses following amniocentesis, 61.5% were singleton fetuses; only 33.3% of the losses following CVS were of single fetuses.

- Whereas none of the perinatal losses in the amniocentesis group had abnormal karyotypes, five such losses in the CVS group involved fetuses or placentas having a chromosomal abnormality, two of which (possibly three) would not have been identified by amniocentesis.

- Because aneuploidy confined to the placenta may be an independent cause of perinatal loss, this raises the question of whether some postamniocentesis losses of single fetuses could have been a consequence of an undiagnosed abnormal placental cell line.

- CVS is as effective as amniocentesis in providing sufficient tissue for accurate diagnosis.

- One must caution that unlike amniocentesis, in which dye injection allows confirmation that individual samples were retrieved, CVS provides no such aid.

- In cases of same sex twins sampled by CVS, there is no guarantee that each twin was individually sampled.

- Each chorion frondosum must be accurately and meticulously identified before and during CVS sampling.

- A combination of sagittal and transverse scanning to confirm appropriate location of the needle or catheter tip before its withdrawal will assure accurate placement.

- If instrument insertion into distinctly separate placental sites is not certain, resampling either immediately by repeat insertion or later by amniocentesis is required.

- CVS in multiple gestations takes significant experience and skill by both the operator and the ultrasonographer and should be restricted to those centers performing the procedure on a regular basis.

- Before the initial CVS sampling session, patients should be counseled as to the potential need for an additional procedure.

- Further evaluation by amniocentesis was performed in nine women (5.6%) from the CVS group.

- Patients required additional testing by amniocentesis either to confirm that individual frondosum sites were sampled or to delineate further questionable CVS results.

- The need for backup amniocentesis to add to the interpretation of mosaic or questionable CVS results continues to be required.

- As knowledge about the clinical significance of mosaic CVS results has been refined, the need for further testing has decreased.

- In most first-trimester cases, the membrane dividing dichorionic gestations is thick and easily visualized, allowing easy demarcation of individual sampling sites.

- Tissue retrieval near this dividing membrane may occasionally lead to contamination of one twin sample with villi from the coexisting twin.

- Knowledge of this potential by the laboratory should prevent misinterpretation when two distinct karyotypes are present in one sample.

- Twin-twin contamination may still present difficulty in the analysis of biochemical results, as normal and abnormal villi will be pooled.

- To avoid this development, analysis of several individual villi from each twin rather than pooled villi is recommended for biochemical analysis.

- To minimize twin-twin contamination and to assure retrieval of villi from individual sacs, both transabdominal and transcervical sampling should be used.

- For this reason, experience and expertise with both techniques is essential in centers where twin pregnancies are sampled.

- Two errors unrelated to twin-twin contamination developed in this series; one followed a CVS and the other followed an amniocentesis.

- The amniocentesis error involved a normal amniocentesis result done as a backup to a 46,XX,r(11) mosaic CVS culture.

- The fetus was confirmed at birth to carry the abnormal cell line in peripheral blood.

- This false-negative amniocentesis, which failed to confirm a mosaic CVS culture, is consistent with similar findings in other rare cases.

- The misinterpretation in the CVS group involved a false-negative laboratory result in a pregnancy at risk for Fanconi anemia. {Fanconi's hypoplastic anemia is a pancytopenia (anemia, neutropenia, thrombocytopenia) associated with congenital anomalies such as short stature, renal deformities, skeletal defects, hyperpigmentation, and microphthalmia. The diagnosis can be confirmed by the presence of an excessive number of chromosomal breaks in peripheral lymphocyte cultures. The inheritance is autosomal recessive.}

- There were no cases of false-negative results secondary to either inadequate sampling or confined placental mosaicism.

- Sampling monochorionic twin pregnancies presents unique problems.

- Although theoretically, most monochorionic pregnancies require only a single sampling, exceptions do occur, as in the case of heterokaryotic twins or when the ultrasound impression of a single chorion is incorrect.

- To prevent misinterpretation, two samples should be obtained, if possible, by selecting sampling sites near individual cord insertions.

- Nevertheless, there were seven cases in this series in which only one sampling attempt was made.
- All of these pregnancies were confirmed at delivery to be monochorionic.
- Although selective termination for discordant results was not required following amniocentesis, eight potential cases followed CVS.
- It is critical that an accurate map of fetal and placental relationships be prepared at the time of sampling.
- Information about the location of the affected fetus will remain reliable for at least 2 to 3 weeks following CVS.
  ° Should the location of the affected fetus be uncertain, a repeat CVS and rapid tissue study can be done a few hours before a requested selective termination to confirm that the correct fetus has been identified.
  ° Recent information has suggested that selective termination is safer if performed before 16 weeks' gestation.
  ° Two small series have found an increased risk of preterm delivery following second trimester selective termination procedures.
  ° Preliminary analysis of a large multicenter registry of selective termination procedures has confirmed the increased prematurity rate following selective termination performed after 16 weeks and has also found a decreased risk of pregnancy loss when reduction procedures are performed before 14 weeks.
  ° These results suggest an additional advantage to the earlier diagnosis afforded by CVS.
- Conclusion: CVS is a safe and effective alternative to amniocentesis for sampling multiple gestations.
- Care must be taken to ensure that individual sites are sampled.
- This is possible when the procedure is carried out in a center experienced and knowledgeable in such techniques.
- Care must also be taken in interpreting test results to avoid errors caused by twin-twin contamination.
- Chorionic villus sampling has the advantage of providing an earlier diagnosis than amniocentesis, and should the results be discordant, elective termination can be done at an earlier gestational age.]

Items 34-36.

In the treatment of pregnancy-induced hypertension:

    A. nicardipine
    B. nifedipine
    C. both
    D. neither

34. more selective dihydropyridine derivative   Ans: A

35. can be infused IV   Ans: A

36. reduced rate of fetal growth retardation   Ans: D

p. 918 (Carbonne B, Jannet D, Touboul C, Khelifati Y, Milliez J. Nicardipine treatment of hypertension during pregnancy. Obstet Gynecol 1993; 81:908)

34-36. [F & I: •Background: **Nifedipine**, a dihydropyridine derivative, is a calcium channel blocker used during pregnancy in the treatment of hypertension.

    •It is used to control preterm labor and to treat hypertension of pregnancy.

    •Nifedipine does **not** reduce uteroplacental or fetal blood flow.

    °It is not always well tolerated and may induce headaches and hot flushes.

•**Nicardipine**, another dihydropyridine-derivative calcium entry blocker, is also a potent antihypertensive drug.

    °Animal experiments suggested that the hemodynamic effects of nicardipine could be responsible for severe fetal acidosis and fetal death.

    °Nicardipine has never been used in pregnant women.

    °The doses used in animal studies are extremely high compared to those used in nonpregnant hypertensive humans.

    °In the sheep, no deleterious effect of the drug was evident after direct injection to the fetus.

•Nicardipine has advantages over nifedipine in that it acts more selectively on the blood vessels than on the myocardium, has less of a negative inotropic effect, and produces less reflex tachycardia.

•Objectives: To determine the tolerance of hypertensive pregnant women to oral and intravenous (IV) nicardipine and to evaluate the effect of the drug on the fetus and neonate.

•Methods: Twenty patients, 12 nulliparas and eight multiparas received IV nicardipine.

•All had previously been treated with oral antihypertensive drugs (alphamethyldopa, hydralazine, metoprolol, or atenolol).

•All had severe preeclampsia, including five with chronic hypertension and superimposed preeclampsia.

•For these patients in whom oral treatment had failed, the idea was to gain a few days using IV therapy in order to favor fetal lung maturation and/or cervical ripening if labor induction was necessary.

- Before treatment with IV nicardipine, the diastolic BP, as assessed by two successive determinations, was 116 ± 6.7 mmHg, systolic BP was 180 ± 16.5 mmHg, and proteinuria was 2.7 ± 1.8 g/24 h.

- Intravenous nicardipine was delivered through a continuous infusion pump, at three different rates according to body weight: 2 mg/h (body weight less than 80 kg, nine patients), 4 mg/h (80-to-90 kg, eight patients), and 6 mg/h (greater than 90 kg, three patients).

- Maternal blood pressure and heart rate were automatically recorded every 15 min until IV nicardipine was discontinued.

- Efficacy of IV nicardipine treatment was evaluated by the time required to steadily decrease the diastolic BP below 90 mmHg.

- Nicardipine and nifedipine, both dihydropyridine calcium entry blockers, are efficient antihypertensive drugs.

- Nicardipine offers theoretical advantages over nifedipine:

  ° It acts more selectively on the vessels,

  ° it has less of a negative inotropic effect,

  ° it produces less reflex tachycardia, and

  ° it induces fewer undesirable side effects, headaches, hot flushes, or edema.

- Being soluble in water, nicardipine can be infused IV.

- Assays in maternal and fetal tissues showed that tissue concentrations are nearly undetectable only a few hours after oral ingestion, suggesting that nicardipine does not accumulate in the placenta, membranes, and umbilical cord.

- Nicardipine did not induce fetal compromise.

- As reported for nifedipine, umbilical Doppler velocimetry remained stable with oral or IV nicardipine, as did cerebral Doppler velocimetry on oral treatment.

- The neonatal outcome further substantiates the good fetal tolerance to nicardipine.

- Despite sometimes severe hypertensive disease, no perinatal deaths occurred.

- The rates of prematurity, growth retardation, and cesarean delivery are also in keeping with the data reported in the literature for other antihypertensive drugs and for nifedipine.

- No definitive conclusion can be drawn about safety without a control group.

- Neonatal calcemia was always found to be normal.

- Maternal tolerance to nicardipine was assessed by the absence of undesirable side effects under oral treatment.

- Uteroplacental blood flow, evaluated by uterine artery Doppler velocimetry, remained stable after 6 weeks of oral nicardipine, confirming the data reported with nifedipine.

- Data on uterine artery Doppler velocimetry both before and after IV nicardipine were too few to analyze.

- Nine patients receiving IV nicardipine complained of headaches, but the respective influences of treatment or preeclampsia are difficult to assess.

•Nicardipine proved to be efficient for treating hypertension in pregnant women and the oral dose used, 20 mg three times a day, seems to be appropriate.

•In only two patients did oral nicardipine fail to control hypertension.

°Labor was induced because both pregnancies were close to term.

°Otherwise, alternative management with a second antihypertensive agent or with IV nicardipine may be indicated.

•Intravenous nicardipine effectively controlled hypertension, at least temporarily, in all 20 pregnant patients treated.

•The progressive decline in BP over more than 1 h seems appropriate in order to avoid the fetal hazards entailed by a precipitous fall in BP.

•Four patients escaped therapeutic control, with diastolic BPs rising again above 120 mmHg after 5 days of IV nicardipine, and it was elected to terminate pregnancy.

•Whether the infusion rate of nicardipine can be safely increased or a second antihypertensive drug added in these cases remains to be determined by further studies.]

Items 37-39.

In the affected fetus:

   A. septated cystic hygroma
   B. nonseptated cystic hygroma
   C. both
   D. neither

37. usually 1 to 5 centimeters   Ans: A

38. regresses before the 16th week of gestation   Ans: B

39. non-immune hydrops   Ans: A

---

p. 686   (Bronshtein M, Bar-Hava I, Blumenfeld I, Bejar J, Toder V, Blumenfeld Z. The difference between septated and nonseptated nuchal cystic hygroma in the early second trimester. Obstet Gynecol 1993; 81:683)

37-39. [F & I: •Background: Cystic hygroma colli can be detected in one in 120 ultrasound examinations performed in early pregnancy, its birth occurrence is quite rare (one in 6000 deliveries).

•Associated chromosomal abnormalities and a variety of other congenital malformations occur in the vast majority of cases.

•It is generally believed that antenatal identification of cystic hygroma carries a grave prognosis and that prenatal death can be expected in more than 90% of the cases.

•Intrauterine regression of cervical cystic hygroma occurs and survival in a small percentage of neonates who were not seriously handicapped.

•Objective: To present experience concerning antenatal identification of nonseptated nuchal cystic hygromas.

•This study evaluated the ultrasonographic characteristics, natural history, chromosomal analysis, and pregnancy and neonatal outcome of fetuses with **nonseptated** nuchal cystic hygromas.

- Cystic hygroma is a well-known lymphatic malformation occurring most commonly in the **posterior** cervical (nuchal) area.

    ° Other locations for cystic hygroma include the anterior cervical, mediastinal, axillary, abdominal-wall, inguinal, and retroperitoneal areas.

- During organogenesis, lymphatic vessels initially drain into two large sacs lateral to the jugular veins and eventually, at 40 days' gestation, connect to the venous system as the terminal portion of the right lymphatic duct and the thoracic duct.

- When this communication fails or is delayed, the jugular lymphatic obstruction sequence may occur: The jugular lymph sacs enlarge and lymph accumulates in the tissues.

- Cystic hygromata colli was initially considered to be associated only with Turner syndrome.

- It occurs with other chromosomal aneuploidies, single-gene disorders, familial inheritance, and large varieties of other congenital syndromes.

- Normal karyotype can be found in 22 to 32% of cystic hygromas.

- Cystic hygromata colli are associated with various anomalies in 60% of cases.

- The cystic masses in the cervical area should not be considered a uniform group but rather heterogeneous lesions.

- Whereas the **septated or reticular cystic hygromas are usually large** (1 to 5 cm) multiloculated cystic masses located in the **posterior cervical area**, the nonseptated cystic hygromas are smaller unilocular sonolucent sacs that are usually located bilaterally in the anterolateral cervical region.

- Their **incidence** is quite different: Septated cystic hygromas occur in one in 677 ultrasound examinations, and nonseptated cystic hygromas can be found in one in 60 fetuses by transvaginal ultrasound examination (125 of 7582).

- Their **time of occurrence** is also different; whereas the septated cystic hygromas can be identified as early as the 10th week, nonseptated cystic hygroma has not been identified before the 13th gestational week.

- The **prognosis** is quite different between nonseptated cystic hygromas and septated cystic hygromas.

    ° **Nonseptated cystic hygromas usually regress before the 16th week**, and a relatively good neonatal outcome can be expected.

    ° **Septated cystic hygromas commonly progress to nonimmune hydrops**, even when there is a normal karyotype.

- Fetal death (in two of 25) or termination of pregnancy (in 20 of 25) occurred in 88% of the cases in this series.

    ° In a small percentage of septated cystic hygromas, regression can occur even from the hydropic state, probably by lymph-vessel recanalization.

    ° When the septated cystic hygroma does regress, it often leaves its mark as variable degrees of nonspecific localized nuchal tissue edema or a thickening called webbed neck (**pterygium colli**).

- The **histologic appearance** differs between septated and nonseptated cystic hygromas.

    ° The latter show no subcutaneous edema on histologic examination, and two well-defined empty cystic lymphatic cavities can be detected in the nuchal region.

°In the septated cystic hygromas, diffuse **subcutaneous edema** is noticed, and the borders of the dorsal cystic hygroma are poorly defined.

•The differences between the septated cystic hygromas and the nonseptated cystic hygromas raise two main possibilities.

°First, the two types of cystic hygroma may be different degrees of the same pathologic process.

°Whereas septated cystic hygroma is due to the complete jugular lymphatic obstruction sequence the nonseptated cystic hygroma represents a transient, short-lived obstruction or delayed communication of the jugular lymphatic sacs to the venous system

°Second, septated and nonseptated cystic hygroma could represent two different entities.

°Septated cystic hygroma could result from lymphatic obstruction with subcutaneous edema, and nonseptated cystic hygroma could represent a delayed form of the physiologic process of lymphatic accumulation that occurs in most fetuses for a short period of time without associated subcutaneous edema.

°For poorly understood reasons, this process is delayed in about 1% of fetuses, and resolution may take longer in dyskaryotic fetuses.

•According to the data, a **normal pregnancy and outcome** (with a mean neonatal follow-up of 20 months) can be expected in **94% of nonseptated cystic hygroma** cases, which supports the latter theory.

•Septated cystic hygromas are commonly associated with various renal and cardiac anomalies.

•**The dilated lymphatics in Turner syndrome may be responsible for the development of coarctation of the aorta and other congenital heart defects.**

•There was a 15% association of nonseptated cystic hygromas with various anomalies, 80% of which were **cardiac and renal.**

•One can postulate that a disturbance in fluid distribution during organogenesis might play a role in the pathogenesis of these malformations.

•Although the antenatal identification of nonseptated cystic hygromas carries a relatively good prognosis in the vast majority of cases, it should be emphasized that 5.7% of the fetuses will have a chromosome abnormality and 15% will have other structural anomalies.

»A detailed sonographic examination and karyotyping are recommended.]

Items 40-42.

    A. dihydralazine
    B. labetalol
    C. both
    D. neither

40. effective antihypertensive in pregnancy   Ans: C

41. antiarrhythmic   Ans: B

42. decreases diastolic filling time   Ans: A

p. 1296 (Bhorat I E, Naidoo D P, Rout C C, Moodley J. Malignant ventricular arrhythmias in eclampsia: A comparison of labetalol with dihydralazine. Am J Obstet Gynec 1993; 168:1292)

40-42. [F & I: •Background: Serious ventricular arrhythmias are a common occurrence in hypertensive crises during pregnancy and may contribute to the high mortality and morbidity associated with the disease.

•Eclampsia is characterized by markedly altered cardiovascular dynamics, and the occurrence of serious ventricular arrhythmias may lead to hemodynamic instability.

•Hypertensive crises in preeclampsia are associated with high circulatory levels of catecholamines, which alone or in combination with myocardial ischemia may lead to ventricular tachycardia and pulmonary edema.

•The resultant tachycardia and elevated systemic vascular resistance could contribute to increased left ventricular stroke work and myocardial ischemia, leading to ventricular tachycardia and pulmonary edema.

•Incorporation of a ß-blocker before delivery for the hemodynamic control of severely hypertensive parturients may effectively block these effects of catecholamines on the myocardium.

•Because labetalol, a combined α and ß-receptor blocker, is known to be a safe and effective antihypertensive in preeclampsia, its effect on arrhythmias in hypertensive crises in pregnancy was investigated.

•Objective: To assess the influence of an intravenous infusion of labetalol on the incidence and severity of ventricular arrhythmias in a group of eclamptic subjects, in comparison with the standard regimen of intermittent intravenous injection of dihydralazine.

•Methods: Blood pressure and heart rate were measured and recorded every 10 min.

•Control subjects received a standard antihypertensive regimen consisting of a slow (4 min) intravenous injection of dihydralazine, 6.25 mg, diluted in 10 ml of 0.9% saline solution.

°This was repeated if necessary at 30-min intervals (maximum three doses) until the diastolic pressure was <100 mm Hg.

•Labetalol was administered to patients in the study group as a constant intravenous infusion of 200 mg in 200 ml 0.9% saline solution beginning at a rate of 20 mg/hr.

°The infusion rate was doubled every 30 min until the diastolic pressure was <100 mm Hg (maximum rate 160 mg/hr) and adjusted to maintain a diastolic pressure between 90 to 100 mm Hg.

•In all patients antihypertensive therapy was used intravenously for 24 hours after delivery, after which oral therapy was begun if necessary.

•Continuous electrocardiographic recording was obtained on a four-channel Holter recorder and continued for 24 h, to include predelivery, delivery, and postdelivery periods.

•Arrhythmia detection and analysis were performed on a Holter analysis computer.

•Electrocardiographic abnormalities were confirmed by visual inspection and arrhythmias graded according to the **Lown grade classification** for ventricular arrhythmias.

•The Lown classification consists of grades 0 to IVB.

°Grade 0 denotes no observed arrythmias.

°Grade I denotes isolated unifocal premature ventricular contractions occurring less frequently than 30 per hour in any hour of recording.

°Grade II denotes isolated unifocal premature ventricular contractions occurring more frequently than 30 per hour.

°Grade III denotes multifocal premature ventricular contractions occurring at any frequency.

°Grade IVA denotes coupling of premature ventricular contractions, and grade IVB denotes runs of three or more premature ventricular contractions (i.e., ventricular tachycardia)

- Results: A high incidence of serious ventricular arrhythmias in hypertensive crises in pregnancy was found and its incidence can be significantly reduced by incorporating labetalol into the peripartum management of hypertension in these patients.

- Labetalol offers both α- and ß-blockade in a ratio of 1:7 in its intravenous preparation.

  °It results in good blood pressure control with a decrease in heart rate.

  °It has powerful antiarrhythmic effects, which are the result of its ß-adrenergic blocking action, i.e., inhibition of ectopic pacemakers and prolongation of the atrioventricular refractory period.

  °The simultaneous α-blocking action effectively antagonizes the widespread vasoconstriction characteristic of eclampsia, thus lowering systemic vascular resistance and achieving effective blood pressure control.

  °In the three patients with ventricular tachycardia who received labetalol, complete abolition of all arrhythmias was obtained.

- Dihydralazine, which has no antiarrhythmic properties, was associated with the persistence of serious ventricular arrhythmias throughout the peripartum period, in spite of adequate blood pressure control.

- The reduction in the incidence of ventricular tachycardias during the delivery period probably relates to the use of general anesthesia for the cesarean section.

- The pathogenesis of these arrhythmias is uncertain.

- A sudden increase in ventricular afterload in these patients, together with raised levels of catecholamines, may contribute to increasing ventricular irritability.

- Intense sympathetic activity with release of catecholamines, such as seen in severe preeclampsia, can produce coronary vasospasm leading to arrhythmias and even myocardial infarction.

- In the presence of myocardial ischemia or toxic myocardial depression, arrhythmias can readily develop.

- Sympathetic stimulation can produce myocardial necrosis in the experimental animal.

  °Autopsy data revealed diffuse myocardial necrosis in patients treated with large doses of ß-sympathomimetics and in patients dying from pheochromocytoma.

  °The adrenochrome metabolite of catecholamines is capable of producing arrhythmias and coronary spasm.

- Myocardial ischemia could be caused directly as part of the microvascular pathologic condition seen with preeclampsia, (i.e., focal vasospasm, fibrin deposition, and platelet aggregation).

- Other factors that alone or in combination with sympathetic activity could cause ventricular rhythm disturbances include hypoxia, acidosis, hypocarbia, and electrolyte disturbances, all of which were observed.

- Serious arrhythmias are associated with sudden death in patients with essential hypertension and are related to the presence of left ventricular hypertrophy.

•In acute hypertensive states in which there is a nonhypertrophoid ventricle sudden increases in afterload and cathecholamine excess are potent factors in the genesis of ventricular arrhythmias and cardiac compromise.

•Whatever the cause of the arrhythmias, the use of an agent such as dihydralazine that acts by reduction of ventricular afterload is **not** appropriate in situations of potential myocardial ischemia, because the drug reduces aortic root pressure and decreases the diastolic filling time, both of which will reduce myocardial perfusion.

•ß-Adrenergic receptor blockade not only decreases heart rate, thereby increasing diastolic filling time, but also reduces myocardial oxygen requirements by its negative inotropic effect and directly antagonizes the arrhythmogenic effects of catecholamines.

•Conclusion: Ventricular arrhythmias in eclampsia are amenable to ß-adrenergic receptor blockade.

•This could be because of its antiadrenergic effect with improvement in the myocardial oxygen supply and demand ratio.]

Items 43-44.

    A. acute fatty liver of pregnancy
    B. HELLP syndrome
    C. both
    D. neither

43.   periportal necrosis   Ans: B

44.   numerous fat droplets   Ans: A

p. 1542   (Barton J R, Riely C A, Adamec T A, Shanklin D R, Khoury A D, Sibai B M. Hepatic histopathologic condition does not correlate with laboratory abnormalities in HELLP syndrome (hemolysis, elevated liver enzymes, and low platelet count. Am J Obstet Gynec 1992; 167:1538)

43-44. [F & I: •Background: Preeclampsia is a complication of pregnancy characterized by the triad of elevated blood pressure, proteinuria, and generalized edema.

•Weinstein coined the term "HELLP syndrome" to describe a special group of preeclamptic pregnant women with evidence of hemolysis ("H"), elevated liver enzymes ("EL"), and low platelet ("LP") count.

•Maternal and perinatal morbidity and mortality are increased in these patients and their progeny.

•The histopathologic condition of hepatic lesions associated with HELLP syndrome has been described.

•An association may exist between the clinical laboratory abnormalities and the histopathologic findings.

•A pathologic continuum may exist between HELLP syndrome, preeclamptic liver disorders in general, and acute fatty liver of pregnancy.

°If such a continuum is proved, conservative management of HELLP syndrome may be unjustified and potentially life-threatening.

•Objectives: To categorize the microscopic findings from liver biopsies obtained under direct visualization after cesarean delivery from pregnancies complicated by HELLP syndrome and to correlate these microscopic findings with the severity of the concurrent clinical and laboratory abnormalities.

•The classic hepatic lesion associated with the HELLP syndrome is periportal or focal parenchymal necrosis in which hyaline deposits of fibrin-like material can be seen in the sinusoids.

°Immunofluorescence studies show fibrin microthrombi and fibrinogen deposits in the sinusoids in areas of hepatocellular necrosis and in sinusoids of histologically normal parenchyma.

°These histopathologic findings may be related to the elevated liver enzymes and the right upper-quadrant pain and tenderness seen in patients with this syndrome.

•Results: Steatosis was noted in several of the liver biopsy specimens from this study population.

•Although there is overlap both clinically and pathologically between acute fatty liver of pregnancy and the HELLP syndrome, these syndromes can be distinguished histopathologically.

•On light microscopy in acute fatty liver of pregnancy, the vacuolization and necrosis is most prominent in the central zone, whereas in HELLP syndrome the necrosis is predominantly periportal.

•Although fat droplets may be present on electron microscopy in hepatocytes from patients with the HELLP syndrome, fat droplets are much more numerous in acute fatty liver of pregnancy.

•Because of the invasive nature of this study, the strict entry criteria, and the low incidence of HELLP syndrome, the study population is small.

°This obviously increases the possibility for type II statistical errors.

°Further, core biopsy specimens of the liver may not adequately reflect the extent, or absence, of hepatic involvement.

•The variability in severity of hepatic histopathologic conditions in HELLP syndrome is clear even with the limited sample number in this study.

• Some consider HELLP syndrome to be an indication for immediate cesarean delivery, whereas others recommend a more conservative approach, to prolong pregnancy in cases of fetal immaturity.

•Occasionally some patients without the true HELLP syndrome may develop antepartum reversal of hematologic abnormalities after bed rest, the use of steroids, or plasma volume expansion.

°The majority of these patients have deterioration in either maternal or fetal condition within 1 to 10 days after conservative management.

•The potential risks associated with conservative management of HELLP syndrome include abruptio placentae, pulmonary edema, acute renal failure, and ruptured liver hematoma.

»All patients with the true HELLP syndrome should be treated aggressively, primarily with delivery.

°This is because the severity of the clinical and laboratory abnormalities in HELLP syndrome do **not** adequately reflect the seriousness of the hepatic histopathologic conditions; experience suggests that limited pregnancy prolongation will **not** result in improved perinatal outcome.]

Directions: For each of the questions or incomplete statements below, ONE or MORE of the answers or completions given is correct. In each case select:

A. if only 1, 2, and 3 are correct
B. if only 1 and 3 are correct
C. if only 2 and 4 are correct
D. if only 4 is correct
E. if all are correct

---

45. Elective cesarean section in cases of antenatally diagnosed gastroschisis decreases neonatal morbidity by

    1. avoiding intestinal ischemia during labor.
    2. decreasing bacterial contamination of the exposed intestines.
    3. decreasing physical damage to the intestine during delivery.
    4. decreasing the incidence of fetal distress if vaginal delivery is anticipated.

p. 1052   Ans: E   (Sakala E P, Erhard L N, White J J. Elective cesarean section improves outcomes of neonates with gastroschisis. Am J Obstet Gynec 1993; 169:1050)

45. [F & I: Background: Gastroschisis is a full-thickness abdominal wall defect, usually to the right of the umbilical cord insertion, that allows the small bowel and other viscera to extrude from the abdominal cavity and float freely in the amniotic sac, exposed to the amniotic fluid, until delivery.

• It is an uncommon fetal structural anomaly having its origin early in embryonic life; it occurs in one in 10,000 live births.

• Associated structural and chromosomal anomalies are found less frequently than in the other major ventral wall defect, omphalocele.

• Surgical repair in the immediate neonatal period is imperative.

• Gastroschisis is being diagnosed prenatally more often because of wider use of maternal serum α–fetoprotein screening and increased use of high-resolution obstetric ultrasonography.

• The optimal method of delivery for fetuses with gastroschisis has been a controversial intervention.

• Avoidance of labor and delivery by elective cesarean section before onset of labor has been proposed to improve neonatal outcome.

• Most published reports have not shown a benefit.

• Objective: To compare the neonatal postoperative morbidity for the fetus with prenatally diagnosed gastroschisis delivered vaginally with that for the fetus delivered by elective cesarean at or before the onset of labor.

• Emergency cesarean section **in labor for obstetric indications appears to have no apparent advantage to the neonate with gastroschisis.**

• The advantages of elective cesarean delivery may arise from avoiding three potentially adverse intrapartum events related to labor and vaginal delivery.

• First, the tenuous mesenteric blood supply could be jeopardized by the compression, stretching, or twisting of the eviscerated bowel by the prolonged repetitive uterine contractions of labor.

° The resulting relative intestinal ischemia may cause bowel injury and edema.

° Although in milder cases prolonged return of bowel function would be the main morbidity noted, in severe cases extensive bowel resection and short bowel syndrome may be a consequence.

• Fact   ° Detail   » issue   * answer

°This hypothesis appears to be supported by the data.

°The study did demonstrate a statistically longer ($p < .01$) return of normal bowel function (more days on total parenteral nutrition, longer days to oral feedings, and thus longer hospital stay) in the vaginal delivery infants compared with the elective cesarean group.

°These findings are consistent with the operating surgeons assessment of normal appearing bowel being significantly higher ($p < .05$) in the cesarean section cases.

°The absence of short bowel syndrome in these cases, compared with a 33% incidence in the vaginal delivery infants, was statistically significant ($p < .05$).

•Second, because no membrane covers the viscera, they may be exposed to any bacterial flora present in the genital tract at labor, which may contribute to postoperative **infectious complications**.

•This second hypothesis also appears confirmed.

°One third of the vaginal delivery infants experienced sepsis compared with none in the elective cesarean section group ($p < .05$).

°This difference was statistically significant.

°There was a nonsignificant trend ($p = .09$) to higher wound infections in the vaginal delivery cases than in the elective cesarean section cases.

•The third hypothesis suggests the extracorporeal viscera are at risk for **avulsion and tear injuries** during vaginal delivery.

•This thesis was **not** confirmed because none of the 22 cases had visceral trauma.

•Although this study does suggest a benefit for fetuses with gastroschisis by avoiding labor, the conclusions must be taken tentatively because the study has a number of limitations.

•First, the cases were not randomized in a prospective manner.

°Although the birth-to-operation interval was similar in both groups, it is possible the higher proportion of neonatal transport babies in the vaginal delivery group made a difference in the outcome.

•Second, because the number of cases is small, it is possible that including a larger number of cases might alter the outcomes.

°The finding of statistically significant differences between the groups in spite of small numbers argues against this.

•Last, the retrospective nature of the data collection makes some assessment parameters less firm than could be identified in a prospective study.

•The final answer to the question of optimal delivery management of the gastroschisis pregnancy awaits a randomized, prospective study.]

46. Sources of amniotic fluid platelet activating factor include

   1. fetal lung.
   2. fetal liver.
   3. fetal kidney.
   4. maternal macrophages.

p. 531 Ans: B (Narahara H, Johnston J M. Effects of endotoxins and cytokines on the secretion of platelet-activating factor-acetylhydrolase by human decidual macrophages. Am J Obstet Gynec 1993; 169:531)

46. [F & I: •Background: Platelet-activating factor (1-O-alkyl-2-acetyl-sn-glycero-3-phosphocholine, PAF) is involved in ovulation, sperm motility, implantation, fetal lung maturation, and initiation and maintenance of parturition.

•PAF is increased in amniotic fluid obtained from women in labor.

•The origin of PAF in amniotic fluid is thought to be fetal lung and kidney.

•PAF stimulates prostaglandin E2 production in fetal membranes.

•PAF is one of the most potent stimuli of uterine myometrial contraction.

•PAF receptors are in human myometrium and at concentrations between 10^{-12} to 10^{-10} mol/l it stimulates Ca^{2+} uptake and myosin light-chain phosphorylation in isolated human myometrial cells.

•PAF metabolism in fetal and maternal compartments may be important throughout gestation.

•PAF is metabolized to ethanolamine plasmalogens, a rich source of arachidonate, in amnion tissue.

•At term in labor the arachidonate released from this lipid fraction by a phospholipase A2 could be used in the formation of eicosanoids.

•The resulting lysoplasmalogens might stimulate PAF synthesis by the transacylation reaction of the remodeling pathway.

•Inactivation of PAF by the enzyme PAF-acetylhydrolase provides another regulation of PAF metabolism.

•During the latter stages of pregnancy PAF-acetylhydrolase activity is significantly decreased in maternal plasma.

•The decrease in PAF-acetylhydrolase in maternal plasma occurs at a time when certain fetal tissues (e.g., the fetal lung and kidney) have an increased capacity for PAF biosynthesis.

•The source of the plasma PAF-acetylhydrolase is thought to be the liver, the macrophages, or both.

•Human peripheral blood-derived macrophages secrete PAF-acetylhydrolase activity of the plasma type.

•The enzyme is secreted by human decidual macrophages and there may be autocrine or paracrine regulation of PAF concentration in the decidual tissue.

•Gram-negative organisms elicit an inflammatory reaction that is largely induced by one of their cell wall constitutents, endotoxin (lipopolysaccharide).

- Lipopolysaccharide potently activates cells in the monocyte-macrophage system, resulting in the production of inflammatory mediators like tumor necrosis factor (TNF), interleukin-1 (IL-1), and eicosanoids.

- PAF is a key mediator of the inflammatory reaction caused by lipopolysaccharide.

- Evidence to date suggests that lipopolysaccharide, cytokines, eicosanoids, and PAF are involved in preterm delivery or premature rupture of membranes associated with bacterial infections.

- Objective: To define the mechanism of PAF action and clarify further the role of PAF in parturition, preterm labor, and premature rupture of membranes, by inverstigating the effects of lipopolysaccharide and cytokines on PAF-acetylhydrolase secretion by decidual macrophages.

- Bacterial endotoxins induce the release of host mediators, including TNF-α, interleukins, interferons, colony-stimulating factors, arachidonate metabolites (eicosanoids), and PAF.

- Host mediators released from activated decidual monocytes and macrophages by endotoxins may initiate labor associated with infection.

- PAF is present in the amniotic fluid of women at term and in labor but only present in trace quantities in women at term and not in labor.

- PAF is present in the amniotic fluid of women with preterm labor and premature rupture of membranes.

- In view of these observations, PAF may be elevated at the fetalmaternal interface in response to bacterial infections that lead to preterm labor or premature rupture of membranes.

- PAF metabolism in the fetal membranes, especially in amnion, may be important to regulate eicosanoids and PAF concentrations.

    ° This is true, because PAF in the amniotic fluid may be metabolized to ethanolamine plasmalogens, a rich source for arachidonate in amnion.

    ° This lipid fraction might be formed in increased amounts in the tissue before labor, as PAF of fetal lung and kidney origin increases.

- At term in labor arachidonate released from the storage of the lipid fraction by a phospholipase A2 could be used for eicosanoid formation.

- The resulting lysoplasmalogens might stimulate PAF synthesis through the transacylation reaction of the remodeling pathway.

- Thus the increased production of eicosanoids and PAF would be closely related.

- The inactivation of PAF produced in the fetal and maternal compartments before its contact with the myometrium would also be of considerable importance, because PAF is a potent stimulator of myometrial contraction.

- Decidua may be the tissue site of the PAF inactivation.

- PAF produced in the fetal and maternal compartments would be inactivated by maternal plasma PAF-acetylhydrolase because of its abundant blood supply, thus preventing PAF from reaching the myometrium.

- Besides the PAF inactivation by plasma PAF-acetylhydrolase in the decidua, a local regulatory mechanism may control the autocrine or paracrine action of PAF, in which PAF-acetylhydrolase secreted by decidual macrophages regulatres the local metabolism of PAF.

•Various lipopolysaccharides inhibited the secretion of PAF-acetylhydrolase by decidual macrophages.

•The inhibitory potency was affected by the stimulation index per microgram of lipopolysaccharide, a marker for the capacity of lipopolysaccharide to induce inflammatory reactions.

•The decrease in PAF-acetylhydrolase production by decidual macrophages may directly relate to the degree of the inflammatory responses caused by various lipopolysaccharides.

•Lipopolysaccharide stimulates the monocyte-macrophage system to induce the release of cytokines such as TNF-α, IL-1α, and IL-1ß.

•These cytokines might mediate the inhibitory effect of lipopolysaccharide on the PAF-acetylhydrolase secretion by decidual macrophages.

•The observations that the lipopolysaccharide-induced inhibition was partially reversed by IL-1 receptor antagonist or by neutralizing antibodies against IL-1α, IL-1ß or TNF-α would be consistent with such a mechanism.

•In addition, the failure of treatment with excess concentrations of these blocking agents, singly or in combination, to obtain a complete reversibility of the lipopolysaccharide-induced inhibition suggests the presence of other lipopolysaccharide-induced mediators.

•These mediators might include other cytokines, eicosanoids, and PAF, because they also act as lipopolysaccharide-induced inflammatory mediators.

°For example, in addition to the presence of cytokines and PAF in the amniotic fluid of women with preterm labor, the concentrations of an arachidonate metabolite, 5-hydroxyeicosatetraenoic acid, are increased in the amniotic fluid of women in preterm labor leading to delivery.

°This observation is of particular importance, because 5-hydroxyeicosatetraenoic acid, and PAF stimulate human uterine contractility.

•The findings that TNF-α, IL-1α, and IL-1ß might participate in the lipopolysaccharide-induced inhibition of PAF-acetylhydrolase secretion directed examination of the role of these cytokines in the PAF-acetylhydrolase secretion by decidual macrophages.

•TNF-α, IL-1α, and IL-1ß decreased the PAF-acetylhydrolase secretion by decidual macrophages.

•Antibodies against TNF-α or IL-1ß specifically and completely neutralized the inhibitory effects of the corresponding cytokines on the PAF-acetylhydrolase secretion, supporting further the specific action of these cytokines.

•The observation that the inhibitory effect of IL-1α or IL-1ß on the secretion was completely reversed by IL-1 receptor antagonist is an indication that the inhibitory effect of IL-1 is receptor mediated.

•IL-1 receptor antagonist, a naturally occurring one, is physiologically present in human amniotic fluid.

•The reversibility suggests the possible modulation of PAF metabolism by the IL-1 receptor antagonist in the intrauterine tissue: the antagonist might decrease PAF concentration by antagonizing the action of IL-1, a cytokine that not only stimulates PAF production but also inhibits PAF-acetylhydrolase secretion.

•Although monocytes and macrophages are one of the major target cells for the action of lipopolysaccharide, synergy between cell types with distinct functions should also be considered important in the induction of bacterial infection in vivo.]

47. Likely to be associated with aneuploidy in the early second trimester fetus with cystic hygroma

   1. septation.
   2. multiple structural anomalies.
   3. size greater than 15 mm.
   4. "space suit" sign.

p. 46 Ans: E   (Nadel A, Bromley B, Benacerraf B R. Muchal thickening or cystic hygromas in first- and early second-trimester fetuses: Prognosis and outcome. Obstet Gynecol 1993; 82:43)

47. [F & I: •Background: Nuchal thickening or cystic hygromas of the second trimester fetus are a congenital malformations of the lymphatic system associated with a high incidence of aneuploidy, particularly Turner or Down syndrome.

•Thirty to 70% of fetuses with cystic hygromas have chromosomal aberrations, and lymphatic abnormalities in the second trimester are associated with a poor prognosis.

•High-resolution and transvaginal sonography now permit recognition of nuchal thickening and cystic hygromas as early as the first trimester.

•Although there is a high association between abnormal karyotypes and various types of nuchal thickening in the first-trimester fetus, resolution of nuchal edema or cystic hygromas, with subsequent good outcomes has been described.

•The prognosis for fetuses with nuchal fluid collections may be uncertain and appropriate antenatal management of these pregnancies is unknown.

•Objective: To describe karyotypic abnormalities, other structural anomalies, and postnatal outcome in 71 fetuses found by sonography to have nuchal thickening or cystic hygromas at 10-to-15 weeks' gestation.

•Although nuchal thickening in the first trimester ranges between 2.5-to-4 mm, 4 mm was chosen as the limit to avoid any pitfalls.

•The pseudo-membrane in the nuchal region seen in some first-trimester fetuses can represent the normal skin surface with specular reflections but also can be confused with nuchal thickening.

•Methods: The criterion for nuchal thickening was a 4 mm or greater measurement of the soft tissues in the posterior occipital region.

•The presence or absence of generalized hydrops or any other structural anomaly was documented at the time of the scan.

•The criterion for hydrops was a "space-suit" appearance of the fetus, with the edema in the nuchal area extending over the entire trunk anteriorly and posteriorly.

•Fetuses were not considered to have hydrops if the edema was confined to only the occipital, nuchal, and upper back area.

•Results: There was a high association between nuchal thickening or cystic hygroma and aneuploidy.

•Forty-three of 63 fetuses (68%) with nuchal thickening and available karyotypes had Turner syndrome; trisomies 13, 18, or 21; or triploidy.

•Fetuses with associated hydrops (space-suit appearance) had an extremely poor outcome and a particularly high incidence of Turner syndrome and trisomy 18.

- Eighty-four percent of fetuses with generalized hydrops had abnormal karyotypes, and there were no surviving infants from this group.

- Even fetuses with normal karyotypes in this group had abnormal fetopsies.

- The smaller, nonseptated nuchal lucencies without hydrops occurred among fetuses with trisomy 21, trisomy 18, and normal karyotypes, but rarely were associated with Turner syndrome.

- The importance of fetal nuchal septations is a confusing issue because some investigators have found a greater association with aneuploidy when septations are present, and others have found no differences between fetuses with and without septations.

- **The presence of septations indicates a far worse prognosis and a higher incidence of Turner syndrome or trisomy 18.**

- **The presence of hydrops or septated cystic hygromas was universally fatal or associated with multiple structural anomalies.**

- Although the absence of septations was associated with a better outcome (36% survival), the increased risk of trisomies 21 and 18 and triploidy still requires karyotyping.

- The survivors had no nuchal septations or hydrops, suggesting that a nonseptated simple nuchal lucency in the setting of a normal karyotype may be encouraging.

- There seems to be a difference in the sonographic appearance of the cystic nuchal lucency in the first versus second trimester.

- There is a far larger number of very large, traditional septated cystic hygromas associated with Turner syndrome in the second-trimester versus first trimester fetus, although the explanation for this is unknown.

- Fetal cystic hygroma or nuchal dilatation probably results from delayed communication of the fetal lymphatics to the venous circulation via the thoracic duct, by several different mechanisms.

- Examination of fetal cystic hygroma reveals a paucity of lymphatic vessels in fetuses with **Turner syndrome**, suggesting that the mechanism for the edema is **lymphatic hypoplasia**.

- **Non-Turner fetuses** with cystic hygromas have abnormal **proliferation and dilatation** of the lymphatic channels leading to nuchal swelling.

- Although nuchal thickening is associated with a greater than 50% incidence of aneuploidy, a normal karyotype in the absence of hydrops seems to carry a good prognosis.

  ° There are occasional syndromes, such as pterygium and Noonan syndrome, in which lymphatic abnormalities of the neck can occur with a normal karyotype and may still lead to an abnormal outcome. {Noonan syndrome: the male phenotype of Turner syndrome, with short stature, webbed neck, low nuchal hairline, low-set ears, and cubitus valgus; valvular pulmonary stenosis rather than coarctation of the aorta is present.}

  ° Four cases of cystic hygromas associated with Noonan syndrome with a normal karyotype have been reported.

  ° These rare syndromes should be mentioned as part of the counseling of patients during the prenatal workup of fetal nuchal lucency.

  ° Resolution of nuchal thickening in fetal life does not represent evidence against trisomy, as nuchal lucencies can resolve even when the karyotype is abnormal.

- One of the limitations of this study is the lack of follow-up on the 29 patients who underwent pregnancy termination without available karyotyping or fetopsy.

°Of the remaining 71 pregnancies with available karyotype, pathologic evaluation, or newborn follow-up represent a large enough proportion of the fetuses with nuchal lucencies to be representative of the outcome for this abnormality.

•Until recently, the presence of cystic nuchal abnormalities was considered to signify a poor prognosis regardless of karyotype.

•These nuchal lucencies can resolve, as they did in at least ten of the 71 fetuses in this study, resulting in normal neonates.]

48. Early surveillance (before 32 weeks) of pregnant diabetic patients should be undertaken if there is concomitant

1. proteinuria.
2. hypertension.
3. systemic lupus erythematosus.
4. diabetics of at least class R or F.

p. 1824   Ans: A   (Lagrew D C, Pircon R A, Towers C V, Dorchester W, Freeman R K. Antepartum fetal surveillance in patients with diabetes: When to start? Am J Obstet Gynec 1993; 168:1820)

48. [F & I: •Background: Pregnancies complicated by maternal diabetes mellitus are at increased risk for intrauterine fetal death.

•Various methods of antepartum fetal surveillance have been advocated in an attempt to identify the compromised fetus before fetal death.

•There are very little data suggesting when testing should begin.

•Objective: To examine when fetal testing should begin in pregnant diabetic women.

•Antepartum fetal surveillance has been advocated for patients at risk for antepartum fetal death.

•This includes patients whose pregnancies are complicated by medical disorders such as diabetes mellitus or hypertension.

•Fetal well-being assessment should be started before the onset of fetal compromise.

•Recent reviews have suggested routine testing be started by 34 weeks in the patient with insulin-dependent diabetes mellitus.

•The onset of fetal compromise is variable and depends on the specific clinical situation.

•Compromise was defined as an intrauterine fetal death, a positive CST, or intervention because of abnormal antepartum fetal testing.

•Results: Forty-nine percent of positive CSTs occurred before 34 weeks.

•Intervention for an abnormal test before 34 weeks occurred in 21%.

•There was one intrauterine fetal death, which occurred at 33 weeks' gestation, before the onset of testing.

•To begin testing at 34 weeks is not early enough for some patients.

•Diabetes linked with hypertension, vascular complications, and growth retardation is associated with earlier compromise.

•In hypertension growth retardation, systemic lupus erythematosus, diabetes, and proteinuria were found to be markers for earlier deterioration.

•The combination of multiple risks leads to compromise of the fetus sooner than in uncomplicated diabetic and hypertensive patients.

•Diabetic class alone was **not** predictive of early compromise, because 32% of patients with an early positive CST and 53% of those with early intervention were class A2 or B.

•Patients with class R or F diabetes had early compromise in a significant number of cases.

•Fifty percent of those with class R or F diabetes who had intervention because of abnormal antepartum fetal testing were delivered at or before 34 weeks' gestation.

•Delivery of an LGA infant did **not** appear to be predictive of early fetal compromise; fetal **growth retardation**, when present, **was** associated with an increased incidence of intervention for an abnormal test.

•When intervention was required, it frequently occurred early.

•In the majority of cases requiring intervention because of an abnormal test, fetal growth retardation was associated with a concomitant diagnosis of maternal hypertension.

•Maternal **hypertension** associated with diabetes mellitus appeared to be a significant risk factor for the development of early compromise.

•Sixty-seven percent of diabetic patients with early intervention because of abnormal antepartum fetal testing had a concomitant diagnosis of hypertension.

•When hypertension is present, some form of antepartum fetal evaluation should be considered when the fetus is considered viable.

•For class A2 to D diabetics without concomitant hypertension, the risk of fetal compromise requiring intervention before 32 weeks' gestation appears small.

°The only three patients with evidence of fetal compromise among nonhypertensive class A2 to D diabetics before 32 weeks had false positive CSTs.

•In patients with class A2 to D insulin-dependent diabetes mellitus without hypertension or clinical intrauterine growth retardation testing can be delayed until **32 weeks'** gestation with little risk of intrauterine fetal death.]

---

49. Rapid intravenous crystalloid infusion into a pregnant patient causes increased blood flow to

    1. skin.
    2. kidney.
    3. skeletal muscle.
    4. placenta.

p. 1607   Ans: E   (Crino J P, Harris A P, Parisi V M, Johnson T R B. Effect of rapid intravenous crystalloid infusion on uteroplacental blood flow and placental implantation-site oxygen delivery in the pregnant ewe. Am J Obstet Gynec 1993; 168:1603)

49. [F & I: •Background: Maternal intravascular volume expansion is advocated to improve both the maternal and the fetal status in conditions such as severe preeclampsia with oliguria, abnormal fetal heart rate patterns, and oligohydramnios.

Obstetrics and Gynecology: Review 1994-Perinatal Medicine References

- Rapid intravenous crystalloid infusion is recommended before the initiation of spinal or epidural anesthesia for labor or cesarean section to avoid an exaggerated hypotensive response to sympathetic nerve blockade.

- Acute intravascular volume expansion significantly increases total uteroplacental blood flow in the pregnant ewe, as measured at the common internal iliac artery.

- Some components of uteroplacental blood flow do not supply the placental implantation site (i.e., myometrial flow); thus their increase would not benefit the fetus.

- Concurrent hemodilution may occur during rapid crystalloid infusion in pregnant women at term, potentially resulting in a decreased oxygen-carrying capacity of the blood, which may be detrimental to the fetus.

- Objective: To investigate the effect of rapid intravenous crystalloid infusion on placental implantation-site blood flow and oxygen delivery in chronically instrumented near-term pregnant ewes.

- The control of placental blood flow and oxygen delivery is not yet completely understood partly because of the difficulties inherent in obtaining accurate dynamic measurements of placental blood flow in human beings as well as the lack of knowledge concerning changes in maternal arterial oxygen content and their effect on placental blood flow.

- Maternal placental vascular bed may be maximally dilated at rest and thus unable to respond to vasodilatory agents.

- Subsequently, placental vasodilatation has been demonstrated in response to both endogenous and exogenous substances, namely, 17ß-estradiol, forskolin, and atrial natriuretic factor.

- Reversible decreases in placental perfusion have also been found, both actively, as in response to maternal stress, and passively, as with decreased venous return to the heart.

- Despite the importance of understanding the physiologic nature of placental blood flow, insight into the conditions under which alterations occur in placental implantation-site oxygen delivery, and oxygen delivery to the fetus, may be of greater importance in the clinically.

- In situations in which maternal hemoglobin concentration changes dynamically, with resulting changes in the oxygen content of maternal arterial blood, the determination of placental oxygen delivery is of critical importance when conclusions are drawn regarding the effect of observed changes in uteroplacental blood flow on fetal well-being.

- It is only the placental implantation-site component of total uteroplacental blood flow, not the myometrial or endometrial components, that contributes to placental oxygen delivery.

- Rapid intravenous crystalloid infusion is one setting in which both the oxygen-carrying capacity of maternal arterial blood and placental blood flow may be altered.

- Results: Using radiolabeled microspheres to measure blood flows, uteroplacental blood flow was separated into placental implantation-site and myometrial components while also measuring blood flows to the maternal kidneys, skin, and skeletal muscle.

- The data showed a 40% increase in placental implantation-site blood flow and a 23% increase in myometrial blood flow after saline infusion.

- Significant increases in maternal MAP as well as in renal, skin, and skeletal muscle blood flows after saline infusion were found.

- Because of the concurrent increase in maternal MAP, the decrease in calculated placental implantation-site vascular resistance did not reach statistical significance.

- This lack of significant decrease in placental implantation-site resistance despite a significant increase in placental implantation-site blood flow suggests that the increase in maternal MAP played a role in the increase in placental implantation-site blood flow.

- Similarly, the mean maternal hemoglobin concentration **decreased** significantly after saline infusion; placental implantation-site oxygen delivery did not increase significantly when the entire group of animals was analyzed.

- As defined by an observed decrease in hemoglobin concentration, six of the nine animals showed evidence of hemodilution after acute crystalloid infusion.

- The remaining three animals showed no change or only a slight increase in postinfusion hemoglobin concentration.

- Presumably the lack of decrease in hemoglobin concentration in these three animals was due to either (1) rapid equilibration or elimination of the infused crystalloid from the maternal circulation without volume expansion in animals that were normovolemic at baseline or (2) the release of noncirculating red blood cell stores from the maternal spleen.

  ° The latter explanation would appear to be less likely because these animals demonstrated none of the blood flow responses, such as decreases in renal, skin, or placental blood flows, typical of those seen during periods of stress.

- The group of six animals in which hemodilution, and therefore volume expansion, occurred had a greater increase in placental implantation-site blood flow (66% vs 40% for the entire group) so that placental implantation-site oxygen delivery increased significantly despite hemodilution.

- Interestingly, placental implantation-site blood flow increased in this group to a much greater degree than MAP, resulting in a significant decrease in calculated placental implantation-site resistance.

- These results suggest that

  ° (1) vasodilation occurred in the maternal placental vascular bed in response to rapid intravenous crystalloid infusion, causing placental blood flow to increase above the baseline state,

  ° (2) a reversal of a vasoconstrictor influence occurred, causing placental blood flow to return toward the baseline state, or

  ° (3) hemodilution resulted in a decrease in blood viscosity sufficient to cause an increase in vascular conductance independent of a change in vascular tone.

- With respect to the third possible explanation, the expected magnitude of increase in placental blood flow for the degree of hemodilution observed in these animals would have been on the order of 10% to 20%, according to studies of whole-animal blood flow during hemodilution, rather than the 66% increase found.

- One or both of the first two possible explanations may indeed be contributory.

- A rise in postinfusion fetal PO_2 was not observed despite the significant increases in placental implantation-site blood flow and oxygen delivery.

- There are several possible explanations for this finding:

  ° (1) The increase in placental perfusion may have caused an increase in placental oxygen consumption with no increase in oxygen availability to the fetus;

  ° (2) the additional placental blood flow may have been shunted in the placental cotyledons so that it did not reach an exchange membrane where oxygen transfer to the fetus could take place;

°(3) maternal volume infusion may have resulted in expansion of fetal blood volume with a redistribution of blood flow in the fetus, causing an increase in fetal oxygen consumption and no net change in fetal PO_2.

•The improvement seen in oligohydramnios and correction of certain abnormal fetal heart rate patterns in response to acute expansion of maternal plasma volume may be due in part to an increase in uterine perfusion.

•Fluid loading before induction of regional anesthesia may directly benefit the fetus by independently increasing placental blood flow and oxygen delivery in addition to reducing the risk of decreased placental blood flow caused by maternal hypotension.

•The beneficial effect of acute crystalloid infusion may be of particular importance in patients who have been given nothing by mouth during labor or before scheduled cesarean section, inasmuch as such patients may have a depleted intravascular volume and may be more likely to demonstrate postinfusion hemodilution.

•A single fluid challenge to has been advocated in an attempt to improve urine output in severely preeclamptic patients with oliguria.

•Patients in this clinical setting almost invariably show evidence of hemodilution after intravenous hydration.]

---

50. True statements about diabetes and vascular function during pregnancy include

1. Blood vessels from nonpregnant diabetic women produce less prostacyclin than blood vessels from healthy subjects.
2. Platelets from nonpregnant women and women with gestational diabetes produce greater amounts of thromboxane than platelets from nondiabetic women and nondiabetic pregnant women.
3. Hydrogen peroxide produces a prostaglandin mediated contraction that is larger in placental vessels from women with gestational diabetes compared to normal women.
4. Responses to hypoxia in the diabetic patient originates and changes in the production of vasoactive mediators produced by the endothelium.

p. 1619   Ans: A   (Figueroa R, Omar H A, Tejani N, Wolin M S. Gestational diabetes alters human placental vascular responses to changes in oxygen tension. Am J Obstet Gynec 1993; 168:1616)

50. [F & I: •Background: In vivo studies using umbilical artery velocimetry as a measure of the placental role in resistance to fetal umbilical artery blood velocity showed that diabetic women with poor glycemic control were more likely to have abnormal umbilical artery velocimetry indicating increased vascular resistance.

•An explanation for the reduced placental blood flow as a result of hyperglycemia could be attributed to alterations in eicosanoid production, since an imbalance in prostacyclin and thromboxane production has been observed in placentas of both women with gestational diabetes and women with insulin-dependent diabetes.

•Posthypoxic reoxygenation induced a contraction in human placental arteries and veins of women with normal pregnancies.

•This response was similar to that caused by exposure to hydrogen peroxide.

•Responses to both reoxygenation and addition of hydrogen peroxide were eliminated by indomethacin, thereby showing the contribution of cyclooxygenase products.

•A prostaglandin-independent hypoxic relaxation of these vessels was also observed.

- •None of these responses seemed to depend on the endothelium, since the responses were observed in endothelium-denuded vessels.

- •Objectives: To investigate whether responses to changes in oxygen tension observed in isolated human placental arteries and veins of women with normal pregnancies were present in similar vessels of women with pregnancies complicated by gestational diabetes.

- •To examine the effects of hypoxia, posthypoxic reoxygenation, and exposure to hydrogen peroxide.

- •To determine whether the responses observed were dependent on endothelium or prostaglandins.

- •Results: In human placental arteries and veins from women with gestational diabetes and those with normal pregnancies, reoxygenation after a period of hypoxia induced **contractions** that were significantly larger in **vessels from placentas** affected by gestational diabetes as compared with normal vessels.

- •This contraction seems to be mediated by cyclooxygenase products in both normal and gestational diabetic placental vessels, since it was eliminated by indomethacin.

- •**Hydrogen peroxide** produces a prostaglandin-mediated **contraction** that is larger in **placental vessels** from women with gestational diabetes as compared with normal vessels.

- •In placental vessels from both gestational diabetic and normal pregnancies, the contractile response to reoxygenation was similar to the contractile response to hydrogen peroxide.

- •This similarity in responses is consistent with the hypothesis that increases in oxygen tension after exposure to hypoxia result in a **prostaglandin-mediated vascular contraction** through the generation of hydrogen peroxide and suggests that this mechanism is also of importance in placental vessels of women with gestational diabetes.

- •The enhancement of contraction to reoxygenation and to hydrogen peroxide does not appear to originate from such processes as a change in endothelial cell function or alteration in the relaxation component of the response to hydrogen peroxide observed after indomethacin treatment.

- •Because similar contractile responses to reoxygenation and to hydrogen peroxide were observed in both the presence and absence of endothelium in vessels from diabetic placentas, the observed enhancement of these responses in the diabetic patient does not originate from changes in the production of vasoactive mediators produced by the endothelium.

- •Alternatively, the enhanced prostaglandin-mediated contraction in response to hydrogen peroxide (or reoxygenation) could originate from an impairment in the prostaglandin independent mechanism of relaxation in response to hydrogen peroxide.

- •This does not appear to be the cause of the enhancement of contractile responses, since a comparable relaxation was observed in the presence of indomethacin in response to hydrogen peroxide or reoxygenation in both control and diabetic patients.

- •Peroxide metabolism may be impaired at sites of arachidonic acid release contractile prostaglandins.

- •A selective increase elicited by reoxygenation or hydrogen peroxide in contractile prostaglandin production or reactivity appears to occur in placental vessels of diabetic patients.

- •Pregnancies complicated by preeclampsia is also associated with decreased uteroplacental blood flow.

- •An imbalance in thromboxane and prostacyclin production favoring the constrictive effects of thromboxane occurs in the placentas of women with preeclamptic pregnancies.

»This pathophysiologic mechanism may be present in diabetic pregnancies because, in addition to the decreased uteroplacental blood flow, there are similarities between preeclamptic and diabetic pregnancies, namely, the development of hypertension and alterations in coagulation.

•Blood vessels isolated from nonpregnant **diabetic** women produce **less** prostacyclin than vessels from healthy control subjects.

•Platelets obtained from nonpregnant women and women with gestational diabetes produced greater amounts of thromboxane than platelets from normal control subjects and nondiabetic pregnant women.

•Studies on placentas from women with gestational diabetic pregnancies showed that although there was no difference in thromboxane production, there was a significant decrease in prostacyclin production in these placentas as compared with placentas of nondiabetic women.

•The larger contractile response observed in the gestational diabetic vessels as compared with the normal vessels could be a reflection of this imbalance.

•The placental vessels of women with gestational diabetes also showed a significantly **larger relaxation** than the vessels from normal pregnant women when exposed to severe **hypoxia**.

•The exact mechanism of this relaxation is not known, although in diabetic vessels it is not mediated by prostaglandins because the relaxation was not significantly altered by indomethacin.

•Conclusions: Posthypoxic reoxygenation produces a prostaglandin-mediated contractile response in isolated human placental arteries and veins, which is enhanced in vessels from diabetic pregnancies.

•This reoxygenation after a period of hypoxia leads to increases in hydrogen peroxide generation, which appears to induce prostaglandin production, leading to the observed contraction.

•Because placentas from gestational diabetic pregnancies have decreased production of relaxant prostaglandins (prostacyclin), the increased generation of contractile prostaglandin activity may explain the enhanced contractile responses observed in the placental vessels from women with gestational diabetes.

•This increased tone generation could contribute to the decreased placental blood flow and pregnancy morbidity in women with diabetic pregnancies.]

---

51. Effects of acoustic stimulation on fetal behavior include

    1. tachycardia.
    2. increased swallowing.
    3. decreased breathing.
    4. fetal heart rate acceleration.

---

p. 549   Ans: E   (Petrikovsky B M, Schifrin B, Diana L. The effect of fetal acoustic stimulation on fetal swallowing and amniotic fluid index. Obstet Gynecol 1993; 81:548)

51. [F & I: •Background: Fetal acoustic stimulation is used for antepartum fetal evaluation to reduce the testing time by changing the fetal behavioral state from sleep to wakefulness and converting a nonreactive nonstress test into a reactive one.

•Concern over the potential risk of fetal acoustic stimulation have been raised, specifically, hearing problems in later life.

•No differences in auditory and brain stem-evoked potentials were found in neonates exposed to acoustic stimulation in utero compared with a control group.

•Auditory studies in 478 children at 4 years of age who were exposed to fetal acoustic stimulation in utero seemed to reveal no negative impact of the vibroacoustic stimulus.

Obstetrics and Gynecology: Review 1994-Perinatal Medicine References

- Fetal responses to acoustic stimulation begin after 24 to 25 weeks' gestation and manifest as startle reflex, increased body movements, decreased breathing, tachycardia, and accelerations of the fetal heart rate (FHR).

- Immediate complications including prolonged changes in FHR, variability, and activity have all been documented in response to fetal acoustic stimulation.

- Objective: To elucidate the potential influence of fetal acoustic stimulation on two immediate behavioral responses—fetal swallowing and amniotic fluid (AF) dynamics.

- Fetal acoustic stimulation is used frequently despite lack of standardization of the stimulus applied, absence of uniform nomenclature to assess test results, and limited data on safety and efficacy.

- The effects of vibroacoustic stimulation on fetal behavior include excessive movements, prolonged tachycardia, and disorganization of fetal behavioral states.

- The FHR pattern changed from 1F (quiet sleep with absent eye movements and occasional brief gross body movements) to 4F (active awake with both eye and gross body movements), which has never been observed in healthy fetuses.

- A sudden FHR acceleration in response to an acoustic stimulus may not harm a healthy fetus but could be potentially dangerous to preterm or compromised fetuses, in whom temporary blood flow changes may cause intracranial bleeding.

- Observations were restricted to changes in fetal swallowing and AF index in response to fetal acoustic stimulation.

- Fluctuations in both of these indices can be associated with severe fetal bradycardia and abnormal decelerations after fetal acoustic stimulation.

- Fetal swallowing is the major mechanism for disposal of AF and may be responsible for the progressive diminution of fluid near term and beyond.

- Seven of 17 subjects with a borderline AF index developed oligohydramnios (index less than 5) after fetal acoustic stimulation.

    ° Four of these fetuses had variable decelerations, which persisted in two and served as an indication for delivery.

    ° The increase in fetal swallowing activity after fetal acoustic stimulation can lead to a decrease in AF.

    ° These findings can be even more significant in fetuses with preexisting oligohydramnios, who are prime candidates for fetal acoustic stimulation.

    ° In these cases, intensive fetal swallowing in response to vibroacoustic stimulation may be another potential mechanism for the development of fetal compromise caused by fetal acoustic stimulation.

    ° It can lead to active disposal of AF and cord entanglement.

  » The AF index should be assessed in each case before fetal acoustic stimulation and if the volume is low, acoustic stimulation should be used with extreme caution.]

- Fact   ° Detail   » issue   * answer

52. Common aneuploidies in newborns include

1. monosomy X
2. trisomy 13
3. trisomy 18.
4. trisomy 21

p. 1524 (Evans M I, Klinger K W, Isada N B, Shook D, Holzgreve W, McGuire N, Johnson M P. Rapid prenatal diagnosis by fluorescent in situ hybridization of chorionic villi: An adjunct to long-term culture and karyotype. Am J Obstet Gynec 1992; 167:1522)

52. [F & I: •Background: Prenatal detection of chromosomal abnormalities relies on analysis of banded metaphase chromosoms.

•Such analysis is accurate and reliable for the detection of aneuploidies and for more subtle abnormalities.

•Standard cytogenetic analysis is technically demanding and can require 1 to 2 weeks to complete.

•There is a need for simple methods for the rapid detection of chromosome abnormalities.

•**Fluorescence in situ hybridization** has the potential to significantly decrease the time required to identify chromosomal abnormalities by allowing the analysis of interphase chromosomes.

•Each human chromosome occupies a discrete focal domain in the interphase nucleus.

•The idea of using interphase chromosome analysis began with the analysis of the Barr and Y bodies to detect sex chromosome aneuploidies.

•Advances in molecular biology have now made it possible to generate a variety of chromosome-specific deoxyribonucleic acid probes, opening up the field of interphase cytogenetics.

•Rapid cytogenetic assays on the basis of hybridization to cell or chromosome preparations of chromosome-specific DNA probes that can be visualized by fluorescence methods have been developed.

•A variety of probe sets were used in these studies, including

°(1) complex probes composed of the inserts from an entire chromosome library,

°(2) a-satellite repeat probes, and

°(3) composite probes composed of single-copy subclones and single cosmids and cosmid contigs.

•Considerable success has been achieved with fluorescence in situ hybridization for identification of marker chromosomes and translocations in metaphase analysis.

•In contrast, early attempts at aneuploidy detection in uncultured amniotic fluid cells had limitations caused by probe design and assay conditions and did not result in clinically useful assays.'

•DNA probe sets, that are based on cosmid contigs that are chromosome specific, have high signal-to-noise ratios, and have good spatial resolution of the fluorescent signals, allow efficient prenatal detection of chromosomal aneuploidies in uncultured amniotic fluid cells.

•Chorionic villus sampling is used to obtain cells for genetic analysis in the first trim ester.

•Objective: To report the results of a preliminary study using the probe set described above, to detect the major clinically relevant chromosomes present in uncultured chorionic villi and thereby demonstrate the potential clinical use of fluoresence in situ hybridization for prenatal diagnosis in the first trimester.

- **Results:** Fluorescence in situ hybridization provides efficient and accurate prenatal detection of the five relevant chromosomal probes in uncultured cells from chorionic villi.

- In this preliminary study the one aneuploidy tested was easily identified.

- The frequencies were determined with which each hybridization pattern would occur in normal and trisomic samples, which allowed the establishment of baseline performance criteria for the assay.

- High efficiencies can be achieved with uncultured chorionic villi used as target cells.

- Hybridization efficiency and the extent to which the hybridization pattern reflects the correct genotype are a product of probe design, hybridization efficiency, and signal detection.

- The impact of sample fixation, cell permeability, probe size, and complexity may vary with cell type, as has been shown for lymphocytes, uncultured amniocytes, and tumor tissue.

- Hybridization efficiencies obtained with uncultured chorionic villi were higher than those obtained with uncultured amniocytes.

- This result is similar to that seen in studies comparing Barr body detection in buccal epithelium and hair root cells and most likely represents the difference in analyzing a population of healthy, viable cells compared with a population of terminally differentiated epithelial cells, many of which are shed decidua.

- High hybridization efficiencies must be achieved for in situ hybridization assays to have clinical use in prenatal diagnosis because the hybridization detection efficiency of the assay greatly impacts the ability to detect the third signal in trisomic cells and therefore to accurately diagnose trisomies.

    ° If the aggregate probability of detecting a target chromosome is 0.9, then the probability of detecting two chromosomes in a nucleus is 0.9 x 0.9, or 0.81, while the probability of detecting three chromosomes is 0.9 x 0.9 x 0.9, or 0.729.

- This study shows that high efficiencies can be achieved with uncultured chorionic villi used as target cells.

- The most common chromosomal abnormalities in newborns are:

    ° trisomy 21, with an incidence of 1 in 800;

    ° trisomy 18, with an incidence of 1 in 8000;

    ° trisomy 13, with an incidence of 1 in 20,000;

    ° monosomy X (Turner syndrome), with an incidence of 1 in 10,000; and

    ° other sex chromosome aneuploidies, with a combined incidence of 1 in 1000.

- Together aneuploidies of the five chromosomes studied can account for up to 95% of chromosome abnormalities in live births accompanied by birth defects in the child, and 67% of all chromosomal abnormalities, if balanced translocations are included.

- Probe sets were designed and tested targeted to these five chromosomes.

- The same hybridization conditions yield equivalent performance characteristics for all five probe sets, allowing them to be used for multicolor analysis when combined with multicolor fluorescence.

- Probe sets for other target chromosomes could be designed, broadening the number of abnormalities detected by the assay.

•Methods that allow rapid and accurate detection of fetal aneuploidies provide additional time for thoughtful consideration of the test results and can aid in clinical decision-making when fetal abnormalities are seen on ultrasonography, when preterm labor occurs, etc.

•Analysis of interphase chromosomes with fluorescence in situ hybridization is extremely rapid.

•Given that there are two technologies for extremely rapid results (fluorescence in situ hybridization and direct chorionic villus sampling), which is likely to be better?

°Direct chorionic villus sampling has the advantage of a complete karyotype, albeit of poor quality, but most experienced centers would be extremely cautious about acting clinically on a nontypical abnormality on the basis of a direct chorionic villus sampling alone.

°Fluorescence in situ hybridization will certainly miss those unusual karyotypes, and its main question will center on the development of thorough statistics as to its reliability.

»The results support the use of fluorescence in situ hybridization technology as an adjunct to enhance standard cytogenetics, allowing accurate identification of trisomic chromosome constitution in uncultured chorionic villi in significantly less time.

°Analysis of the complete karyotype ensures that less common chromosomal abnormalities will also be detected.]

---

53. Associated with the development of peripartum cardiomyopathy

    1. increased maternal age
    2. twin gestation
    3. preeclampsia
    4. terbutaline

---

p. 494   Ans: E   (Lampert M B, Hibbard J, Weinert L, Briller J, Lindheimer M, Lang R M. Peripartum heart failure associated with prolonged tocolytic therapy. Am J Obstet Gynec 1993; 168:493)

53. [F & I: •Background: ß-Adrenergic receptor agonists (terbutaline, ritodrine, isoxuprine, or salbutamol), extensively used to treat preterm labor, may provoke maternal pulmonary edema.

•This complication develops after 12 to 96 h of intravenous or oral tocolysis and is believed to be the result of noncardiogenic causes.

•The direct and adverse effects of this therapy on the heart are less appreciated.

•Objective: To review the clinical course of 4 patients who had undergone tocolytic therapy and developed peripartum cardiomyopathy.

•Peripartum cardiomyopathy, an unusual complication of pregnancy, is of unknown etiology.

•Factors associated with the development of this entity include increased maternal age, multiparity, twin gestation, preeclampsia, and hypertension.

•Prolonged use of the ß-adrenergic receptor agonist terbutaline may be a factor in provoking peripartum cardiomyopathy.

•Other cardiovascular events associated with ß-sympathomimetic therapy in pregnancy include pulmonary edema and chest pain, which occur after short-term treatment.

•The proposed mechanisms for pulmonary edema formation include such noncardiogenic causes as ß-sympathomimetic induced **sodium retention** leading to volume overload, increased pulmonary capillary permeability, and decreased plasma oncotic pressure.

•Invasive hemodynamic evaluation, performed in some of these patients, corroborated these findings.

•In contrast, pulmonary edema was caused by a **dilated cardiomyopathy** and occurred after prolonged tocolytic therapy.

•Prolonged ß-adrenergic receptor stimulation results in receptor down-regulation in models of tachyphylaxis and heightened neurohormonal tone.

•In addition, incessant tachycardia, pheochromocytoma, and catecholamines are associated with reversible cardiomyopathies.

•In the setting of heart failure the importance of this mechanism is highlighted by the improvement in hemodynamics associated with ß-adrenergic receptor blocker therapy, which leads to ß-adrenergic receptor up-regulation.

•Prolonged ß-adrenergic receptor activation such as tocolysis may lead to both receptor down-regulation and desensitization, which mimics the ß-adrenergic receptor alterations observed in idiopathic dilated cardiomyopathy.

•Some of these women may have harbored a preexisting subclinical cardiomyopathy that was exacerbated by prolonged ß-adrenergic receptor stimulation.

»Patients receiving prolonged tocolytic therapy for preterm labor should undergo frequent clinical evaluation, with a focus on cardiopulmonary abnormalities.]

---

54. Viruses which may be responsible for triggering the development of diabetic mellitus in genetically susceptible patients include

    1. Coxackie B
    2. mumps
    3. rubella
    4. CMV

p. 1568　　Ans: E　　(Lee G, Shamma F N, Diamond M P, Lee J T D. HLA-DQß57 in Hispanic patients with insulin-dependent diabetes mellitus Am J Obstet Gynec 1992; 167:1565)

54. [F & I: •Background: In the Caucasian population class II major histocompatibility complex determinants (HLA-DR3 and HLADR4) are associated with increased susceptibility to insulin-dependent diabetes mellitus.

•Approximately 95% of patients with insulin-dependent diabetes mellitus have HLA-DR3 or 4 as opposed to 50% of the general population.

•Close linkage between DR and DQ loci previously obscured antigen contribution from DR versus DQ as determined serologically.

•With the advent of molecular analysis DQ subtypes are easily distinguished.

•There is growing evidence that the DQ locus is more important in determining susceptibility to insulin-dependent diabetes mellitus in Caucasians.

•In particular, amino acid residue 57 of the DQ ß-chain is strongly associated with susceptibility or resistance to insulin-dependent diabetes mellitus in Caucasians.

•As high as 96% of diabetic probands homozygous for a nonaspartate amino acid at DQß57 have been found in the Caucasian population.

- A single aspartate for residue 57 is postulated to confer a protective effect from insulin-dependent diabetes mellitus.

- The greatest susceptibility to insulin-dependent diabetes mellitus is presumed to be in individuals with both DQ alleles at position 57 encoding non-aspartate amino acids.

- Previous studies in non-Caucasian groups found that HLA-DR3 or 4 association in insulin-dependent diabetes mellitus does not hold across all racial groups.

- DR and DQ linkage disequilibrium also give haplotype associations that can vary depending on the population studied.

- If the DQß57 residue is a genetic marker for insulin-dependent diabetes mellitus common to all individuals, it would be an important marker for the identification of individuals who would be predisposed to insulin-dependent diabetes mellitus.

- Alternatively, DQß57 may be a relevant marker only for a particular segment of the general population; consequently, its general clinical significance would be more limited.

- Objectives: To investigate the distribution of this residue in Hispanic patients with insulin-dependent diabetes mellitus in order to better understand the influence of the DQß57 marker on resistance or susceptibility to insulin-dependent diabetes mellitus in non-Caucasian subjects.

- To determine whether the extreme homozygosity for a nonaspartate amino acid at this position in Caucasians with insulin-dependent diabetes mellitus reflected an ethnic HLA antigen distribution or whether a single aspartate would truly confer a protective effect in other populations as well.

- A single aspartate conferring protection from insulin-dependent diabetes mellitus in the Hispanic population would establish a common mechanism for residue 57 of DQß in determining susceptibility to insulin-dependent diabetes mellitus.

- Type I diabetes or insulin-dependent diabetes mellitus may be regarded as a disease expressed in individuals with genetic susceptibility after triggering by environmental agents.

    ° These environmental agents have included viruses such as Coxsackie virus B, mumps, rubella, and cytomegalovirus.

    ° Chemicals such as alloxan, vactor (rodenticide), pentamidine, and cyclosporine have also been implicated as causes.

- HLA as a genetic marker was initially identified in the B locus in 1974 (HLA-B8 and Bw15).

- After class II HLA loci were later recognized, HLA-B locus association with insulin-dependent diabetes mellitus was noted to be the consequence of linkage disequilibrium with the DR locus.

- HLA-DR3 and DR4 have an even stronger association with insulin-dependent diabetes mellitus susceptibility than any HLA-B antigen.

- DR and DQ loci linkage disequilibrium now points to the DQ locus, specifically the DQß57 residue as a marker of insulin-dependent diabetes mellitus susceptibility in Caucasians.

- In the search for a genetic marker for insulin-dependent diabetes mellitus, the pathogenesis of insulin-dependent diabetes mellitus is also being elucidated.

- Monozygotic twins are only 25% to 50% concordant for insulin-dependent diabetes mellitus.

- The combination of genetic susceptibility and an environmental trigger ultimately determines the disease state.

•Major histocompatibility complex interaction with T lymphocytes is divided into class I-CD8 T cell and class II-CD4 T cell recognition.

•In autoimmune disease class II major histocompatiblity complex molecules have strong disease association and have an immunoregulatory effect.

•In insulin-dependent diabetes mellitus class II HLA (DR/DQ) disease association implies that islet cell-specific autoimmunity is T-cell dependent.

•A theoretic model for the class II major histocompatibility complex structure places DQß chain residue 57 at the position corresponding to residue 14 of the class I α–2 domain.

•This residue is part of the α–2 domain helix that forms one side of the presumed antigen-binding cleft.

•Abnormal binding of foreign peptide was one mechanism proposed to explain the high degree of non-aspartate homozygosity found in Caucasian populations with insulin-dependent diabetes mellitus.

•Homozygosity for a non-aspartate, amino acid is likewise increased in Hispanic insulin dependent diabetes mellitus.

•The high rate of heterozygosity (53.3%) indicates that a single residue for aspartate is not protective at this site.

•Thus the location of the residue near the binding site can at best be a partial explanation of the influence of this single residue in Caucasians.

•The lack of total influence by HLA-DQß57 in Hispanic insulin-dependent diabetes mellitus indicates that genetic susceptibility for insulin-dependent diabetes mellitus is exerted by more than one element of HLA expression.

•Conclusion: Hispanic insulin-dependent diabetes mellitus, as opposed to Caucasian insulin-dependent diabetes mellitus, has a different distribution of HLA haplotypes.

°In particular, the distribution of DQ,B57 amino acid residues varies.

°A single aspartate at this position is not protective from insulin-dependent diabetes mellitus because approximately half of all Hispanic insulin-dependent diabetes mellitus in the patient cohort examined were heterozygous for aspartate.

•Low-level expression of class I major histocompatibility complex determinants was found in a small group of patients with long-term, juvenile-onset, insulin-dependent diabetes and subsets of prediabetics categorized as most likely to become hyperglycemic.

•Interestingly, class II susceptibility was not predictive of the low-level class I expression.

•Genetic susceptibility or insulin-dependent diabetes mellitus as determined by class II major histocompatibility complex association probably encompasses a variety of immune mechanisms in antigen presentation, recognition, and response, ultimately resulting in a common pathologic pathway.

•Markers such as DQß57 aspartate are only valid for specific patient populations.]

55. Associated with fetal chylothorax

1. Down syndrome
2. Turner syndrome
3. Noonan syndrome
4. generalized lymphangiectasis

p. 1295   Ans: E   (Mandelbrot L, Dommergues M, Aubry M, Mussat P, Dumez Y. Reversal of fetal distress by emergency in utero decompression of hydrothorax. Am J Obstet Gynec 1992; 167:1278)

55. [F & I: •Background: Prenatal therapy of fetal hydrothorax consists of either thoracocentesis or chronic pleural drainage.

•An improvement in perinatal survival has been suggested but has not been found because of

°(1) the lack of controls and

°(2) the possibility of a spontaneous favorable outcome, including cases of spontaneous in utero disappearance of pleural effusions.

•Without therapy the fetal and neonatal mortality in prenatally diagnosed hydrothorax is nearly 50%.

•In cases with fetal hydrops, the mortality is as high as 100%; among 13 previously published cases of hydropic fetuses managed with thoracoamniotic shunting, eight survived.

•Hydrops after in utero decompression can resolve.

•Objective: To report four cases of hydrothorax with evidence of fetal distress for which prenatal decompression was performed.

•Cardiotocographic findings have not been reported on fetal hydrothoroax.

•Severe fetal pleural effusions can be responsible for fetal distress and severely altered cardiotocogram patterns can be reversed in utero by emergency pleural decompression.

•The cases presented had common features:

°(1) marked skin edema predominating on the upper half of the body,

°(2) polyhydramnios, and

°(3) large pleural effusions.

•Such a pattern supports the hypothesis that the upper vena cava and mediastinum were compressed by pleural effusions, resulting in polyhydramnios, fetal edema and, finally, fetal distress.

•The first case illustrates that cardiotocogram alterations can occur rapidly and lead to a premortem stage at which prenatal therapy is no longer effective.

•In the three other fetuses pathologic cardiotocograms were identified at an earlier stage and the fetal heart rate showed immediate or progressive improvement after emergency in utero decompression.

•Prenatal therapy is an alternative to prompt cesarean delivery in cases of fetal distress associated with compressive hydrothorax.

•In utero decompression has two potential advantages over immediate delivery of severely compromised fetuses.

°First, postponing delivery allows a complete evaluation when it has not already been performed.

°Even when ultrasonographic findings suggest primary hydrothorax, pleural effusions may result from other causes of hydrops requiring specific and urgent therapy, such as in utero transfusion for severe fetal anemia.

°Primary hydrothorax is most often a prenatal expression of **chylothorax**; this diagnosis can be confirmed only postnatally.

°Chylothorax itself carries an association with chromosome abnormalities, mostly **Turner's** and **Down's syndrome**, for which perinatal management may be quite different.

°Chylothorax may also be caused by a variety of conditions, such as generalized lymphangiectasis or **Noonan's syndrome**.

°Differential diagnosis between primary and secondary hydrothorax may be difficult.

°A polymalformative complex could be suspected on the basis of short femurs and slightly enlarged lateral ventricles; C syndrome, which is not classically associated with pleural effusions, may be considered postnatally.

•A second potential advantage of performing decompression before delivery could be an improvement in postnatal management.

•Resuscitation of stabilized, nonhydropic infants may be less hazardous than it is for neonates born with severe hydrops and acute distress.

•Pleural decompression can be achieved by thoracocentesis or by pleuroamniotic shunting.

•Thoracocentesis is technically simple and can be a life-saving emergency procedure; the effusions tend to reaccumulate rapidly.

•Thoracocentesis may be useful in the late third trimester followed by prompt delivery before the fluid reaccumulates.

•Such management would be most appropriate in fetuses who have already had diagnostic procedures before the onset of fetal distress.

•Pleuroamniotic shunting is more invasive but has the advantage of a potentially long-lasting effect.

°It may be indicated early in the third trimester and when fetal distress occurs before thorough biologic evaluation.

•For patients who are initially referred in a compromised state, pleuroamniotic shunting should be performed rapidly along with a complete diagnostic evaluation.]

---

56. In pregnancies complicating diabetic nephropathy

    1. the fetus has hematologic changes and alterations in fetal heart rate patterns similar to the intrauterine growth retarded fetus secondary to decreased placental perfusion
    2. there is not hypoxia induced redistribution in the fetal circulation
    3. the diagnosis of fetal hypoxemia may be obscured
    4. there is impedance to flow in the uterine artery

p. 1300   Ans: A   (Salvesen D R, Higueras M T, Brudenell J M, Drury P L, Nicolaides K H. Doppler velocimetry and fetal heart rate studies in nephropathic diabetics. Am J Obstet Gynec 1992; 167:1297)

56. [F & I: •Background: In pregnancies complicated by preeclampsia or intrauterine growth retardation (IUGR) there is histologic evidence of abnormal trophoblastic invasion of the maternal spiral arteries.

•Doppler studies in such cases have documented increased impedance to flow in the uterine arteries, which may precede the development of growth retardation or pregnancy-induced hypertension.

•Hypoxemic IUGR is associated with pathologic fetal heart rate (FHR) patterns and Doppler evidence of redistribution of the fetal circulation in favor of the brain and at the expense of the viscera.

•In women with diabetic nephropathy the incidence of both proteinuric hypertension and IUGR is increased.

•Objectives: To determine

°(1) if impedance to flow in the uterine artery and or umbilical artery of pregnant diabetics with nephropathy is increased and

°(2) if these fetuses are hypoxemic and acidemic and have appropriate changes in FHR variation and Doppler evidence of redistribution in their circulation.

•Results: In pregnancies complicated by diabetic nephropathy, some fetuses are acidemic and hypoxemic.

•The fetuses have hematologic changes and alterations in FHR patterns similar to those observed in IUGR as a result of impaired placental perfusion.

•In contrast to findings in growth retardation, there is no evidence of increased impedance to flow in the uterine arteries.

•Evidence of hypoxia-induced redistribution in the fetal circulation in favor of the brain and at the expense of the viscera was observed in only one of the six cases.

•The implications of these findings in pregnant diabetic patients with nephropathy are as follows:

°(1) Worsening proteinuric hypertension and fluid retention may be a consequence of pregnancy-associated impairment in renal function rather than evidence for the onset of superimposed preeclampsia;

°(2) fetal hypoxemia or acidemia is unlikely to be the consequence of impaired placental perfusion;

°(3) the noninvasive diagnosis of fetal hypoxemia or acidemia may be obscured by apparent normal growth and failure of the fetuses to have blood flow redistribution.

•Proteinuric hypertension is a common feature of pregnancies complicated by diabetic nephropathy.

•It may be difficult to distinguish between superimposed preeclampsia and proteinuric hypertension of renal origin.

•In preeclampsia histologic studies of placentas have shown impaired trophoblastic invasion of maternal spiral arteries.

•Impedance to flow in the uterine artery is determined by the degree of dilatation of the maternal spiral arteries caused by trophoblastic invasion of these vessels.

•The finding of normal impedance to flow in the uterine artery suggests that in pregnancies complicated by diabetic nephropathy the observed worsening in the triad of hypertension, proteinuria, and edema may not be caused by superimposed preeclampsia.

• Because impedance to flow in the uterine and umbilical arteries was normal in all but one case, the cause of the observed hypoxemia and acidemia is unlikely to be impaired uteroplacental or fetoplacental perfusion.

• The fetal hypoxemia and acidemia may be a consequence of poor glycemic control.

• Animal studies have shown that mild hyperglycemia is associated with acidemia alone, whereas higher degrees of hyperglycemia are associated with both acidemia and hypoxemia.

• Another reason for the fetal hypoxemia is that in maternal nephropathy the hypoproteinemia and fluid retention are accompanied by intervillous edema and consequent impaired placental transport in the presence of normal perfusion.

• Although IUGR is more common in nephropathic than nonnephropathic diabetics, in spite of hypoxemia and acidemia antenatal fetal growth was normal and the birth weight was appropriate for gestation in four of the six cases, providing further support for normal placental perfusion.

• In IUGR the metabolic disturbance extends beyond hypoxemia and acidemia, and the fetus may have deranged carbohydrate, lipid, amino acid, and endocrine function.

• The lack of blood flow redistribution may indicate that metabolic derangements other than blood pH and PO_2 are important in the pathogenesis of this hemodynamic alteration.]

---

57. Conditions associated with nonimmune hydrops include

 1. congenital heart block
 2. fetomaternal hemorrhage
 3. twin-twin transfusion syndrome
 4. fetal hypoproteinemia

p. 1310   Ans: E   (Johnson P, Sharland G, Allan L D, Tynan M J, Maxwell D J. Umbilical venous pressure in nonimmune hydrops fetalis: Correlation with cardiac size. Am J Obstet Gynec 1992; 167:1309)

57. [F & I: • Background: The antenatal diagnosis of nonimmune hydrops fetalis remains a considerable challenge to the practicing clinician.

• Fetal blood sampling under ultrasonographic guidance is an integral part of the investigation, and its use has served to highlight the diversity of fetal and maternal conditions associated with this diagnosis.

• Uncertainty as to the underlying pathophysiologic conditions gives rise to difficulty in management.

• Numerous causes of nonimmune hydrops includes congenital heart disease, fetal infections, and association with other structural and karyotypic anomalies.

• Nonimmune hydrops is associated with high rates of fetal and neonatal loss, although successful prenatal therapy has been reported.

• Therapy usually involves the treatment of fetal heart failure or drainage of fluid collections but may include intrauterine transfusion of blood or albumin.

• Treatment has often been empiric and has not been based on the results of investigations, but with the invasive fetal investigation now available appropriate therapy can be offered in some cases.

• **The majority of cases of hydrops fetalis represent intrauterine cardiac failure.**

• Postnatally cardiac failure is accompanied by an increase in cardiac size and an elevation of central venous pressure.

- In the fetus cardiomegaly can be assessed by measurement of the cardiothoracic ratio.

- Umbilical venous pressure, which is believed to reflect central venous pressure, can be measured at the time of fetal blood sampling.

- Objective: To report the venous or atrial pressures and the cardiothoracic ratio for the investigation of nonimmune hydrops in a series of 14 fetuses.

- The pathogenesis of nonimmune hydrops fetalis is unknown and is probably a combination of two or more factors.

- The three main pathologic conditions involved in the development of hydrops are cardiac failure, anemia, and hypoproteinemia.

- Cardiac failure is the most common mechanism whereby hydrops develops.

- Supportive evidence has so far been based on noninvasive assessment of cardiac function and postmortem studies, although elevation of umbilical pressure has been noted.

- The diagnosis of intrauterine cardiac failure is made in the presence of cardiac dysfunction without evidence.

- Invasive fetal investigation has confirmed anemia and hypoproteinemia to be present in a number of cases.

- Anemia may lead to high-output cardiac failure.

- The effect of hypoproteinemia is less clear.

- Many fetuses with hydrops have reduced plasma protein levels, but the cause of this is obscure.

- Hypoproteinemia may occur as a result of the loss of protein into the extravascular space, therefore being a secondary effect of the hydrops rather than a contributing factor.

  ° Low fetal plasma protein levels would be expected to lead to a reduction in plasma colloid oncotic pressure and aid the formation of extravascular fluid collections.

- In extrauterine life cardiac failure is associated with an increase in cardiac size and elevation of central venous pressure.

- The umbilical venous pressure can be expected to reflect central venous pressure in the human fetus.

- Elevation of umbilical venous pressure in hydrops fetalis has been found.

- Results: The significant relationship between cardiac size and venous pressure provides direct evidence of cardiac failure in some cases of fetal hydrops.

  ° Only when ascites is present are cardiac size and venous pressure increased.

  ° In no case **without** ascites was there evidence to suggest that cardiac failure was present.

  ° One possible explanation for the elevation of venous pressure in the presence of ascites is compression of the intraabdominal portion of the umbilical vein.

  ° The associated increase in cardiac size in these cases suggests that this is not the primary mechanism.

- Cardiac failure seems to be one of the mechanisms underlying hydrops associated with ascites.

•There are two populations of nonimmune hydrops fetalis: those with cardiac failure and those without.

•There is a marked difference in the outcome of these two groups.

•Seven of the 10 fetuses with ascites survived, whereas three of the four without ascites died, the fourth case undergoing elective termination of pregnancy.

°This suggests a better prognosis when cardiac failure is present, particularly because therapy for some causes of fetal cardiac failure is available prenatally.

•The statistically significant relationship between umbilical venous pressure and the cardiothoracic ratio validates this noninvasive test of cardiac function, both in initial assessment of the fetus and in monitoring therapy.

•Thorough investigation of all cases of nonimmune hydrops fetalis is an essential prelude to sensible management.

•Ultrasonographically guided fetal blood sampling helps diagnose associated conditions and, when combined with measurement of the cardiothoracic ratio and measurement of umbilical venous pressure, can identify cases where cardiac failure is present.

•If prenatal therapy is instituted, measurement of the cardiothoracic ratio is likely to be of considerable value in monitoring the fetal condition.]

---

58. Platelet activating factor

    1. increases PGE2 function in the amnion.
    2. stimulates myometrial contraction.
    3. is a proinflammatory agent.
    4. is responsible for the vascular refractoriness to pressor agents during pregnancy.

---

p. 51   Ans: E   (Maki N, Magness R R, Miyaura S, Gant N F, Johnston J M. Platelet-activating factor-acetylhydrolase activity in normotensive and hypertensive pregnancies. Am J Obstet Gynec 1993; 168:50)

58. [F & I: •Background: Normal pregnancy is associated with increases in cardiac output, heart rate, and blood volume and decreases in systemic and uterine vascular resistance.

•The mean arterial blood pressure decreases to a nadir during the second through early third trimesters and then increases slightly during the last trimester of pregnancy.

•In pregnancies complicated by pregnancy-induced hypertension-preeclampsia, these cardiovascular changes are significantly modified.

•The underlying mechanism controlling these normal and pathologic changes in the cardiovascular system during normal and hypertensive pregnancies may be that normal pregnancy is associated with an increase in the production of a hypotensive agent relative to that of a vasoconstrictive agent.

•Prostacyclin (PGI2) and prostaglandin E2 (PGE2) are possible candidates of the vasodilatory prostanoids and that thromboxane A2 or angiotensin may be the vasoconstrictive agents.

•Antiplatelet therapies such as low-dose aspirin may have a beneficial effect on the severity of pregnancy-induced hypertension-preeclampsia because it inhibits thromboxane A2 synthesis to a greater extent than PGE2 production in pregnancy.

•An additional factor that may modulate blood pressure and platelet function in normal and hypertensive pregnancies is platelet-activating factor (PAF).

°This very potent autacoid is an ether-containing glycerophospholipid which at very low doses stimulates platelet aggregation, increases PGE2 production in a variety of cells including amnion, stimulates smooth-muscle contraction including myometrium, and is one of the most potent proinflammatory and hypotensive agents described.

•PAF can cause its physiologic and pathologic action at concentrations as low as 10 to 12 mol/L.

°The metabolism of PAF is markedly altered in mid- to late pregnancy in several species.

°PAF biosynthesis is increased in the fetal lung and kidney.

°Biologically active PAF is converted to the inactive lysoPAF by the enzyme PAF-acetylhydrolase.

°Plasma and intracellular forms of the enzyme can exhibit different properties.

•A decrease in PAF-acetylhydrolase may occur during normal human pregnancy resulting, in turn, in higher levels of PAF possible in the endothelial lining of the blood vessels.

»The resulting increase in PAF may be responsible, in part, for the vascular refractoriness to various pressor agents that characterizes normal pregnancy.

•The reciprocal response would likely result in hyperreactivity to these pressor agents as noted in patients with preeclampsia.

•This latter theory is supported by the observations that plasma PAF-acetylhydrolase activity is increased in patients with essential hypertension.

•These observations support the hypothesis that higher PAF-acetylhydrolase activity results in a lower plasma PAF level and that ultimately a lower PAF level could result in vasoconstriction and hypertension.

•Objectives: To ascertain (1) whether plasma PAF-acetylhydrolase activity is decreased in normal pregnant women compared with normal nonpregnant controls;

•(2) the changes in PAF-acetylhydrolase that occur in pregnancies complicated by pregnancy-induced hypertension-preeclampsia;

•(3) the effect of oral contraceptives on PAF-acetylhydrolase activity; and

•(4) whether the activity of PAF-acetylhydrolase is different between women and men.

•Results: Maternal plasma PAF-acetylhydrolase activity decreased.

•This decrease was observed at approximately 60% to 65% of gestation.

•The decrease in PAF-acetylhydrolase in maternal plasma occurs at a time when certain fetal tissues such as the fetal lung have an increased capacity for PAF biosynthesis.

•Early in gestation a limited synthesis of PAF occurs in the fetal tissues, and any PAF that escapes this compartment is rapidly inactivated by the high plasma PAF-acetylhydrolase activity in the maternal circulation.

•The decidua may be the tissue site of inactivation of PAF because of its "lush" blood supply.

•Late in gestation as PAF synthesis is increased in fetal tissues, PAF would escape inactivation by the decidua because of the low PAF-acetylhydrolase activity in the maternal plasma.

•If this proves to be the case, PAF could reach the myometrium, where is has potent actions as a stimulator of myometrial contraction.

- PAF-acetylhydrolase is closely associated with the lipoprotein fraction, that is, in the human 70% and 30% with the low-density lipoprotein and high-density lipoprotein fractions, respectively.

- In normal human pregnancy the low-density lipoprotein fraction increases <36 weeks and the high-density lipoprotein concentration increases until week 25, followed by a decrease until week 32 of gestation.

- PAF is one of the most potent hypotensive compounds described.

- The site of the increase in PAF is most likely the vascular endothelial cells because these cells are capable of PAF synthesis.

- The PAF in the plasma membrane of these cells can also serve as substrates for the plasma PAF-acetylhydrolase.

- Pregnant women with normotension and with hypertension can be distinguished on the basis of the pressor response to agents such as angiotensin II at approximately 26 weeks of gestation.

» The refractoriness at the normotensive group to pressor agents may be in part the result of the increase in the potent hypotensive agent PAF.

- The hormone responsible for the decrease in plasma PAF-acetylhydrolase activity may be **estrogen**.

- Consistent with this view is the observation that the decrease in PAF-acetylhydrolase activity occurs at a time in pregnancy in which estrogen production is increasing rapidly and the enzyme activity is low in fetal plasma, where the estrogen levels are quite high.

- Additional support for a role for estrogen in the regulation of PAF-acetylhydrolase in human beings is provided in that the PAF-acetylhydrolase activity is lower in nonpregnant women than in men.

- Further support is provided by the finding that an inverse relationship exists between plasma estradiol-17ß concentration and PAF-acetylhydrolase activity in a group of women undergoing superovulation in preparation for an in vitro fertilization procedure.

- Hypertension is associated with an increased plasma PAF-acetylhydrolase activity.

- Results: PAF-acetylhydrolase activity was similar in patients with pregnancy-induced hypertension-preeclampsia compared with the nonpregnant group.

- When the PAF-acetylhydrolase activity from this group of women was compared with that determined in a similar gestational age-matched normotensive pregnant control group, the activity of PAF-acetylhydrolase was significantly greater.

- The women with pregnancy-induced hypertension preeclampsia may have an increase in PAF-acetylhydrolase activity similar to that observed in other hypertensive groups.

- One reason women with this disease have an increased responsiveness to pressor agents such as angiotensin II and catecholamines is the decrease in PAF, possibly in the vascular endothelial cells.

- The mechanism of PAF-acetylhydrolase regulation in women with pregnancy-induced hypertension-preeclampsia is of major importance.

- Although it could be suggested that the decreased blood volume in preeclampsia may account for the higher PAF-acetylhydrolase activity, this does not appear to be the case because relationships in PAF-acetylhydrolase activity were observed with the data expressed per unit of protein or volume.

- Further support for a role of platelet-activating factor in the development of pregnancy-induced hypertension-preeclampsia was provided by the reported increase in platelet-activating factor concentration in the blood of both young and aged **smokers**.

•In addition, plasma PAF-acetylhydrolase is inhibited by a factor in cigarette smoke.

•In most instances cigarette smoking caused an adverse effect on pregnancy outcome with one exception: **preeclampsia**.

°Both in the mild and severe forms of the disease, the incidence of pregnancy-induced hypertension-preeclampsia was decreased in smokers in direct proportion to the number of cigarettes smoked.

°One reason for the decrease in the incidence of pregnancy-induced hypertension-preeclampsia in pregnant women who smoke may be that PAF-acetylhydrolase activity has been artificially lowered by smoking to a level similar to that observed in normal pregnant women.

•The combined effect of estrogens and smoking on the activity of PAF-acetylhydrolase may also contribute to the increased incidence of thrombotic episodes in women taking oral contraceptives who also smoke.]

---

59. Protein S is known to be decreased in

    1. warfarin therapy
    2. chronic liver disease
    3. seminated intravascular coagulation
    4. pregnancy

---

p. 141   Ans: E   (Tharakan T, Baxi L V, Diuguid D. Protein S deficiency in pregnancy: A case report. Am J Obstet Gynec 1993; 168:141)

59. [F & I: •Background: Thromboembolism is an important complication of pregnancy, and pulmonary embolism is a leading cause of maternal death.

•Pregnancy is a hypercoagulable state because of increased coagulation factors, venous stasis, and release of tissue thromboplastins.

•Normally, the plasma anticoagulant system of protein S, protein C, and antithrombin III counters this tendency, but in congenital or acquired deficiencies this protection is lost.

•Protein S deficiency may be a cause of stillbirth, as a result of a hypercoagulable state associated with thrombosis of major vessels.

•Protein S is a vitamin K dependent, naturally occurring inhibitor of hemostasis.

•It is a cofactor for protein C in the neutralization of activated factor V and in fibrinolysis.

•It is synthesized and released from the endothelium.

•Congenital deficiency occurs, as are acquired deficiencies, which may result from decreased production caused by chronic liver disease or increased consumption, as in disseminated intravascular coagulation.

•About 40% of protein S is in the free, active form, whereas the remainder is bound to C4b binding protein, an inhibitor of the complement system, and is inactive.

•A decrease in total and free protein S is seen in pregnancy and the postpartum period.

•The free protein S level falls significantly and progressively during pregnancy although in only one third of patients did the level fall below the normal range.

•Protein S is an inhibitor of hemostasis, and its deficiency leads to recurrent venous thrombosis.

60. Effects of ritodrine include

    1. fetal tachycardia
    2. neonatal hypoglycemia
    3. maternal tachyarrhythmias
    4. increase in maternal glycogenolysis

p. 149   Ans: E   (Collins P L, Zink E, Moore R M, Roberts J M, Maguire M E. Moore J J. Ritodrine: A ß-adrenergic receptor antagonist in human amnion. Am J Obstet Gynec 1993; 168:143)

60. [F & I: •Background: Ritodrine is a ß2-adrenergic receptor agonist widely used to treat premature labor.

•Ritodrine interacts with ß-adrenergic receptors on myometrium, causing uterine relaxation and an increase in intracellular cyclic adenosine 3'5'-monophosphate.

•Generally, ritodrine inhibits labor successfully only for short periods of time.

•This may be due to tachyphylaxis of the ß-adrenergic response system in the myometrium.

•Effects of ritodrine on other reproductive tissues may also be a contributing factor.

•Ritodrine crosses the placenta and is found unchanged in amniotic fluid in equimolar concentrations with umbilical blood.

•Amniotic fluid bathes the amnion, a presumed target tissue for hormonal messages from the fetus to affect the timing of labor.

•Prostaglandin production in the amnion increases with gestation and with labor.

•Although the specific activity of enzymes required for prostaglandin production in amnion increases near the end of gestation, the hormonal control of this process has not been characterized.

•Endogenous catecholamines and other ß-adrenergic agonists increase prostaglandin production in amnion membranes and dispersed amnion cell preparations.

•Because catecholamine levels are very high in the fetus near parturition and ß-adrenergic agents are commonly used to inhibit the labor process, investigation of the response of the amnion to these agents through the ß-adrenergic receptor-cyclic adenosine 3'5'-monophosphate (cAMP) intracellular cascade system is of interest.

•Catecholamines and ß-adrenergic agents exert their effects by binding to membrane receptors and activating adenylate cyclase through an intermediary coupling protein complex (Gs).

•Activated adenylate cyclase then produces cAMP, which binds to and activates cAMP-dependent protein kinase; cAMP-dependent protein kinase phosphorylates specific cell proteins, constituting the effect of the hormone in the cell.

•All major components of the ß-adrenergic receptor and adenylate cyclase cascade system are in human amnion.

•Amnion ß-adrenergic receptors are coupled to catecholamine-sensitive adenylate cyclase.

•cAMP-dependent protein kinase and specific cAMP-dependent phosphoprotein substrates have been partially characterized.

•cAMP has physiologic effects in this tissue, that is, to affect the production of prostaglandins.

•Objective: To study the interaction of ritodrine with the ß-adrenergic response system in human amnion.

•Ritodrine acts as an **antagonist** rather than an agonist in this tissue.

•Ritodrine inhibited the catecholamine mediated release of prostaglandins from the amnion.

•Ritodrine, unlike isoproterenol, did not cause tachyphylaxis.

•Ritodrine not only failed to stimulate prostaglandin E2 production in amniocytes but also inhibited isoproterenol-stimulated prostaglandin E2 production.

•Ritodrine is a partial agonist in a number of tissues.

•ß-receptor coupling is minimal in amnion, such that the reduced efficacy of ritodrine results in no activation of adenylate cyclase in this tissue.

•Ritodrine is widely used for the inhibition of premature labor.

•The postulated site of action of this agent is myometrium, causing an intracellular increase in cAMP and relaxation.

•There is also some evidence in rat uterine muscle that ritodrine causes a decrease in prostaglandin E2 production that could not be mimicked by dibutyryl cAMP.

•In addition to uterus other tissues in both the mother and fetus are affected by ritodrine.

•Effects on the fetus include **tachycardia and hypoglycemia** after delivery.

•Maternal cardiovascular effects such as tachycardia, tachyarrhythmias, myocardial ischemia, and pulmonary edema and metabolic effects such as increases in hepatic glycogenolysis and hyperglycemia are encountered.

•Maternal serum, umbilical vein, and amniotic fluid compartments have ritodrine concentrations ranging from 50 to 200 nmol/l after a short intravenous infusion.

•Because the fetus does not metabolize ritodrine and ritodrine is excreted unchanged in fetal urine, it is reasonable to assume that ritodrine bathes the fetal membranes in vivo.

•Amnion may be involved in the onset of labor by producing prostaglandins.

•Catecholamines increase the prostaglandin release by amnion and decidua.

•If ritodrine were to act as a ß-adrenergic receptor agonist in amnion, prostaglandin output could increase, which would oppose an inhibitory action on the myometrium.

•From these studies the effect of ritodrine on the amnion is as an **antagonist**, and the effect on amnion may be additive with its tocolytic effect on myometrium.]

61. True statements about glycated hemoglobin and glycated albumin during pregnancy include

   1. glycated albumin is increased in the first to the third trimester
   2. fructosamine begins to fall in the second trimester
   3. glycated hemoglobin of light erythrocytes is lower in the second and third trimester
   4. glycated hemoglobin of dense erythrocytes is low in the first and second trimester and elevated in the third trimester

p. 1374   Ans: E   (Kurishita M, Nakashima K, Kozu H. Glycated hemoglobin of fractionated erythrocytes, glycated albumin, and plasma fructosamine during pregnancy. Am J Obstet Gynec 1992; 167:1372)

61. [F & I: •Background: Gestational diabetes mellitus, defined as glucose intolerance of variable severity first recognized during pregnancy, occurs in approximately 1% to 5% of pregnancies.

•Because the metabolic abnormality in gestational diabetes mellitus is relatively mild and most patients are asymptomatic, screening is required to identify the disorder.

•The Second International Workshop Conference on Gestational Diabetes Mellitus recommended the glucose challenge test, a 50 gm oral glucose load, for screening.

•Glycated proteins such as glycated hemoglobin, fructosamine, and glycated albumin have been used as measurements of the long-term glycemic status in diabetes mellitus.

•There have been two practical improvements to the method of assaying glycated hemoglobin.

°First, it has become possible to easily eliminate labile glycated hemoglobin, which is directly influenced by the glucose level of the sample, to measure stable glycated hemoglobin.

°Second, it has been possible to easily measure the glycated hemoglobin of fractionated erythrocytes, which are separated by centrifugation.

°The stable glycated hemoglobin of the different cell populations, young or old, is expected to give additional information for evaluating glucose metabolism in pregnancy.

•Objective: To examine the fructosamine, glycated albumin, and stable glycated hemoglobin of the fractionated erythrocytes in pregnant patients with normal and abnormal glucose tolerance.

•In normal pregnancy glycated hemoglobin displays biphasic excursions with nadir levels at 24 weeks' gestation, followed by a subsequent slow reascension to peak levels near term.

°This change may reflect the biphasic alterations in the mean blood sugar occurring 4 weeks earlier.

°The changes in glycated hemoglobin may be due to changes in both carbohydrate metabolism and **erythrocyte dynamics**, and interpretation of this biphasic change should be cautious, because the changes in mean diurnal plasma glucose with the progression of pregnancy are small and the data concerning erythrocyte dynamics are confusing.

•Results: In normal pregnancy the stable glycated hemoglobin of the young erythrocyte fraction (glycated hemoglobin of the light erythrocytes) was lowered in the second and third trimesters, whereas the stable glycated hemoglobin of the old erythrocyte fraction (glycated hemoglobin of the dense erythrocytes) was lowered in the first and second trimesters but elevated in the third trimester.

•Only the stable glycated hemoglobin of the light-middle fraction showed a biphasic pattern.

•If the glycated hemoglobin concentrations depend only on the ambient glycemic state, the glycated hemoglobin values of every erythrocyte fraction should have a biphasic pattern.

Obstetrics and Gynecology: Review 1994-Perinatal Medicine References

- This study does not support the concept that the biphasic change of glycated hemoglobin of nonfractionated erythrocytes reflects the glycemic conditions of the preceding 4 weeks.

- The biphasic change of glycated hemoglobin is the result of the **summation of lower young-cell glycated hemoglobin in the second and third trimesters and higher old-cell glycated hemoglobin in the third trimester.**

- Glycation of hemoglobin increases progressively during late pregnancy.

- During the latter half of pregnancy carbohydrate metabolism must be influenced by many factors, such as nutritional requirements, limited activity, and hormonal changes (the rising level of human placental lactogen from the placenta, prolactin decidual and possibly of pituitary origin, cortisol, glucagon, estrogen, and progesterone).

  ° These changes contribute to decreased glucose tolerance, increased insulin resistance, a decreased store of hepatic glycogen, and an increase in production of hepatic glucose.

  ° These combined effects occur in **accelerated starvation** during fasting and facilitated anabolism during feeding which results in higher postprandial glucose levels, although fasting blood glucose is lowered.

- The significantly higher level of glycated hemoglobin of the dense erythrocytes in the third trimester is caused by these pregnancy-associated physiologic changes.

- In the postpartum period the mean value of glycated hemoglobin of the **light** erythrocytes tended to recover to the value of nonpregnant women, suggesting a sudden reduction of erythropoiesis and a slow recovery of carbohydrate metabolism after delivery.

- On the contrary, the mean value of glycated hemoglobin of the **dense** erythrocytes showed a slight but statistically insignificant increase.

  ° The survival of old cells with higher glycated hemoglobin and the sudden reduction of erythropoiesis might relatively increase older cells in the dense fraction and result in an overshoot of glycated hemoglobin of the dense erythrocyte levels in the postpartum period.

- Viewed overall throughout pregnancy, glycated hemoglobin of the light erythrocytes reflects short-term glycemic status and glycated hemoglobin of the dense erythrocytes reflects long-term glycemic status influenced by pregnancy-associated physiologic changes.

- In cases with abnormal glucose tolerance, there were statistically highly significant differences in the glycated hemoglobin of the light erythrocytes in the first and third trimesters and in the glycated hemoglobin of the dense erythrocytes in the second and third trimesters, compared with normal pregnancies.

- This suggests that glycated hemoglobin of the light erythrocytes is a prompt reflector of glycemic status in the first trimester and that glycated hemoglobin of the dense erythrocytes is a good indicator of glycemic status in late pregnancy.

- Fructosamine is a parameter of the glycation of plasma proteins.

  ° Its estimation involves measurement of the reducing activity of the serum or plasma, and it is reported to reflect blood glucose levels during the previous **2 to 3 weeks**.

  ° The assay is of limited specificity for the exact measurement of glycated protein and is influenced by many things such as the serum protein concentration, which is changed by dilution during pregnancy.

  ° Fructosamine begins to fall in the second trimester and remains reduced until the end of pregnancy.

•Fact   °Detail   »issue   *answer

°This test may be useful for the severely diabetic pregnant patient.

•Glycated albumin was measured automatically by the high-performance liquid chromatographic method with double columns.

°The method is rapid and precise and requires only a small sample (5 µl).

°Because albumin has a shorter circulating half-life than hemoglobin, the glycated albumin may be expected to reflect the short-term glycemic status.

°Glycated albumin was slightly reduced during normal pregnancy and statistically higher in the first trimester than in the second or third trimesters.

°In late pregnancy increasing blood volume accelerates albumin production, resulting in an increase of newly generated albumin, and the glycated albumin reflects the glycemic status over a much shorter period than in nonpregnant woman.

°This low level in the third trimester may also be due to the influence of the lower fasting glucose level produced by accelerated starvation.

°Although the differences in the mean values of each trimester were small, the pattern was the same as that of glycated hemoglobin of the light erythrocytes and fructosamine, indicating that these tests reflect the recent glycemic state.

°In the abnormal glucose tolerance group, glycated albumin was significantly elevated in all trimesters.

°This suggests that glycated albumin may indeed be a sensitive indicator of mild hyperglycemia.

°But it remains questionable whether this is also a good parameter to monitor the glycemic condition late in a pregnancy with an abnormal glucose metabolism, because it might reflect too short a term of glycemic status to reveal the total glucose metabolic change, which is much accelerated by other pregnancy-associated physiologic changes late in the normal pregnancy.

•The stable glycated hemoglobin of fractionated erythrocytes and the glycated albumin directly reflect maternal glucose metabolism.

•They provide additional information for the detection and control of abnormal glucose tolerance, and both have advantages in different stages of pregnancy.]

---

62. Substances with a strong affinity for collagen include

    1. hyaluronic acid
    2. dermatan sulfate
    3. chondroitin sulfate
    4. fibronectin

---

p. 91 Ans: C (Osmers R, Rath W, Pflanz M, Kuhn W, Stuhlsatz H, Szeverenyi M. Glycosaminoglycans in cervical connective tissue during pregnancy and parturition. Obstet Gynecol 1993; 81:88)

62. [F & I: •Background: Cervical ripening during pregnancy is not a function of passive stretch accomplished by uterine contractions, but rather an active and dynamic process associated with significant structural and biochemical alterations within the cervical connective tissue.

•Investigations of the structural alterations of cervical connective tissue during pregnancy and labor have focused predominantly on quantitative changes of the collagen content and the role of collagen-degrading enzymes.

Obstetrics and Gynecology: Review 1994-Perinatal Medicine References

- There are indications that other macromolecular components of the cervix, such as proteoglycans, may also be involved.

- Proteoglycans are core proteins with covalently attached, unbranched polysaccharide chains (glycosaminoglycans).

  ° The carbohydrate portion may represent up to 90% of the total mass of these compounds.

  ° In addition to hyaluronic acid, dermatan sulfate, heparan sulfate, chondroitin, chondroitin-sulfate, and chondroitin-6-sulfate have also been isolated from the human cervix.

  ° The absolute amounts of glycosaminoglycans increase during pregnancy.

- A significant decrease of dermatan sulfate has been shown, occurring before the fall in collagen content.

- Dermatan sulfate and its interactions with collagen play an important role in preserving the rigid cervical consistency in nonpregnant women and women in early pregnancy.

- A marked increase in hyaluronic acid concentration associated with increased water uptake and, finally, an increase in the concentration of heparan sulfate have been demonstrated.

- These data are based on measurements taken at only a few points during pregnancy.

- There is no information about the changes in the distribution pattern of glycosaminoglycans in the human cervix in relation to cervical consistency.

- Objective: To elucidate the role of changes in glycosaminoglycan content and distribution pattern by cross-sectional determinations throughout pregnancy and parturition.

- Results: Changes in glycosaminoglycan concentrations play a role in the structural alterations of the cervical connective tissue during pregnancy and parturition.

- The highest glycosaminoglycan level in cervical tissue samples were obtained at the beginning of labor, which coincides with a ripe cervix.

  ° This peak coincides with the appearance of a ripe, soft cervix just before the onset of labor.

  ° At the chosen time point in the latent phase of labor with a cervical dilatation of 2 to 3 cm, the maximum glycosaminoglycan concentration may already have occurred.

  ° These considerable changes in glycosaminoglycan concentrations in the cervical connective tissue at the end of pregnancy indicate that cervical ripening is primarily an anabolic process controlled by glycosaminoglycan synthesis.

  ° A distinct decrease in glycosaminoglycan content also makes enzymatic degradation probable.

- The possible relationship between increased elastase concentrations in cervical tissue and glycosaminoglycan degradation is as yet unclear.

- Proteoglycans may be a specific substrate for elastase, but can also be degraded by several other enzymes.

- Although the absolute amount of dermatan sulfate, the most important cervical glycosaminoglycan, was substantially higher in nonpregnant than in postmenopausal women, the relative amounts were nearly the same.

  ° Both groups have a rigid and closed cervix.

- Dermatan sulfate proteoglycan, because of its ability to bind in orthogonal positions at the d and e-bands of collagen fibrils, is the most important stabilizer of cervical consistency.

- Dermatan sulfate proteoglycan binds to fibronectin, which also has a strong affinity to collagen.

- These close interactions between collagen, fibronectin, and dermatan sulfate proteoglycan could explain the rigid consistency in nonpregnant cervices.

- The progressive cervical dilatation seen during parturition is associated with a distinct decrease in the absolute and relative content of dermatan sulfate.

- The rapid fall in dermatan sulfate did not occur during pregnancy, but rather with the onset of cervical ripening in late pregnancy.

  ° The loss of dermatan sulfate may facilitate flexibility and distensibility in the ripened cervix associated with destabilization of collagen fibrils.

- Hyaluronic acid, along with dermatan sulfate, is the most interesting of the glycosaminoglycans found in cervical tissue.

- In contrast to dermatan sulfate, hyaluronic acid and chondroitin sulfate have only a weak affinity to fibronectin and collagen.

- Both glycosaminoglycans are assigned a "space-filling" function between the collagen fibrils.

- Increasing hyaluronic acid concentrations weaken the affinity of fibronectin to collagen, thus contributing to the loosening of the collagenous framework at term.

- Hyaluronic acid itself has a high water-binding capacity.

- In comparison to a triple helical collagen molecule of comparable weight, a hyaluronic acid molecule has a much higher volume, which may explain the increased water content of the human cervix at term.

- Together, these findings explain the soft, swollen, and fragile consistency of the ripened cervix.

- These theoretical aspects correspond well with these findings:

  ° 1) The "space-filling" chondroitin sulfate concentrations peak at the end of pregnancy before cervical ripening.

  ° 2) This peak is followed by a decrease of dermatan sulfate content during cervical ripening, before the onset of labor.

  ° 3) At the same time, cervical softening is intensified by the increase in hyaluronic acid.

- Chondroitin sulfate is one of the key elements in the **early** stage of cervical ripening.

- Hyaluronic acid, on the other hand, is responsible for the **later** phase.

- Hyaluronic acid may trigger cervical dilatation.

- Hyaluronic acid is an endogenous inductor of interleukin-1, a potent substance for capillary adhesion and migration of polymorphonuclear leukocytes.

- Polymorphonuclear leukocytes may play a fundamental role in cervical dilatation.

- Heparan sulfate behaves differently during pregnancy and parturition.

- Heparan sulfate is located predominantly in vessel walls.

°Consequently, an increase in this glycosaminoglycan may reflect improved cervical vascularization in early pregnancy, particularly in the fully ripened cervix at term.

°The vascular system is not subject to the same degree of degradation as the tissue in which it is embedded.

•The quantitative and qualitative changes of the different glycosaminoglycans are important regulators of human cervical function.]

---

63. Clinically useful in the management of pulmonary edema secondary to left ventricular contractile dysfunction

    1. diltiazem
    2. captopril
    3. propranolol
    4. furosemide

p. 233 Ans: C (Mabie W C, Hackman B B, Sibai B M. Pulmonary edema associated with pregnancy: Echocardiographic insights and implications for treatment. Obstet Gynecol 1993; 81:227)

63. [F & I: •Background: A variety of cardiac and noncardiac derangements have been described in pulmonary edema associated with pregnancy.

•Noncardiac factors, such as reduced plasma oncotic pressure and increased capillary permeability, are often reversible and, despite causing significant in-hospital morbidity, usually do not require long-term intervention.

•Cardiac disease causes pulmonary edema by impairing either left ventricular contractile function (systolic dysfunction) or filling (diastolic dysfunction).

•These two basic abnormalities differ significantly in their specific treatment and in impact on morbidity and mortality.

•Routine clinical investigation (i.e., history, physical examination, and chest roentgenography) frequently fails to discriminate between pulmonary edema caused by systolic dysfunction, diastolic dysfunction, or isolated noncardiac factors.

•Echocardiography is a readily available diagnostic procedure that allows simultaneous assessment of ventricular dimensions, mass, and function, as well as valvular morphology and function.

•It has become the pivotal tool for evaluating heart failure and pulmonary edema in general medical populations.

•Objective: To demonstrate the usefulness of echocardiography in determining the etiology of pulmonary edema in a pregnant population and the impact this information has on the management of these patients.

•Given a patient with pulmonary edema, the clinician needs to know whether the heart is normal or abnormal.

•If abnormal, is the problem valvular or myocardial?

•If myocardial, is the problem systolic dysfunction, diastolic dysfunction, or both?

•None of the patients had primary valvular disease.

•Echocardiography is excellent at detecting and gauging the severity of such disease.

- Several patients with dilated cardiomyopathies did have functional mitral or tricuspid regurgitation.

- Conclusion: Echocardiography provides an accurate diagnosis, which is essential for rational long-term therapy of obstetric patients with pulmonary edema.

- Nearly half the time, the echocardiographic diagnosis is different from the clinical impression obtained from the history, physical examination, and chest x-ray.

- Three groups were identified, whose management and long-term outcomes may be significantly different

  ° 1) those with abnormal left ventricular systolic function,

  ° 2) those with normal systolic function but increased left ventricular mass and probable diastolic dysfunction, and

  ° 3) those with no identifiable cardiac abnormality ("noncardiogenic").

- Pulmonary edema occurs when the forces favoring fluid retention within the pulmonary intravascular space (plasma oncotic pressure and interstitial hydrostatic pressure) are overwhelmed by those driving fluid from the vascular to the interstitial space (pulmonary capillary hydrostatic pressure and interstitial oncotic pressure).

- Accordingly, decreases in plasma oncotic pressure by relative (dilutional) or absolute reduction of plasma colloids, transfer of plasma colloid to the interstitial space (capillary leak), or increases in capillary hydrostatic pressure (volume expansion or cardiac dysfunction) are frequently causative, singly or in combination.

- All have been implicated in the genesis of pulmonary edema associated with pregnancy.

- Heart failure and pulmonary edema due to primary cardiac disease are mediated by impaired left ventricular systolic (contractile) function.

- Reduced systolic function results in incomplete left ventricular emptying, elevated left ventricular end-diastolic pressure, and ultimately increased pulmonary capillary hydrostatic pressure.

- Over one-third of cardiogenic pulmonary edema is due to abnormal left ventricular diastolic filling with normal or even hyperdynamic systolic function.

  ° In these cases, increases in residual left atrial volume raise the left atrial pressure, which is in turn transmitted to the pulmonary capillary bed.

  ° Impaired filling may be due to impaired ventricular relaxation in early diastole, reduced myocardial compliance (the "stiff heart" syndrome), or a combination of the two.

  ° Isolated diastolic dysfunction in particular has been associated with the hypertrophic cardiomyopathies.

- Based on echocardiographic classification, the largest group (group 1: 42%) consisted of patients with impaired left ventricular systolic function; all but two had dilated chambers consistent with dilated cardiomyopathy.

  ° The etiology and duration of cardiomyopathy in these patients were often unknown.

  ° A paucity of congestive and exertional symptoms have been noted in some patients despite severe ventricular dysfunction.

- Twelve patients gave a history of chronic hypertension.

° Although long-standing, uncontrolled hypertension may eventually lead to dilated myopathic hearts, it is unusual at this young age and in the absence of other end organ involvement, particularly of the kidney and the eye.

° Only two women with a history of chronic hypertension had evidence of renal insufficiency.

° Six had a prior history of idiopathic dilated cardiomyopathy and heart failure with previous pregnancies.

° Hence, most subjects in group 1 had newly diagnosed heart disease and fit the pattern for "peripartum" cardiomyopathy, i.e., all presented between 4 weeks antepartum and 5 months postpartum with no identifiable valvular, ischemic, or infiltrative processes.

° This form of dilated cardiomyopathy is pathologically indistinguishable from other forms.

• Proposed causes include immunologic mechanisms caused by autoimmunity to myocardial proteins released during viral myocarditis, or cross-reactivity with myometrial proteins during parturition.

• Whether "peripartum" cardiomyopathy is even a distinct entity is controversial.

• In many cases, preexisting heart disease is probably unmasked by the hemodynamic stresses of pregnancy, especially when associated with obstetric complications.

• Patients with heart failure due to **impaired left ventricular contractile function** have a relatively **poor** prognosis both in pregnant and general medical populations.

• Progressive heart failure and early death are common outcomes.

• Recently, enalapril or the combination of isosorbide dinitrate and hydralazine has been shown to prolong life in patients with dilated cardiomyopathy and moderate to severe heart failure.

° Institution of early therapy may slow the progression of disease in less symptomatic patients.

• Based on this assumtpion, all postpartum patients with systolic dysfunction were given captopril or enalapril in addition to furosemide and digoxin.

• **Beta-blockers and most calcium-channel agents may have significant negative inotropic effects and should generally be avoided in patients with depressed contractile function.**

• Seventeen patients had normal left ventricular systolic function in conjunction with increased left ventricular mass.

° These patients tended to be obese (mean body mass 92 kg) and had significant left ventricular hypertrophy on echocardiography (mean 159 gm^2).

° In this group, diastolic dysfunction, which is frequently associated with left ventricular hypertrophy, probably played a significant role in the genesis of pulmonary edema.

° When ventricular filling is impaired, relatively small increments in intravascular volume translate into relatively large increases in left ventricular end-diastolic and pulmonary capillary hydrostatic pressures.

° This makes these patients extraordinarily sensitive to volume loading and changes in capillary permeability, which are commonly encountered during complicated pregnancies.

• Patients with **isolated diastolic dysfunction** as a cause of heart failure have a **better** prognosis than do those with systolic dysfunction.

•Diuresis must be closely monitored because excessive reduction in central blood volume may reduce preload below that necessary to fill the stiff ventricle adequately and thereby maintain forward cardiac output.

•Tachycardia is also detrimental because it shortens the time available for diastolic filling, which is already retarded.

•Treatment with beta-blockers or central alpha-agonists is often useful to control blood pressure and to slow heart rate.

•Most antihypertensive agents, except the vasodilators hydralazine and minoxidil, have been shown to reverse left ventricular hypertrophy and may have a salutary effect on long-term survival.

•**Digitalis has essentially no role in these patients.**

•Most of the patients with normal hearts received tocolytics before developing pulmonary edema.

•The mechanism of tocolytic-induced pulmonary edema is incompletely understood.

•Augmented ADH release combined with iatrogenic volume overload will raise pulmonary capillary hydrostatic pressure and may contribute to the problem.

•Increased capillary permeability and direct myocardial toxicity have also been proposed.

•The echocardiographic findings are important in several ways:

°1) They changed the clinical concept of the disease in all 21 patients;

°2) digoxin and angiotensin-converting enzyme inhibitors were added in eight patients with **systolic dysfunction**;

°3) digoxin was avoided in six with left ventricular hypertrophy and good systolic function; and

°4) digoxin and angiotensin-converting enzyme inhibitors were avoided in two women suspected of having systolic dysfunction.

•From a therapeutic and prognostic standpoint, the patients who benefited most from echocardiographic diagnosis were the eight with unanticipated systolic dysfunction.

•The etiology of pregnancy-associated pulmonary edema is usually a combination of cardiac and noncardiac abnormalities.

•**Underlying cardiac disease, which was present in most of the patients, may be the most potent predictor of outcome.**

•Echocardiography was used to define subgroups and to tailor therapy according to cardiac structure and function.

•Extrapolation from other patient populations suggests that these subgroups have different clinical courses and that specific treatment may favorably alter long-term outcomes.]

64. Anticonvulsant drugs which induce microsomal enzymes to degrade vitamin K1 include

   1. phenobarbital.
   2. phenytoin.
   3. carbamazepine.
   4. valproic acid.

p.887   Ans: A   (Cornelissen M, Steegers-Theunissen R, Kollee L, Eskes T, Motohara K, Monnens L. Supplementation of vitamin K in pregnant women receiving anticonvulsant therapy prevents neonatal vitamin K deficiency. Am J Obstet Gynec 1993; 168:884)

64. [F & I: •Background: The activity of vitamin K-dependent coagulation factors in neonates is lower than in adults.

•Severe hemorrhagic disorders have been reported in young infants suffering from vitamin K deficiency.

•The Committee on Nutrition of the American Academy of Pediatrics has recommended that prophylactic vitamin K be administered to all newborns.

•The incidence of hemorrhagic disease of the newborn declined dramatically in Japan because of vitamin K prophylaxis.

•Newborns exposed in utero to **anticonvulsant drugs** are most at risk for vitamin K deficiency.

•PIVKA-II (protein induced by vitamin K absence for factor II; precursor prothrombin; decarboxylated prothrombin), which is a biochemical symptom of vitamin K deficiency, was significantly more frequently detectable in cord blood of newborns prenatally exposed to anticonvulsant drugs than in controls, especially if enzyme-inducive drugs were involved.

•Cord blood concentrations of vitamin K1 were predominantly below the detection limit.

•Hemorrhage in infants from mothers taking anticonvulsant medication during pregnancy can occur in spite of vitamin K prophylaxis at birth.

•Intrapartum or early neonatal hemorrhages may not be prevented by postnatal administration of vitamin K.

°Prenatal administration might be worthwhile.

•Objective: To study the effect of vitamin K1 supplementation by measuring plasma vitamin K1 and PIVKA-II concentrations in mother-neonate pairs on anticonvulsant therapy who were supplemented with extra vitamin K1 during the last month of pregnancy, and compare these levels with controls.

•Placental transfer of vitamin K is hampered.

•A high maternal-fetal concentration gradient is required for diffusion across the placental barrier.

•In cord blood of unsupplemented neonates exposed in utero to anticonvulsant drugs, vitamin K1 levels were predominantly below the detection limit, as in control newborns.

•Maternal supplementation with an oral dose of 10 mg of vitamin K, daily raised the median maternal vitamin K1 level some sixtyfold and the median cord level at least fifteenfold.

°The median maternal-cord ratio was 44.

•Other studies confirm placental transfer of vitamin K1 after supplementation of the mother, unless it is administered at least 4 h before delivery.

- Duration of therapy seems not important to the elevation of vitamin K1 concentrations in cord blood.
  - The correlations between the time elapsed since last vitamin K ingestion and maternal or cord vitamin K1 levels demonstrate that vitamin K1 plasma levels decline rapidly after administration of pharmacologic doses of vitamin K1.
- Another parameter for defining vitamin K status is determination of PIVKA-II.
- Detection of this protein indicates that not all prothrombin is carboxylated completely.
- Because of a long disappearance time, PIVKA-II can still be present after the deficiency has been corrected.
- Vitamin K supplementation abolishes the presence of PIVKA-II, so detection of PIVKA-II seems a specific indicator of vitamin K deficiency.
- Low levels of PIVKA-II have no clinical consequences, but identify which group of infants is most at risk for vitamin K deficiency.
  - An additional burden may lead to bleeding diathesis and hemorrhage.
- The current study is the first to report PIVKA-II levels in mother-infant pairs on anticonvulsant therapy with and without supplementation of vitamin K1.
  - PIVKA-II was detected in none of the supplemented neonates as compared with 20% of the control newborns.
  - The incidence was 20% PIVKA-II detectability in control newborns.
  - In neonates exposed to anticonvulsant drugs the incidence was increased to 54%.
    - Excluding medication with valproic acid, the frequency was an even 65%.
  - Except for a higher frequency of PIVKA-II detectability, PIVKA-II levels were higher in infants exposed to enzyme-inducing anticonvulsant drugs than in controls.
- After antenatal vitamin K1 supplementation PIVKA-II was not detectable in cord plasma.
  - Consequently, under these conditions all prothrombin seems to be carboxylated completely.
- Antenatal vitamin K prophylaxis will diminish the risk of neonatal hemorrhages related to vitamin K deficiency.
- Administration of vitamin K resulted in high maternal vitamin K1 blood levels, but adverse effects were not reported.
- It remains unknown what would be the best dosage to prescribe.
- The existence of elevated vitamin K1 cord blood levels and disappearance of PIVKA-II after maternal ingestion of vitamin K1 confirms that prenatal prophylaxis of hemorrhagic disease of the newborn is reliable.
- Such treatment is indicated to protect fetuses and newborns whose mothers receive medications that induce vitamin K deficiency.
- The pathogenetic mechanism by which anticonvulsants induce vitamin K deficiency is not established yet.

•Phenobarbital, phenytoin, and carbamazepine induce **microsomal mixed-function oxidase enzymes** in the fetal liver, and it is hypothesized that these enzymes **increase degradation of vitamin K**.

•The degree of enzyme induction might be higher in fetuses, which normally have low activity of microsomal enzymes, as compared with adults.

•Because fetal plasma levels of vitamin K1 are extremely low, it is conceivable that some extra degradation of vitamin K results in vitamin K deficiency.

•Which of the cytochrome P450 isozymes is involved in vitamin K's metabolism is not known.

•Valproic acid did not increase the rate of PIVKA-II detection in cord blood of exposed neonates.

°This is in agreement with the fact that valproic acid is not enzyme inducive.

•Other hypotheses by which anticonvulsants could induce vitamin K deficiency are **hampering of placental transfer** of vitamin K and **inhibition of the carboxylase system**.

•Although recommendations on antenatal vitamin K therapy may result in unnecessary treatment of many, each intracranial hemorrhage with fatal or serious sequelae in otherwise normal children must be prevented.

»Conclusion: Vitamin K1 supplementation during the last days of pregnant in mothers on a regimen of enzyme-inducive anticonvulsant medication, to prevent vitamin K deficiency in their neonates.]

---

65. Causes of hypertension developing in patients following orthotopic liver transplants include

    1. use of corticosteroids
    2. use of cyclosporin A
    3. nulliparity
    4. graft rejection

p. 899   Ans: A   (Ville Y, Fernandez H, Samuel D, Bismuth H, Frydman R. Pregnancy in liver transplant recipients: Course and outcome in 19 cases. Am J Obstet Gynec 1993; 168:896)

65. [F & I: •Background: More than 4000 orthotopic liver transplants have been performed since 1967, mostly (3000) in the United States; between 10% and 30% of recipients are children.

•The number of orthotopic liver transplants is increasing with the improving 1 (32% in 1979, 80% in 1988) and 5-year survival rates (60% to 70% in 1988).

•More often patients are able to resume a normal lifestyle, and, in spite of concern over the long-term use of immunosuppressive medication, many women are choosing to become pregnant.

•In contrast to the large number of successful pregnancies in kidney transplant recipients, only 35 pregnancies in orthotopic liver transplant recipients have been reported.

•In one such case, orthotopic liver transplantation was performed during pregnancy, with a successful outcome for both mother and child.

•Objective: To report the outcome of the 19 pregnancies that have occurred among 775 patients who have undergone orthotopic liver transplantation and propose specific measures for the management of pregnant liver transplant recipients.

•With regard to the course of pregnancy, spontaneous abortion occurred at the same rate as in the normal hospital population.

•The incidence of elevated liver enzyme activities, particularly alkaline phosphatase, is about 35% during normal pregnancy, but these abnormalities resolve in 80% of cases during the postpartum period.

- Liver biopsy was performed because of suspected rejection in three previously reported cases during the last trimester; rejection was confirmed in two and hepatitis was diagnosed in one.

- The annual rate of graft rejection in this population of 775 patients with liver transplants is 35% during the first year and <10% thereafter.

	NORMAL	INTRAHEPATIC CHOLESTASIS	FATTY LIVER
MAJOR SIGNS AND SYMPTOMS		Pruritis, jaundice	Nausea, vomiting; abdominal pain;confusion, coma; ±fever, ±preeclampsia; ±coagulopathy
TRANSAMINASE	normal	↑ 5 x	↑ 10 x
ALK P'ASE	↑ 2 x	↑ 7 to 10 x	↑ 3 x
BILIRUBIN (MG/100ML)	1.0	<5.0 (mostly direct)	10
PROTHROMBIN TIME	normal	2 x	↑ 2 x
WBC	↑ 10-15,000		↑ 20-30,000
BILE ACIDS		10-100 x	
BIOPSY		dilated bile canaliculi	centrilobular microvascular fat and cholestasis

- One patient developed severe cholestasis associated with hypertension, but this was probably caused by a coincidental association of preeclampsia and intrahepatic cholestasis of pregnancy, although acute fatty liver of pregnancy could not be ruled out.

- There were no other suspected or confirmed episodes of graft rejection, suggesting that pregnancy does not increase the risk of this complication.

- The frequency of graft impairment does not seem to vary with the time elapsing between orthotopic liver transplantation and conception.

- The incidence of clinical toxemia in pregnant orthotopic liver transplant recipients is 10% to 20%.

- Hypertension before 36 weeks of gestation was significantly more frequent in this series (27.3%) than in the general pregnant population (3.3%) and in the country (9.3%), whereas the overall incidence of hypertension in nonpregnant orthotopic liver transplant recipients is of the order of 30%.

- Corticosteroids are known to enhance the renin-angiotensinaldosterone system, and in up to 40% of patients taking **cyclosporin A**, a nephrotoxic drug, hypertension develops during pregnancy.

° Most of pregnant orthotopic liver transplant recipients were primiparous.

- Immunosuppressive drug-induced suppression of maternal antibodies that block antipaternal antigen recognition is also associated with preeclampsia.

- Orthotopic liver transplant recipients are more susceptible to various infections because of the immunosuppressive regimen.

- **CMV infection**, a frequent complication of liver transplantation, occurred in one patient in this series and caused a miscarriage.

- Patients undergoing transplantation before the introduction of screening tests of donor blood were exposed to the risk of HIV infection, which carries a rate of vertical transmission of the order of 20% to 25%.

- In this series the only HIV-infected woman opted for termination.

- The risk of mother-to-infant transmission of **hepatitis B virus** (of the order of 10%) may be reduced by the use of immunoglobulins weekly throughout pregnancy, together with neonatal immunoprophylaxis; none of the infants born to the HBsAg-seropositive women in this series had evidence of hepatitis B virus infection.

- **Toxoplasma, rubella,** and **parvovirus** infections, which are likely to be reactivated in immunosuppressed patients, were not seen in this study.

- None of the neonatal complications of immunosuppressive therapy described in the literature were seen in this series, and the infants are developing well at 9 months to 5 years of age.

- Fetal respiratory distress, adrenal insufficiency, and neonatal lymphocytopenia are unlikely at the daily doses generally administered in this setting.

- Theoretically, the fetus should be protected from the effects of **azathioprine**, a drug first used during pregnancy in 1973.

    ° Although azathioprine crosses the placenta in early pregnancy, the fetus lacks the enzyme that converts azathioprine into its active metabolite.

    ° Anomalies have been reported in seven of 110 babies whose mothers had been taking a significantly higher daily dose of azathioprine than those who had normal babies (2.64 vs 2.02 mg/kg).

    ° These are the only cases of birth anomalies among more than 1600 pregnancies; this could be a coincidence.

    ° Doubts remain as to the long-term side effects of azathioprine, particularly regarding reproductive potential and the risk of malignancy.

- Cyclosporin A crosses the placenta passively according to Fick's law, but the toxicity of cyclosporin A metabolites is unknown.

    ° No large series is available, but isolated anomalies have been reported in the offspring of 116 women who had taken cyclosporin A throughout pregnancy, although none were observed more than once.

- **Intrauterine growth retardation** has been reported in up to 50% of pregnant orthotopic liver transplant patients, and there has been one reported case of intrauterine death due to cyclosporin-induced vasoconstriction.

- Cyclosporin A levels are 10 to 20 times higher in an electively aborted 10-week-old embryo than in the maternal serum, whereas others have reported lower levels in the fetus at 33 weeks' gestation.

    ° Some of the explanations regarding the high level of cyclosporin A in the fetal kidneys and liver is that these organs are capable of accumulating the drug and are unable to excrete it at 10 weeks.

    ° Alternatively, these organs could have special receptors for cyclosporin A, and immunologic implications for the fetus need further evaluation.

- Of the 11 viable pregnancies in this study, none gave rise to preterm births, although preterm delivery has been reported in 70% of orthotopic liver transplant recipients (mean 36 weeks).

- The main causes were interventions because of maternal complications (30%) and untoward events such as premature rupture of membranes or premature labor (40%).

- One possible explanation for this difference is that the French National Health Service provides for careful management of pregnant women from 22 weeks' gestation.

- Four cesarean sections were performed for maternal complications, all after 37 weeks' gestation.

- There were no cases of premature rupture of membranes or preterm labor.

- Long-term steroid therapy favors premature rupture of membranes by weakening connective tissue and reducing resistance to local infection.

- The reported average birth weight of infants born to liver transplant recipients is low (2500 gm) because most deliveries have been preterm.

  - The incidence of small-for-gestational-age babies is 8% to 45% in kidney recipients and up to 60% in liver recipients.

  - Low birth weight is not necessarily related to liver impairment or hypertension because half the mothers of small-for-gestational age babies have normal blood pressure.

- Immunogenetic disparity between the conceptus and mother is advantageous, with bigger placentas and fetuses; nonspecific depression of the maternal immune system by immunosuppressive drugs might thus contribute to fetal growth retardation, as may undiagnosed viral infection of the fetus.

- Spontaneous vaginal delivery should be the aim.

- Primary cesarean section was necessary only for purely obstetric reasons.

  - The reported rate of 70% (40% in this series) reflects the high rate of fetal distress and both maternal and obstetric complications in this setting.

- Although most congenital or genetic defects primarily affecting the liver (mainly Wilson's disease) are rare, couples must be aware that the risk to the fetus is unpredictable given the different modes of transmission and the variable clinical expression of these diseases.

- Childbearing in orthotopic liver transplant recipients should be planned and managed as a high-risk situation at as early a stage as possible, for two main reasons:

  - 1. Pregnancy is not advised in patients with poor liver function or active viral infection.

    - A 12-month interval from orthotopic liver transplantation to conception is thus recommended.

  - 2. Couples must be fully informed of the risks to the fetus, and genetic counseling should be provided when the primary liver disease is hereditary.

- Post-transplant immunosuppressive therapy should be maintained throughout pregnancy unless liver function impairment occurs.

- Pregnancy is not only feasible but also successful in a large proportion of orthotopic liver transplant recipients.]

66. Effective in relaxing human myometrium

   1. cyclooxygenase inhibitors.
   2. ß agonists.
   3. calcium channel blockers.
   4. potassium channel openers.

p. 953   Ans: E   (Cheuk J M S, Hollingsworth M, Hughes S J, Piper I T, Maresh M J A. Inhibition of contractions of the isolated human myometrium by potassium channel openers. Am J Obstet Gynec 1993; 168:953)

66. [F & I: •Background: In spite of the advances in obstetric management and neonatal intensive care, preterm delivery continues to be a major cause of perinatal mortality and morbidity.

•ß-Adrenoceptor agonists are the drugs most extensively used in the suppression of preterm uterine contractions.

•Their uterine relaxant effects are well documented, and there is no doubt that these drugs can postpone delivery.

•Beneficial effects on perinatal morbidity and mortality are less clear.

•Insufficient tissue selectivity, with resultant serious metabolic and cardiovascular side effects, and the development of tolerance in the myometrium after continuous exposure are among the major factors limiting efficacy.

•The treatment of dysmenorrhea is also not ideal.

•Cyclooxygenase inhibitors (e.g., aspirin, naproxen) are the mainstay of treatment but are not sufficiently emicacious in all patients.

•Potassium channel openers are a novel class of smooth muscle relaxants.

•They act by opening potassium channels in the plasma membrane so that the membrane potential of the smooth muscle cell is moved to a more negative potential close to the potassium equilibrium potential.

•This potential is more negative than the threshold potential at which calcium channels open, reducing calcium influx.

•These compounds produce relaxation or inhibition of excitation of the smooth muscle.

•Potassium channel openers are being intensively investigated as potential antihypertensive and antiasthmatic agents.

•Such a group of compounds may have therapeutic potential in preterm labor or dysmenorrhea.

•Objective: To determine the relaxant properties of two potassium channel openers, aprikalim (RP 52891) and BRL 38227, in isolated myometrium from both nonpregnant and pregnant women.

•Characteristic findings of potassium channel openers in nonhuman isolated tissues are their ability to inhibit contractions to low but not high potassium chloride concentrations and to be antagonized by glibenclamide, a purported blocker of adenosine 5'-triphosphate-sensitive potassium channels.

•Results: Two potassium channel openers (aprikalim and BRL 38227) are potent relaxants of the isolated human myometrium.

•These effects were observed both in the nonpregnant and pregnant states and their actions were rapid in onset and reversible.

•The compounds were antagonized by glibenclamide, a purported blocker of adenosine 5'-triphosphate-sensitive potassium channels.

•More direct evidence for a potassium channel opening action of BRL 38227 was provided in the myometrium of a pregnant woman, where the drug increased K efflux.

•These two sets of data support an action of the two drugs to open membrane potassium channels in human myometrium.

•Glibenclamide is a blocker of adenosine 5'-triphosphate-sensitive potassium channels in pancreatic cells and in smooth muscle.

•Glibenclamide produced rightward shifts of the concentration-effect curves for aprikalim and BRL 38227 against oxytocin-induced contractions, suggesting that these two potassium channel openers have an action involving glibenclamide-sensitive mechanisms in the human myometrium, possible adenosine 5'-triphosphate-sensitive potassium channels.

•It should be recognized that glibenclamide has pharmacologic properties other than blockade of these potassium channels at high concentrations.

•Electrophysiologic studies of the human myometrium are limited.

•Electrical spike activity has been described and the properties of sodium, calcium, and calcium-activated potassium channels characterized.

•In many smooth muscles potassium channels serve to regulate excitability.

•Aprikalim, BRL 38227, and glibendamide will be useful pharmacologic tools to probe the functional roles of potassium channels in the human myometrium.

•The two potassium channel openers were more potent in myometrium from nonpregnant than pregnant women.

•Hormonal status can modify the properties of channels with which the potassium channel openers interact.

•An alternative explanation is that the myometrial samples in the two groups were collected from different regions of the uterus.

•Potassium channel openers may have therapeutic potential in the management of preterm labor and dysmenorrhea.

•Potassium channel openers are known to lower blood pressure and produce a small reflex tachycardia in human and nonhuman species.]

---

67. Amino acid N-methyl-D-aspartate receptors are involved in

    1. epilepsy.
    2. ischemic brain damage.
    3. Huntington's disease.
    4. Alzheimer's disease.

---

p.975   Ans: E   (Cotton D B, Hallak M, Janusz C, Irtenkauf S M, Berman R F. Central anticonvulsant effects of magnesium sulfate on N-methyl-D-aspartate-induced seizures. Am J Obstet Gynec 1993; 168:974)

67. [F & I: •Background: The empiric efficacy of magnesium sulfate in the treatment and prevention of eclamptic convulsions is well established.

- The mechanism by which it exerts anticonvulsant activity is less clear.

- Magnesium sulfate is clinically effective in the absence of neuromuscular blockade; implying a central mode of action.

- Magnesium sulfate does have central anticonvulsant activity in a rat hippocampal seizure model.

- Magnesium sulfate might exert its anticonvulsant activity by blockade of the excitatory amino acid N-methyl-D-aspartate (NMDA) receptor.

- Excitatory amino acid receptors are now generally accepted as the main transmitter receptors mediating synaptic excitation in the mammalian central nervous system.

- The NMDA receptor serves as an amplifier of excitatory synaptic responses, such that a small input in the proper circumstance can lead to a large response.

- There is also a body of evidence that suggests that the NMDA receptor is involved in the pathophysiologic characteristics of a variety of neurologic disorders, including epilepsy, ischemic brain damage, and possibly neurodegenerative disorders such as Huntington's and Alzheimer's disease.

- Objective: To evaluate magnesium sulfate's ability to inhibit seizure activity resulting from direct injection of NMDA into the rat hippocampus, an area with a low seizure threshold and one of the highest concentrations of NMDA receptors in the brain.

- Results: Magnesium sulfate's anticonvulsant activity may be partially mediated by suppression of NMDA receptor activation.

- The NMDA receptor has been identified as one of the excitatory amino acid receptors that, when stimulated, can lead to electroencephalographic seizures and tonicclonic convulsions.

- Magnesium under a variety of experimental conditions has an inhibitory action on activation of the NMDA receptor.

- In this model of NMDA-induced seizures both peripheral and direct intracranial administration of magnesium sulfate prolonged the time of onset to seizure activity.

- In 40% of those animals treated with magnesium sulfate, no seizure activity occurred after administration of NMDA.

- This is in contrast to the saline solution control group in which all animals had seizures and 30% of the animals had status epilepticus-type seizures.

- Investigations that used hyperbaric oxygen to induce seizures have also shown a protective effect of magnesium sulfate injections.

  ° The anticonvulsant efficacy in eclampsia may be mediated through NMDA receptor suppression.

  ° The results of the current study are consistent with that suggestion.

- Excitatory amino acid receptors consist of at least five subtypes, three of which (NMDA, kainate, and AMPA [a-amino-3-hydroxy-5-methyl-4-isoxazole propionic acid]) incorporate a nonspecific cation channel within the receptor complex, which is permeable to both Na^+ and $K+$.

- The NMDA receptor is also permeable to Ca^{++}.

- One proposed mechanism for magnesium's suppressive action on the NMDA receptor is that $Mg++$ enters the channel and blocks the passage of more permeable ions, such as Ca^{++}, in a voltage dependent manner.

• Magnesium sulfate's central anticonvulsant effect may extend beyond just simple suppression of the postsynaptic NMDA receptor.

• A second possibility is that Mg^{++} competes with Ca^{++} uptake presynaptically, reducing calcium-dependent neurotransmitter release.

• This generalized inhibition of neurotransmitter release could also account for magnesium's anticonvulsant effects.

• A recent study of chronic NMDA receptor blockade in hippocampal cultures identified an undesirable homeostatic effect.

° After a several-week exposure followed by sudden withdrawal of NMDA receptor blockers, neurons underwent intense seizure activity and many subsequently died.]

---

68. The tachyphylaxis that occurs with ritodrine infusion during the treatment of preterm labor is secondary to

    1. decline in ß2-receptor density
    2. production of $PGF2\alpha$
    3. uncoupling of the receptor with adenylyl cyclase
    4. production of PGE

---

p. 325   Ans: A   (Rauk P N, Laifer S A. The prostaglandin synthesis inhibitor ketoralac blocks ritodrine-stimulated production of prostaglandin $F2\alpha$ in pregnant sheep. Obstet Gynecol 1993; 81:323)

68. [F & I: • Background: The effectiveness of ritodrine as a labor-inhibiting drug is limited by the tachyphylaxis that occurs with continuous infusion.

• Mechanisms for the loss of the relaxing properties of ritodrine have largely concerned on the ß-adrenergic receptor signaling system.

• Tachyphylaxis may result from the local production of uterotonic mediators, e.g., prostaglandins (PGs), which by stimulating uterine contractions oppose the relaxing properties of ritodrine.

• Ritodrine infusion to pregnant sheep increases uteroplacental production of $PGF2\alpha$.

• Prostaglandin $F2\alpha$ is a potent uterine stimulant, and is the predominant PG released into the maternal plasma during cortisol-induced labor in sheep.

• If the release of $PGF2\alpha$ contributes to ritodrine tachyphylaxis, then blocking PG synthesis might preserve the relaxing properties of ritodrine.

• Objective: To determine whether infusion of the PG synthesis inhibitor **ketorolac** would block ritodrine-induced production of $PGF2\alpha$ when the two agents were administered in combination to pregnant sheep.

• Results: An increase in uterine venous $PGF2\alpha$, concentrations during ritodrine infusion in the pregnant sheep was found.

• This increase is completely blocked by concurrent systemic infusion of the PG synthesis inhibitor ketorolac.

• ß-adrenergic agonists used to relax the uterine muscle may paradoxically stimulate production of stimulatory PGs.

• Previous studies using pregnant sheep have shown that inhibition of contractions during ritodrine infusion is lost by 24 h.

°The elevation in uterine venous PGF2 concentrations that observed at 1 to 4 h may be unrelated to the tachyphylaxis that has been observed at 24 h.

•PGF2, concentrations remain elevated after 24 h of continuous ritodrine infusion.

°Prostaglandin F2 concentrations also returned to baseline values within 24 h of discontinuation of the infusion.

°The concurrent infusion of ketorolac continued to inhibit PGF2α synthesis at 24 h.

•Beta-adrenergic agonists such as ritodrine act by interacting with membrane ß-receptors.

•The agonist-receptor complex physically couples to a guanine nucleotide-binding protein, leading to activation of adenylyl cyclase and generation of cyclic adenosine monophosphate.

•Cyclic adenosine monophosphate mediates smooth-muscle relaxation.

•The guanine nucleotide-binding protein exists as a heterotrimer of alpha (α), beta (ß), and gamma (γ) subunits.

•The guanine triphosphate-bound α subunit stimulates adenylyl cyclase.

•In cardiac muscle, retina, and neuronal tissue the ßγ complex can stimulate phospholipase A2, which results in the release of arachidonic acid from membrane glycerophospholipids.

•Arachidonic acid can then be metabolized by cyclooxygenase to PGs.

•In this model, ß-adrenergic agonists could lead to PG production through stimulation of phospholipases and mobilization of arachidonic acid.

°Arachidonic acid, released from astrocytoma cells after isoproterenol treatment, is completely blocked by mepacrine, a phospholipase A2 inhibitor.

°The precise tissue of origin of PGF2α production cannot be determined.

°In human and ovine tissues both amnion and decidua produce PGE and PGF after ß-adrenergic stimulation.

°It is likely that ketorolac blocks uteroplacental production of PGF2α by inhibiting cyclooxygenase in these tissues.

•Recent evidence indicates that although prolonged infusion of ritodrine to pregnant sheep results in a decline in ß-receptor density and an uncoupling of the receptor with adenylyl cyclase, these changes may not correlate with loss of contraction inhibition

•Stimulatory PGs such as PGF2α, may underlie the tachyphylaxis associated with prolonged ß-agonist infusions.

°Several studies have indicated that inhibition of PG synthesis prevents tachyphylaxis to ß-agonists.

°In rat myometrium, flurbiprofen enhances the contraction inhibitory response to salbutamol.

°Indomethacin blocks isoproterenol-stimulated PGE2 production in guinea pig bronchial smooth muscle and prevents tachyphylaxis.

°Indomethacin also restores adenylyl cyclase activity.

»The results of this study may have important implications for the treatment of preterm labor in humans.

•If ritodrine stimulates uteroplacental PG production in humans as it does in sheep, then inhibition of PG production may improve the efficacy of ritodrine.

•A regimen combining ritodrine with a PG synthesis inhibitor may reduce the tachyphylaxis observed in humans with ß-agonist tocolysis.]

69.　Changes which accompany preeclampsia include

　　1.　altered platelet membrane function
　　2.　reduced antioxidant systems in red blood cells
　　3.　endothelial cell dysfunction
　　4.　platelet aggregation

---

p. 339　　Ans: E　　(Garzetti G C, Tranquilli A L. Cugini A M, Mazzanti L, Cester N, Romanini C. Altered lipid composition, increased lipid peroxidation, and altered fluidity of the membrane as evidence of platelet damage in preeclampsia. Obstet Gynecol 1993; 81:337)

69. [F & I: •Background: Fluidity is a chemical-physical property of the cell membrane that favors cell functions such as cation and substance transport, enzymatic activities deformability, and aggregation.

•Membrane fluidity is dependent on the amount of phospholipids and unsaturated fatty acids, and is inversely related to the amount of cholesterol and saturated fatty acids in the phospholipids.

•Cell aging and different stresses cause oxidation of membrane lipids, altering membrane fluidity and function.

•Unsaturated fatty acids are the larger substrate for oxidation and for thromboxane synthesis, whereas peroxides deriving from lipid oxidation in the membrane may inhibit prostacyclin synthesis.

•An imbalance between platelet thromboxane A2 and prostacyclin production has been postulated as one of the pathogenetic determinants of **gestational hypertension**, and platelet membrane function has been modified by low-dose aspirin and dietary prophylaxis.

•Platelets may be an experimental model for the smooth periarteriolar myocytes, which are also involved in the pathogenesis of preeclampsia, and hypertension per se may determine platelet lesions.

　°Platelet lesions can maintain hypertension through inhibition of prostacyclin synthesis deriving
　　from the oxidation of membrane lipids.

•Objective: To study the lipid composition, lipid peroxidation, and membrane fluidity in platelets from preeclamptic women to assess these factors in this disease.

•Results: Indicate that a structural abnormality of the platelet membrane accompanies preeclampsia.

•The significant increase in cholesterol and in the cholesterol-to-phospholipid molar ratio demonstrates a rearrangement of the lipid composition of the platelet membrane.

•This structural alteration may also account for the impairment of certain functions, such as ion transport across the membrane, that has been noted in gestational hypertension.

•The altered membrane structure can also favor platelet aggregation and destruction, increasing the liberation of arachidonic acid derivatives, which may produce vasoconstriction.

•Lipid peroxidation products, besides inhibiting prostacyclin synthesis, stimulate smooth-muscle contraction.

•Fact　　　　　°Detail　　　　　　　　　　　»issue　　　　*answer

- The vasoconstriction thus produced can worsen hypertension by means of ischemic injury to the cells and subsequent peroxidation, leading to a vicious cycle.

- The increased peroxidation should be considered in low-dose aspirin prophylaxis because its effect on cyclooxygenase inhibition, which lowers thromboxane production, may be outweighed by the direct prostacyclin synthetase inhibition exerted by the peroxides.

- The increased cholesterol concentration and cholesterol-phospholipid ratio are not consistent with decreased polarization and increased membrane fluidity, because cholesterol has the effect of increasing membrane rigidity.

- Despite the lack of change in the amount of phospholipids in the membrane, the qualitative changes observed in the phospholipid composition may offset the effect of the increased cholesterol content.

- An increased concentration of unsaturated fatty acids in the bilayer of the membrane increases the substrate for peroxidation and decreases polarization and enhances fluidity of both intact platelets and platelet membranes.

  ° Analogous fatty acid changes in the trophoblast membrane in hypertensive women have been found.

  ° Other cell lines such as periarteriolar myocytes, of which platelets may represent the circulating experimental model, may share the same alterations, thus contributing more extensively to the pathophysiology of preeclampsia.

  ° Endothelial cell dysfunction associated with pregnancy-induced hypertension may come from **oxidative stress.**

- The findings are consistent with previous observations on increased circulating lipid peroxides as a measure of the increased free radical activity during hypertension in pregnancy.

- The ultimate reason for the increased peroxidation of the platelet membrane is still obscure.

- Some antioxidant systems, such as the superoxide dismutase and the lysate thiol, are reduced in red blood cells in preeclampsia; and such antioxidant changes occur in platelets, as well.

- Pregnancy and preeclampsia are conditions of increased intrinsic oxidative stress for the cells; increased free radical activity or reduced antioxidative defenses may contribute to this.

- Whichever the cause, the involvement of the platelet membrane may confirm the role of cell damage in the onset and the development of gestational hypertensive diseases.]

INDEX

abdominal incision
    lymphadenectomy 229
abortion
    second trimester 106
    spontaneous
        donor insemination 139
        histology 81
        recurrent
            immunotherapy 136
abruptio placentae 287, 353
    D-dimer test 330
Accuprobe 361
acetaminophen 413
    pregnancy 371
acoustic stimulation
    amniotic fluid index 518
acute fatty liver of pregnancy 549
acute renal failure 285
add back therapy 122
adhesions
    colchicine 54
adnexal torsion 87
adrenal hyperandrogenism 118
adrenal gland
    steroid secretion 171
adriamycin 201
adult respiratory distress syndrome 383
alcohol abuse 467
alpha-fetoprotein 20
    congenital nephrosis 481
alphamethyldopa 496
alprazolam 413, 414
Alvarez waves 404
Alzheimer's disease 554
amnioinfusion 347
amniotic bands
    ultrasound identification 463
amniotic fluid 424
amniotic fluid index
    acoustic stimulation 518
amniotomy 346
amoxicillin 94, 107, 307
amphetamine 367
ampicillin 307, 386
aneuploidy
    congenital heart disease 363
angiography 443
angiotensin 438
anticardiolipin antibodies 355
anticonvulsant therapy
    vitamin K 546
antiphospholipid antibodies 158
antithrombin III 66, 111, 534
aortic stenosis
    congenital
        pregnancy 319
ARDS 451
argon beam coagulator 209
arsenic 367

aspirin 477, 552
    preeclampsia 367
    prophylaxis 355
asthma 411
atenolol 496
atherosclerosis 454
autoantibodies
    pregnancy 143
azithromycin 7, 94

ß-endorphin 141
ß-hCG 239 (See also human chorionic gonadotropin)
ß2-microglobulin 474
bacterial vaginosis
    treatment 11
Ballard examination 324
balloon valvuloplasty 320
bilateral cortical necrosis 451
birth defect
    chylothorax 526
    congenital nephrosis 481
    cystic hygroma 498
    urinary 474
bladder exstrophy 301
breast feeding
    maternal drug ingestion 412
breast
    cancer 34
        tamoxifen 216
    sex hormones 161
Brodhead packer 335

CA 125 192, 197
    ovarian cancer 208
calcium carbonate 7, 99
carboplatin 186
carcinoembryonic antigen 239
carcinoid 52
carcinoma of the fallopian tube
    second-look laparoscopy 182
cardiomyopathy
    pregnancy 522
cardioversion 444
Cavitron ultrasonic surgical aspirator 209
cefaclor 413
cefotetan 374
cell tissue factor 108
ceruloplasmin 66
cervical intraepithelial neoplasia 35, 89
    human immunodeficiency virus 218
cervix
    adenocarcinoma 225
    cancer
        cesarean hysterectomy 190
        flow cytometry 214
        prognosis 230
        radical hysterectomy 240
        surgery 223
        treatment 193
        unsuspected 209

cervix (continued)
    conization 28
    dysplasia 55
    glycosaminoglycans 539
    LLETZ 68
cesarean hysterectomy 79
    cervical cancer 190
cesarean section
    endometritis 338
chemotherapy
    ovary 186
chlamydia 16
    antibiotics for 94
    break-through bleeding 21
    pregnancy 304
chorioamnionitis 402
choriocarcinoma 61
chorionic villus sampling 380
    fluorescent in situ hybridization 520
    twins 492
chronic villitis 490
chylothorax 527
    fetal 526
cigarette smoking 35, 137, 442
    urine incontinence 43
ciprofloxacin 89
cisplatin 186, 254
climacteric 52
clindamycin 95, 307, 386
clomiphene challenge test 133
cloxacillin 413
coarctation of the aorta 320
cocaine 342, 355
    myometrial binding 316
    preeclampsia 366
    pregnancy 417
    presence in amniotic fluid 454
codeine 413
colchicine 54
    adhesions 54
collagen
    parturition 539
colony-stimulating factor-1
    ovary
        cancer 249
colposcopy 71
condom 140
congenital heart disease
    aneuploidy 363
congenital nephrosis 481
conization 28, 77
conjunctivitis 304
creatine kinase 442
cryotherapy 69
cyclooxygenase 371
cyclophosphamide 182
cyclosporine 453
cystic hygroma 484, 498, 510
cytochrome P450 548
cytology
    reporting difficulties 30

cytomegalovirus 298

D-dimer test 330
danazol 13, 176
    endometriosis 160
decidual vasculitis 83
diabetes mellitus 442
    Doppler 419
    etiology 523
    glycolated proteins 537
    induction of labor 314
    nephropathy 527
    preeclampsia 277
    pregnancy 374, 476
    pregnancy surveillance 512
    screening in pregnancy 295
diastolic notch 446
Didronel 100
dihydralazine 500
diphenhydramine 414
direct egg injection 164
disseminated intravascular coagulation 285, 450
DNA index 203, 247
donor insemination
    spontaneous abortion 139
Doppler color flow 331
Doppler flow velocimetry
    uterine artery 436
Doppler ultrasonography 477
Down syndrome 380, 510
    prenatal detection 387
doxorubicin 182
doxycycline 107
drug abuse 220 (*See also* individual substances).
dual-energy x-ray absorptiometry 100
ductus arteriosus
    indomethacin 302
duplex Doppler ultrasonography 58
dyspareunia 13, 49
dystocia 296

echocardiography 443
    pregnancy 542
ectopic pregnancy
    laparoscopy 51
    medical management 84
    ovarian 112
    persistent 51
    serum markers 20, 96
    ultrasound 47
electrocardiogram
    pregnancy 440
embryotoxins
    pregnancy loss 153
enalapril 544
endocervical brush 71
endocervical curettage 71
endothelin 390
endometrial stripe
    ultrasound 41
endometriosis 127, 140

endometriosis (continued)
   goserelin 13
   infertility 173
   treatment 160, 175
endometritis 21
   cesarean section 338
   postpartum 386
endometrium
   cancer
      diagnosis 195
      DNA analysis 246
      lymph node sampling 236
      lymphadenectomy 220
      risks 36
   receptors in neoplasia 250
   sampling and ultrasound 41
endothelial-derived relaxing factor 369
endothelin 377, 405, 412
endotoxin 383
enterococcus
   endometritis 386
epidermal growth factor receptor
   ovary
      cancer 258
epididymitis 304
epidural anesthesia 402
Erb's palsies 346
erythromycin 94, 304, 413
erythropoietin 466
   intrauterine growth retardation 469
   isoimmunization 482
estradiol 122
estrogen replacement therapy
   breast cancer 92
estrogens
   exercise 105
etidronate 7, 99, 100
exercise
   estrogens 105
external cephalic version 325

Fanconi anemia. 494
fecundability 140
fentanyl 107
Ferguson reflex 323
fetal hydrops 449
fetus
   distress 477
   growth retarded 436
   large for gestational age 487
   obstructive uropathy 433
   urinary biochemistry 433
   very low birth weight
      survival 324
fibrinogen uptake test 58
fibronectin
   labor 384
fine-needle aspiration 162

5-fluorouracil 220, 253
flow cytometry 214

fluidity 557
fluorescence in situ hybridization 380
flurbiprofen 556
fructosamine 538

gamete fusogens 164
gastroschisis
   cesarean section 505
   prenatal diagnosis 472
gentamicin 386
gestational diabetes
   two hour blood test 328
gestational trophoblastic disease 206
   polymerase chain reaction 60
GIFT 129
glibenclamide 552
glycohemoglobin 278
glycosaminoglycans
   cervix 539
GnRH
   ovarian carcinoma 234
GnRH agonist
   effects on pregnancy 168
   osteoporosis 122
goiter 52
gonadal dysgenesis 113
goserelin
   endometriosis 13
Gram stain 396, 424
GTT periodicity 375

hCG 145
headache
   menstrual 70
hearing loss 298
heart transplant
   pregnancy 453
HELLP syndrome 284, 503
   renal failure 450
hemizona assay 134
heparin 57
   pregnancy 151
heroin 367
hirsutism 170
   lipoprotein 120
HIV 549
HLA-DQβ57 523
HLA-DR
   pregnancy-induced hypertension 479
Holmes packer 334
human immunodeficiency virus 139
   cervical intraepithelial neoplasia 218
   pregnancy 280
human papilloma virus
   cervix 260
   DNA testing 183
Huntington's 554
Hutterites 143

hydatidiform moles
    karyotype 243
hydralazine 285, 451, 496, 544
hydramnios 329 (*See also* polyhydramnios)
3ß-Hydroxysteroid dehydrogenase deficiency 170
17ß,20α-hydroxysteroid dehydrogenase 456
hypercholesterolemia 442
hyperstimulation syndrome 150
hypertension 442
hypothyroidism 442
    pregnancy 376
hysterectomy
    radical 212
    sexuality 103
hysteroscopy 242
    post-menopausal bleeding 9

ibuprofen 414
iliococcygeus muscle 45
Iloprost 377
immotile cilia syndrome 165
immunotherapy
    recurrent spontaneous abortion 136
impedance plethysmography 58
in vitro fertilization 155, 164
    complications 148
in vitro fertilization-embryo transfer 148
indomethacin 268, 303, 357, 368, 378, 517
infertility 133
    intrauterine insemination/hMG treatment 127
inhibin 133
insulin growth factor binding protein-1 487
insulin resistance 120
interferon gamma 458
interferon therapy 220
interferons 258
interleukin-6 292
interstitial cystitis 49
intervillositis 83
intrahepatic cholestasis of pregnancy 549
intrauterine growth retardation 399
    aneuploidy 275
    erythropoietin 469
intrauterine insemination 127
isoproterenol 556
isosorbide dinitrate 544

Kegel exercise 102
ketorolac 555
kidney
    fetal
        function 461

labetalol 444, 500
labor
    active management 401
    diabetes mellitus 314
lactate dehydrogenase 442
lactation
    metabolic changes 308

laminaria tents 107
laser 68
learning deficits 399
LEEP
    toxic shock syndrome 89
leiomyomata uteri
    indications for removal 24
    progesterone receptor 90
leiomyosarcomas 33
leukemia 52
leukocyte esterase 398
leuprolide 100, 168
    endometriosis 160
LH kit
    post-coital test 22
lichen sclerosis 75
lidocaine 367, 443
lipoproteins
    hirsutism 120
liver transplants
    hypertension 548
LLETZ see below
loop excision of the transformation zone 73
    cervical neoplasia 68
Lorazepam 414
Lown grade classification 501
lupus anticoagulant 109, 158, 355
luteal phase defects 140
luteinizing hormone 63
lymphadenectomy
    abdominal incision 229
lymphangiectasia 484

macrosomia 374
magnesium sulfate 285, 390
    myometrial inhibition 349
    preeclampsia 415
magnetic resonance imaging
    pregnancy 279
male infertility 164
mammography 15
mastocytosis 52
McRoberts maneuver 270, 344
meconium aspiration syndrome 408
medroxyprogesterone acetate 7, 99
megacystis 435
Mehring denervation 74
melphalan 187, 200
menopause 52
    endometrial cancer 63
    estrogen replacement therapy 137
methadone
    pregnancy 340
methotrexate 52, 84
methyldopa 444
metoprolol 496
metronidazole 307
microalbuminuria 278
minoxidil 545
Mueller-Hillis maneuver 268, 296
multicystic kidney dysplasia 301

multiple births 129
mycoplasma
    cesarean morbidity 372
myocardial infarction
    pregnancy 440
myomectomy 80
myometrium
    inhibition by magnesium 349

N-methyl-D-aspartate 554
N-methyl-D-aspartate receptors
    seizures 553
nadolol 70
Naegele's rule 274, 420
naloxone 142
naltrexone
    polycystic ovarian disease 141
naproxen 273, 412, 414, 552
nephrotic syndrome 394
newborn
    asphyxia 422
nicardipine 429, 496
nifedipine 285, 429, 451, 496
nitroprusside 285, 451
nonimmune hydrops fetalis 529
    umbilical pressure 483
Noonan's syndrome 484, 527
norepinephrine 406, 438, 439
norethindrone 7, 99
norethisterone 122
Norlutin 100

oligohydramnios 304, 434, 461, 462
omphalocele 505
oral contraception
oral contraceptives 21
    coagulation 110
    fibrin 65
orthostatic uterovascular syndrome 403
osteoporosis 151
    GnRH agonist 99
    transdermal estradiol 116
ovarian hyperstimulation syndrome 129
ovarian masses
    transvaginal ultrasound 204
ovary
    cancer 227
        CA 125 208
        chemotherapy 186, 200
        Colony-stimulating factor-1 249
        cytokines 254
        epidermal growth factor receptor 258
        GnRH 234
        prior hysterectomy 23
        prognosis 201
        restaging 264
        taxol 256
        tumor markers 238
    cyst fluid 192
    ectopic pregnancy of 112

ovary (continued)
    evaluation for malignancy 197
    steroid secretion 171
ovulation induction 150
oxytocin 392
    nocturnal activity 321

Paget disease 100, 101
partial thromboplastin time 111
parturition 392
parvovirus 485
Pedersen-Freinkel hypothesis 489
pelvic infection 129
pelvic inflammatory disease
    detection of 18
    transvaginal ultrasound 38
pelvic muscle exercises 101
pelvic radionuclide scintigraphy
    diagnosis of pelvic inflammatory disease 18
perineoplasty 51
pheochromocytoma 52, 523
phospholipase C 406
pipelle 41
placenta
    blood flow 513
    retained
        treatment 379
    vasculopathy 490
placenta accreta 334
placenta previa 334
placental lactogen 239
placental protein 14 138
plasmapheresis 287, 449, 452
platelet activating factor 531
platelet-derived growth factor 412
platinum 182
pneumatic calf compression 57
pneumonia 304
polycystic ovarian disease 114, 118
    naltrexone 141
polyhydramnios 461, 462
polymerase chain reaction 16, 17, 166, 184, 299
    gestational trophoblastic disease 60
post-coital test
    LH kit 22
posterior urethral valves 434
postmenopausal bleeding 195
postpartum hemorrhage 335
    uterine packing 333
potassium channel openers 552
Potter sequence 434
Potter syndrome 302
prednisolone may work by decreasing maternal
antibody levels 449
preeclampsia 329, 377, 442, 476, 532, 534
    aspirin 367
    asthma 411
    cocaine 366
    donor insemination 140
    endothelial activators 405
platelets 557

preeclampsia (continued)
    uterine artery Doppler study 445
pregnancy
    diabetes
        glycolated proteins 537
    diabetic nephropathy 527
    heparin 151
    hypertension 531
    hypothyroidism 376
    length 420
    pulmonary edema 542
pregnancy-induced hypertension
    HLA-DR 479
    nifedipine 496
pregnancy loss
    embryotoxins 153
    recurrent 40
premature rupture of the membranes 292
    diagnosis 396
prenatal diagnosis 492
    cytomegalovirus 298
preterm labor 353, 364
    indomethacin 357
    relaxin 130
    sequelae at 24 weeks 342
procainamide 443
procaine 367
progesterone receptor
    leiomyomata 90
prolactin 308
promethazine 444
propranolol 70, 318
prostacyclin 358
prostaglandin F2a 555
prostaglandin synthetase 371
prostanoids
    pregnancy 470
prostate cancer 168
protein C 66, 108, 534
protein S 66
    deficiency in pregnancy 534
proteinuria
    preeclampsia and diabetes 277
    pregnancy 393
prothrombin time 111
^{32}P 200
pudendal nerve 75
pulmonary edema 285, 542
pulmonary embolism 58
pulmonary maturation 288
pulsatility index 204
pyelonephritis
    labor 382

quinidine 443

radiation 187
radical hysterectomy 240
    obesity 212
ramiprilat 438

rapid eye test 418
    cocaine 417
receiver-operator characteristic curves 398
relaxin
    preterm labor 130
Rely tampon 89
renal failure
    HELLP syndrome 450
resistance index 204
respiratory distress syndrome 288
Rh immune globulin 326
Rhenium 186-labeled monoclonal antibody 186
ritodrine 389, 466, 467
    amnion 535
robertsonian translocations 387
RU 486 90, 261

salbutamol 413, 556
salicylate 414
saralasin 438
Schauta-Amreich vaginal hysterectomy 223
second-look laparoscopy
    carcinoma of the fallopian tube 182
serotonin 412
sexuality
    hysterectomy 103
short bowel syndrome 506
shoulder dystocia 344
Sjogren syndrome 448
somatomedin inhibitory substance 489
sonography
    ovarian cancer 197
sperm penetration assay 134
stress urinary incontinence 101
"stiff heart" syndrome 543
sulfonamide creams 307
sumatriptan 70
    menstrual migraine 70
supine hypotensive syndrome 404
surfactant 325
Swyer syndrome 114
syphilis 442
systemic lupus erythematosus 143, 442, 448
    congenital heart block 448

tamoxifen 216, 242
    uterine effects 242
taxol 256
    ovary cancer 256
terbutaline 389, 467
    glucose tolerance in pregnancy 388
testicular determining factor 113
tetracycline 304, 307
tetralogy of Fallot 486
thrombomodulin 108
thromboxane 405, 476
tibolone 123
Tissue factor, 108
tissue plasminogen activator 66

tocolysis 522
    potassium channel openers 552
Torpin packer 334
toxemia 549
toxic shock syndrome
    LEEP 89
toxic shock syndrome toxin-1 89
transvaginal ultrasound
    ovarian masses 204
traveler's diarrhea 89
trisomy 18, 380, 460, 510
Turner syndrome 499, 510
twin-twin transfusion syndrome 460, 464, 485
    umbilical artery flow velocimetry 460
twins
    fetal presentation 352
    ideal outcome 310
    surveillance 351

ultrasound 197
    abortion 32
    detection of fetal uropathy 433
    fetal bladder visualization 300
    pregnancy loss 40
    survival of very low birth weight fetus 324
umbilical artery waveform velocity 449
under zona insemination 164
unexplained infertility 134
unruptured tubal pregnancies 112
ureaplasma
    cesarean morbidity 372
urethral instability 49
urethral syndrome 49
urinary incontinence 75
    levator ani 97
urine incontinence
    cigarette smoking 43
uropathy
    fetal 474
uterine artery velocity waveforms
    preeclampsia 445
uterine atony 334
uterine packing 333
uterus
    rupture
        VBAC 290

vagina
    cuff suspension 45
vaginal delivery after cesarean section
    uterine rupture 359
vaginosis
    treatment 306
valproic acid 547
vasopressin 51, 406, 439
velamentous cord insertion 464
venous thrombosis 57
ventilation-perfusion lung scan 58
ventricular arrhythmia 500
villous infarct 83

vitamin D
    preeclampsia 415
vitamin K
    anticonvulsant therapy 546
vulva
    cancer
        secondary neoplasms 263
        staging 211
    carcinoma
        recurrent 252
    pruritis 73
    vestibulitis 49

yttrium 90 189

Zavanelli maneuver 270, 344
Zoladex 14, 122